BASIC PHARMACOLOGY IN MEDICINE

EDITORS

Joseph R. DiPalma, M.D., Professor, Editor

Richard G. Sample, Ph.D., Assistant Professor, Editorial Coordinator

CONTRIBUTING EDITORS

Benjamin Calesnick, M.D., Professor

Warren S. Chernick, D.Sc., Professor and Chairman

Edward I. Ciaccio, Ph.D., Associate Professor

G. John DiGregorio, Ph.D., Associate Professor

Andrew P. Ferko, Ph.D., Assistant Professor

Alexander Gero, Ph.D., Professor

Department of Pharmacology
Hahnemann Medical College and Hospital
Philadelphia, Pennsylvania

BASIC PHARMACOLOGY IN MEDICINE

JOSEPH R. DiPALMA, M.D.

Editor
Professor of Pharmacology
Vice President and Dean
Hahnemann Medical College and Hospital, Philadelphia

McGRAW-HILL BOOK COMPANY
A Blakiston Publication

New York   St. Louis   San Francisco   Auckland   Düsseldorf
Johannesburg   Kuala Lumpur   London   Mexico
Montreal   New Delhi   Panama   Paris
São Paulo   Singapore   Sydney   Tokyo   Toronto

NOTICE

Medicine is an ever-changing science. As new research and clinical experience broaden our knowledge, changes in treatment and drug therapy are required. The editors and the publisher of this work have made every effort to ensure that the drug dosage schedules herein are accurate and in accord with the standards accepted at the time of publication. Readers are advised, however, to check the product information sheet included in the package of each drug they plan to administer to be certain that changes have not been made in the recommended dose or in the contraindications for administration. This recommendation is of particular importance in regard to new or infrequently used drugs.

Library of Congress Cataloging in Publication Data

Main entry under title:

Basic pharmacology in medicine.

"A Blakiston publication."
Based on the 4th ed. of V. A. Drill's Pharmacology in medicine.
Bibliography: p.
Includes index.
1. Pharmacology.   I.   DiPalma, Joseph R.   II. Drill, Victor Alexander, date   ed. Pharmacology in medicine. [DNLM: 1. Pharmacology. QV4 D596b]
RM300.B29   615'.7   75-43614
ISBN 0-07-017010-X

BASIC PHARMACOLOGY IN MEDICINE

1234567890   VHVH   7832109876

This book was set in Times Roman by Monotype Composition Company, Inc.
The editors were J. Dereck Jeffers and Michael LaBarbera;
the cover was designed by Nicholas Krenitsky;
the production supervisor was Thomas J. LoPinto.
The drawings were done by J & R Services, Inc.
Von Hoffmann Press, Inc., was printer and binder.

CONTENTS

LIST OF CONTRIBUTORS

The original authors of the corresponding chapters in *Drill's Pharmacology in Medicine,* Fourth Edition, which have been edited for this text are listed below, together with the chapter numbers as they appear in the new text.

Raymond P. Ahlquist, Ph.D.
Professor of Pharmacology, University of Texas, Medical Branch, Galveston—Chapter 13

Evangelos T. Angelakos, Ph.D., M.D.
Professor and Chairman, Department of Physiology and Biophysics, Hahnemann Medical College and Hospital—Chapter 23

Domingo M. Aviado, M.D.
Professor of Pharmacology, University of Pennsylvania School of Medicine—Chapter 19

Allan D. Bass, M.D.
Professor and Head, Department of Pharmacology, Vanderbilt University School of Medicine—Chapter 37

Samuel B. Beaser, M.D.
Clinical Associate Professor in Medicine, Harvard University Medical School—Chapter 30

William S. Beck, M.D.
Associate Professor of Medicine and Tutor in Biochemical Sciences, Harvard University; Chief of the Hematology Unit and Director of the Clinical Laboratories, Massachusetts General Hospital—Chapter 26

Frederick Bernheim, Ph.D.
Professor of Pharmacology, Duke University School of Medicine and Medical Center—Chapter 37

J. Thomas Bigger, Jr., M.D.
Assistant Professor, Department of Medicine, Columbia University College of Physicians and Surgeons—Chapter 22

John R. Boring, III, Ph.D.
Associate Professor of Preventive Medicine and Community Health and Associate Professor of Medicine (Infectious Diseases), Emory University College of Medicine—Chapter 35

Arthur H. Briggs, M.D.
Professor and Chairman, Department of Pharmacology, University of Texas Medical School at San Antonio—Chapter 25

Elmer B. Brown, M.D.
Associate Professor of Medicine, Washington University School of Medicine—Chapter 26

Benjamin Calesnick, M.D.
Professor of Pharmacology, Hahnemann Medical College and Hospital—Chapter 5

Warren S. Chernick, D.Sc.
Professor and Chairman, Department of Pharmacology, Hahnemann Medical College and Hospital—Chapter 7

Edward I. Ciaccio, Ph.D.
Associate Professor of Pharmacology, Hahnemann Medical College and Hospital—Chapter 4

Thomas Clarkson, Ph.D.
Associate Professor of Radiation Biology and Biophysics and Associate Professor of Pharmacology and Toxicology, University of Rochester School of Medicine and Dentistry—Chapter 38

George A. Condouris, Ph.D.
Professor and Chairman, Department of Pharmacology, New Jersey College of Medicine and Dentistry—Chapter 1

Harry Cullumbine, M.D.
Corporate Medical Director
Narco Scientific Industries
Fort Washington, Pennsylvania—Chapter 14

Clarke Davison, Ph.D.
Senior Research Biochemist and Section Head in Metabolic Chemistry, Sterling-Winthrop Research Institute, Rensselaer, New York—Chapter 14

Stanley Deutsch, Ph.D., M.D.
Chairman, Department of Anesthesiology, Michael Reese Hospital and Medical Center; Professor of Anesthesiology, The University of Chicago, Pritzker School of Medicine—Chapter 6

Victor DiStefano, Ph.D.
Associate Professor of Pharmacology and Toxicology, University of Rochester School of Medicine and Dentistry—Chapter 38

Edward F. Domino, M.D.
Professor of Pharmacology, University of Michigan School of Medicine; Michigan Neuropsychopharmacology Research Program—Chapter 10

Roger C. Duvoisin, M.D.
Associate Professor of Neurology, Columbia University Colllege of Physicians and Surgeons —Chapter 12

W. Edmund Farrar, Jr., M.D.
Associate Professor Preventive Medicine and Associate Professor of Medicine, Emory University School of Medicine—Chapter 35

Robert B. Forney, Ph.D.
Professor of Pharmacology and Toxicology, Indiana University School of Medicine— Chapter 8

Peter C. Gazes, M.D.
Professor of Medicine (Cardiology) and Pharmacology, Medical College of South Carolina—Chapter 21

Alexander Gero, Ph.D.
Professor of Pharmacology, Hahnemann Medical College and Hospital—Chapters 2 and 21

Mehran Goulian, M.D.
Professor of Medicine, University of California at San Diego—Chapter 26

R. N. Harger, Ph.D.
Professor of Biochemistry and Toxicology, Emeritus, Indiana University School of Medicine —Chapter 8

Gavin Hildick-Smith, M.A., M.D., M.R.C.P.
Director of Clinical Research, Johnson & Johnson—Chapter 36

Harold Hodge, Ph.D.
Professor of Pharmacology, Department of Pharmacology, University of California, San Francisco—Chapter 38

Brian R. Hoffman, M.D.
Professor and Chairman, Department of Pharmacology, Columbia University College of Physicians and Surgeons—Chapter 22

William C. Holland, M.D.
Profesor and Chairman, Department of Pharmacology and Toxicology, University of Mississippi School of Medicine—Chapter 25

Leo E. Hollister, M.D.
Medical Investigator, V.A. Hospital, Palo Alto, California, Associate Professor, Department of Medicine, Stamford University School of Medicine—Chapter 11

Duncan E. Hutcheon, M.D., D.Phil. (Oxon.)
Professor of Pharmacology and Associate
Professor of Medicine, New Jersey College of
Medicine and Dentistry—Chapter 24

Irwin H. Krakoff, M.D.
Division of Chemotherapy Research, Sloan-
Kettering Institute for Cancer Research—
Chapter 34

David Kritchevsky, Ph.D.
Wistar Institute of Anatomy and Biology; Wistar
Institute of Biochemistry in the School of Veteri-
nary Medicine at the University of Pennsylvania
—Chapter 23

Herbert S. Kupperman, M.D., Ph.D.
Associate Professor of Medicine, New York
University Medical Center—Chapters 31 and 32

Leonard J. Leach, B.S.
Assistant Professor of Radiation Biology and
Biophysics, University of Rochester, School of
Medicine and Dentistry—Chapter 38

Harold A. Levey, Ph.D.
Associate Professor of Physiology, State
University of New York, Downstate Medical
Center—Chapter 29

Bernard Levy, Ph.D.
Professor of Pharmacology, University of Texas,
Medical Branch, Galveston—Chapter 17

Ted A. Loomis, Ph.D., M.D.
Professor of Pharmacology, University of Washington Medical School—Chapter 27

H. George Mandel, Ph.D.
Professor and Chairman, Department of Phar-
macology, George Washington University
School of Medicine—Chapter 14

William R. Martin, M.D.
Chief, Addiction Research Center, National
Institute of Mental Health—Chapter 15

Everett W. Maynert, M.D., Ph.D.
Professor and Chairman, Department of
Pharmacology, University of Illinois College of
Medicine—Chapter 8

Robert A. Maxwell, Ph.D.
Head of Pharmacology Department, Wellcome
Research Laboratories, Research Triangle Park,
N.C.—Chapter 18

Lewis C. Mills, M.D.
Professor of Medicine and Associate Dean,
Hahnemann Medical College and Hospital—
Chapter 33

Paul L. Munson, Ph.D., M.A. (hon.)
Professor and Chairman, Department of Phar-
macology, University of North Carolina School of
Medicine—Chapter 29

Henry B. Murphree, M.D.
Professor, Department of Psychiatry, Rutgers
University Medical School—Chapters 9 and 13

Martin Perlmutter, M.D.
Clinical Associate Professor of Medicine and
Attending Physician, State University of New
York, Downstate Medical Center; Endocrine
Consultant and Former Director of Endocrine
Division, Maimonides Hospital, New York—
Chapter 29

John T. Potts, Jr., M.D.
Chief, Endocrine Unit, Massachusetts General
Hospital, Boston—Chapter 29

Franklin E. Roth, Ph.D.
Head, Department of Pharmacology; Associate
Director, Biological Research Division, Schering
Corporation—Chapter 28

Lewis S. Schanker, Ph.D.
Professor of Pharmacology, University of
Missouri-Kansas City Schools of Pharmacy and
Dentistry—Chapter 3

Thomas F. Sellers, Jr., M.D.
McAlister Professor and Chairman, Department
of Preventive Medicine and Community Health,
Emory University School of Medicine—Chapters
36 and 37

Ralph Shaw, M.D., Ph.D.
Associate Professor of Medicine, Hahnemann
Medical College and Hospital—Chapter 30

Jonas Shulman, M.D.
Associate Professor of Preventive Medicine and
Community Health and Associate Professor of
Medicine and Assistant Dean, Emory University
School of Medicine—Chapter 35

Frank A. Smith, Ph.D.
Associate Professor of Pharmacology (Toxicology) University of Rochester School of Medicine
and Dentistry—Chapter 38

William H. Strain, Ph.D.
Research Associate in Radiology, University of Rochester School of Medicine and Dentistry—Chapter 38

Irving I. A. Tabachnick, Ph.D.
Associate Director, Division of Biological Research, Schering Corporation—Chapter 28

Donald R. Taves, Ph.D., M.D.
Associate Professor of Pharmacology and Toxicology and Associate Professor of Radiation Biology and Biophysics, University of Rochester School of Medicine and Dentistry—Chapter 38

Leroy D. Vandam, M.D.
Professor of Anesthesia, Harvard Medical School; Director of Anesthesia, Peter Bent Brigham Hospital—Chapter 6

Robert W. Virtue, Ph.D., M.D.
Professor of Anesthesiology (Retired), University of Colorado Medical Center—Chapter 6

Robert L. Volle, Ph.D.
Professor and Chairman, Department of Pharmacology, University of Connecticut, School of Medicine—Chapters 16 and 19

Robert P. Walton, Ph.D., M.D. (deceased)
Professor and Chairman, Department of Pharmacology, Medical College of South Carolina—Chapter 21

B. E. Waud, M.D.
Instructor in Anesthesia, Department of Anesthesiology, Peter Bent Brigham Hospital, Harvard University Medical School—Chapter 20

Douglas R. Waud, Ph.D., M.D.
Associate Profesor, Department of Pharmacology, Harvard University Medical School—Chapter 20

Richard W. Whitehead, M.A., M.D.
Professor of Pharmacology, Emeritus, University of Colorado Medical Center—Chapter 6

Melvin D. Yahr, M.D.
Professor of Neurology and Associate Dean, Columbia University College of Physicians and Surgeons—Chapter 12

PREFACE

The faculty of the Department of Pharmacology at Hahnemann Medical College, from long experience in teaching a core curriculum using a number of major textbooks, has concluded that the medical student of today needs a book which is brief but also encourages exploration of each subject in depth. The purpose of the work would be to provide a concise presentation of the general theories and pertinent facts of pharmacology as they apply to medicine. To this end we have written this textbook as a companion volume to *Drill's Pharmacology in Medicine*. It has been abbreviated, edited, brought up to date, and simplified directly from the 4th edition of *Drill's Pharmacology*.

In the past two years we have written abbreviated chapters for our pharmacology course to supplement the major text. The enthusiasm of the students and the course's general overall success have encouraged us to undertake the task of an abbreviated textbook for the entire course in fresh-man medical school pharmacology. We believe we have learned how to handle the material so as to make it most useful to the student while still permitting the level of instruction to remain high.

It is quite evident that the present accretion of knowledge makes it impossible to compress all available information into the same number of hours which ten years ago sufficed. The question is what to include and what to delete. Our editors felt that all material on the nature and mechanisms of drug action which is reasonably established must be included. Certainly, a classical exposition of the major drug groups such as antibiotics, autonomic drugs, cardiovascular drugs, and central nervous system drugs could not be left out. However, many areas more peripheral to pharmacology, such as the vitamins and convulsive drugs, could be omitted. Toxicology of specific agents and less commonly used drugs, such as those for tropical diseases, can be taught in subsequent courses. Once the student has mastered the major drugs, it should not be difficult to acquire information on other therapeutic agents by self-instruction.

The editors found that some sections of *Drill's Pharmacology in Medicine* could be included verbatim, and some sections had to be completely rewritten. All have undergone a critical process of reduction and reclassification. In all instances speculative and debatable material was eliminated. Many of the illustrations are from the major text. A bibliography, subdivided by chapter, appears at the end of the text.

The basic course in pharmacology must be one which can be built upon in subsequent courses in clinical medicine and applied basic science. The serious student can of course use the major text for a complete and exhaustive treatise. The minor text remains as a convenient summary of the basic facts he must know to go on to clinical medicine and to review for examinations. This method of study encourages self-instruction and provides the means for continuing education.

Editing this work has included many stages. A particular topic was initially prepared by one editor, then reviewed by a second group of editors (and usually torn apart). A rewriting in most instances made the grade. This was then subjected to review by graduate students in order to get a different and pertinent point of view. After these corrections and additions a final version was produced, which we consider to be direct, clear, and succinct.

For their very appreciable aid in the preparation of this text we wish to extend our sincere thanks to David M. Ritchie, Barbara T. Nagle, Robert J. Capetola, Emil Bobyock, and Margot Newman.

The Editors

Part One

Modern Approaches
to Pharmacology

Chapter 1

The Natural Laws Concerning the Use of Drugs in Man and Animals

The quantitative aspects of drug action constitute one of the principal fields of study in pharmacology, providing a basis for analytic investigation of the mechanisms of action and for a rational use of drugs in therapeutics.

A drug produces a pharmacologic effect when the concentration or quantity of the drug at the site of a responsive tissue attains some critical minimum level. The magnitude of this "effective" level is determined by four general factors: (1) the affinity between the drug and the tissue receptors; (2) the intrinsic potential of the drug to cause cellular changes; (3) the responsiveness of the target tissue at the time the cellular changes occur; and (4) the effectiveness of cellular and systemic reflexes in resisting or modifying the changes induced by the drug.

In disease, tissue responsiveness may be even more variable. The reflexes provoked by drug action are also in a dynamic state and are subject to considerable variations. Since the final outcome of drug action depends upon the interaction of all of these factors, it is apparent that pharmacology is beset with an inordinate amount of quantitative variability. The following sections deal with the problem of pharmacologic variability and the methods used to cope with it.

THE NATURE, EXTENT, AND CAUSES OF PHARMACOLOGIC VARIABILITY

Quantitative variability in pharmacology may be expressed in terms of either the *size of the effect* (intensity or duration) elicited by a standard quantity of a drug or the *size of the dose* needed to produce a standard response. Quantitative variability may be observed between individuals in a group of organisms or even within a single organism when it is examined repeatedly with the same drug and dose.

The underlying reasons for pharmacologic variability may be ascribed to two major causes: (1) the variation in the purity or composition of the drug, and (2) the constantly changing physiologic and biochemical state of an organism.

The vast majority of drugs used in medicine are chemically pure and reasonably stable and therefore make only a minor contribution to pharmacologic variability. However, there is a relatively small number of drugs, mainly of biologic origin, with a significant potential for causing considerable variability in drug effects. This group includes drugs of unknown composition (such as some hormones) and drugs composed of mixtures of active ingredients in proportions that are not uniform (such as digitalis powder). The standardization of the potencies of insulin and digitalis powder are typical examples of the successful reduction of pharmacologic variability through biologic assay.

Most of the variation attending the use of drugs, especially in therapeutics, lies in the wide ranges of physiologic, biochemical, and pathologic conditions that confront the drug when it is administered to a living organism. The physiologic and biochemical states of an organism at systemic, tissue, cellular, and subcellular levels have a great influence in the final outcome by determining the amount of drug that reaches the site of action, the rate at which it accumulates at that site, the rate and extent of biotransformation of the active drug to an inactive form, and the rate of elimination of the drug from the body. In this regard, age, sex, body weight, body surface area, basal metabolic rate, and other biologic characteristics of living organisms are all known to affect quantitatively the results of drug action. Moreover, the pathologic state of a subject can influence all of the above conditions and, in addition, may even have a major role in determining the maximum extent of pharmacologic effect that can be obtained.

The recently developed field of pharmacogenetics reveals yet another source contributing to pharmacologic variability. The genetic modification of pharmacologic responses can be attributed to receptor site abnormalities, drug metabolism disorders, tissue metabolism disorders, or anatomic abnormalities.

STATISTICS OF DRUG ADMINISTRATION

Conventional statistics such as the mean and standard deviations are basic statistics that can be

used to describe the quantitative aspects of drug action.

Perhaps the most fundamental principle of pharmacology is that which states that the magnitude of a drug effect is a function of the dose administered. There are two basic types of dose-response relationships: (1) the *graded*, or *quantitative*, type which relates the dose of a drug to the size of the response in a single biologic unit; and (2) the *quantal*, or *all-or-none*, type in which the relationship is between the dose of the drug and the *proportion* of biologic objects displaying a given pharmacologic effect. The biologic material may be an intact organism, an isolated tissue, or even a single cell.

Dose-Response Curves (Graded)

An example of the graded curve is given in Fig. 1-1. As the dose administered to a single subject or to a discrete organ or tissue is increased, the pharmacologic response will increase in a gradual, smooth fashion, provided the dose has exceeded a critical level called the *threshold dose*.

The upper end of the curve has essentially the same properties as the lower end. The degree of effect produced by increasing doses of a drug will

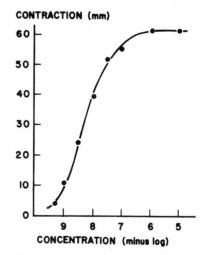

Figure 1-1 A graded response of an isolated aortic strip to increasing concentrations of norepinephrine. The isotonic contractions of the aorta are expressed in millimeters on the ordinate; the concentrations are shown on the abscissa as the negative values of the exponents of the concentrations; that is, $8 = -\log 10^{-8}$ g/ml.

eventually reach a steady level, the so-called "ceiling effect." Doses beyond the one that produced the ceiling effect, that is, the ceiling dose, do not elicit any further increase in effect. In fact, doses exceeding the ceiling dose may actually provoke different and possibly undesirable responses. In spite of this disadvantage of vagueness, the ceiling dose has a considerable importance in therapeutics where the aim often is the achievement of a maximum pharmacologic effect. It is interesting that the ceiling dose has served as the basis for a systematic comparison of the therapeutic "efficacy" of drugs.

The main body of the graded curve lies between the threshold dose and the ceiling dose. The graded curve may describe a symmetric sigmoid curve, an asymmetric sigmoid curve where either end may be distorted, or even one-half of a sigmoid curve (the upper half), which would then make it a hyperbolic function. Knowledge of the general shape of the graded curve for a given drug has practical use in medicine when a patient has to be virtually titrated with the drug in order for the optimum result to be achieved. It is usual that the central part of the graded curve is linear for a range so that the rate of change of response is directly related to the rate of change of dose. Since a linear function of dose on effect offers convenience, the boundaries of linearity have been considerably extended by means of a mathematical transformation of the units of measure of either the dose, the response, or both.

Dose-Response Curves (Quantal)

The quantal, or all-or-none, curve relates the frequency with which any dose of a drug evokes a stated, fixed (all-or-none), pharmacologic response. It is therefore essentially a curve describing the distribution of minimum doses that produce a given effect in a population of biologic objects. Minimum (or threshold) doses for the effect can be obtained either directly by titrating the subject with the drug until the desired effect is produced or, alternatively, by giving a series of doses to different groups of subjects and noting the proportion of subjects responding to each dose. In either case, the frequency of occurrence of threshold doses can be plotted against the actual dose on any of several different coordinate systems.

In its most basic form, the quantal dose-response

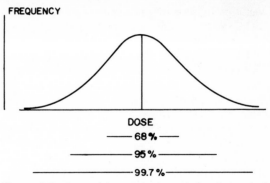

Figure 1-2 A graphic expression of the theoretical normal distribution of doses needed to elicit a quantal response in subjects from a large sample. The horizontal bars delineate the borders of ±1, 2, and 3 standard deviations from the mean dose, which is shown by the vertical bar. The proportion of subjects requiring doses within the boundaries is indicated as a percentage of the sample. The dose units are unspecified.

curve takes the shape of a gaussian or normal distribution (Fig. 1-2). The gaussian distribution suggests that the observed variation in doses needed to produce the response is due to simple random variation.

It is usual to obtain dose distributions that are imperfect normal distributions, either because one or the other end of the distribution is not available (truncation) or because some extraneous drug effect or other experimental limitation is opposing or modifying the main action of the drug.

In a symmetric normal or bell-shaped curve, the value that has the greatest frequency is called the *mode*; it is equal to the mean (average value) and median (the value that bisects the population of values into equal halves). Furthermore, the two inflection points on the curve occur at values which are ± one standard deviation from the mean value and therefore enclose 68 percent of the values in the distribution. Because the bell-shaped curve is not a convenient form for the analysis of quantal dose-effect data, other graphic forms have been developed. Three of the graphic forms are illustrated in Fig. 1-3, which shows the data for two dose-response curves.

Every drug has at least two quantal dose-response curves, one for the desired pharmacologic response and one for some unwanted toxic manifestation. The data in Fig. 1-3 were obtained by

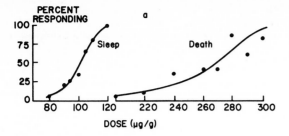

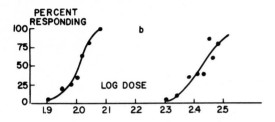

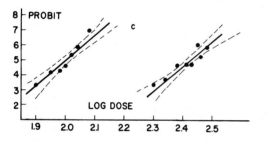

Figure 1-3 Three graphic forms, showing data for two dose-response curves. (See discussion in text.)

injecting groups of 20 mice with different doses of a central nervous system depressant, phenobarbital, and observing the presence or absence of the righting reflex. If the animals lost the righting reflex, they were regarded as being ''asleep''; if they died within 24 h, the dose was considered lethal. This is an example of the indirect method for determining the individual threshold doses for the quantal responses sleep and death.

The observed proportion (percentage) responding to the drug with either sleep or death can be plotted against the dose of the drug, as in Fig. 1-3a. This is the form the normal curve shown in Fig. 1-2 takes when the number responding is integrated from the lowest to the highest doses; it is referred to as the *accumulated* or *integrated normal curve*. In Fig. 1-3a, the dose-response curve for sleep is a reasonably good sigmoid curve, but the lethal curve

is not. This amount of variation is not uncommon in pharmacology when the end point (death in 24 h) is subject to an extraneous factor such as the development of bacterial infection as a sequel to prolonged central nervous system depression. Many quantal curves often show a definite skewing in one end of the curve, usually the higher end. The skew must first be corrected with an appropriate mathematical transformation of the dose unit (metameter). The one most often used is the logarithmic transformation in which the dose is simply converted to the log-dose.

Replotting the same data using the log-dose improves the shapes and the symmetry of the curves (Fig. 1-3b).

The extremes of the integrated normal curve, however, are usually nonlinear and in fact approach the upper and lower limits of response only asymptotically. In order to make the quantal dose-response curves linear over a wider range of doses, the data can be replotted on coordinates in which the ordinate is expressed simply in multiples of the standard deviation called *normal equivalent deviates* (NED). Normal equivalent deviates and their corresponding percent response values are tabulated in Table 1-1.

The use of the NED as an expression of the percentage response in quantal dose-response curves was further refined by the elimination of the positive and negative signs by the expedient of adding 5 algebraically to each NED. This unit of response is termed *probit* (from the contraction of the phrase *probability unit*). The concepts of the NED and probit, which were developed independently, con-

Table 1-1 Normal Equivalent Deviates and Their Percentage Values and Probits

Normal equivalent deviates	% Responding	Probit
+3	99.9	8
+2	97.7	7
+1	84	6
0	50	5
−1	16	4
−2	2.3	3
−3	0.1	2

siderably facilitate statistical computations. The relationship of probits to NED and percentage response is also given in Table 1-1.

The advantage in the use of the probit is seen in Fig. 1-3c, where the same data as in Fig. 1-3a and b are plotted linearly over a wider range of log-doses.

The quantal curve, expressed in this manner, can be used to determine whether a set of data follows a normal distribution; to estimate, graphically, the mean dose and the standard deviation of doses about the mean; or to serve as the basis for biologic assays.

Statistics Derived from the Quantal Dose-Response Curve

Arithmetic Mean Dose   The arithmetic mean (average) dose of a drug is the dose computed as the sum of all the doses required to produce a stated response, divided by the number of such doses in the summation $\bar{x} = [S(x)]/N$.

The arithmetic mean has two important properties. The sum of all deviations from the mean is equal to zero and the sum of the squares of these deviations (that is, error of estimation) is a minimum. These two properties make the arithmetic mean an "efficient" and "sufficient" statistic to describe the central tendency of drug doses.

Median Dose   The median dose is the smallest dose that is effective in 50 percent of individuals.

The median effective dose, expressed symbolically as ED_{50} for *effective dose, 50 percent*, is in common use in pharmacology because of several favorable properties: (1) The entire population of doses need not be known for its estimation because it is obtained simply by interpolation between two doses, one to which 50 percent of organisms respond and one which elicits more than a 50 percent response. (2) It is unaffected by extreme values and hence is stable even in a skewed distribution. (3) The ED_{50} readily allows for the expression of the phenomena of synergism and antagonism when the interaction of two drugs is studied (see Chap. 2). (4) The error associated with its estimation is smaller than the error of any other estimated dose of the quantal dose-response curve.

Confidence Limits   Every statistic derived from experimental data is only an estimate of the "true"

value of the statistic in a population of infinite size, and each estimate is associated with an error which is expressed generally as the standard error for the statistic. Another more meaningful way of indicating the precision of a statistic is through the use of confidence limits. These are boundaries which are expected to contain the "true" value of a statistic at some selected level of probability. To illustrate, when the 95 percent confidence limits are calculated for an ED_{50}, the assertion is made that the true ED_{50} for the drug in an infinite population of animals will be found within these limits with a probability of 95 percent and will lie outside these limits, by chance, only 5 times out of 100 repeated experiments.

The confidence limits for an ED_{50} of high precision will have a narrower range than will those for a less precise statistic at the same level of probability. But since confidence limits are a function of the standard error of the statistic, the limits can always be narrowed to give greater confidence by increasing the number of animals used in arriving at the statistic.

Therapeutic Index   The therapeutic index of a drug is an approximate statement of the relative safety of the drug expressed as the ratio of the lethal or toxic dose to the therapeutic dose. The larger the ratio, the greater the relative safety.

It is not sufficient merely to state the therapeutic index in terms of "lethal dose" and "therapeutic dose" without specifically defining where on the quantal dose-response curves these doses occur. One could, for example, speak of the *minimum lethal dose* and the *minimum therapeutic dose* or the *maximum therapeutic dose* and the *maximum lethal dose*. Most often the therapeutic index is based on the estimates of the ED_{50} and the median lethal dose (LD_{50}) of a drug, for the reasons presented in the discussion of the properties of the median dose. But the use of the median effective and median lethal doses is not without disadvantage, since median doses tell nothing about the slopes of the dose-response curves for therapeutic and toxic effects.

One method suggested to overcome this deficiency uses the ED_{99} or ED_{95} for the desired drug effect and the LD_1 or even the $LD_{0.1}$ for the undesired effect. Using these levels of response, the therapeutic index is denoted, for example, by the ratio $LD_{0.1}:ED_{99}$. A better notation to use instead of therapeutic index is *safety margin* or *standard safety margin*, which is a more descriptive use of the index.

The *standard safety margin* is defined as the percentage increase of a dose above the therapeutic dose that is lethal to a given proportion of subjects. The standard safety margin in item 4 of Table 1-2, for instance, states that the dose of phenobarbital that is effective in producing sleep in 99 percent of mice needs to be increased 34 percent before 1 percent of the mice die. Similarly (item 5), the dose that is effective in 999 out of 1,000 mice has to be increased only 8 percent in order to be lethal for 1 out of 1,000 animals. In this index of safety, therefore, the statement on safety is more precise and is in terms of actual therapeutic doses used.

Time-Action Curves

The relationship between dose and response is usually established when the drug effect at a particular dose has reached a maximum or a steady level. Naturally, drug effects do not develop instantaneously or continue indefinitely; they change with time. Thus, the magnitude of a drug effect at any given moment is a function not only of the *dose* but also of the amount of *time* elapsed since the drug has made contact with the reactive tissues. These three factors, dose, time, and effect, can most accurately and completely be represented in a three-dimensional system of coordinates, but for convenience the three factors are treated as two separate pairs on binary coordinates, dose response (at equilibrium) and time action (at one-dose level).

The time-action properties of drugs have considerable importance in experimental pharmacology, where they are used in the analysis of mechanism of action, and in applied pharmacology, where they form the basis for selection of the best drug and the optimum dosage schedule either for sustained therapeutic effect or, in some instances, for a transient effect.

The basic ideas of time action have been concisely summarized in the diagram shown in Fig. 1-4. There are three distinct phases in all time-action curves; a fourth phase is present and pronounced with some drugs and absent with others.

Table 1-2 Safety Margins or Therapeutic Indices Calculated by Different Methods for the Data in Fig. 1-3

Therapeutic index and symbol	Value of index
Conventional index LD_1/ND_1*	2.35
Conventional index LD_5/ND_5	2.43
Median index $\quad LD_{50}/ND_{50}$	2.62
Standard safety margin $[(LD_1/ND_{99}) - 1] \times 100$	$34 \pm 12\%$
Standard safety margin $[(LD_{0.1}/ND_{99.9}) - 1] \times 100$	8%

* ND_1 = narcotic dose 1 percent, or minimum effective dose.

Phase I: time for onset action Following the administration of a drug to an organism or to isolated tissues, there is a delay in time before the first signs of drug effect are manifested.

Phase II: time to peak effect The maximum response will occur when the most resistant cell has been affected to its maximum or when the drug has reached the most inaccessible cells of the responsive tissue.

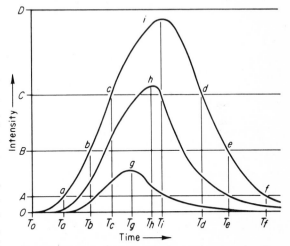

Figure 1-4 The intensity of effect related to the time of administration of a drug and the influence of dosage on the time-effect relationship. Three different doses of the same drug are given at time T_0. A is the threshold effect; B is the therapeutic effect; C is the toxic effect; D is the maximal effect of the drug. The peak effects of the three doses occur at times T_c, T_b, T_i. The other lower-case letters refer to other end points. For example, T_a = latency time; T_i = peak time; T_f = persistence time.

Phase III: duration of action   The duration of action of a drug extends from the moment of onset of perceptible effects to the time when an action can no longer be measured.

Phase IV: residual effects   Even after its primary actions are terminated, it is possible for a drug to exert a residual action that is unmasked only when another dose of the same drug is administered and an exaggerated response is evoked or when another entirely different drug is given and the phenomenon of synergism or antagonism is manifested (Chap. 2). Residual effects are also referred to as *carry-over*.

The first three phases of the temporal course of drug action are closely dependent on the size of the dose administered. In general, the larger the dose, the shorter the time to onset and time to peak effect, and the longer the overall duration of action. Of course, the higher the dose, the greater the maximum effect.

BIOLOGIC ASSAY

Bioassay is defined as "a determination of the potency of a physical, chemical, or biological agent by means of a biological indicator." Physical agents may include such forces as ionizing radiation; chemical and biologic agents include drugs, hormones, vitamins, toxins, and antitoxins. The indicators of biologic activity are the measurable responses provoked by these agents in a surviving organism or tissue. Numerous indicators exist; blood pressure, blood glucose level, muscle tension, and inhibition of microorganism growth are some examples. A variety of biologic objects supply the biologic responses. These may be whole organisms, isolated organs or tissues, and populations of cells. The objective of a bioassay is to establish the relative potency of a drug and to supply an estimate of the reliability of the potency.

When the drug that is bioassayed is composed of a mixture of ingredients with varying individual activities, it is not possible from a bioassay against a standard preparation to make any conclusion on the *quantity* of drug present in the test sample. Digitalis powder, for example, is a mixture of several active digitalis compounds that are found in varying proportions in digitalis plants from different areas. It is assayed against a standard such as the U.S.P. (United States Pharmacopeia) Digitalis

Reference Standard. If the amount of activity of a sample of digitalis is found to be equal to 0.1 g of the reference standard, it does not follow that the sample contains 0.1 g of digitalis compounds, since the presence of excess amounts of a very weak, or a very active, digitalis compound could significantly affect the total amount of digitalis in an equieffective dose of the mixture. To circumvent this obstacle, official reference standards are assigned arbitrary units of activity for a specified weight of the standard. The U.S.P. Digitalis Reference Standard is assigned 1 unit of activity for 0.1 g of powder. Thus, when a quantity of digitalis sample of unknown potency gives pharmacologic activity equal to that observed with 0.1 g of standard, the sample is said to contain 1 U.S.P. unit of digitalis activity per quantity of material. If, for instance, 1 unit of activity resided in 0.08 g of the sample powder, the sample would have 20 percent greater relative potency than the standard and could be diluted with inert material in order to make its potency equal to that of the U.S.P. standard.

BIOLOGIC ASSAY VERSUS CHEMICAL ASSAY

The estimation of relative potency of a drug by bioassay generally is less precise than the determination of the quantity of a drug by chemical assay. Nevertheless, biologic assay is still the method of choice in the standardization of a substantial number of drugs, largely because of the following advantages of bioassay over chemical assay: (1) The active principle does not have to be known. (2) The active principle may be known, but its chemical composition does not have to be established. (3) The active principle does not have to be in a pure state. (4) The sensitivity of bioassay methods may be far greater than that of chemical methods; for example, in the microbiologic assay of vitamin B_{12}, concentrations can be detected as low as 0.00002 μg/ml, whereas the chemical method requires 5 μg/ml, a 250,000-fold difference in sensitivity. (5) Drugs which are chemically pure but chemically unstable may sometimes be bioassayed without loss of the drug activity. (6) Bioassay can often reveal the active isomer of a drug which has active and inactive isomers.

Biologic assay has the disadvantages of lower precision and costliness in time and animals. Wherever possible, chemical assay is preferred over biologic assay.

Chapter 2

Mechanisms of Molecular Drug Action

It must be realized that drug action represents artificial interference with the natural functioning of
the organism. This interference may result in either
enhancement or diminution of the existing function
which may take a variety of forms. For example,
drug action includes replacement therapy, chemical
antagonism, or physicochemical environmental
alteration. The physicochemical environmental alteration may be the result of a specific or nonspecific interaction.

Replacement therapy, administration of a missing or deficient substance, may consist of prescribing some essential component of the body, such as
a vitamin, hormone, or metal. For example, diabetes mellitus (insulin deficiency) is treated by
administering insulin and iron-deficiency anemia by
administering iron.

Chemical antagonism is the addition of a drug
substance to counteract chemically a physiologic
imbalance that may be caused by an excess of some
normal, even essential, ingredient of the organism.

Thus, if gastric acidity is excessive, an antacid will
raise the pH of the gastric juice.

Nonspecific drugs are agents which bring about
a physicochemical alteration simply by their physical presence rather than by their interaction with
any specific chemical agent in the organism. Such
an alteration results from general anesthetics, ethanol, or barbiturates which, by virtue of their affinity
for lipid material, tend to accumulate in nerve membranes and so depress nerve function, particularly
in the central nervous system.

Specific drugs are agents which enter into actual
chemical reaction with a receptive chemical structure in the organism. Sites of reactive chemical
groupings on the surface or within the cell are
termed *receptors*. These may be very complex in
their structural nature and in the arrangement of
their electrical charges. A drug may alter the properties of a receptor when it combines either reversibly or irreversibly with the receptor. The forces of
attachment between the drug and receptor may be

9

covalent, ionic, hydrogen, or van der Waals bonds. The final outcome of most drug effects depends upon a drug-receptor interaction. For example, a drug can react with one or another of the enzymes involved in some essential metabolic pathway. The administered drug may compete with the normal substrate, interfering with, and possibly blocking completely, the metabolic pathway it enters and then serves as an antimetabolite. In this way, sulfonamides and antibiotics inhibit essential biologic processes of microorganisms and can be used as antimicrobial agents.

Inhibition of an enzyme is not the only way in which drugs can block synthesis of an essential intermediate of metabolism. Inhibition of an enzyme may exacerbate, not depress, a biologic event when the function of the enzyme is to stop such an event. An example of this is acetylcholinesterase which serves the function of hydrolyzing acetylcholine and thus stopping acetylcholine-mediated activity in the autonomic nervous system. If acetylcholinesterase activity is blocked, the acetylcholine generated by the organism will survive and remain active far beyond its normal intensity and duration of action.

Another very important type of specific drug action is that of *mimetic agents*. These are compounds that mimic the action of some chemical transmitter in the organism. Such a transmitter can be a neurohormone, for instance, norepinephrine. Mimetic agents are able to react with the particular structures (receptors) specifically devoted to the transmitters in the organism. It is the interaction of the mimetic agent and the receptor which results in a pharmacologic effect. It is this effect of their interaction which defines the compounds as drugs.

RECEPTOR THEORY

The majority of drugs are specific and participate in actual chemical reactions within the organism. Drug action is an interaction between the drug and the organism where the drug is one reagent and the other is a component of the organism.

The receptor concept allows us to order our factual knowledge and to apply thermodynamic principles to gain a more profound understanding of drug action. The reader may appreciate the difficulties of such an undertaking since we are at-

tempting to make reasoned statements about a reaction of which we know only the identity and concentration of one reagent and some possibly remote observable effect. Small wonder that pharmacologists have not yet agreed on one comprehensive theory! Only one theory is presented here in some detail (without prejudice to the possibility that future developments may change the situation and force preference for some other theory). The theory is based on three assumptions: (1) Drugs react reversibly with their receptors. (2) One drug molecule reacts with one receptor molecule. Therefore, symbolizing the receptor as R and the drug as A, we can write their reaction as

$$R + A \rightleftharpoons RA$$

where RA represents a complex formed from drug and receptor. (3) The effect is proportional to the concentration of the drug-receptor complex and may be expressed as

$$E_A = \alpha[RA]$$

where E_A is the effect of drug A, and α is a proportionality constant linking the effect to the concentration of the drug-receptor complex. The proportionality constant is termed the *intrinsic activity* or the *efficacy* of the drug.

From these two algebraic formulations, a great many deductions can be made by simple mathematical reasoning. In this brief text, however, only the most important results of the algebraic reasoning are presented in words and graphs.

From the two equations presented above, it follows that

$$E_A = \frac{\alpha[R]_t}{K_A/[A] + 1}$$

where $[R]_t$ is the total receptor concentration, and K_A is the dissociation constant of the drug-receptor complex. One practical virtue of this formulation is that the only variables it contains are the experimentally accessible magnitudes $[A]$ and E_A. All other magnitudes are constants. Although of these constants only K_A is generally measurable, to some extent we can test the theory even if we assign only arbitrary values to the constants α and $[R]_t$. Thus we find that, at arbitrary values of the constants, a plot of E_A against the logarithm of [A] has a sigmoid shape (Fig. 2-1), and such sigmoid semilogarithmic dose-response curves are indeed characteristically obtained in experiments whenever the magnitude of the effect lends itself to measurement. From the last equation above, it also follows that by plotting the reciprocal value of the effect against the reciprocal value of the drug concentration, a straight line should result. Experiment confirms this expectation.

DRUG-RECEPTOR INTERACTIONS

The theory is best demonstrated when examining the simultaneous action of two drugs, A and B, on the same organism. The first instance of such drug interaction discussed is where A and B act on the same receptor, with the respective efficacies α and β.

There are two important cases, depending on the relative magnitudes of α and β. When $\alpha = \beta$, the effects of the two drugs are *additive*. When one of the two drugs, perhaps B, has only affinity for the common receptor of the two drugs but no efficacy (that is, when $\beta = 0$), then B will be a *competitive antagonist* of the *agonist* A. The theory predicts that in this case, when the effect of varying concentrations of A is determined in the presence of a constant concentration of B, the log-dose-versus-effect curve of A will be displaced to the right parallel to itself, as much more to the right as the concentration of B is greater (Fig. 2-2). The theory also predicts that, in the presence of a constant concentration of B, the double-reciprocal plot should still be linear and have the same intercept on the $1/E$ axis as it had in the absence of B, but its slope should be steeper, as much steeper as the concentration of B is greater (Fig. 2-3). All of these conclusions have been proved by experiment.

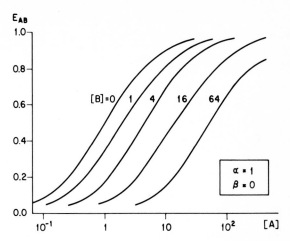

Figure 2-2 Theoretical dose-response curves for combinations of several constant concentrations of B (0, 1, 4, 16, 64) with varying concentrations of A.

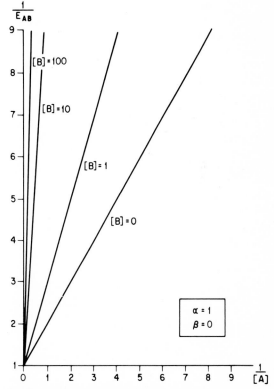

Figure 2-3 Double-reciprocal plots calculated for combinations of several constant concentrations of B with varying concentrations of A.

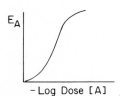

Figure 2-1 Theoretical dose-response curve.

In addition, competitive antagonism can be symbolized by

$$R \rightarrow E_{AB}$$
$$\diagup \quad \diagdown$$
$$A \qquad B$$

where R is the receptor, A is the agonist, B is a drug which lacks efficacy but has affinity, and E_{AB} is the effect of A and B. As the concentration of B is increased, the magnitude of the pharmacologic response produced by drug A is diminished. However, according to the law of mass action, this inhibition caused by a concentration of drug B can be overcome merely by increasing the dosage level of A in the system. A specific example of competitive antagonism is the interaction between acetylcholine and tubocurarine at the neuromuscular junction. Tubocurarine causes skeletal muscle paralysis by reducing the accessibility of acetylcholine to the receptor site. As mentioned previously, if the concentration of acetylcholine is increased in this region, a reduction in the tubocurarine-induced inhibition will result.

The phenomenon of *noncompetitive antagonism* is another type of drug interaction. Noncompetitive antagonism arises when two drugs act on separate but not independent receptors, the effect of the reaction of drug B with its receptor being to decrease the efficacy of the drug-receptor complex RA. The drug interaction between an agonist and a noncompetitive antagonist at receptors can be symbolized by

$$E_{AB}$$
$$\uparrow$$
$$R - R'$$
$$| \qquad |$$
$$A \qquad B$$

where R, A, and E_{AB} are the same as for competitive antagonism, but B is a noncompetitive antagonist and R' is a separate but interdependent receptor. The theory predicts that, in contrast with competitive antagonism, here the dose-effect curves obtained at constant concentrations of the antagonist are not parallel: they begin to rise at the same point where the dose-effect curve for drug A alone begins to rise, but they rise to a lower maximum, as much lower as the concentration of the antagonist B is greater (Fig. 2-4). Double-reciprocal

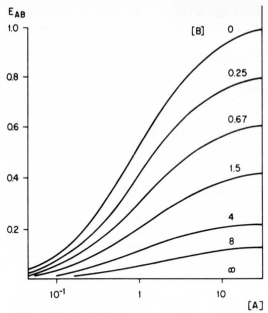

Figure 2-4 Theoretical dose-response curves for combinations of several constant concentrations of the noncompetitive antagonist B with varying concentrations of the agonist A.

plots are linear, but both the slope and the intercept are altered (Fig. 2-5). The foregoing examples illustrate the power and usefulness of the theory: simply, the aspect of the log-dose-versus-effect curves obtained for drug A in the presence of several constant concentrations of drug B reveals the mechanism of their interference with each other.

An interesting theoretical possibility is *functional interaction*, defined as the phenomenon whereby two drugs act on different receptors, but the effect of both drug-receptor interactions manifests itself in the same way on the same effector organ. To differentiate the two cases between noncompetitive interaction and functional interaction, we resort to curves known as *isoboles* which are loci of identical effects of a combination of two drugs. Such curves are drawn by plotting [A] against [B], as in Fig. 2-6. The point P_1 represents a certain concentration of A; P_2, an equiactive concentration of B; the straight line I connecting the two points is an isobole denoting strict additivity of the actions of A and B. Isoboles of the type of curve II, lying above I everywhere between P_1 and P_2, signify that higher doses

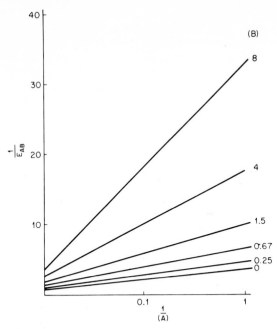

Figure 2-5 Double-reciprocal plots for noncompetitive antagonism, constructed from the curves in Fig. 2-4.

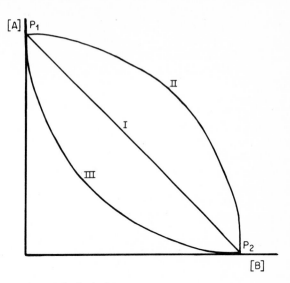

Figure 2-6 Isoboles.

of A and B are required to obtain the same effect—A and B antagonize each other. Curve III is a case not encountered before: It is a hyperbola which lies entirely *below* curve I, indicating that for any given effect of the two drugs in combination, less of the mixture is needed than calculated from additivity, or to put it differently, the magnitude of the effect of the drug mixture is greater than the sum of the individual effects of the components of the mixture. This phenomenon is known to pharmacologists as *synergism* or *potentiation*.[1]

RECEPTORS FOR ACETYLCHOLINE

The *cholinergic transmitter*, acetylcholine (ACh), has a vast spectrum of activity within the organism. ACh functions as the transmitter in the para-

[1] Linguistic usage is uncertain on this point. Some authors use the term *synergism* for all cases in which two drugs give similar effects, and speak of "additive synergism" instead of additivity and of "synergism with potentiation" instead of synergism or potentiation as defined here.

sympathetic nervous system; in all ganglia, both sympathetic and parasympathetic; at the neuromuscular junction; and, together with norepinephrine, in the cardiovascular system and in the central nervous system. Acetylcholine strongly interacts with acetylcholinesterase, which serves the function of limiting ACh action by hydrolyzing the transmitter and thus quenching the transmitted signal. It would certainly be an oversimplified view to assume a unique ACh receptor in all the systems just enumerated, and in fact it was found that ACh analogues and antagonists are more specific than ACh itself, that is, more selective in their effect on one or another of the objects of ACh action. It is quite possible, therefore, that we are dealing with a number of different receptors, and if ACh can act on all of them, this may be only because its simple, flexible molecule can adapt itself to the topography of more than one receptor. Therefore, we must distinguish at least three ACh receptors, located at the smooth-muscle effectors such as the gut, the autonomic ganglia, and the skeletal neuromuscular junction. As a fourth receptor may be added the enzyme acetylcholinesterase.

Acetylcholine,

$$CH_3—COO—CH_2—CH_2—N^+(CH_3)_3,$$

has only two functional groups, an ester and a quaternary ammonium group, to offer to a receptor.

Very likely, therefore, all ACh receptors will have an anionic site to bind the cationic "head" of ACh by electrostatic attraction. In addition, at least the ester-hydrolyzing acetylcholinesterase must also have an "esteratic" site, adapted specifically to the task of splitting the ester group. We now think of the esteratic site as a bifunctional site G—H, composed of a nucleophilic part G and an electrophilic part H, to react by concerted acid and base catalysis with the C=O group of the ester (see Fig. 2-7). Here the enzyme forms with ACh a complex which then breaks up into choline and acetyl enzyme, the latter subsequently hydrolyzed to acetic acid and free enzyme. The function of the anionic site is to hold on to the cationic head of ACh and force it to remain in place long enough to be hydrolyzed.

Smooth-muscle ACh receptors also have an anionic site, but instead of the esteratic site (which attacks the C=O group), they are more likely to be fitted with sites binding the two oxygen atoms of ACh, probably by hydrogen bonds. Evidence for the conclusion that the smooth-muscle receptor contains an oxygen-binding site includes the fact that choline HO—CH₂—CH₂—N⁺(CH₃)₃ and its ethers are weak parasympathomimetic agents, and that muscarine,

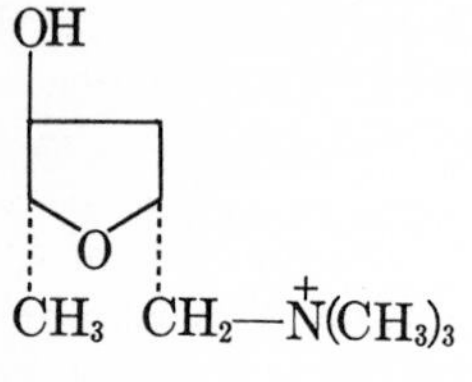

which holds the two O atoms and the quaternary N rigidly in the most favorable mutual orientation, is more selective in its action than ACh, and on organs on which it acts is more potent than ACh, while several of its stereoisomers are less potent. (The high activity of muscarine on ACh receptors in smooth muscle and in glands has caused these ACh receptors to be termed *muscarinic* receptors.)

Muscarinic drugs of asymmetric structure often show greater potency in one enantiomorph than in the other. The obvious conclusion is that the receptor which attaches them is also asymmetric, and various proposals have been made to incorporate such asymmetry in the receptor in addition to the anionic site and oxygen-binding site.

Replacement of the ether oxygen in muscarine by sulfur, thus enlarging the molecule while decreasing its capacity for hydrogen bonding, reduces the activity of muscarine to $\frac{1}{4,500}$. This points up the importance of the right size of the component parts of a drug molecule for accurate fit to the receptor. Similarly, the potency of ACh decreases when ethyl is substituted for methyl in the cationic head. Replacement of one methyl by ethyl cuts potency in half, which becomes plausible on the assumption that only two of the three *N*-methyl groups actually have to fit the receptor.

Similar observations have been made in the ester group of ACh. Replacement of the acetyl group of ACh by propionyl, butyryl, and valeryl reduces the ACh action to $\frac{1}{33}$, $\frac{1}{400}$, and $\frac{1}{5,000}$, respectively. This phenomenon is clearly correlated with the increas-

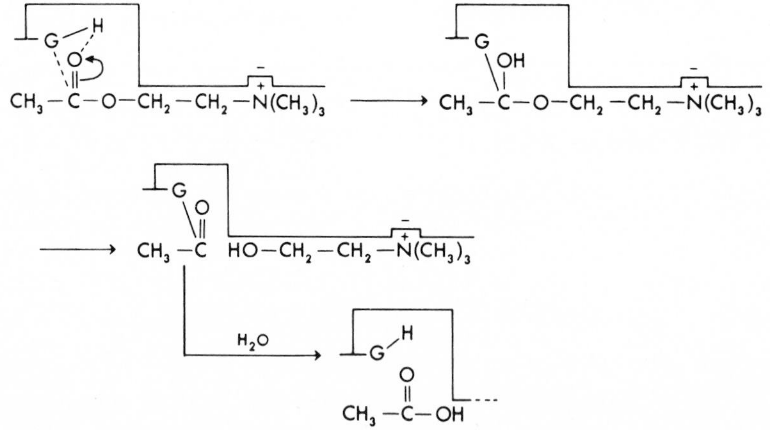

Figure 2-7 Mechanism of the hydrolysis of acetylcholine by acetylcholinesterase.

ing size of the acyl group, which makes it increasingly difficult for the drug to approach the receptor to reactive distance. It is quite in keeping with this conclusion that replacement of the acetyl group by the even smaller carbamoyl group NH_2CO— does not impair activity.

The ACh derivatives, being specific drugs, depend for their action on accurate fit to their receptors; successively larger molecules in their homologous series, which still fit the receptor sufficiently for some binding but no longer for full efficacy, are first weaker agonists, then antagonists.

THE MORPHINE RECEPTOR

Morphine is an alkaloid with a complex ring system

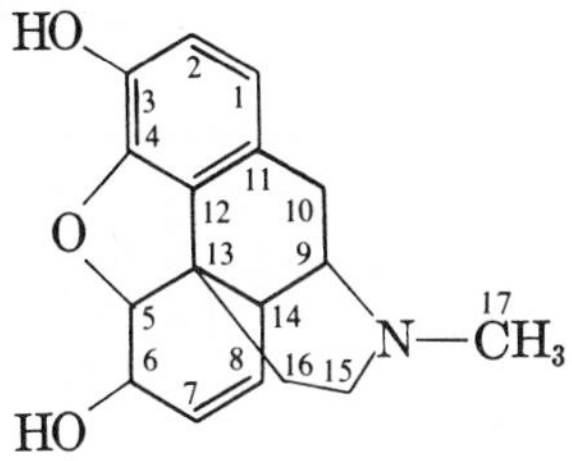

which, however, certainly is not essential in its entirety for the characteristic analgesic action of the drug. Of the many simpler synthetic drugs which share this action, the following are representative examples:

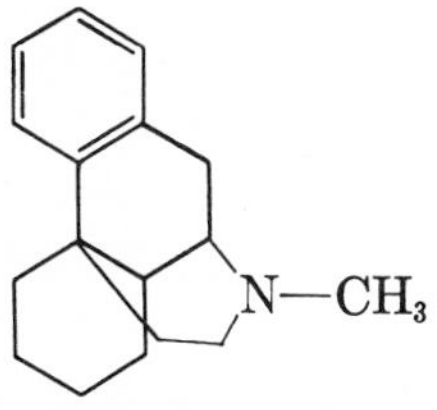

N-Methylmorphinan

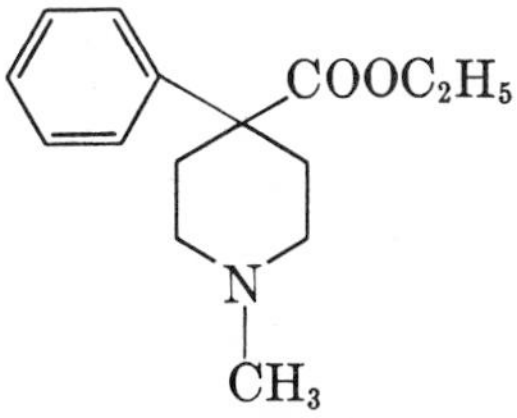

Meperidine

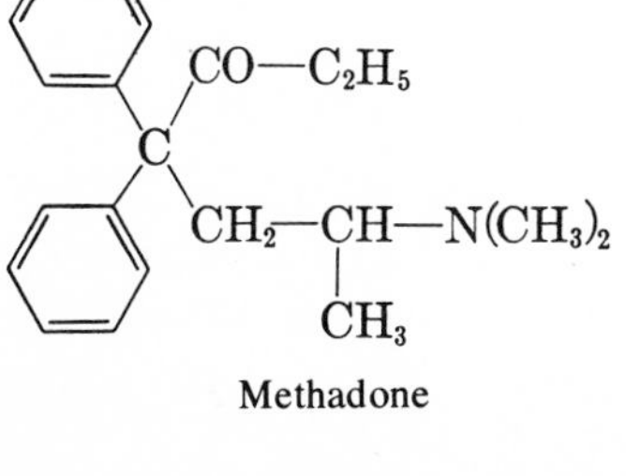

Methadone

Of these three compounds, only *N*-methylmorphinan shows immediate structural similarity to morphine, and it also lacks the furan ring, the OH groups, and the 7-8 double bond of the natural drug. We conclude that all these groups, although possibly helpful for affinity to the receptor, play no role in efficacy. The cyclohexane rings also seem to be dispensable, as shown by the analgesic activity of meperidine, so that the essential structure for action on the morphine receptor appears to be *N*-methyl-γ-phenylpiperidine:

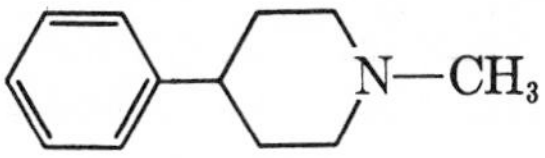

True, in methadone even the piperidine ring is absent, but steric and hydrogen-bonding interactions within the methadone molecule force it into a conformation simulating a piperidine ring:

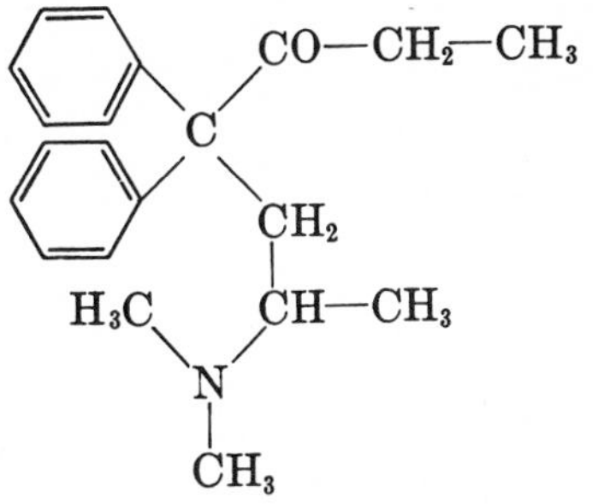

On the other hand, it has been argued that the piperidine ring per se is not important, but rather that the tertiary nitrogen should be held more or less fixed in a determined position in relation to the benzene ring. This aim is achieved by the steric and hydrogen-bonding interactions referred to in discussing methadone, and by a piperidine ring in all the other morphine-like compounds shown above; but it can be achieved in other ways as well, for instance, by a seven-membered ring in a homologue of meperidine which is quite active:

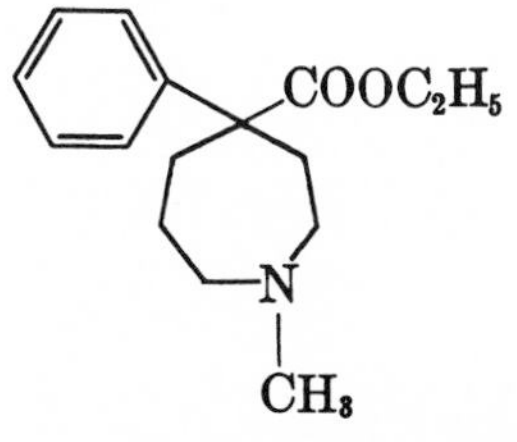

Thus, in general, morphine-like analgesics have somewhat rigid molecules containing at least one benzene (or in some cases not shown here, other aromatic) ring and a cationic nitrogen atom, the latter pointed up by the observation that weakly basic morphine analogues are pharmacologically inactive. Therefore, the morphine receptor must have two sites specifically receptive to these two features, presumably a flat nonpolar bonding site to accommodate the flat benzene ring and an anionic site for the cationic nitrogen. Moreover, usually morphine-like drug molecules are asymmetric, and one enantiomorph is generally more potent than the other. This situation, reminiscent of that observed with the muscarine stereoisomers, leads to the conclusion that there must be a third point of attachment to the receptor. As is shown in Fig. 2-8, if the rectangular area represents the receptor surface and X is the postulated third point of contact required of a drug for maximally productive interaction with the receptor, then only the enantiomorph shown on the right will have full efficacy; the one on the left can attach only to two of the three points of attachment and will produce poorer results.

On this basis, a tentative structure for the morphine receptor was proposed as early as 1954. However, we now know that the situation is more complicated. First of all, we have learned the absolute configuration of morphine as well as that of other morphine-like analgesics, and in several pairs of enantiomorphs, the more potent one does not always have the same configuration. Moreover, when the structure of morphine is noted with due attention to conformation (Fig. 2-9), it may be seen that the benzene ring is fixed in an axial position relative to the piperidine ring, whereas it has been shown that in various derivatives of meperidine the more potent stereoisomer has the benzene ring in equatorial conformation; the two conformations differ considerably in the relative distances of the

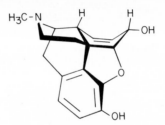

Figure 2-9 Perspective image of the morphine molecule.

cationic nitrogen from the benzene ring. Thus the initial postulate of a flat area and an anionic site at fixed distance from each other in the morphine receptor must be eliminated. There has been speculation that there may be two or more morphine receptors, one for one conformation and one for the other; but surely an equally attractive hypothesis may be based on the concept of conformational mobility which appears to be generally accepted for enzymes and which might be equally valid for receptors. On this assumption, the same receptor may accommodate all morphine-like analgesics by being flexible enough to adapt to all of them.

PROSPECTS FOR THE FUTURE

Present-day knowledge of specific drug action is based largely on hindsight with some experimental confirmation, and many of the ideas which now appear so persuasive may have to be modified or discarded in coming years. But that is the natural course of events in any science at the stage where a coherent theory takes shape. It is nevertheless true that a picture of drug action is emerging which is well grounded in biochemistry, physical chemistry, organic chemistry, physiology, and not least —in experiment.

At the same time, the results so far obtained raise an overwhelming number of questions. Just what is that second event which transforms drug binding into drug action? What is the complete structure of receptors? Why and how does this structure, in its interaction with drugs, result in that modification of normal physiology which is called drug action? These and many other questions will have to be answered separately for each receptor which will ultimately make it possible to design drugs with a specific selectivity and a specific purpose.

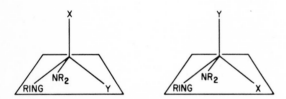

Figure 2-8 Attachment of L and D enantiomorphs of morphine-type drugs to their receptor.

Chapter 3

Absorption, Distribution, and Excretion

Some of the physiologic factors that influence the concentration of a drug at its site of action are depicted in Fig. 3-1. To begin with, a drug must be absorbed from its site of administration. Once within the blood plasma, drug molecules may become reversibly bound to plasma proteins in an inactive form. Free drug molecules, however, move to sites of action, biotransformation, excretion, and tissue storage.

Not shown clearly in Fig. 3-1 are perhaps the most important of the physiologic factors that determine the absorption, distribution, and excretion of a drug: the membranes that separate biologic sites from one another. Membranes enclose sites of drug action, absorption, biotransformation, excretion, and storage. Our first concern, then, will be the body membranes and how they are penetrated by drugs.

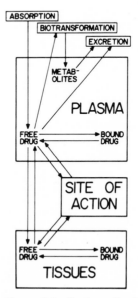

Figure 3-1 Factors affecting the concentration of a drug at its site of action.

PASSAGE OF DRUGS ACROSS MEMBRANES

Nature of Body Membranes

Electron microscopic studies of tissues suggest that all body membranes are composed of a fundamental structure called the *unit membrane* or *plasma membrane*. This boundary, which is about 80 Å thick, surrounds single cells, such as the erythrocyte, epithelial cell, and neuron, and also subcellular structures, such as the mitochondrion and cell nucleus. More complex membranes, like the intestinal epithelium and the skin, are composed of multiples of the fundamental structure. Chemical analysis of cell membranes has shown that they are composed mainly of lipids and proteins, with about 70 molecules of lipid for each molecule of protein.

Previous studies had led to the view that the cell boundary is a lipidlike layer interspersed with small, aqueous channels or pores; lipid-soluble substances penetrate the membrane by dissolving in the lipoid phase, and lipid-insoluble molecules penetrate only if they are small enough to pass through the pores. Later workers recognized that the cell membrane also possessed specialized transport processes, since certain large, lipid-insoluble molecules, such as sugars and amino acids, could penetrate cells readily.

Processes by Which Drugs Cross Membranes

The diverse ways in which solutes move across membranes can be grouped under two general headings: passive transfer and specialized transport.

Passive Transfer   Many drugs penetrate body membranes by *simple diffusion*; that is, their rate of transfer is directly proportional to their concentration gradient across the membrane. Some of the substances traverse the membrane as though it were a layer of lipoid material, the relative speed of passage being determined by the lipid solubility, or more precisely, the lipid-to-water partition coefficient, of the substances. In contrast, a number of lipid-insoluble compounds of relatively low molecular weight diffuse across the membrane as though it were a sieve made up of small water-filled channels, the smaller molecules crossing more rapidly than the larger ones. With lipid-insoluble ions, however, the speed of transfer may be determined

more by the ionic charge than by the size; for example, in the red cell, anions penetrate much more rapidly than cations.

Compounds can also cross membranes by hydrodynamic flow, or *filtration*. In this passive process, when a hydrostatic or osmotic pressure difference exists across a membrane, water flows, in bulk, through the membrane pores, dragging with it any solute molecules whose dimensions are less than those of the pores. As an example, the water that filters through the relatively large pores of the renal glomerular membrane is accompanied by all the solutes of plasma except the protein molecules.

Effect of pH and Protein Binding on Passive Transfer   In considering the diffusion of drugs across membranes, it is necessary to take into account that most drugs are weak acids or bases which exist in solution as a mixture of the ionized and nonionized forms. This complicates the problem of describing the passage of drugs across a lipoid-pore membrane, since usually only the un-ionized form of a drug is lipid-soluble, and the ionized moiety is too large to pass readily through the pores. Accordingly, the un-ionized form of a drug penetrates many body membranes at a rate related to its lipid-to-water partition coefficient and its concentration gradient across the membrane, whereas the ionized form penetrates at a very slow rate. This process is sometimes called *nonionic diffusion*.

The proportion of drug in the un-ionized form depends on the dissociation constant of the drug and on the pH of the medium in which it is dissolved, a relationship shown by the Henderson-Hasselbalch equation.

For an acid:

$$pK_a = pH + \log\frac{\text{concentration of un-ionized acid}}{\text{concentration of ionized acid}}$$

For a base:

$$pK_a = pH + \log\frac{\text{concentration of ionized base}}{\text{concentration of un-ionized base}}$$

In these equations, the dissociation constant of both acids and bases is expressed as a pK_a, which is the negative logarithm of the acidic dissociation constant. From the equations, it can be seen that barbital, an acid with a pK_a of 7.5, is approximately 91 percent ionized at pH 8.5, 50 percent ionized at pH 7.5, and 9 percent ionized at pH 6.5. Quinine, a base with a pK_a of 8.4, is about 91 percent ionized at pH 7.4, 50 percent ionized at pH 8.4, and 9 percent ionized at pH 9.4. While most drugs have pK_a values between 3 and 11 and are accordingly partly ionized and partly un-ionized over the range of physiologic pH values, some are at the extreme ends of the scale. For instance, acetanilide, a weak base with a pK_a of 0.3, is almost completely un-ionized at all body pH values. Sulfonic acids, with a pK_a below 1, are almost completely ionized at all pH values, and quaternary ammonium compounds exist only as cations at any pH.

Drugs that penetrate a biologic membrane by simple diffusion become distributed across the membrane according to their degree of ionization, the charge of their ionized form, and the extent to which they are bound to proteins or other macromolecules in the solutions bathing the membrane. A difference in pH on the two sides of a membrane affects the distribution of a partly ionized substance because of the preferential permeability of membranes to the lipid-soluble, un-ionized form of compounds. This is illustrated in Fig. 3-2, which shows the distribution of a weak acid ($pK_a = 6$) between solutions of pH 7 and 5; the solutions are separated by a membrane permeable only to the un-ionized form of the compound. At the steady state, the concentration of the un-ionized solute is the same in both solutions; but the concentrations of the ionized form are unequal because of the difference in pH of the two fluids. Accordingly, the total concentration of solute (ionized plus un-ionized) on both sides of the membrane is a function of the pH of the two fluids and the pK_a of the solute.

Since biologic membranes are virtually impermeable to protein molecules, the degree of protein binding of a drug can markedly influence its distribution across a membrane. For example, a drug that is highly bound to plasma albumin has a much greater concentration in plasma than in fluids relatively free of protein such as the glomerular filtrate or the cerebrospinal fluid. Moreover, very few drugs become distributed evenly between plasma and tissues because the degrees of intracellular and extracellular binding are different. An example of the effect of protein binding on the distribution of a drug is shown in Fig. 3-3.

Specialized Transport Although passive transfer across a lipoid-pore boundary adequately describes the penetration of body membranes by many drugs and other foreign organic compounds, it does not explain the rapid penetration and peculiar kinetic behavior of certain large, lipid-insoluble

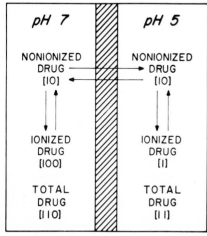

Figure 3-2 Distribution of a weak acid ($pK_a = 6$) between aqueous solutions of pH 7 and pH 5. The solutions are separated by a membrane that is permeable only to the un-ionized form of the weak acid. Concentrations at the steady state are shown in brackets.

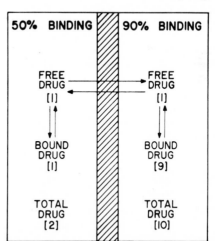

Figure 3-3 Distribution of a drug between two protein solutions. In one solution the drug is 50 percent bound to protein, and in the other it is 90 percent bound. The solutions are separated by a membrane that is permeable only to free drug. Concentrations at the steady state are shown in brackets.

molecules and ions. For example, glucose and a number of other monosaccharides are readily absorbed from the small intestine and renal tubule and penetrate most cells at a rapid rate; moreover, the same is true of the highly ionized amino acids. In addition, a number of sulfonic acid anions and quaternary ammonium cations are rapidly transported across cell membranes of the liver, renal tubule, and choroid plexus. Not only are the rates of transport rapid, but in most cases the substances can move across membranes in an "uphill" direction, that is, from a solution of low concentration into one of higher concentration. The concept of membrane *carriers* has arisen as a tentative explanation for the unique permeability of membranes to these substances.

Membrane carriers are viewed as components of the unit membrane, which are capable of combining with a solute at one surface of the membrane; the carrier-solute complex moves across the membrane, the solute is released, and the carrier then returns to the original surface where it can combine with another molecule of solute.

Two main types of carrier transport are recognized: *active transport* and *facilitated diffusion*. Active transport signifies a process in which the solute crosses the membrane against a concentration gradient, or if the solute is an ion, it crosses against an electrochemical potential gradient. Facilitated diffusion denotes a transport process that is similar to active transport, except that the solute is not transferred against a concentration or electrochemical potential gradient.

Although proteins and other macromolecules move across most body membranes at rates that seem almost insignificant compared with the rates of transfer of lipid-soluble drugs and carrier-transported substances, it is important to emphasize that they are transported. Two forms of specialized transport, *pinocytosis* and *phagocytosis*, may account for this movement. In these complex processes, the cell engulfs a droplet of extracellular fluid (pinocytosis) or a particle of solid material such as a bacterium (phagocytosis).

BINDING OF DRUGS TO MACROMOLECULES

Binding of drugs to proteins and other macromolecules is known to occur in almost every tissue of the body. It has been demonstrated with albumin,

mucopolysaccharides, nucleoproteins, and other substances.

Binding is generally a reversible process and therefore arrives at an equilibrium in which only the unbound fraction of the drug is free to act and to be metabolized and excreted, while the bound fraction functions as a depot from which the drug is regenerated as the equilibrium is reestablished after removal of the free fraction. The forces responsible for the binding are weak bonds of the van der Waals, hydrogen, and ionic types. The position of the equilibrium, and the rate at which the free fraction of the drug is removed by metabolism and excretion, determines the biologic half-life of the drug which can vary widely. For example, the trypanocidal drug suramin is tightly bound, and a single dose protects against infection for as long as 3 months.

Thus the reversible binding of drugs to various intracellular and extracellular substances is important in determining how long a drug remains in the body. Without these storage pools, many drugs would be metabolized and excreted so rapidly that they would hardly have time to exert their pharmacologic action.

Binding to Plasma Proteins

The plasma protein binding of drugs is usually expressed as a percentage, that is, the percent of total drug bound. Most drugs show some degree of binding in plasma, and much of this is accounted for by the plasma albumin. Examples of highly bound compounds include phenylbutazone, bishydroxycoumarin, quinine, and thiopental (75 to 98 percent bound); compounds with moderate degrees of binding include salicylic acid, pentobarbital, and mecamylamine (20 to 40 percent bound). Drugs such as barbital, guanethidine, and sulfaguanidine exhibit a low degree of plasma binding (1 to 8 percent).

Because albumin and other plasma proteins possess a limited number of binding sites, two drugs with an affinity for the same site will compete with one another for binding. Furthermore, if one of the drugs is administered after the other, the second will displace a portion of the first from the binding sites, and the organism suddenly will be faced with a markedly increased plasma concentration of pharmacologically active compound. With a drug that is normally highly bound, the usual therapeutic dose may become lethal when followed by administration of a drug that displaces it from its storage sites.

Competition between drugs for binding sites can also bring about significant changes in the distribution of drugs between plasma and tissues. For example, sulfinpyrazone displaces a highly bound sulfonamide, sulfaethylthiadiazole, from plasma albumin; as a result, the free sulfonamide diffuses into tissues such as brain and muscle, thereby causing the plasma concentration to decline.

The influence of protein binding on the passive transfer of drugs across membranes has already been mentioned (Fig. 3-3). When binding to plasma proteins creates an equilibrium mixture of free and protein-bound drug, only the free fraction can diffuse across membranes. It is true that, as these processes remove free drug, more is liberated as the equilibrium is reestablished, but when the equilibrium is strongly on the side of binding, only a very meager portion of the total drug may leave the blood on a single passage of the blood through an organ. This situation is modified when a drug is actively transported across a membrane or crosses by some other form of specialized transport. As an example, phenol red and penicillin, both tightly bound in plasma, are actively transported into urine by the renal tubular epithelium and are almost completely cleared from plasma in one passage through the kidney. The speed of reversibility of the drug-protein interaction is apparently great enough to keep pace with the rapid removal of free drug from plasma by the membrane carriers.

Binding to Tissues

The binding of drugs to components of various tissues is difficult to measure quantitatively. Certain drugs show a much greater affinity for tissues than for plasma proteins, and in some instances, the affinity for one tissue is considerably greater than for another. Tetracycline has an unusual affinity for bone; quinacrine, for the nuclei of liver cells; and guanethidine, for heart and skeletal muscle.

MECHANISMS OF DRUG ABSORPTION, DISTRIBUTION, AND EXCRETION

Before considering the routes of drug administration and the various dosage forms used, let us ana-lyze the movement of dissolved drug molecules through the body in terms of the general principles outlined above.

Alimentary Canal

The passage of drugs and other foreign compounds across the epithelial lining of the oral cavity, stomach, small intestine, colon, and rectum is explainable for the most part in terms of simple diffusion across a lipoid membrane. Drugs in true solution are readily absorbed in their lipid-soluble un-ionized form and very slowly absorbed in their lipid-insoluble ionized form. Moreover, with most compounds that exist mainly as un-ionized molecules, the relative rates of absorption are directly related to the lipid-to-water partition coefficients of the molecules.

The stomach is a significant site of absorption for many acidic and neutral compounds but not for basic compounds. For example, acidic drugs like the salicylates and barbiturates, which exist as un-ionized lipid-soluble molecules in the acid gastric contents, are readily absorbed, whereas basic drugs like the plant alkaloids, which exist largely as ions, are hardly absorbed at all. In other portions of the alimentary canal, where the intraluminal pH is closer to neutrality, many weak acids and bases are to a considerable extent un-ionized and are absorbed at rates related to their lipid-to-water partition ratios. At all levels of the canal, slowest rates of absorption are found with completely ionized drugs, such as the quaternary ammonium compounds and sulfonic acids, and with lipid-insoluble neutral molecules, such as sulfaguanidine and mannitol. Certain quaternary amines may be absorbed in part in the form of chemical complexes.

The rate of absorption of most drugs is directly proportional to drug concentration in accord with the process of simple diffusion. If the intraluminal concentration is raised threefold, 3 times as much drug will be absorbed per unit of time, the percentage absorption remaining constant.

The absorption of drugs is increased by changes in pH which increase the fraction of drug in the lipid-soluble un-ionized form. For example, raising the gastric pH to a value of 8 with sodium bicarbonate results in a markedly increased rate of absorption for many basic drugs; conversely, the gastric absorption of most acidic compounds is decreased at the elevated pH value. A similar relationship between pH and absorption rate occurs in the mouth, small and large intestines, and rectum.

In the small intestine, weak acids and bases become distributed between intestinal fluid of pH 6.6 and plasma of pH 7.4 (see Fig. 3-2) as though the intestinal pH were 5.3. Thus the pH at the absorbing surface appears to be lower than that of the intestinal contents, and it is this lower pH value that may determine the degree of ionization and hence the rate of absorption of weak electrolytes. The colonic and rectal mucosae also show an apparent surface pH somewhat lower than that of the luminal contents.

While most drugs cross the intestinal boundary by a process of simple diffusion, a drug can be absorbed by specialized active transport if its chemical structure is similar enough to that of a substrate which is naturally transported. For example, the antitumor compounds 5-fluorouracil and 5-bromouracil are actively transported across the intestine by the process which transports the natural pyrimidines uracil and thymine.

Skin

Many drugs and other organic compounds diffuse across mammalian skin at rates directly related to their lipid-to-water partition coefficients. In addition, the skin is more permeable to the lipid-soluble, un-ionized form of drugs than to the ionized form. Because of the relatively great thickness of the skin, drugs penetrate this boundary much more slowly than they do most other body membranes.

Lung

Drugs administered as gases penetrate the respiratory-tract epithelium with great rapidity. These substances have high lipid-to-water partition coefficients and small molecular sizes.

Blood Capillary

Most drugs traverse the capillary wall by a combination of two processes, diffusion and filtration (hydrodynamic flow). In addition, most drugs, whether lipid-soluble or not, cross the capillary wall at rates which are extremely rapid in comparison with their rates of passage across many other body membranes. Thus, the supply of drugs to the various tissues may be limited more by the rate of blood flow than by the restraint imposed by the capillary endothelium.

Brain and Cerebrospinal Fluid

The passage of drugs into and out of the central nervous system involves transfer between three major compartments: brain, cerebrospinal fluid (CSF), and blood. The boundary between blood and brain consists of several membranes: those of the blood capillary wall, those of the glial cells closely surrounding the capillary, and that of the neuron. The so-called "blood-brain barrier," which provides the main hindrance to the diffusion of drugs, is located at the capillary wall–glial cell region. After a drug penetrates this barrier and enters the extracellular fluid of the brain, it must then cross the neuronal cell membrane to enter nervous tissue. The *blood-CSF barrier* consists mainly of the epithelium of the choroid plexuses located within the cerebral ventricles.

Drugs pass from blood into brain and CSF at rates related to the lipid-to-water partition coefficients and degrees of ionization of the compounds. Lipid-soluble, un-ionized substances penetrate readily, whereas lipid-insoluble molecules and ions penetrate with great difficulty. For example, a highly lipid-soluble compound such as thiopental passes from blood into CSF thousands of times more rapidly than do certain quaternary ammonium compounds or sulfonic acids.

The exit of drugs from the central nervous system involves more pathways than the entrance. Drugs can diffuse across the blood-brain and blood-CSF barriers in the reverse direction at rates determined by their lipid solubility and degree of ionization. Moreover, all drugs, whether lipid-soluble or not, pass from CSF into blood at similar rates as CSF drains into the dural blood sinuses by flowing through the wide channels of the arachnoid villi. In addition, certain organic anions and cations are rapidly transferred from CSF to blood by active transport across the choroid plexuses; anions such as penicillin and phenol red are transported by one process, and cations such as hexamethonium and choline by another. Because of the ready removal of certain poorly lipid-soluble drugs from the CSF by active transport as well as by the CSF drainage mechanism, many of these substances never attain a concentration in CSF equal to that in plasma.

Eye

The ocular fluid is similar to CSF with regard to the entry and exit of drugs. Thus the blood-ocular fluid boundary, which consists mainly of the ciliary body epithelium and the capillary walls and surrounding connective tissue of the iris, behaves as a lipoid barrier to most organic compounds.

Drugs applied to the corneal surface of the eye penetrate into the aqueous humor at rates related to the lipid-to-water partition coefficient of their un-ionized form.

Mammary Gland, Salivary Glands, and Sweat Glands

Many drugs are excreted in milk, saliva, and sweat by a process of simple diffusion of the un-ionized drug form. Since the pH of milk is usually about 0.7 unit below that of plasma, basic drugs appear in milk in a concentration greater than that in plasma, and acidic drugs in a concentration less than that in plasma (see Fig. 3-2). Completely un-ionized substances such as ethanol and antipyrine become distributed evenly between the two fluids.

Sweat also has a pH somewhat below that of plasma, and a number of acidic drugs accordingly appear in this fluid in a concentration less than that in plasma.

Liver

The hepatic parenchymal cell is readily penetrated by most drugs. In addition to the rapid penetration of many un-ionized compounds, which presumably pass through lipoid areas as well as pores in the cell membrane, a wide variety of organic anions and cations are readily taken up by the parenchymal cell by carrier-type transport processes.

The liver has at least three active transport processes for the biliary excretion of certain poorly lipid-soluble organic compounds. One process excretes a variety of organic anions including sulfonic acid dyes, bile acids, bilirubin, penicillin, and probably many drug metabolites such as glucuronides and other acidic conjugation products. A second process is responsible for the biliary excretion of organic cations, including certain quaternary ammonium compounds and tertiary amines. A third process excretes a number of un-ionic, poorly lipid-soluble cardioactive glycosides such as oua-

bain, scillaren A, and lanatosides A and C. In these processes, compounds are transported from plasma into bile against a large concentration gradient, the excretion mechanism becomes saturated at high plasma levels of the compound, and compounds that are excreted by the same process inhibit the transport of one another in a competitive manner.

After a drug has been excreted into the intestine via the bile, it may be partly reabsorbed and partly excreted in the feces. Glucuronides or other conjugated forms of drugs may be split within the intestinal lumina to release the free, lipid-soluble drug molecules; the drug is readily reabsorbed, conjugated in the liver, and again excreted into bile. This enterohepatic cycle can delay considerably the elimination of a drug from the body.

Lipid-soluble, un-ionized drugs do not appear in the bile in high concentrations. During their passage through the bile duct, these molecules can diffuse readily across the bile duct epithelium and thereby remain in equilibrium with the drug concentration in plasma.

Kidney

All drugs cross the highly porous glomerular membrane at similar rates by a process of filtration. As the renal tubular fluid becomes more concentrated, un-ionized drug molecules are reabsorbed by diffusion across the tubular epithelium at rates related to their lipid-to-water partition coefficients. Accordingly, compounds of low lipid solubility, which are poorly reabsorbed, are excreted in urine more readily than are compounds of high lipid solubility.

In accordance with the principles governing the distribution of weak electrolytes across a lipoid membrane (see Fig. 3-2), when the tubular urine is made alkaline, weak bases become less concentrated in urine than in plasma and, as a result, are excreted more slowly; when the urine is made acidic, the bases become concentrated in the urine and are excreted more rapidly. Conversely, weak acids are excreted more readily in an alkaline urine and more slowly in an acidic urine.

The tubular epithelium has at least two specialized processes which actively transport (secrete) organic ions into urine. One process transports a variety of organic anions, such as penicillin, phenol red, iodopyracet, and p-aminohippurate, and the other a wide array of organic cations, such as tetraethylammonium, mepiperphenidol, and N^1-methyl-nicotinamide, to mention only a few of the compounds. These substances are transported against a concentration gradient; the processes show a transport maximum; and there is competition for transport among various anionic compounds and similar competition for transport among various cationic compounds. Since the ionized form of lipid-soluble drugs, for example, salicylate anion and quinine cation, are actively transported by these processes, the renal excretion of many weak acids and bases involves three mechanisms: glomerular filtration, active tubular secretion of the ionized drug form, and passive tubular reabsorption of the un-ionized form.

REDISTRIBUTION OF DRUGS IN THE BODY

The pattern of distribution of drugs is governed by two factors: (1) the affinity of the drug for the various tissues (i.e., the equilibrium between the blood and each tissue) and (2) the rate of blood flow to each tissue. Those tissues with the best blood supply come into equilibrium with the blood almost immediately; those with the poorest blood supply, very slowly. As a result, the tissues with good blood supply initially accumulate an inordinately high proportion of the total drug present, which is then gradually redistributed in the body as other tissues also come into equilibrium with the blood. The final situation, where all tissues are in equilibrium with each other by the intermediary of the blood which supplies them, may take many hours.

Thiopental, a highly lipid-soluble drug that penetrates all cells readily and has an especially high affinity for body fat, does not initially become localized in fat. Rather, after intravenous administration, it first reaches high concentrations in brain, liver, kidney, and other tissues that have high rates of blood flow. The concentration of drug in muscle rises slowly because of the slower rate of delivery to that tissue, and the concentration in fat rises even more slowly for the same reason. As thiopental is taken up by the large muscle mass of the body as well as by fat, the plasma concentration declines, and the drug begins to diffuse out of the brain and other early sites of deposition. Body fat, with its high affinity for the barbiturate, gradually accumulates the drug, and after some time, the bulk

of the drug has moved out of the muscle and into fat depots.

ROUTES OF ADMINISTRATION AND DOSAGE FORMS

Alimentary Canal

The alimentary tract is by far the most common site of administration when a drug is intended for systemic action. The dosage forms include tablets, capsules, specially formulated tablets or capsules for prolonged action or other uses, suspensions, powders, emulsions, various flavored or unflavored solutions (elixirs, syrups, solutions, tinctures, fluidextracts), and rectal suppositories.

Gastrointestinal Tract   The oral route of administration is the safest, most convenient, and most economical. However, it has a number of disadvantages: (1) irritation to the gastric mucosa with resultant nausea or vomiting; (2) destruction of some drugs by gastric acid or digestive enzymes; (3) precipitation or insolubility of some drugs in gastrointestinal fluids; (4) formation of nonabsorbable complexes between drugs and food materials; (5) variable rates of absorption due to physiologic factors such as gastric emptying time, gastrointestinal motility, and mixing; (6) too slow an absorption rate for effectiveness in an emergency situation; (7) inability to use the oral route in an unconscious patient; and (8) the unpleasant taste of some drugs.

Some of the disadvantages of the oral route can be overcome in various ways. Gastric irritation, as well as the destruction, precipitation, or complexing of drugs in the stomach, can be avoided by using an enteric-coated tablet or capsule which resists gastric acid but dissolves in the higher pH range of the intestine or in the presence of intestinal enzymes. In some cases, gastric irritation can be minimized or avoided simply by administering a drug at mealtime or immediately after a meal.

Conversely, for rapid absorption, a drug should be taken with the stomach empty; a glass of water should accompany the dose to dissolve the drug and wash it into the intestine.

The "prolonged-action" dosage forms for oral administration have been developed with the idea of supplying in one capsule, tablet, or teaspoonful all the drug that will be needed over a period of many hours. For a particular drug, the objective might be to produce quickly a desired plasma concentration of drug and then supply additional drug to maintain this concentration for a number of hours. Or the objective might be to release various doses of one or more drugs at widely spaced intervals. A major obstacle to the use of these dosage forms is the high variability of physiologic factors in patients.

An important point to be emphasized in considering absorption after oral administration is that a drug must be dissolved before it can be absorbed. The drug administered in solid form will be absorbed at a rate limited by the rate at which it dissolves in the intestinal fluids. Many factors influence the rate of solution, or the *dissolution rate* as it is sometimes called; these include (1) solubility, particle size, crystalline form, and salt form of the drug; (2) the rate of disintegration of the solid-dosage form in the gastrointestinal lumina; and (3) gastrointestinal pH, motility, and food content.

Oral Mucosa   Since many drugs are readily absorbed from the oral cavity, the *sublingual* route offers a simple, convenient method of administration. A small tablet is placed under the tongue and allowed to dissolve. Drugs may also be given by the *buccal* route, in which the tablet is placed between the cheek and gingiva. Advantages of these routes include (1) delayed degradation of drug by avoiding early passage through the liver and (2) avoidance of many of the disadvantages of gastrointestinal-tract administration. Disadvantages of the sublingual and buccal routes include the unpleasant taste and irritating effects of some drugs.

Rectal Mucosa   Drugs are administered rectally in the form of suppositories which melt at body temperature. The rectal route is useful when unconsciousness or vomiting preclude use of the oral route. As with the sublingual route, the absorbed drug enters the general circulation before passing through the liver. Disadvantages include irritation to the mucosa by some drugs and inconvenience.

Skin

For local effects on the skin, drugs may be applied in the form of ointments, liniments, lotions, creams, and pastes. The skin is not ordinarily used as a site of absorption for drugs. The percutaneous absorption of ionized drugs can be enhanced by the method of *iontophoresis*, in which drug solution in contact with an electrode is placed against the skin and a galvanic current applied to both the drug electrode and another electrode placed elsewhere on the body. Absorption through the skin can also be enhanced by dissolving a drug in oil, an ointment base, or other organic solvent and rubbing it into the skin, a procedure known as *inunction*.

Respiratory Tract

Although many drugs and other chemicals appear to be rapidly absorbed when inhaled as sprays, aerosols, or dusts, this route of absorption has had very limited use in therapeutics. A major problem is the difficulty of administration and retention of exact quantities of drug. Physiologic variables may include respiratory-tract infections and other pathologic states, ciliary action, and the mucous coating of the tract.

An *aerosol* is an air suspension of liquid or solid particles so small that they do not readily settle out under the force of gravity. Particles with a diameter greater than 10 μm become deposited mainly in the nasal passages, whereas particles less than 2 μm in diameter penetrate deeper into the respiratory tract before deposition occurs. For significant penetration into the alveolar ducts and sacs, it is probably necessary to have particles less than 1 μm in diameter.

Aerosols can be used for the administration of drugs intended to act locally in the lung.

Injection Routes

Administration of drugs by injection, sometimes called *parenteral* administration because it is not via the intestine, includes the subcutaneous, intramuscular, intravenous, intraarterial, bone marrow, and intrathecal routes. Each of these avenues has its own merits and pitfalls, but a number of features are shared by all. Generally, parenteral administration produces a more prompt response than that obtained after oral administration. More accurate dosage is usually attained with the parenteral route than with the oral route. Injection routes are valuable when vomiting or unconsciousness preclude use of the oral route.

Parenteral administration has several drawbacks. Because of the generally rapid rate of absorption, there often is not much time to combat adverse drug reactions and accidental overdoses. Moreover, parenteral administration requires sterile dosage forms and aseptic procedures; it may be painful; it is relatively expensive; and patients cannot readily administer the drug to themselves.

Subcutaneous Route   Absorption of drugs from aqueous solutions injected at this site is rapid and depends mainly on the ease of penetration of the capillary wall, the area over which the solution has spread, and the rate of blood flow through the area. Accordingly, the rate of absorption can be influenced by a number of procedures. Absorption can be hastened by massage or application of heat to the injected area, or it can be slowed by reducing circulation to the injected area, for example, by local cooling or by inclusion of a vasoconstrictor agent in the drug solution.

To obtain a slow, continuous rate of absorption from a subcutaneous site, drugs may be injected as a suspension of poorly soluble crystals or implanted under the skin in the form of a compressed pellet.

Irritating drugs should not be injected subcutaneously. They can produce severe pain and local necrosis.

Intramuscular Route   Drugs injected into skeletal muscle in the form of aqueous solutions are absorbed rapidly. The rate of absorption is determined mainly by the speed of penetration of the capillary wall, the area of solution exposed to the circulation, and the rate of blood flow.

The intramuscular route is often used for depot forms of drugs, for example, aqueous or oil suspensions or poorly soluble salts.

Intravenous Route   Injection of drugs directly into the bloodstream avoids all the delays and variables of absorption. Penetration to the site of drug action is usually very rapid, and this factor affords certain advantages: (1) rapid drug action in emergency therapy and (2) continuous control of the degree of pharmacologic action (for example, in general anesthesia) because the drug can be given slowly and the rate of administration varied as necessary. Other advantages of the intravenous route include (1) greatest accuracy in drug dosage; (2) ability to give large volumes of solutions over a long period of time; and (3) ability to administer irritating, hypertonic, acidic, or alkaline solutions, since, when given slowly, these become diluted in a large volume of fluid; however, it is important to avoid extravasation of these solutions into tissue surrounding the vein.

The intravenous route is the most dangerous of all avenues of administration because of the speed of onset of pharmacologic action. An overdose cannot be withdrawn, nor can its absorption be retarded. If a safe dose is given too rapidly, toxicity can result from the undesired high drug concentration which initially perfuses reactive sites.

Drugs which precipitate readily at the pH of blood and drugs suspended or dissolved in oily liquids should not be given intravenously because of the danger of embolism.

Intrathecal Route   Injection of drugs into the spinal subarachnoid space is used for producing spinal anesthesia with local anesthetic agents. It is also used for treating infections or tumors of brain and spinal tissues with drugs that do not penetrate well into the central nervous system.

Other Routes of Administration

Drugs can be absorbed from sites other than those described above, for example, the conjunctiva, urethra, vagina, and nasal mucous membranes. Although medicinals are applied at these sites, the purpose is almost always for local action.

Chapter 4

Drug Metabolism

The duration and intensity of action of various drugs and other foreign substances depend largely on the ability of the mammalian metabolic systems to metabolize (biotransform) the compounds and on the excretory system of the kidney to excrete the end products of metabolism. In regulating these two aspects of drug action, the metabolic systems perform two *major* functions: (1) inactivation of various drugs or foreign substances through enzymatic reactions (detoxication) and (2) an increase in the water solubility of the drug and its metabolites for clearance through the various excretory systems. The majority of metabolic reactions occur within the liver, particularly the liver microsomes which contain the *drug microsomal metabolizing system*. The remainder of the metabolic reactions occur within various systems of the body such as blood or kidney.

BIOTRANSFORMATION REACTIONS

Lipid-soluble, nonpolar foreign compounds introduced into the body are usually not excreted until they undergo one or more chemical changes that result in an increase in polarity. Ordinarily they are metabolized in one or both of two general phases of metabolism. Phase I consists of oxidations, reductions, and cleavages or hydrolysis. Phase II consists of synthetic or conjugation reactions.

$$\text{Drug} \xrightarrow{\text{phase I}} \begin{array}{c} \text{oxidation,} \\ \text{reduction,} \\ \text{and/or} \\ \text{cleavage} \\ \text{products} \end{array} \xrightarrow{\text{phase II}} \begin{array}{c} \text{conjugated} \\ \text{products} \end{array}$$

Phase I reactions tend to increase the polarity of drug molecules and thereby usually change the pharmacologic activity. With most drugs, phase I biotransformation reactions result in a decrease or loss in pharmacologic activity. In some instances, however, an inactive precursor may be biotransformed into a pharmacologically active drug,

$$\text{Parathion} \xrightarrow{\text{desulfuration (oxidative)}} \text{paraoxon}$$

or an active drug may be biotransformed to a metabolite which is also active,

$$\text{Aspirin} \xrightarrow{\text{hydrolysis}} \text{salicylic acid}$$

or, in other instances, the pharmacologic activity may be changed to another type,

$$\text{Phenylbutazone} \xrightarrow{\text{side-chain hydroxylation}} \text{hydroxy-phenyl-butazone}$$

or the product may be rendered more toxic than the precursor

$$\text{Methanol} \xrightarrow{\text{alcohol oxidation}} \text{formaldehyde and formic acid}$$

Phase II synthetic reactions usually involve polar functional groups on the drug molecules such as those introduced in the phase I reactions. In synthesis or conjugation, the drug is combined through its polar group with a substrate endogenous to the body, such as glucuronic or amino acids or, occasionally, methyl and other alkyl groups. These phase II synthetic reactions usually render the conjugated molecule more polar, less lipid-soluble, and therefore more readily excretable. Phase II reactions usually result in loss of pharmacologic activity and have been called *detoxication reactions*.

Drug biotransformations by phase I and II reactions have been found to be mediated by enzymes in various components of the cell. The level of lipid-solubility generally determines whether a drug is biotransformed primarily by the "soluble fraction," mitochondrial fraction, or microsomal fraction. Those drugs resembling the less lipid-soluble, more water-soluble, and natural substrates of the body are usually metabolized by the soluble or mitochondrial fractions of homogenates. Highly

lipid-soluble drugs are usually biotransformed by enzyme systems in the microsomal fraction. The microsomal enzyme systems differ functionally from those found in the mitochondria and soluble systems, in that the microsomal enzyme systems can vary greatly because of the previous conditions to which the body is subjected. Pathologic, nutritional, other environmental conditions, or previous drug intake may induce drug biotransformation of either nonspecific or specific types to become much more active in some instances or, in other instances, may drastically reduce nonspecific or specific drug biotransformations.

SPECIFIC DRUG BIOTRANSFORMATION REACTIONS

Table 4-1 lists the more prominent oxidations of the nonmicrosomal and microsomal systems and, in addition, illustrates the general reaction mechanisms and examples of specific drugs that can be biotransformed. Many drugs may be biotransformed simultaneously or serially in more than one reaction. The predominant biotransformation sequence is determined by metabolic conditions and species differences.

I Oxidations

A Nonmicrosomal Oxidations (Soluble and Mitochondrial Fractions)
1 Alcohol Oxidation The oxidation of primary or secondary alcohols is mediated by NAD-linked alcohol dehydrogenase found in liver, kidney, and lung. Methanol is biotransformed at a slower rate in the presence of ethanol as a result of substrate competition, and because methanol toxicity is due to its metabolic products, formaldehyde and formic acid, the claim is made that ethanol decreases the toxicity of methanol.

2 Aldehyde Oxidation An *aliphatic aldehyde* such as chloral hydrate is biotransformed by the NAD-linked aldehyde dehydrogenase. This enzyme can reduce, as well as oxidize, aldehydes. Inhibition of aldehyde dehydrogenase by disulfiram or by calcium carbamide after ethanol ingestion results in the accumulation of acetaldehyde to toxic levels in the body.

3 Monoamine and Diamine Oxidation Short-

Table 4-1 Drug Biotransformation Reactions: I Oxidations

Reaction type	General biotransformation mechanism	Examples
A Nonmicrosomal oxidations (soluble and mitochondrial fractions)		
1 Alcohol dehydrogenation	$\begin{smallmatrix}R\\R\end{smallmatrix}\!CHOH + NAD^+ \rightarrow \begin{smallmatrix}R\\R\end{smallmatrix}\!C{=}O + NADH + H^+$	Ethanol, methanol
2 Aldehyde dehydrogenation		
a Aliphatic aldehydes	$R{-}C\!\!\overset{O}{\underset{H}{<}} + NAD^+ \rightarrow R{-}C\!\!\overset{O}{\underset{OH}{<}} + NADH + H^+$	Chloral hydrate
b Purines	$C_5H_2N_4{-}OH + H_2O + O_2 \rightarrow$ Hypoxanthine $C_5HN_4{-}(OH)_2 + H_2O_2$ Xanthine	6-Mercaptopurine
3 Monoamine oxidation and diamine oxidation	$R{-}CH_2NH_2 \xrightarrow{O_2} R{-}CH{=}NH + H_2O_2 \xrightarrow{H_2O} R{-}CH{=}O + NH_3$	Dopamine, norepinephrine, tyramine, serotonin, histamine
B Microsomal oxidations		
1 Carbon oxygenation		
a Hydroxylation of carbon		
(1) Side-chain hydroxylation	$R{-}CH_2CH_2CH_2CH_3 \rightarrow$ $R{-}CHOHCH_2CH_2CH_3$ / $R{-}CH_2CH_2CHOHCH_3$ / $R{-}CH_2CH_2CH_2CH_2OH$	Barbiturates, phenylbutazone
(2) Ring hydroxylation	$R{-}\bigcirc \rightarrow R{-}\bigcirc{-}OH$	Quinine, hexobarbital
(3) Oxidative deamination	$R{-}CH_2{-}\overset{CH_3}{\underset{}{CH}}{-}NH_2 \rightarrow R{-}CH_2{-}\overset{CH_3}{\underset{}{C}}{=}O$	Amphetamine, other α-methylated amines
b Dealkylation		
(1) N-Dealkylation	$R{-}N\!\!\overset{CH_3}{\underset{CH_3}{<}} \rightarrow R{-}N\!\!\overset{H}{\underset{CH_3}{<}} + HCHO$	Imipramine, morphine
(2) O-Dealkylation	$Ar{-}O{-}CH_3 \rightarrow Ar{-}OH + HCHO$	Codeine
2 N-Oxygenation		
a N-Oxidation	$\begin{smallmatrix}R\\R'\\R''\end{smallmatrix}\!N \rightarrow \begin{smallmatrix}R\\R'\\R''\end{smallmatrix}\!N \rightarrow O$	Chlorpromazine
3 S-Oxidation	$R{-}S{-}R' \rightarrow R{-}\overset{O}{\underset{}{S}}{-}R'$	Phenothiazines
4 Desulfuration	$\begin{smallmatrix}R\\R'\end{smallmatrix}\!C{=}S \rightarrow \begin{smallmatrix}R\\R'\end{smallmatrix}\!C{=}O$	Thiobarbiturate
	$\begin{smallmatrix}R{-}O\\R'{-}O\\R''{-}O\end{smallmatrix}\!P{=}S \rightarrow \begin{smallmatrix}R{-}O\\R'{-}O\\R''{-}O\end{smallmatrix}\!P{=}O$	Parathion, malathion

chain monoamines (catecholamines, tyramine, tryptophan) and long-chain diamines not substituted on the α carbon, are oxidized by monoamine oxidase (MAO). Short-chain α-substituted amines, such as amphetamines, are not readily metabolized by MAO and may be inhibitors. Amphetamine is biotransformed by a microsomal enzyme system. MAO inhibitors have been used to elevate mood; however, if a food product rich in amines such as tyramine (as in cheese) is ingested when a patient is taking MAO-inhibitor drugs, a hypertensive crisis may occur, resulting in an intracranial hemorrhage.

B Microsomal Oxygenation Microsomal oxygenations differ mechanistically from the usual soluble fraction and the mitochondrial oxidations described above in that the oxygenases of these microsomes fix molecular oxygen into the substrates. In mitochondrial respiration, the reduction equivalents (electrons or hydrogen atoms) are removed from the substrate by dehydrogenases. These reduction equivalents are then transferred through various carriers to molecular oxygen which is reduced to either H_2O or H_2O_2. This transfer of reduction equivalents through the electron transport system of mitochondria may be coupled to energy production [adenosine triphosphate (ATP)]. However, in the microsomal mixed-function oxygenase (or monooxygenase) reactions, reduction equivalents from NADPH (possibly also NADH) are used to reduce molecular oxygen so that it can

be carried by a cytochrome called P-450 to the substrate to be oxygenated. This "active oxygen" is then fixed into the organic substrate, usually as a hydroxyl group (i.e., hydroxylation). The microsomal system does not produce useful energy, but instead requires reduction equivalents (NADPH) formed in other reactions. Table 4-1 illustrates carbon and nitrogen oxygenation, sulfur oxidation, and desulfuration. It is sufficient to emphasize at this point that in microsomal oxygenation (1) NADPH (and possibly NADH) are required to activate molecular oxygen, and (2) molecular oxygen is fixed into a portion of the drug molecule. Figure 4-1 shows the mixed function of the oxygenase system in greater detail.

II Reductions

A Nonmicrosomal Reductions (Soluble and Mitochondrial Fractions) Reductions are less common in drug biotransformation than are oxidations. Table 4-2 illustrates the reduction reactions, the most important of which is mediated by alcohol dehydrogenase.

III Hydrolysis (Table 4-3)

A Ester Hydrolysis Procaine is hydrolyzed by plasma esterases and also by a liver microsomal esterase. Different substrate specificities exist for these two enzymes, since meperidine is also hydrolyzed by the microsomal enzyme but not by the

Table 4-2 Drug Biotransformation Reactions: II Reductions

Reaction type	General biotransformation mechanism	Examples
A Nonmicrosomal reductions (soluble and mitochondrial fractions)		
1 Aldehyde reduction	$R_2C{=}O + NADH + H^+ \rightarrow R_2CHOH + NAD^+$	Chloral hydrate, *trans*-retinene
B Microsomal reductions		
1 Nitro reduction	$Ar{-}NO_2 \rightarrow ArNH_2$	*p*-Nitrobenzoic acid, nitrobenzene, chloramphenicol
2 Azo reduction	$Ar{-}N{=}N{-}Ar' \rightarrow ArNH_2 + Ar'NH_2$	Prontosil, azobenzene, 4-dimethylazobenzene
3 Reductive dehalogenation	$R{-}CCl_3 \rightarrow R{-}CHCl_2$	DDT, carbon tetrachloride, methoxyflurane, halothane

soluble enzyme. A number of different soluble enzymes also exist, including acetylcholinesterase and pseudocholinesterase.

B Amide Hydrolysis Procainamide, the amide analogue of the ester procaine, is not hydrolyzed by plasma enzymes but is metabolized slowly by tissue enzymes, which prolongs its action and makes it a more useful agent in the treatment of arrhythmias.

IV Conjugations

A number of small endogenous compounds can react with polar functional groups on drugs. These reactions are called conjugations or syntheses be-cause cofactors are usually involved and energy is used to form these bonds. Conjugation with glu-curonic acid is by far the most important conjuga-tion reaction in human beings. The reaction type and general biotransformation mechanism are shown here.

Formation of "activated" glucuronic acid:

$$Glucose\ 1\text{-phosphate} + UTP \rightarrow UDPG + P_2O_7^{4-}$$

$$UDP\text{-glucose}$$

$$UDPG + 2NAD^+ \rightarrow UDPGA + 2NADH$$

$$UDP\text{-glucuronic acid}$$

Conjugation:

$$UDPGA + ROH \rightarrow RO\text{---glucuronide} + UDP$$

ELECTRON TRANSPORT IN THE DRUG MICROSOMAL METABOLIZING SYSTEM

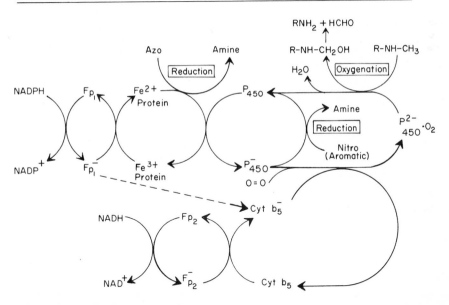

Figure 4-1 NADPH reduction equivalents are passed on to a flavoprotein (Fp) similar to a cytochrome c reductase. The reduced flavoprotein (Fp*) then passes its reduction equivalents to a nonheme iron-containing protein (Fe^{3+} protein) which in turn reduces P*-450. Reduced P*-450 picks up atoms of oxygen from molecular oxygen and reacts with the drug mono-oxygenase complex to place an atom of oxygen into the drug, usually as a hydroxyl group. P*-450 can also react with carbon monoxide (CO) and form a P*-450·CO complex which absorbs at 450 mμ and which gives this cytochrome its name. Strong light can break the P*-450·CO complex. This microsomal electron transport chain can conceivably reduce atoms other than oxygen, and it does. Azo compounds are reduced to amines at the level of the nonheme iron-containing protein, while aromatic nitro compounds are reduced by the P*-450. As expected, aerobic conditions (oxygen) interfere at the level of the P*-450, but not at the Fe^{2+} protein level. Recently, it has been claimed that in some reactions NADH can substi-tute for NADPH, as shown in the diagram.

Table 4-3   Drug Biotransformation Reactions: III   Hydrolysis

Reaction type	General biotransformation mechanism	Examples
A Ester hydrolysis	$R-\overset{O}{\overset{\|}{C}}-O-\overset{H}{\underset{H}{C}}-R' + H_2O \rightarrow R-\overset{O}{\overset{\|}{C}}-OH + HO-\overset{H}{\underset{H}{C}}-R'$	Acetylcholine, carbachol, succinylcholine, procaine
B Amide hydrolysis	$R-\overset{O}{\overset{\|}{C}}-NH-R' + H_2O \rightarrow R-\overset{O}{\overset{\|}{C}}-OH + NH_2-R'$	Procainamide, nicotin- amide, benzamide
C Other hydrolysis Glycoside hydrolysis	Nicotinamide—Ribose—Phosphate—Phosphate—Ribose—Adenine (βNAD$^+$) + H$_2$O + Acetylpyridine or another pyridine Adenine Ribose Ribose Acetylpyridine Adenine Phosphate—Phosphate Ribose Ribose + Nicotinamide Phosphate—Phosphate + Nicotinamide	

The synthetic or conjugation reactions are classified in Table 4-4. Glucuronide conjugation is always a detoxication reaction. Newborn infants have a very low glucuronyl transferase activity, because this enzyme usually develops after the first few weeks of life. If these infants are given large doses of the antibiotic chloramphenicol, they are unable to detoxify and excrete it, and a toxic manifestation called "gray baby" syndrome develops. Other infants are born with a syndrome of high bilirubin plasma levels (icterus neonatorum), whereby high levels of bilirubin are formed and conjugation with glucuronic acid is too slow to detoxify the bilirubin. Both these syndromes respond to low levels of barbiturates such as phenobarbital. Phenobarbital stimulates the proliferation (induction) of microsomal enzymes and hence the glucuronyl transferase activity. A genetic defect (congenital nonhemolytic jaundice, Crigler-Najjar syndrome) has been ascribed to a lower glucuronyl transferase activity. In this defect, children as well as adults are unable to conjugate bilirubin and drugs normally excreted as glucuronides.

Table 4-4   Drug Biotransformation Reactions: IV   Conjugations

Reaction type	Examples
A Glucuronide	Bilirubin, many drugs and biotransformation products of drugs, chloramphenicol, chloral hydrate, disulfiram (Antabuse), phenacetin
B Acylation	Sulfonamides, histamine, isoniazid
C Methylation	Norepinephrine and other phenylethanolamines, serotonin, tryptamine, histamine, nicotinamide, dimercaprol, H$_2$S, thiouracil
D Sulfate ester synthesis	Estrone, androsterone

V   Spontaneous Reactions

A number of drugs are transformed not by the enzyme systems but spontaneously in aqueous solutions at various pH's. These spontaneous degradation products may then react with some of the biological constituents of the cell, such as proteins, ribonucleic acid (RNA), and deoxyribonucleic acid (DNA), and are called *alkylating agents*. Others, like thalidomide, may form more water-soluble polar compounds from lipid-soluble parent compounds and these polar products may be toxic.

DRUGS NOT BIOTRANSFORMED

Highly polar compounds such as moderately strong acids or bases are not likely to be metabolized to any great extent. These compounds are not likely to penetrate through the lipid layers of the microsomes where much of the biotransformation of drugs takes place and, in many cases, are more rapidly excreted than nonpolar compounds. Examples of polar compounds not metabolized are hexamethonium salts and methotrexate. Some less polar compounds such as chlorothiazide are only very slowly metabolized and are also excreted unchanged. Nonpolar compounds which are very slowly metabolized, if at all, include barbital, diethyl ether, and halothane. Diethyl ether and halothane are readily excreted via the lung.

THE METABOLIC FATE OF DRUGS

Drugs are biotransformed according to the active chemical groupings they contain. Since many drugs contain more than one functional group, and since each functional group may undergo more than one biotransformation, multiple products may be formed. For instance, salicylic acid is primarily excreted unchanged; however, some of it is biotransformed and excreted as the ether-glucuronide or the ester-glucuronide, or as a glycine conjugate, salicyluric acid. Some individuals may excrete half the dose as salicyluric acid, some may excrete none; some individuals may excrete 10 percent as unchanged salicylic acid, some 85 percent. Because modification of substituent groups may drastically change the biotransformation pattern of analogues, empirical determination is the only safe method. For example, barbital is very slowly metabolized, but hexobarbital is rapidly biotransformed. A knowledge of the major metabolic fates of some functional groups, however, can provide insight into the products most likely to be formed.

FACTORS AFFECTING THE DRUG MICROSOMAL METABOLIZING SYSTEM

The level of activity of the drug microsomal metabolizing system determines the duration and intensity of action of many drugs. The activities of these enzymes can be altered by:

The drugs themselves
Genetic factors
    Comparative patterns
    Genetic differences in man
Physiologic factors
    Age and development
    Nutrition
    Hormones
    Disease
Environmental factors
    Stress
    Light
    Foreign lipid-soluble compounds

The most important parameter affecting drug metabolism is the drug itself.

The Drugs Themselves as Factors Affecting the Drug Microsomal Metabolizing System

Stimulating and Inhibiting Drugs in Man More than 200 drugs and environmental chemicals are known to stimulate the activity of the drug biotransforming enzymes in hepatic microsomes. Examples in humans are: Phenobarbital stimulates the metabolism of diphenylhydantoin, cortisol, bishydroxycoumarin, warfarin, and digitoxin, as well as serum bilirubin. Glutethimide stimulates metabolism of warfarin; meprobamate, of meprobamate; phenylbutazone, of tolbutamide and cortisol; diphenylhydantoin, of cortisol; chloral hydrate, of bishydroxycoumarin; bishydroxycoumarin, of tolbutamide; and ethanol, of barbiturates. However, even though ethanol finally induces the drug microsomal metabolizing system when present in the system with barbiturates, it inhibits the metabolism of these barbiturates. Thus, in an alcoholic when ethanol is not present, the general hypnotic dose may not be effective, but in the presence of alcohol the same dose may be toxic (double depressant action).

Consequences of Stimulation and Inhibition of Biotransformation of Drugs When the system that biotransforms a drug is induced, the drug is metabolized more quickly, that is, the metabolite is formed more rapidly. The relative activity of the drug and the metabolite determine the consequences to the organism. When the metabolite has little effect of its own, then enzyme induction accelerates inactivation of the drug. A usually effective dose of a drug may thereby be completely ineffective. This is probably a factor in many types of tolerance phenomena. The opposite effect can occur, however, when the metabolite is a pharmacologically active drug or a toxic product.

Genetic Differences in Man

Small yet significant differences may exist in the genetic control of certain drug levels in man. Genetic differences exist in man in the acetylation conjugating enzymes, pseudocholinesterase, glucuronide conjugating enzymes, glucose 6-phosphate dehydrogenase deficiency with hemolysis and methemoglobin formation, O-dealkylating enzymes, and in other genetic variations. Obviously, it is the practicing physician in these instances who is the valuable reporter of unusual drug reactions and who thereby exposes unusual genetic differences in man.

Physiologic Factors in Drug Biotransformation

Age and development, nutrition, hormones, and disease all have profound effects on drug metabolism in humans. Newborns are not well endowed with drug-metabolizing enzymes and may be more sensitive to drugs. The effect of nutrition and stress on drug metabolism has been measured by a number of investigators. Most of the information has been gathered by measuring the activity of the microsomal enzymes of the liver in vivo after barbiturate administration. Drug metabolism can be impaired by starvation or by a diet low in ascorbic acid or protein. A calcium-deficient diet will also impair hepatic drug metabolism.

Drug metabolism is usually inhibited by starvation, but depending on the sex of the animal and timing, one can actually increase barbiturate metabolism.

Liver damage in human patients makes them more sensitive to a variety of drugs. Obstructive jaundice, hepatitis, and cirrhosis impair the formation of glucuronide and sulfate conjugates; thus care should be taken in prescribing drugs for these patients.

Environmental Factors in Drug Biotransformation

By far the most important environmental factor in drug metabolism is the intake of lipid-soluble foreign compounds in foods, food additives, pollutants, and pesticides. The defenses of the body are activated by these compounds and, perhaps most important, by the stimulation of the microsomal systems.

Chapter 5

Clinical Pharmacology

The branch of pharmacology that deals directly with the effectiveness and safety of drugs in humans is generally called *clinical pharmacology*. Since particular skills and unusual precautions are required to investigate these drugs, many medical centers maintain specialized units equipped for this purpose.

The nature of drug action is determined by certain characteristic properties, including absorption, distribution, metabolism, and excretion. Of particular importance is the pharmacokinetic profile exhibited by a drug, which establishes the dose required to achieve various blood levels. The incidence of pharmacologic activity and/or toxicity may be associated with concentration of a drug in the blood. The ability to adjust drug blood levels by manipulating the administered dose and thereby to control pharmacologic response is an important aspect of pharmacokinetics.

This chapter primarily deals with the steps involved in preparing a drug for release as a market-able product, including the complications and ethics of drug testing in humans.

NEW DRUG APPLICATION (IND)

Most marketed drugs are developed by pharmaceutical firms which have collected exhaustive data on the chemistry, identity, and pharmacology of a new substance. Studies in humans begin only after a federal Food and Drug Administration (FDA) form 1571 is filed, which is a notice of claimed Investigational Exemption for a New Drug (IND). The FDA reviews the IND and determines whether the drug or chemical may be studied in man and under what restricted conditions. At the minimum an IND will contain the following information: (1) chemistry and biological activity of the drug; (2) specific dosage forms for man; (3) quality control in the manufacture and identification of the drug; (4) description of conditions of manufacture; (5) names and qualifications of individuals who are to be responsible for the investigation; (6) signed statements from each investigator, indicating an intimate knowledge of the drug and a willingness to cooperate fully in all requirements regarding human volunteers; (7) the facilities for the study; (8) protocols indicating the dose, the route of administration, and clinical and laboratory observations to be performed; (9) all pertinent information for the investigation, including predictable toxicity; and (10) any specific observations which should be reported at once.

Phase I Studies

After the IND has been approved by the FDA, clinical trial of the specified chemical may be carefully begun in man. Ultimately, clinical drug trials in humans involve three phases of study designated as phase I, II, and III. The main purpose of the initial pharmacodynamic studies is to determine if the agent has biologic and therapeutic effects that may be useful in therapy. The range of the doses must be established and special attention given to drug toxicity. This can be combined with pharmacokinetic studies which include chemical or radiochemical measurement of absorption, distribution, protein binding, metabolism, and excretion. If a potentially useful therapeutic effect has been observed, additional information must be obtained on dosage, side effects, and therapeutic indications.

Special Problems in Selection of Subjects   Special problems may arise regarding volunteer participation:

Children   Although new agents are evaluated initially in adults, unique pediatric problems require that first trials for efficacy of some drugs be performed in children; for example, mumps and rubella vaccine.

Women of child-bearing age   Women who are known to be or who may be pregnant should not be used for the earliest initial studies because of possible fetal injury. If agents are specifically intended for use by pregnant women, however, the first clinical studies for efficacy will have to be performed on them; for example, toxemia of pregnancy.

Volunteers in special situations   Individuals in a position of dependence, such as students or prisoners, who are asked to volunteer for studies might feel that they are subject to undue pressure. Special care by competent investigators is needed to review the purpose and design of the trial.

Prediction of Toxic Effects   Not all possible effects in man produced by a compound can be predicted solely from in vitro tests or from the results obtained in lower animal experimentation. However, a toxic effect occurring in only one of several species has demonstrated a favorable prognosis for man. Accordingly, Lichtfield's "rules" predict effects in man from animal data: (1) If an effect is noted in both rats and dogs, it has a 79 percent probability of occurring in man. (2) If an effect is noted only in rats or dogs, the probability that it will not occur in man is 74 percent.

These rules indicate that an effect observed in two phylogenetically different species has a greater probability of involving a common physiologic system which may also be common to a third species. An effect observed in only one of several species suggests a system or idiosyncratic phenomenon peculiar to that species.

Animal Versus Human Dose   One of the main problems in the initial human studies is to extrapolate the first dose to be used from the data obtained in lower animals. These data predict the quantitative and qualitative effects that may be expected from a compound. Although there is no set of rules here, the basis of extrapolation must include a comparison of animal species, body weights, metabolic rates, and rates of drug metabolism. One should be conservative in determining the first dose to be administered to people because of possible unexpected reactions. These include idiosyncrasy, hypersensitivity, effects on special brain centers, blood and bone marrow disturbances, and unusual metabolic actions.

Based on the data from acute animal toxicity studies, logarithmically increasing doses of the agent are administered to the selected animal to obtain the minimum effective dose. From these data are made estimates of the therapeutic index and therapeutic range. For example, perhaps a parasympathomimetic agent is studied in a group of animals and the dose-response relationship is as follows:

mg/kg	Pharmacologic response
2.5	No effect
5.0	Mild diarrhea
7.5	Bradycardia
10.0	Hyperpyrexia and achromodacryorrhea

The initial single human dose would be a fraction of the minimum effective dose which in this example is 5.0 mg. If the rat were the test animal, a safe arbitrary suggestion might be $\frac{1}{200}$ of this dose as the total single initial dose for an average-size human, using the same route of administration. If the dog were the test animal, then $\frac{1}{10}$ of this minimum effective dose might be used.

Although mice, rats, rabbits, cats, and dogs are the animal species generally used, it is highly desirable to study nonhuman (monkey) and subhuman primates (orangutan or baboon) because of their physiologic similarity to man. Here, one-half the minimum effective dose might be used in the initial human studies.

If an atropine-like agent is studied in certain rodents, a much smaller fraction of the minimum effective dose would be used in man, since the rodent is resistant to compounds having atropine-like structures, and consequently, man can be expected to be more sensitive. Such preclinical evaluations are important considerations.

Single-Dose Methodology When there is no detectable response in the human to the initial dose (based on the estimated dose suggested by the preceding considerations), the dose is slowly increased until a response appears. The response may or may not be the anticipated one, but all subjective and objective reactions are recorded. A second subject is given the same dose, and the reactions are again observed. When there is no response to these initial human trials using the estimated dosage, the dose is slowly increased until drug activity is manifested. Once this minimum effective dose has been determined, the dose is further increased to establish the *maximum tolerated dose*—or the dose which does not elicit undesirable effects. No individual should be exposed to more than a single dose in a short period of time. Usually a rest period of at least 1 week is allowed to prevent cumulative effects.

Blind and Double-Blind Studies When evaluation of drug efficacy involves personal judgment, either subjective on the part of the patient or objective on the part of the investigator, further controls are necessary to prevent bias. This is particularly true for such drugs as analgesics, sedatives, antianginals, or tranquilizers, which are usually evaluated by their subjective effects. Even in diseases with such objective signs as hypertension, patient reassurance alone may produce a therapeutic effect and thereby mask the effect of the test substance. Because of psychologic influences, proper control is often difficult to achieve. Transference and countertransference between the enthusiastic investigator and subject or patient may lead to a variety of results. To avoid these bias factors, statistical techniques are resorted to, and "blinding" becomes necessary. In "single-blind" trials, the physician and associates—but not the patient—know the substance being used. When a completely dispassionate evaluation is needed, a "double-blind" trial is performed. Here, neither the individual administering the compound nor the patient knows the identity of the substance. All material is coded, including the test substance and a placebo and, if possible, an already known active substance therapeutically similar to the one being tested (standard reference or positive control). Occasionally, negative controls are used to duplicate certain side effects to prevent identification of the test substance. For example, quinine may be used to mimic the taste of a bitter substance. Obviously, the physical appearance and manner of handling the materials should render them indistinguishable.

Placebo Effect Early in this century it was realized that certain drugs which had been used for years for specific conditions actually had no pharmacological effect when studied objectively. Distinction must be made between the placebo and the placebo effect. *Placebo* is a Latin verb meaning "I shall please"; *placebo effect* may or may not occur and is defined as the psychologic or physiologic effect of a therapeutic drug or procedure which is not related to its specific pharmacologic activity. Most observers believe placebo effect can be explained by a psychologic mechanism. Experienced clinicians are well aware that many therapeutic effects are the results of a good sales talk and a pat on the back.

In any population some individuals are more susceptible to placebos than others. It must also be pointed out that while the greater number respond to a placebo with positive effects there are a minority who react negatively. Double-blind and blind studies help to identify placebo effects because the patient does not know when he is receiving the active ingredient or the placebo.

Statistical Studies Obviously, all data must be analyzed by acceptable statistical methods. Therapeutic effects are seldom clear-cut and require analysis of the overall effect in a patient population. Often comparisons with established drugs will show that a new product when analyzed statistically is not superior to the old. This becomes of greater importance in phase II and III studies.

Phase II Studies

Phase II studies begin once initial pharmacodynamics and toxicity observations and determinations of absorption, metabolism, and elimination have been made. The FDA must be kept informed of all data, especially if any serious toxicity becomes evident. In phase II, small numbers of patients are selected with the symptoms or diseases for which the drug is purported to be effective. A design protocol is established which aims to demonstrate conclusively efficacy in relation to safety. Again the design may follow single-blind, double-blind, or indeed any rational approach indicated for a particular drug or disease. As new data accumulate, it is usually advisable to do chronic toxicity studies in animals. Additional metabolic and pharmacokinetic studies may also be indicated. If the drug is to be used for long periods of time in females, special studies of its effects on reproduction and fertility are necessary to forestall teratogenic effects. Usually there will be a late stage in phase II where findings are finalized and any additional observations are performed which are felt to be important.

Phase III Studies

If the drug survives phase II, then—with the approval of the FDA—phase III may be performed. This is actually a broad clinical trial on a large sample of specified patients. Here the attempt is to prove efficacy in the field; the investigation is usually performed by a number of different clinicians in different centers or even under actual medical practice conditions. The protocol of the investigation is designed to be more restrictive about the variability of what can be done. Dosage forms, methods, and routes of administration are clearly defined. The protocol must be approved by the FDA, and any toxicity must be immediately reported. Phase III studies usually require from 1 to 3 years. Following the collection and documentation of all data in humans, the FDA may allow the drug to be marketed for specified therapeutic purposes and applications. In most instances, clear proof must be advanced that the new drug is superior to an established product.

ETHICS OF DRUG INVESTIGATION IN HUMANS

In view of the inevitable toxicity of drugs, it might well be asked, "What are the moral and humanistic aspects of human investigation?" Obviously, when the only object of administering a drug is an attempt to alter a course of a usually fatal disease, considerable toxicity may be justified, for example, cancer chemotherapy. However, systematic medical research may not have as its sole or even major aim the cure of immediate disease but the explanation of mechanisms which may later lead to beneficial therapeutic agents. Under what conditions may an individual serve as "guinea pig?" The code laid down in 1947 by the Nuremberg judges following the atrocities of World War II still stands as a classic document. It clearly states the principles which are still followed today:

1 The voluntary consent of the human subject is absolutely essential.
   a This means that the person involved should have legal capacity to give consent; should be so situated as to be able to exercise free power of choice, without the intervention of any element of force, fraud, deceit, duress, overreaching, or other ulterior form and constraint or coercion; and should have sufficient knowledge and comprehension of the elements of the subject matter involved to enable him to make an understanding and enlightened decision. The latter element requires that before the acceptance of an affirmative decision by the experimental subject, there should be made known to him the nature, duration, and purpose of the experiment; the method and means by which it is to be conducted; all inconveniences and hazards reasonably to be expected; and the effects upon his health or person which may possibly come from his participation in the experiment.
   b The consent of the human subject shall be in writing; his signature shall be affixed to a writ-

ten instrument setting forth substantially the aforementioned requirements which shall be signed in the presence of at least one witness who shall attest to such signature in writing.

c The duty and responsibility for ascertaining the quality of the consent rests upon each individual who initiates, directs, or engages in the experiment. It is a personal duty and responsibility which may not be delegated to another with impunity.

2 The experiment should be such as to yield fruitful results for the good of society, unprocurable by other methods or means of study, and not random and unnecessary in nature.

3 The number of volunteers used shall be kept at a minimum.

4 The experiment should be so designed and based on the results of animal experimentation and a knowledge of the natural history of the disease or other problem under study that the anticipated results will justify the performance of the experiment.

5 The experiment should be so conducted as to avoid all unnecessary physical and mental suffering and injury.

6 No experiment should be conducted where there is *a priori* reason to believe that death or disability injury will occur.

Since this code was promulgated, other declarations have been published. The AMA affirmed the concepts of consent, competence, and care. The British Medical Association, the Medical Research Council, and the World Medical Association have issued guidelines for conduct of experimentation not essentially different in principle.

The World Medical Association approved the Helsinki declaration in 1964, which established:

In the field of clinical research, a fundamental distinction must be recognized between clinical research in which the aim is essentially therapeutic for a patient, and clinical research, the essential object of which is purely scientific and without therapeutic value to the person subjected to the research.

The declaration asserts that where research is combined with professional care "if at all possible, consistent with patient psychology, the doctor should obtain the patient's freely-given consent after the patient has been given a full explanation." The

Helsinki declaration is the current *vade mecum* to guide us through the ethical maze.

In addition, there is the "consent clause" of the FDA law. This statute states that investigators must inform any human being used in the tests or controls that the agent is being used for investigational purposes; it also states that investigators will obtain the informed consent of such individuals or their representatives, except where it is deemed not feasible or, in their professional judgment, contrary to the best interests of the individual.

In all human drug studies performed under a government contract or grant, and in order to comply with the more recent regulations of the FDA, there is the additional requirement that the study be approved by a Human Research Review Committee. Such a committee must be composed of impartial scientists, clinicians, lay people from the community, including at the least, a lawyer and a clergyman. Full disclosure of the drug's chemical and biologic background is required. The risks to the human subjects involved are estimated; the responsibility of the investigation is established; and it is determined that the facilities available for the investigation are adequate and ensure safety. The use of consultants is often made a requirement. Disclosure of the risk involved to the volunteer is mandatory, and informed consent is supervised. The protocol of the investigation is carefully reviewed. Reports of any toxicity are to be immediately reported to the committee.

FATE OF MARKETED DRUGS

Results of the experimental and clinical evaluation of new drugs often become well publicized and may have a tremendous influence on sales; however, the results then obtained by practicing physicians may not be the same as those obtained under experimental conditions. Since the new drug may offer no advantage over the drug already being prescribed, physicians may become reluctant to use the new product, so that its sale diminishes rapidly. On the other hand, because of keen competition among over a thousand companies in the pharmaceutical industry, research programs will be either initiated or intensified to develop a competitive product. Thus, the natural history of many new drug products may be divided into four phases:

(1) enthusiastic reception; (2) qualified use; (3) declining use due to ineffectiveness, side effects, or competitive drugs; and (4) obsolescence.

DRUG FACTORS

Drug Interactions

One of the "spin-off" benefits of careful investigation of drugs in humans by clinical pharmacologists has been the discovery of drug interactions. One drug may influence the action of a second drug (or vice versa) so as to influence the therapeutic response and toxicity of either drug. The mechanisms by which this may occur are suggested below.

Gastrointestinal Absorption Insoluble complexes may be formed when two drugs are given simultaneously, for example, an antacid which chelates tetracycline and prevents its absorption. Antacids may also prevent the absorption of drugs which depend on an acid pH to exist in an unionized form. Other drugs such as anticholinergics may affect gastrointestinal motility, which may actually increase in some cases and decrease absorption in other cases. Diphenylhydantoin may inhibit the activity of conjugase enzymes which in time may prevent the conversion of folic acid to an absorbable form, eventually causing megaloblastic anemia. Other mechanisms may involve changes in intestinal flora and inhibition of vitamin K synthesis or absorption, thus influencing anticoagulant therapy.

Protein Binding Drugs do not exist in a free form in body fluids. The blood proteins bind to a varying degree nearly all drugs, and there is therefore a competition between this site and the receptor site. A second drug which has a greater affinity for binding to plasma proteins may displace the first drug and this leads to a greater effect than might be expected from a particular dose. An example might be displacement of coumarin anticoagulants by clofibrate, leading to enhanced antiprothrombin effect and perhaps bleeding tendencies. Another example is the displacement of methotrexate from plasma protein by salicylates. This has caused increased methotrexate toxicity.

Adrenergic Mechanisms Many active drugs resemble sympathomimetic amines and may interact with the adrenergic receptor so as to displace norepinephrine and prevent its reabsorption at the adrenergic site, or they may cause its release from a storage site. Reserpine, for example, slowly releases norepinephrine from the intragranular pools. Tricyclic antidepressants block the uptake of norepinephrine. Some drugs may compete for the receptor site for norepinephrine and thus become antagonists or blockers.

Another major adrenergic mechanism involves catecholamine metabolism by monoamine oxidase (MAO). Inhibition of MAO results in accumulation of norepinephrine in adrenergic neurons. Administration of secondary-acting sympathomimetic amines such as amphetamine or tyramine (old wine, cheese) can result in an exaggerated hypertensive response.

Thus, a great many interactions are possible at the adrenergic neuron. These may involve drugs such as guanethidine (an antihypertensive), tolbutamide (a hypoglycemic), propranolol (a beta-adrenergic receptor blocking agent), and many others.

Cholinergic Mechanisms Many commonly used drugs have anticholinergic actions in addition to their major pharmacologic action. Examples are meperidine, tricyclic antidepressants, diphenhydramine, and phenothiazines. When given in conjunction with a standard anticholinergic such as atropine, excessive anticholinergic effects may be noted.

Neuromuscular Junction Antibiotics such as neomycin and kanamycin have a blocking action on the neuromuscular junction aside from their antibiotic effect. When used together with anesthetics such as ether, halothane, or methoxyflurane, excessive and prolonged muscle paralysis might occur. Quinidine, another drug with a blocking action at the neuromuscular junction, is capable of intensifying the effects of tubocurarine, gallamine, and other standard neuromuscular blocking agents. Anticholinesterase agents may prolong the action of succinylcholine.

Drug Metabolism The term *drug interaction* arose from studies which implicated the potential of one drug to influence greatly the metabolism of another through an intermediary mechanism. It was observed that phenobarbital and other highly lipophilic drugs caused induction of the microsomal enzyme system of the liver. This increased the amount and activity of this drug-metabolizing enzyme. In consequence, a second drug given during the course of phenobarbital therapy would be rapidly metabolized and thus be relatively less effective for a given dose. An anticoagulant, for example, would be rapidly metabolized under these circumstances, and the attending physician would consequently increase the dose. If phenobarbital therapy were then terminated, the anticoagulant might cause fatal bleeding.

Many examples of this type of interaction have been established experimentally and clinically. In some instances metabolism of the second drug is inhibited instead of enhanced. Some cases are rarely significant clinically, but it is always a mechanism to be kept in mind, since it might be exaggerated in such unusual circumstances as a primary defect in a metabolizing enzyme.

Renal Tubular Transport Some drugs inhibit the excretion of a second drug at the renal tubular level. One of the classic drug interactions is that of probenecid and its blockade of penicillin excretion. This is an example of drug interaction which may be used to achieve a useful purpose—to increase and prolong the therapeutic blood level of an antibiotic. On the other hand, there are instances where probenecid has produced toxic effects by causing the accumulation of a second drug. Indomethacin excretion, for example, is blocked by probenecid.

There are many other drugs which act on the renal tubule. It should be mentioned that dicumarol (bishydroxycoumarin), phenylbutazone, and salicylates inhibit the excretion of oral hypoglycemic drugs, causing an excessive hypoglycemic effect.

Urinary pH and Drug Excretion Altering the pH of the urine has a profound effect on the rate of excretion of many drugs. Creation of an alkaline urine by diet or drug therapy will cause an increased excretion of phenobarbital, salicylic acid, and some sulfonamides. In fact, all drugs that are weak acids (pK_a 3.0 to 7.5) will be increased; conversely, in acid urine their excretion will be decreased.

On the other hand, many drugs which are weak bases (pK_a 7.5 to 10.5) will demonstrate an increased excretion in acid urine and decreased alkaline urine. Examples of these drugs are amphetamine, meperidine, and quinidine.

Toxicities

Single-Drug Toxicity This may be a dose-related extension of therapeutic effects and may occur in all individuals if it is due to overdosage, for example, cycloplegia during anticholinergic therapy, diarrhea during treatment with colchicine, and bleeding tendency with coumarin. Individuals who are at the lower end of the frequency distribution in a quantal log-dose–response curve may be ultrasensitive to a low dose; for example, those with tachycardia when epinephrine is used as a bronchodilator. On the other hand, drug toxicity may manifest as an "untoward" or side effect associated with the total pharmacodynamics of a drug, for example, nausea and vomiting often seen with cardiac glycosides, or sedation by certain antihistamines when used for allergic states.

Drug Allergy A reaction that has an immunologic basis is a drug allergy. Prior sensitization is required with the same or closely related chemical structure, and an antigen-antibody interaction results. The effect is independent of the normal action of the drug and may result in dermatitis, urticaria, conjunctivitis, gastrointestinal disturbances, or fatal anaphylactic shock. This reaction is not dose-related and is characterized by the presence of circulating humoral or tissue antibodies. An example is the high incidence of penicillin allergy.

Idiosyncrasy An abnormal reaction to a drug which is qualitatively different from the effect usually obtained in a majority of the population is said to be an *idiosyncrasy*. Prior sensitization is not required as in drug allergy and may be explained, not by antibodies, but by a biochemical abnormality present in an individual with a genetic defect. One example is the nonthrombocytopenic purpura which develops in a small percentage of individuals receiving quinine. Another is the photosensitivity

Table 5-1 Some Examples of Genetic Defects Which Modify Drug Biotransformation

	Enzymatic reaction	Examples of drugs involved	Effect
1	Glucose 6-phosphate dehydrogenase deficiency in erythrocytes	Acetylsalicylic acid Acetophenetidin Nitrofurans p-Aminosalicylic acid Primaquine and others 8-Aminoquinolines Quinidine Sulfonamides	Acute hemolytic anemia
2	Glucuronyl transferase deficiency (found in Crigler-Najjar syndrome and newborn infants)	Acetophenetidin Chloral hydrate Codeine Chloramphenicol Indomethacin Morphine Nicotinic acid Probenecid	Exaggerated drug toxicity
3	γ-Aminolevulinic acid (ALA)-synthetase stimulation	Barbiturates Chloroquine Estrogens Griseofulvin Sulfonamides	Acute intermittent porphyria
4	Pseudocholinesterase abnormality or deficiency	Succinylcholine	Prolonged apnea
5	Acetylase deficiency	Isoniazid	Peripheral neuropathy
6	Methemoglobin reductase deficiency	Chloroquine Diaminodiphenylsulfone (DDS) Primaquine	Methemoglobinemia

induced by phenothiazines, sulfonamides, griseofulvin, and tetracyclines.

Pharmacogenetics This is the study of hereditary factors that influence responses to drugs and may help to explain hypersensitivity, drug allergy, or idiosyncrasy. Genetic heterogenicity or polymorphism between individuals may modify biotransformation of drugs, as illustrated in Table 5-1.

Iatrogenic Effects of Drugs The great increase in the number of drugs prescribed by doctors, as well as the greatly increased use of drugs, has led to a whole group of conditions which are drug-induced. The public and legislators are seriously concerned that drugs not be used to cause degenerative diseases or carcinogenic and teratogenic effects. A study from a leading teaching hospital has reported that as many as 30 percent of all patients were admitted because of drug-associated toxicity. (This was undoubtedly too high an estimate because of certain deficiencies in the collection of data). Nevertheless, it cannot be denied that there exists a definite and increasing incidence of drug-induced diseases.

Part Two

Anesthetic Agents

Chapter 6

General Anesthetics

Anesthesia is a loss of all modalities of sensation and loss of consciousness. *Surgical anesthesia* is a degree of central nervous system depression sufficient to allow surgical procedures. Therefore, there must be unconsciousness and depression of spinal reflexes adequate for skeletal muscle relaxation.

UPTAKE AND TRANSPORT OF ANESTHETICS AND STAGES OF ANESTHESIA

The inherent safety of inhalation anesthesia lies in this fact: If natural or artificial respiration is maintained, anesthesia can always be reversed by the elimination of anesthetics through the lungs.

The relative inertness of anesthetic vapors and gases implies that they behave like other inert gases under laws governing partial pressure, diffusion, and solubility in liquids. Since uptake and distribution, and perhaps narcosis, depend upon the tension or pressure of the dissolved gas in blood and tissues, these aspects of inhalation anesthesia will

be presented in terms of the *partial* pressures of anesthetics rather than their concentrations. The partial pressure of inhaled anesthetic depends on the vapor pressure and the volume of air or oxygen in which the anesthetic is mixed. Gas flows are measured by accurate flowmeters, and liquids are quantitatively vaporized to provide mixtures of known partial pressure. The inhaled partial pressure is constant in a nonrebreathing system, but varies in rebreathing systems, more or less according to the volume of fresh gas inflow. In any case, the partial pressure of anesthetic obeys Dalton's law: The pressure of a mixture of gases is the sum of the partial pressures of the constituents. In this discussion we shall assume that the inhaled partial pressure remains constant. Practically, however, the anesthetist constantly alters the partial pressure in order to induce anesthesia as rapidly and safely as possible, and then to maintain a steady state and provide the right amount of anesthesia for the operation.

The effect of a given amount of an anesthetic depends on its potency and the manner in which it is handled by the transport mechanism of the body. Here potency is the degree of general anesthesia afforded, ranging from slight to maximum inhibition of neurologic function. Relative potency has been estimated clinically by measuring the minimal alveolar concentration (MAC) of an anesthetic that prevents movement in response to a painful stimulus after a steady state of anesthesia has been reached. As concerns the general anesthetic process, potency has been equated with physical properties, such as solubility in oil and vapor pressure. An anesthetic is administered so that it will reach a tension in the brain sufficient for anesthesia. Each phase of transport follows in sequence from the time the anesthetic is inhaled through the nose and the mouth until the necessary depth of surgical anesthesia is reached, although the several phases actually go on simultaneously, one modifying the other (see Fig. 6-1). An inhaled anesthetic gas is eventually carried to the brain by circulating blood. After intake, the anesthetic agent is mixed in the functional residual air of the lungs. As the concentration or partial pressure of the gas increases in the lungs, diffusion through the pulmonary membrane and solution in pulmonary capillary blood occur (arrow across pulmonary membrane in Fig. 6-1). Subsequent distribution throughout the body is shown by the directional arrows. On the arterial side (A), the tension of the anesthetic reaching organs and tissues is the same. The mass of the brain is pictured as the smallest area, although the volume of blood flow is large. Similarly, the combined mass of the other organs—heart, liver, and kidneys—is smaller compared to the rest of the body tissues, but the volume of circulating blood is larger for these organs. Diffusion of anesthetic gas into and out of the tissues, according to the prevailing pressure gradient, is shown on the venous side (V) of the circulation. On the venous side, the tension of anesthetic represents the average of the tensions of anesthetic returned from the tissues.

Analysis of Variables in the Uptake and Distribution of Anesthetics

Since physiologic and physical constants are operative in uptake and distribution, mathematical equations have been derived to predict the course of

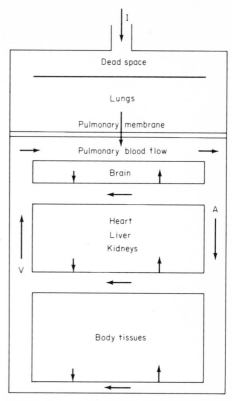

Figure 6-1 Diagram illustrating some of the physiologic and physical factors underlying the uptake of inhalation anesthetics by the body.

anesthesia. Kety derived an equation to predict the behavior of inert gases as they are handled by the body; some of the analyses thus derived describing the mechanisms of anesthetic induction and emergence follow.

In Fig. 6-2, curves demonstrate the increase in arterial partial pressure of several anesthetics expected to occur during administration of anesthetics to humans. The curves show how arterial anesthetic gas tensions approach a constant inhaled tension of the gas or vapor which would be expected to produce anesthesia. The curves also show the partial pressures reached in the brain leading to induction of the anesthetic state. It is assumed that the minute volume of respiration, the size of the lung compartments, and the cardiac output are average normal values for adult humans; the solubility coefficients for blood and tissues are given in Table 6-1. The

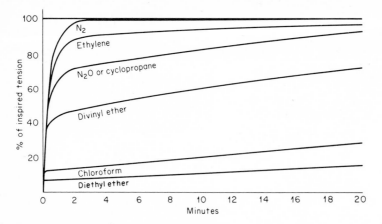

Figure 6-2 Exchange of inert gas at lungs and tissues —graphic representation of how the tension of anesthetic gas in arterial blood approaches inspired tension during the course of inhalational anesthesia (values calculated from a formula derived by Kety). With the inspired tension of anesthetic gas shown as 100 percent, the tension of anesthetic in arterial blood is read from the ordinate as a percentage of the inspired tension. Time in min is shown on the abscissa. The form of the curves for each anesthetic gas or vapor represented is determined by the physiologic and physical factors discussed in the text.

general shape and direction of the curves in Fig. 6-2 are similar for each anesthetic, indicating the constancy of the physiologic conditions. The variations are explained by differences in the physical properties of the anesthetics. Initially, within 2 to 3 min in each case, there is a sharp rise in the arterial curve with leveling off at the knee of the curve, a different height for each anesthetic. The slope and time are manifestations of lung washout which is the same for all anesthetics. The heights reached indicate that nitrogen and ethylene approach the inhaled tension most rapidly. This again is a manifestation of the relative solubilities in blood, those anesthetics with the lesser solubilities maintaining an alveolar pressure close to the inhaled tension. Thus the height of the knee for each anesthetic corresponds to its solubility in blood, so that ethylene may be expected to induce anesthesia quickly, diethyl ether, slowly.

Subsequent sloping plateaus of the arterial curves gradually approaching 100 percent (the inhaled partial pressure required for anesthesia) represent the simultaneous occurrence of uptake in the lungs, circulation to the body compartments, and recirculation of anesthetic to the lungs. The latter is the major factor in attaining the necessary partial

pressure of anesthetic in circulating blood and brain. Recirculation, in turn, is the reciprocal of the blood flows and solubilities in the several body tissues. Where there is greater solubility in certain tissues, the slope of the plateau should be less steep. The greater solubility of chloroform and diethyl ether in fat is therefore shown by the lesser slopes.

It appears from Fig. 6-2 that anesthesia is never reached with the anesthetics most soluble in blood. Practically, however, the anesthetist does not maintain a constant inhaled partial pressure of anesthetic, as the diagram suggests, but increases the partial pressure for a rapid induction and subsequently varies the level according to the patient's reactions and the surgical needs. When saturation of tissues is approached, the arterial anesthetic tension approximates that of the inhaled tension. The process of desaturation and emergence from anesthesia can be followed graphically by inverting the curves shown in Fig. 6-2, but this is true only if equilibration was reached; otherwise, redistribution among tissues could still be going on. Thus emergence from anesthesia will be most rapid with the agents that are least soluble in blood. At the same time, rapid diffusion into the alveoli lowers the

Table 6-1 Partition Coefficients of Some Anesthetic Gases at 37°C ± 0.5°C

Anesthetic gas	Water/gas	Blood/gas	Oil/gas	Tissue/blood	
Ethylene	0.081*	0.140	1.28	1.0	Heart
				1.2	Brain
Xenon	0.102	0.20	1.90	1.25	Brain, white
	0.097*		1.93*	0.7	Brain, gray
Cyclopropane	0.204	0.415	11.2*	0.81	Muscle
				1.36	Liver
Nitrous oxide	0.435*	0.468*	1.4	1.13	Heart
				1.06	Brain
				1.0	Lung
Fluroxene	0.84	1.37	47.7	1.43	Brain
				1.37	Liver
				2.24	Muscle
Halothane	0.74	2.3	224.0	2.6	Brain
		2.36		2.6	Liver
		2.4		1.6	Kidney
				3.5	Muscle
Divinyl ether	1.40	2.8	58.0	60.0	Fat
Trichloroethylene	1.55	9.15	960.0		
		9.85			
Chloroform	3.8	10.3	265.0	1.0	Heart
		8.4		1.0	Brain
Diethyl ether	13.1	12.1	65.0	1.14	Brain
	15.61	15.2	50.2	1.2	Lung
Methoxyflurane	4.5	13.0	825.0	2.34	Brain, white
		11.12		1.70	Brain, gray
				1.34	Muscle

* Bunsen coefficient corrected to 37°C.

blood level quickly, and within the period of lung washout there should be an approach to recovery of consciousness. Even in this case, however, a residual concentration is present in blood as long as the tissues retain the anesthetic, this again being a function of circulation and distribution between blood and tissues.

The most important principle to grasp is that the relative rapidity of induction can be equated with the blood/gas partition coefficient. Anesthetics with low coefficients induce anesthesia more rapidly than do those with higher coefficients. It would seem that greater solubility should lead to more rapid onset of anesthesia, but the crucial point is that the effective inhaled anesthetic pressure must be maintained in the alveoli and pulmonary capillary blood. If alveolar gas pressure is constantly lowered because of a high blood solubility, neither the alveolar nor the arterial tension will be sufficient to induce the necessary anesthetic state.

Signs and Stages of Anesthesia

The discussion of uptake and distribution of anesthetics is based on the premise that anesthetics owe their action to an effect on the central nervous system. A closer analysis of this follows, so that the clinical signs, so important for a safe course during anesthesia, appear more rational. Anesthetists have learned to observe the patient's reactions not only to provide good operating conditions but to avoid or reverse dangerous degrees of circulatory and respiratory depression. With diethyl ether, particularly, the patient passes through several well-defined stages: (1) altered consciousness or analgesia; (2) excitement; and (3) relaxation of muscles

and deep unconsciousness, suitable for operation, where the patient neither experiences pain nor moves when the incision is made. A fourth stage, that of overdosage, is also recognized, where respiratory and circulatory failure occurs.

In Fig. 6-3, the signs of the stages of anesthesia are presented in tabular form, a modification of the chart originally prepared by Guedel. From the beginning, observing the signs and stages has been of great benefit, but newer anesthetics and adjuncts obscure the traditional guidelines so that less attention is paid them. Much can be learned by simple observation for the presence of hypoxia, untoward autonomic effects, and changes in body temperature. To date, almost the only means of assessing circulation have been by auscultatory measurement of blood pressure, counting the pulse beats, ob-

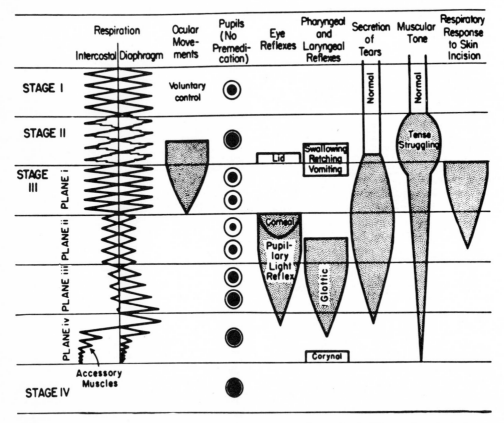

Figure 6-3 The signs and reflex reactions of the stages of anesthesia. The wedge-shaped areas indicate not only patient variability but the factor of variability in disappearance of the signs in the planes of anesthesia.

serving bleeding in the operative field, and recording the ECG; and for respiration, by counting the rate, watching the movement of chest and reservoir bag, and looking for dark blood or peripheral cyanosis. Gradually a change has taken place because of the increasing complexity of the operations performed and the ancillary apparatus used by both anesthetist and surgeon. First, the inhaled concentration of anesthetic is better known because of precision vaporization. A peripheral artery can be cannulated well before operation or just before induction of anesthesia to permit constant recording of mean arterial blood pressure and sampling of blood for analysis of blood gases and alterations in acid-base balance. These measurements are necessary when ventilation is controlled and when a variety of fluids, electrolytes, and osmotic diuretics are given. On the same oscilloscopic screen that displays blood pressure, the ECG and venous pressure can be observed. The bladder is catheterized and urinary output measured as a check on renal perfusion. Central venous catheterization is done to balance the effects of blood loss and replacement against changes in myocardial competence, venous compliance, and circulation capacity. Spot sampling of electrolytes, potassium for example, permits correction of the imbalance often seen during extracorporeal circulation.

VOLATILE ANESTHETIC AGENTS

Diethyl Ether, Ether

Diethyl ether, C_2H_5—O—C_2H_5, was the first general anesthetic accepted as a clinically useful agent. Ether is a clear, colorless, volatile liquid which boils at 34.6°C and has a distinctive, chilling sweet odor.

Effects on Organ Systems

Nervous System With increasing depth of anesthesia, ether produces generalized depression of the central nervous system at all levels. All volatile anesthetics have been observed to depress neuronal membrane excitability. Although the cellular and subcellular actions of anesthetics are still unknown, evidence has been presented which indicates depressant effects at synapses in both brain and spinal cord, the latter being responsible in part for the ex-

cellent muscle relaxation obtained in deeper surgical planes. Depressant effects of anesthetics on the ascending and descending multisynaptic pathways of the brainstem reticular formation concerned with transmitting impulses from the periphery to the cortex are believed to be the basis of the neurophysiology of anesthesia.

Ether is capable of producing stage IV anesthesia without oxygen deprivation, and therefore is referred to as a *complete anesthetic*. The MAC required in humans to prevent a muscular response to a painful stimulus in 50 percent of subjects at equilibrium is 1.90 percent (Table 6-2).

Respiratory System Because of the irritating effect on both the upper and lower respiratory tracts, ether must be added gradually to the mixture of gases inhaled during induction. Failure to do this may result in breath holding, coughing, and laryngospasm as a result of irritation and perhaps stimulation of the sympathetic nervous system, thus delaying the onset of anesthesia. Salivary and bronchial secretions are stimulated by ether and may result in upper respiratory obstruction and interference with gas exchange. Only at relatively high blood-ether concentration is the arterial P_{CO_2} increased without narcotic analgesic premedication, even though central depression is indicated by decreased response to carbon dioxide. The respiratory rate is generally increased until deep levels of anesthesia are reached.

Cardiovascular System Studies with ether have revealed well-maintained cardiac output, and in some instances increased cardiac output, until deeper planes of anesthesia are reached. Increased sympathetic nervous system discharge during ether anesthesia, as evidenced by increased levels of circulating norepinephrine, may explain in part the cardiovascular response to ether in humans. Heart rate is generally increased during ether anesthesia and has been shown to have a positive correlation

Table 6-2 Minimum Alveolar Concentration (MAC), Percent at 1 atm

Methoxyflurane	0.16
Halothane	0.76
Ether	1.90
Cyclopropane	9.20
Nitrous oxide	101.00

with blood-ether concentration. The increased heart rate may be related to a vagolytic effect, as well as sympathetic nervous system stimulation of the heart. Atropine administration during anesthesia produces little increase in heart rate, suggesting a vagolytic action of ether. Arterial pressure is maintained during light surgical planes of anesthesia, but is reduced at deep levels of anesthesia as a result of myocardial depression and effects on the peripheral vasculature.

Serious cardiac arrhythmias, such as premature ventricular contractions and ventricular tachycardia, are rarely observed during well-conducted ether anesthesia. However, a variety of supraventricular arrhythmias are a relatively common observation, including sinus tachycardia, atrioventricular nodal irregularities, and nodal rhythms. Ether does not sensitize the myocardium to catecholamine production of ventricular arrhythmias as do the halogenated hydrocarbons.

Skeletal Musculature By its depressant action on the pyramidal and extrapyramidal pathways of the central nervous system in both the brain and spinal cord, ether produces relaxation of skeletal muscle at depths of anesthesia below plane 2. It has also been shown to reduce the sensitivity of the postjunctional membrane to acetylcholine. When used with ether, the dose of a substance such as curare should be considerably reduced, titrating the effect to secure the desired degree of relaxation.

Gastrointestinal Tract Nausea and vomiting following ether anesthesia are commonly observed, perhaps the result of a central emetic effect, and may persist relatively long into the postoperative period. Induction of anesthesia with ether may be associated with nausea and vomiting as a result of central medullary stimulation and probably local irritation of the stomach by swallowed vapors.

Absorption, Fate, and Excretion Ether is absorbed through the pulmonary epithelium and transported to the brain and other organs. Only a very small percentage of ether administered is metabolized and has no real significance clinically. Most (over 90 percent) is eliminated by the lungs.

Toxicity Acute toxicity of ether is related to overdosage during anesthetic administration. Respiratory arrest generally precedes cardiovascular collapse, so that removal of ether from the inhaled mixture and increasing alveolar ventilation by support of respiration will result in a reduction of ether in the blood going to the brain, subsequent reduction in the concentration in the brain, and return of respiration.

Therapeutic Use Ether is employed primarily for general anesthesia and has been found to be an extremely useful agent for many years. The well-defined neurologic signs and stages, with maintenance of adequate respiration at surgical planes of anesthesia, enables it to be used safely. The mortality rate in patients receiving ether is quite low. The relatively slow induction of diethyl ether, its flammability, and the relatively high incidence of nausea and vomiting in the postanesthetic period have resulted in a marked reduction of its use in modern clinical practice.

Halothane (Fluothane)

Halothane represents one of a number of halogenated hydrocarbons produced in the search for potent, nonexplosive anesthetics. The chemical formula for halothane is CF_3—CHClBr. It has a sweet, nonirritating, not unpleasant odor and is nonflammable in the ranges of concentration used clinically. Halothane, like ether, is capable of producing stage IV anesthesia without oxygen deprivation. Unlike diethyl ether, however, halothane is not a potent analgesic early in anesthesia, and in order to hasten induction, obtain satisfactory anesthesia, and avoid the undesirable cardiovascular effects of deep halothane anesthesia, nitrous oxide in oxygen is generally administered with halothane. The MAC reported for halothane is 0.76 percent (Table 6-2).

Effects on Organ Systems
Central Nervous System Effects of halothane on the reticular activating system account not only for the ability of the agent to alter consciousness but also explain some of the effects of halothane on the cardiovascular system. Halothane is a mild cerebral vasodilator, and at surgical levels of anesthesia, cerebral blood flow is increased slightly above normal. The cerebral vessels exhibit a normal re-

sponse to increased carbon dioxide tensions (vaso-dilatation) and constrict with hypocapnia. A slight decrease in the cerebral metabolic rate of oxygen is observed during halothane anesthesia.

Respiratory System Halothane, unlike diethyl ether, is nonirritating to the upper and lower respiratory tracts; bronchial secretions are therefore not stimulated, and the concentration to be inhaled by the patient may be increased relatively rapidly during induction of anesthesia.

Depression of respiratory centers is evidenced by decreased ventilatory response to carbon dioxide with increased anesthetic depth.

Halothane produces bronchiolar dilatation as a result of direct action on smooth muscle, and this forms the basis for using halothane to control anesthesia in patients with asthma.

Cardiovascular System Cardiovascular depression, evidenced by arterial hypotension, reduction in cardiac output, peripheral resistance, and myocardial contractility, is seen with halothane at surgical levels of anesthesia. The degree of cardiovascular depression increases with increased depth of anesthesia. Action on peripheral circulation is predominantly that of vasodilatation in both skin and skeletal muscle vessels. In the presence of reduced blood volume, severe hypotension may be observed with halothane anesthesia as the result of vasodilatation.

Alterations in cardiac rhythm, including bradycardia and atrioventricular (AV) nodal rhythm, often the cause of hypotension, are frequently observed during halothane anesthesia at light levels and are indicative of increased parasympathetic nervous activity with halothane. Halothane, like other halogenated hydrocarbon anesthetics, sensitizes the myocardium to the arrhythmic effects of catecholamines.

Skeletal Muscle Although halothane has some effect on neuromuscular transmission and spinal mono- and polysynaptic pathways, muscular relaxation is not prominent at light levels of anesthesia. In general, the cardiovascular depression at deeper levels of anesthesia, where muscular relaxation is observed, prohibits use of halothane alone for attaining muscle relaxation during a surgical operation.

Liver Reports of acute hepatic necrosis following halothane administration prompted a retrospec-tive study of the relationship between halothane and hepatic necrosis. The possible occurrence of halothane-induced hepatic necrosis could not be ruled out, although the incidence of necrosis with halothane was no greater than the average for all anesthetics. Repeated exposure to halothane has been related to hepatic necrosis through development of a hypersensitivity causing hepatic damage. A hepatotoxic metabolite of halothane may also explain this phenomenon. It is recommended that patients who have unexplained fever, anorexia, prolonged nausea, or vomiting with or without jaundice following halothane administration not be reexposed to the agent.

Absorption, Fate, and Excretion The pulmonary epithelium is the main area for both absorption and excretion of halothane. A small percentage (12 to 20 percent) of halothane undergoes biotransformation. Trifluoroacetic acid and bromide have been detected as metabolites in the urine.

Toxicity Acute toxicity is related to overdosage. Patients with reduced blood volume are especially vulnerable to halothane in that profound hypotension may be produced early in the induction of anesthesia. Patients with severe cardiac disease and therefore reduced myocardial reserve may respond to the increased myocardial depression produced by halothane with severe hypotension.

Arrhythmias may occur with halothane anesthesia. Reports of malignant hyperpyrexia are associated with halothane and succinylcholine administration. Severe liver damage may develop with repeated use of halothane.

Unpleasant effects related to its use include postoperative shivering to increase body temperature lowered as a result of heat loss during operation.

Its solubility in blood and fat may result in maintained blood levels for prolonged periods with delayed awakening if halothane is not discontinued toward the end of the operation.

Therapeutic Use The relative lack of respiratory irritation and flammability, and the low incidence of postanesthetic nausea and vomiting have made halothane one of the most popular anesthetic agents. By controlling the administered concentration by precision vaporization, supplementing its analgesia with nitrous oxide, and adding neuromuscular blocking drugs, excellent conditions may be obtained for all operations.

Methoxyflurane (Penthrane)

Like halothane, methoxyflurane, $CHCl_2$-CF_2-OCH_3, represents a deliberate effort to synthesize a potent nonflammable agent. It is a clear, colorless liquid having a characteristic fruity odor. The MAC at equilibrium is 0.16 percent (Table 6-2).

Effects on Organ Systems   Analgesia without unconsciousness may be provided as with diethyl ether at very low concentrations (0.6 percent). Progressively greater depths of anesthesia are obtained as the concentration is increased.

At light levels of anesthesia, respiration is apparently not depressed. With increasing depth, definite respiratory depression is noted, so that assistance is necessary to avoid respiratory acidosis during operation. Mild to moderate reductions in arterial pressure accompanied by reduced cardiac output and myocardial contractile force are exhibited at light surgical levels of anesthesia.

Methoxyflurane sensitizes the myocardium to catecholamines, but to a lesser degree than does cyclopropane or halothane. Cardiovascular depression increases with increased depth of anesthesia.

Isolated instances of hepatic necrosis have followed methoxyflurane anesthesia. Routine liver function tests are temporarily abnormal as with all anesthetics.

Administration   Because of the high boiling point, low vapor pressure, and high blood/gas solubility coefficient, induction of anesthesia is prolonged. Thiopental and nitrous oxide in oxygen are frequently administered with methoxyflurane to increase the speed of induction and to permit analgesia at lighter levels of anesthesia with less respiratory and cardiovascular depression. Because of its great fat and tissue solubility, emergence from anesthesia may be prolonged if methoxyflurane is not discontinued well before the end of the operation. Analgesia in the postoperative period is also the result of maintaining analgesic concentrations in the blood for prolonged periods of time.

Trichloroethylene (Trilene)

Trichloroethylene, $CHCl{=}CCl_2$, is a colorless liquid with an odor similar to that of chloroform.

Effects on Organ Systems   Rapid analgesia is produced after a few inhalations of trichloroethylene, and it is relatively nonirritating to the respiratory tract when compared with diethyl ether. Respiratory rate is increased to 2 to 3 times the patient's preoperative rate. Arterial pressure is not generally altered by trichloroethylene. Cardiac arrhythmias, including multiple ventricular extrasystoles and ventricular tachycardia, are observed at deep anesthetic levels. Bradycardia and AV nodal rhythms are common at light planes of anesthesia. Trichloroethylene sensitizes the myocardium to catecholamines.

Absorption, Fate, and Excretion   The respiratory epithelium is the main route of transfer of trichloroethylene. However, it has been estimated that 20 percent or more is metabolized to chloral hydrate and subsequently to trichlorethanol and trichloracetic acid, which are excreted in the urine for as long as 5 days following anesthesia.

Toxicity   Acute toxicities include tachypnea with resultant respiratory acidosis and cardiac irregularities. Delayed poisoning is related to effects on cranial nerves, especially the trigeminal nerve. Hepatotoxicity has also been reported.

Therapeutic Uses   Trichloroethylene is commonly employed for analgesia in obstetrics. It is administered by inhalers that deliver low concentrations, held by the patient and inhaled with the onset of uterine contractions. With nitrous oxide, trichloroethylene is used for such procedures as burn dressing changes and cystoscopy in which muscular relaxation is not required.

Fluroxene (Fluoromar)

Fluroxene ($CF_3{-}CH_2{-}O{-}CH{=}CH_2$) was the first fluorinated ether used clinically. It has a mild, nonirritating, pleasant odor, not unlike that of halothane. Fluroxene is flammable.

Effects on Organ Systems   Salivary and bronchial secretions are not stimulated by fluroxene.

Fluroxene, like halothane, is a respiratory depressant. Respiratory rate and P_{CO_2} increase progressively, while the ventilatory response to carbon dioxide is reduced with increased depth of anesthesia. Cardiovascular effects of fluroxene resemble those of diethyl ether rather than halothane.

At light levels of anesthesia, blood pressure is well maintained. Cardiac rhythm generally is not altered, and AV nodal rhythm is occasionally the only change observed. Like diethyl ether, fluroxene does not sensitize the myocardium to catecholamines; circulating catecholamines are not increased during fluroxene anesthesia. Moderate relaxation of skeletal muscle is obtained at light levels of anesthesia. Deep levels of anesthesia cause moderate to severe hypotension. Neuromuscular blocking drugs are generally administered along with fluroxene to avoid the hypotension observed at deep levels of anesthesia.

Therapeutic Use   Due to its relatively nonirritating property, concentrations of 6 to 8 percent can be delivered early in the induction of anesthesia, resulting in rapid central nervous system depression. Because of high solubility in fat and maintenance of blood level after discontinuance, analgesia may be present for some time after drug cessation. Flammability has limited fluroxene's use in modern clinical anesthetic practice.

Enflurane (Ethrane)

Enflurane (CHF_2—O—CF_2CHFCl) is a potent, stable, nonflammable, halogenated ether. Its properties are similar to those of halothane.

Effects on Organ Systems   Enflurane does not cause excessive secretions in the respiratory tract. Generally, respiration is not seriously depressed until deep anesthesia is achieved, and there is little difficulty in assuming manual control of breathing.

Muscle relaxation produced by this anesthetic is better than with halothane, although muscle relaxants are added to provide adequate paralysis. If tubocurarine or any other nondepolarizing agent is employed, synergism may occur and should be anticipated.

The cardiovascular system remains relatively stable, except at deep levels of anesthesia where marked hypotension results. As with halothane,

enflurane most likely sensitizes the myocardium to catecholamines.

Divinyl Ether (Vinethene)

Because of renal and hepatic toxicity, divinyl ether has generally been used by open-drop technique for brief surgical procedures. However, as with ethyl chloride, it is difficult to defend its use as an anesthetic today.

Chloroform

Hepatic toxicity associated with chloroform as well as the introduction of potent nonflammable agents have caused the almost complete disappearance of chloroform from the armamentarium of the clinical anesthetist. Availability of relatively nontoxic anesthetics make it difficult to justify a well-recognized hepatotoxin for any clinical use.

GASEOUS ANESTHETIC AGENTS

Nitrous Oxide

In current anesthetic practice, the relative lack of potency (MAC at equilibrium is 101 percent, Table 6-2) of nitrous oxide (N_2O) is overcome by the addition of other drugs in what is referred to as *balanced anesthesia*. Today nitrous oxide, because of the analgesia afforded, is probably the most widely used general anesthetic in this country.

Effects on Organ Systems   In general, one may characterize the pharmacologic effects of nitrous oxide administered with adequate oxygen as relatively mild. This fits well with its relative lack of potency and low lipid solubility.

Central Nervous System   In concentrations of 20 to 30 percent, analgesia is easily demonstrable, and the drug is thus used in obstetrics and dental surgery. Administration of 75 to 80 percent nitrous oxide in oxygen without narcotic analgesic or barbiturate premedication is barely sufficient to produce minimal surgical anesthesia at approximately plane 1. Although nitrous oxide has no apparent effect on cerebral blood flow, the cerebral vessels respond to hypocapnia with vasoconstriction. Cerebral oxygen utilization is decreased approximately 15 percent with 70 percent nitrous oxide.

Respiratory System   Nitrous oxide in oxygen has been shown to increase the respiratory minute volume without depressing the response of the respiratory center to carbon dioxide. Following administration of thiopental and narcotics (morphine or meperidine), nitrous oxide depresses the respiratory response to carbon dioxide in a synergistic manner.

Cardiovascular System   In studies on nitrous oxide added to halothane or methoxyflurane anesthesia, varied cardiovascular responses have been observed. Cardiac output, heart rate, and arterial pressure may be further reduced by the nitrous oxide, or a slight increase in total peripheral resistance may be noted. The increase in peripheral resistance has been correlated with increased circulating levels of norepinephrine in peripheral blood. Cardiac arrhythmias are not seen during nitrous oxide anesthesia in the absence of hypoxia and hypercapnia.

Other Organ Systems   Skeletal muscle relaxation is not ordinarily achieved with nitrous oxide alone; therefore, neuromuscular blockers must be administered to obtain optimum conditions in surgical operations requiring relaxation.

Nitrous oxide in oxygen has little effect on uterine muscle tone.

Absorption, Fate, and Excretion   Transport across the pulmonary epithelium accounts for the uptake and excretion of the largest portion of nitrous oxide in the body. Passage into the bowel has been reported, but the greater amount returns to the blood when the drug is discontinued.

Toxicity   Toxicity with nitrous oxide is related to its administration in adequate concentrations of oxygen. Convulsions, delayed return of consciousness, confusion, and in some instances, permanent brain damage as the result of inadequate oxygen concentrations can occur.

Therapeutic Use   Because of its relative low potency, nitrous oxide is administered with other agents such as narcotic analgesics, halothane, methoxyflurane, neuroleptics, and neuromuscular blocking drugs. The analgesic property permits administration of lower concentrations of halothane and methoxyflurane, thereby minimizing their cardiovascular depressant properties.

Cyclopropane

Cyclopropane is the simplest of the cyclic chemical compounds and has the following structure:

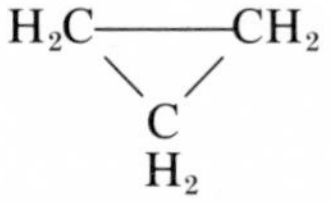

$$H_2C\text{------}CH_2$$
$$\diagdown\diagup$$
$$C$$
$$H_2$$

Uptake of cyclopropane from the alveoli resembles that of nitrous oxide because of similar blood/gas partition coefficients. Its MAC at equilibrium is 9.20 percent (Table 6-2). Recovery from anesthesia is rapid following its discontinuation.

Effects on Organ Systems

Central Nervous System   Cyclopropane is a complete anesthetic, as are halothane, chloroform, and diethyl ether. Because of its potency, the high concentrations used, and its low blood/gas solubility coefficient, unconsciousness may be produced within 60 s to 2 min. Induction excitement is frequently either not observed or mild because of the drug's ability to deliver high concentrations and obtain depth of anesthesia rapidly. Postoperative emergence excitement is commonly observed with cyclopropane and may be averted by the intravenous administration of a small amount of narcotic analgesic prior to discontinuing cyclopropane. Restlessness and excitement may be related to several factors, including pain, preexisting fear, or a stage of excitement comparable to that seen during induction.

Respiratory System   Cyclopropane is a potent respiratory center depressant at surgical levels of anesthesia. With narcotic premedication, respiratory depression produced by the combination of both drugs is demonstrable shortly after induction of anesthesia. Ventilatory assistance must be given to prevent respiratory acidosis at all surgical levels of cyclopropane anesthesia. Cyclopropane is supposed to produce bronchospasm and is therefore not recommended for patients with asthma.

Cardiovascular System   In general, cyclopropane may be said to maintain or even stimulate the circulation. Mean arterial pressure is usually increased or unchanged, and in the absence of narcotic analgesic premedication, cardiac output is generally increased at surgical levels of anesthesia. Cyclopropane causes increased sympathetic nervous system activity resulting in increased circulating catecholamines. The increased sympathetic tone causes augmented cardiac output and an increase in peripheral vascular resistance. Cyclopropane is a direct myocardial depressant, as are other general anesthetics.

Heart rate is either unchanged or slightly lower during anesthesia, suggesting an element of increased cardiac vagal activity. Morphine premedication causes even greater reduction in cardiac rate due to its ability to increase vagal tone, probably on the basis of central nervous system action.

Cardiac rhythm may vary markedly during cyclopropane anesthesia; alterations include AV nodal rhythms, AV nodal dissociation, atrial extrasystoles, ventricular extrasystoles, bigeminy, and multifocal ventricular tachycardia may be observed.

Discontinuance of cyclopropane anesthesia after relatively prolonged operations frequently causes hypotension.

Skeletal Muscle Due to effects on synaptic transmission in the spinal cord, cyclopropane provides adequate relaxation for most abdominal procedures at deep levels of anesthesia. With the tendency to use light levels of anesthesia in clinical practice, neuromuscular blocking drugs, such as *d*-tubocurarine or succinylcholine, are frequently employed in conjunction with cyclopropane to attain muscle relaxation.

Metabolic Effects Oxygen consumption is reduced during cyclopropane anesthesia. Blood glucose levels are transiently elevated early and return to preanesthetic levels as anesthesia progresses. Decreased glucose utilization may occur. Hyperglycemia has been attributed to increased sympathetic activity and to increased glucocorticoid secretion during cyclopropane anesthesia.

Absorption, Fate, and Excretion The pulmonary membrane is the main area of cyclopropane elimination. Because of relative insolubility in blood, it is fairly rapidly exhaled following its removal from the inhaled mixture of gas. Biotransformation accounts for a small degree of cyclopropane elimination.

Toxicity and Therapeutic Uses Aside from the potential for producing cardiac arrhythmias, especially if carbon dioxide is permitted to accumulate or catecholamines are administered, cyclopropane has enjoyed some use in clinical anesthesia, although there is considerable concern for flammability, violence of the explosion it produces, and the need for antistatic precautions. Ability to deliver high concentrations of oxygen and to support the circulation, as well as high potency, have made it a leading choice in patients with compromised cardiovascular status and in those with reduced arterial oxygen tensions. The ability to support the circulation has rendered it useful in the presence of hemorrhage.

Widespread use of electrocautery during operation has been responsible for the decreased use of all explosive agents, including cyclopropane.

Ethylene

Ethylene is little used today and, similar to nitrous oxide, requires concomitant use of thiopental, narcotic analgesics, and neuromuscular blocking drugs. It is used in a few clinics for obstetrical anesthesia. Its flammability and the development of more potent nonexplosive agents are the reasons for ethylene's almost complete abandonment.

INTRAVENOUS ANESTHETIC AGENTS

Ultra-Short-Acting Barbiturates

A large number of barbiturate derivatives have been developed by substituting the hydrogen atoms on the carbon in position 5 (R_1 and R_2) with alkyl, aryl, or aralkyl groups.

Barbituric acid

The thiobarbiturates differ from the barbiturates in that the oxygen atom of the urea portion of the molecule (position 2) is replaced by a sulfur atom.

The chemical relationships of the ultra-short-acting barbiturates most widely used in anesthesia are shown in the following tabulation of substitutions in the barbituric acid molecule:

Barbiturate	R_1	R_2	Other
Thiopental sodium	Ethyl	1-Methylbutyl	2-Thio
Thiamylal sodium	Allyl	1-Methylbutyl	2-Thio
Methohexital sodium	Allyl	1-Methyl 2-Pentenyl	1-Methyl

Thiopental differs from pentobarbital only by the substitution of sulfur for oxygen in position 2, which gives the compound a very short duration of action. Although the thiobarbiturates are generally ultra-short-acting, the sulfur atom is not essential to this action, since methohexital is not a thiobarbiturate. The principal effect of these drugs administered intravenously is the induction of hypnosis leading to surgical anesthesia. The response of the body to the intravenous injection of an effective quantity of a nonvolatile anesthetic such as methohexital or thiopental is the same, but with minor differences, as that occurring after the inhalation of anesthetics. Consciousness is lost first, then the ability to react in a reflex manner to external stimuli; then motor tone is lost. Finally, after excessive doses, the vital medullary centers fail in this order: the respiratory center, the vasomotor centers, and, terminally, the cardiac centers. Furthermore, it has been observed that recovery from the nonvolatile anesthetics follows the same pattern as that noted during recovery from the volatile anesthetics.

When the thiobarbiturates were introduced, they were believed to be ultra-short-acting because of rapid metabolism. With the development of quantitative methods of analysis, rapid emergence from anesthesia was found to be more a matter of rapid diffusion from an initially high concentration in the brain to other areas of high blood flow. The final reservoir was adipose tissue, from which a slow release led to prolonged but low circulating blood levels. The rate of destruction proved to be approximately 15 percent/h of the circulating blood level, a far cry from the concept of an ultra-short-acting drug. Nevertheless, metabolic transformation

should not be overlooked as an important factor in recovery, particularly with more rapidly metabolized compounds such as the barbiturates.

As in the analysis of inhalation anesthesia, similar methods have been applied to the study of the barbiturates. One approach used a digital computer and a compartmental system of variable blood distribution as an analogue (Fig. 6-4). The diagram does not completely take into account several other factors that govern emergence from anesthesia. Furthermore, there is no consistent relationship between the concentration of thiopental in plasma and the depth of anesthesia. However, it can be seen that uptake of barbiturates continues for 30 min both in the lean body tissues and in fat, according to their mass. Thereafter, the adipose compartment is the only site where the concentration of drug continues to rise, the maximum being reached in approximately an hour.

The chief disadvantage of intravenous barbiturates is respiratory depression. Circulatory depression may also occur. Intravenous barbiturates depress the respiratory center so that it will not respond normally to carbon dioxide. Barbiturates depress the reaction of the aortic and carotid bodies (chemoreceptors). This action is in complete contrast to that of diethyl ether which reflexly stimulates respiration. The intravenous use of barbiturates in patients who have had a history of asthma has been followed by acute asthmatic episodes.

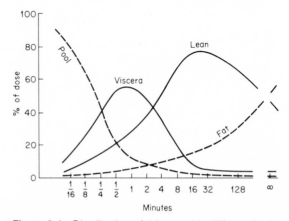

Figure 6-4 Distribution of thiopental in different body tissues at various times after intravenous injection. Time scale (in min) progresses geometrically. Final values are at infinity.

Barbiturates should be used with extreme caution in patients in shock, because they may easily aggravate the already poor circulatory condition.

The ultra-short-acting barbiturates used in anesthesia have come to be recognized as hypnotic rather than analgesic agents. They are rarely used alone for general anesthesia because they afford little analgesia and are poor relaxants of skeletal muscle. Thiopental may be administered rectally as well as intravenously, especially in children.

Preparations and Doses *Sodium thiopental* (Pentothal sodium) for injection is available in ampuls containing 500 mg, 1, 5, or 10 g. Usual dose: Intravenous induction, 2 to 3 ml of 2.5 percent solution at the rate of 1 ml every 5 to 10 s; maintenance, 0.5 to 2 ml as required; rectal, 45 mg/kg body weight in a 5 to 10 percent solution to a total dose of 3 g.

Sodium methohexital (Brevital sodium) is available in ampuls containing 500 mg, 2.5, or 5 g. Usual dose: Intravenous induction, 7.5 ml of 1 percent solution at the rate of 1 ml every 5 s; maintenance, 2 to 4 ml every 4 to 6 min as required.

Sodium thiamylal (Surital) is available in ampuls containing 500 mg and 1.5 and 10 g. Usual dose: Intravenous induction, 3 to 6 ml of 2.5 percent solution; maintenance, 0.15 to 1 ml as required.

Ketamine Hydrochloride (Ketaject, Ketalar)

This agent is neither a narcotic nor a barbiturate. Given intravenously, ketamine promptly causes anesthesia which lasts 8 to 10 min; profound analgesia is induced, but the patient does not appear to be asleep. Under ketamine, the laryngeal and pharyngeal reflexes are maintained. There is moderate increase in pulse rate and blood pressure under ketamine, and it is reported to have an antiarrhythmic effect.

The drug appears to have a wide margin of safety, and organ toxicity is low. Incidence of postoperative vomiting is low. The drug reportedly does not depress the fetus when used in labor.

The main criticism of ketamine is its tendency to cause vivid dreams, especially in adults. Some investigators believe that this can be held to a minimum by proper management during the postoperative period. The drug is contraindicated in patients with hypertension and in those with a history of cerebrovascular accident, as well as in those with cardiac decompensation.

Ketamine is a most unusual drug in that it gives excellent analgesia rapidly, without depression of respiration. It is valuable for external eye surgery. (Since it provides no relaxation, it should not be used for intraocular procedures.) It has been used extensively for debridement of burns and for pneumoencephalography. Children are not bothered by such vivid dreams as are adults, so that its use has been limited in some places to patients under 15 years of age. The drug is of value for operations about the head and face, if one inserts a nasopharyngeal airway. It is an excellent choice for rapid induction in an emergency.

PREANESTHETIC MEDICATION

Choice of preanesthetic drugs depends upon the conditions at the time. In general, patients should be brought to the operating room slightly drowsy, free of apprehension, and able to cooperate in the preliminary preparations for anesthesia.

Drugs commonly used for preanesthetic medication include sedatives, narcotics, anticholinergics, antianxiety agents, phenothiazines, and butyrophenones. These drugs are very often given in combination for several reasons: to allay apprehension; to diminish the amount of general anesthesia required through a basal narcotic effect; to eliminate undesirable reflexes, for example, reflex bradycardia incident to anesthesia and operation; and lastly, to inhibit salivary and respiratory tract secretions. Although these goals constitute a pharmacologic possibility, the properties of the drugs used unfortunately often produce unwanted effects.

ADJUNCTS TO ANESTHESIA

The skeletal muscle relaxant drugs, such as succinylcholine or tubocurarine, are employed with general anesthetics, particularly during abdominal surgical procedures, to provide adequate muscle relaxation and to reduce the depth of anesthesia and the dose of the anesthetic drug (see Chap. 20).

Chapter 7

Local Anesthetics

Local anesthetics are agents which possess the specific ability to reversibly block nerve conduction in low concentrations. Reversibility is the important concept in this process, since a number of substances and procedures, such as metabolic inhibitors and neural damage, are capable of affecting nerve conduction irreversibly. The therapeutic practicality of local anesthetics lies in their ability to quantitatively block nerve conduction for a desired period of time, which is followed by recovery with no apparent residual neural damage.

The prototype local anesthetic, procaine, was synthesized in 1905. Since that time, thousands of local anesthetics have been synthesized and tested, many with substantial advantages over procaine. Nevertheless, this compound reigned as the principal local anesthetic for over 50 years, laying the foundation and permitting the development of our modern approaches to the use of these agents.

Most useful local anesthetics are composed of three structural entities: (A) a carbocyclic or het-erocyclic ring of the aromatic type (lipophilic portion), (B) an intermediate chain, and (C) an amino group (hydrophilic portion) (see Fig. 7-1). Such entities can be readily seen in the formula for procaine. The aromatic ring is essential for anesthetic activity; and therapeutically useful injectable local anesthetics require a delicate balance between the degree of lipid solubility, represented by a particular ringed structure, and the potential water solubility of a compound as expressed by the amine group. In addition to the characterization of local anesthetics on the traditional basis of solubility, most local anesthetics can be classified chemically as to the type of linkage between the aromatic group and the intermediate chain. One group is represented by the esteratic linkage, susceptible to plasma hydrolysis, found in *procaine*, and the other by *lidocaine*, in which the aromatic group is linked to the rest of the molecule by an amide function and is relatively resistant to enzymatic inactivation in the blood.

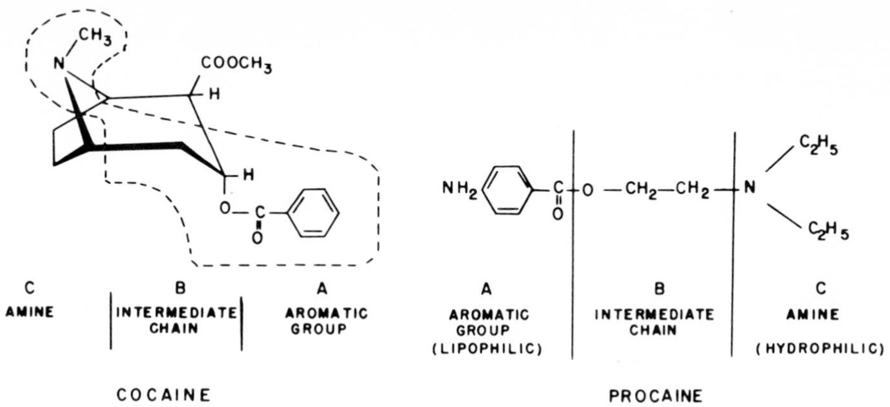

Figure 7-1 Comparison of the chemical structures of cocaine and procaine.

MECHANISM OF ACTION

According to current concepts, the membrane of a resting nerve registers a negative potential produced primarily by the relative concentrations of sodium and potassium ions on either side of this excitable tissue. As the impulse is propagated along the membrane, an alteration in membrane permeability at a particular area occurs followed by a large, transient influx of sodium associated with local depolarization. This rise in the permeability of the membrane to sodium ions sharply changes the potential and generates a nerve action potential (Fig. 7-2). Repolarization is aided by the subsequent efflux of potassium ion and the active "pumping out" of sodium. The adjacent area undergoes depolarization, the sequence is repeated, and conduction of the impulse is thus accomplished.

Local anesthetics have been shown to (1) increase the threshold for electrical excitation in nerve, (2) slow propagation of the impulse, (3) reduce the rate of rise of the action potential, and (4) eventually block conduction of the nerve impulse. Many investigators have indicated that all such effects of local anesthetics can be explained on the basis of a reduction in the carrying capacity of the system which permits sodium ions to be transported across the membrane. Thus the simple blockade of this fundamental sodium influx would inhibit the propagation of the nerve impulse. Inhibition of ion permeability may also explain the

observation that local anesthetics block conduction without depolarization of the nerve and consequently produce little change in potential.

Although blockade of nerve conduction can be said to be primarily accomplished by interference with the fundamental factor necessary for generation of the action potential, namely sodium influx, the intimate mechanisms by which such inhibition is accomplished are still not clearly understood. One of the most intriguing current theories concerns the interaction of local anesthetics and membrane calcium.

It has been suggested for a number of years that calcium ions and local anesthetics act on, or are attached to, the same system, namely, the system which is responsible for conveying sodium ions through the nerve membrane. Theoretically, it has been suggested that phospholipids, present in the nerve membrane, could function as part of the membrane sodium-carrying system and bind the individual ions by a change in conformation, depending on the electric field. The molecule would therefore bind either calcium or sodium ions, and in this manner act as a "gating" mechanism which would control axon membrane permeability changes. On the basis of present knowledge, the following postulations can be presented as a possible mechanism by which certain local anesthetics may antagonize membrane permeability (see Fig. 7-2 *E, F, G*): (1) Calcium is normally bound to the membrane where it confers stability and a certain degree of

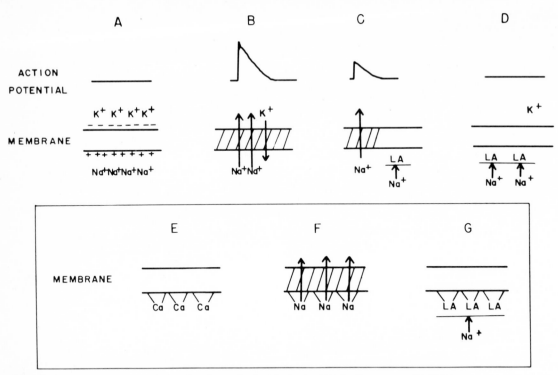

Figure 7-2 Ionic movement during local anesthetic blockade. (*A*) Resting nerve. (*B*) Depolarization with sodium influx and the onset of an action potential. (*C*) Partial reduction in membrane sodium permeability and depression of action potential by local anesthetic. (*D*) Complete block of sodium influx with no potential change. (*E*) Resting nerve; calcium occupies sites on surface membrane. (*F*) Depolarization with sodium exchange for calcium sites and influx through membrane. (*G*) Local anesthetics occupy calcium sites; therefore, no exchange with sodium and blockade results.

impermeability to sodium ions; (2) during depolarization the calcium ion is displaced from its binding site, thus allowing sodium to pass more readily through the membrane; (3) a local anesthetic in the vicinity of the nerve membrane, by virtue of its higher concentration, competitively displaces calcium and is bound to the site; (4) propagation of the nerve impulse fails to initiate depolarization in this area because of the inability of the process to displace the local anesthetic from the binding site as it would normally displace calcium. Thus, sodium ions cannot enter, propagation is halted, and blockade is accomplished.

SEQUENCE OF NEURON BLOCKADE

Generally, small nerve fibers, which are usually nonmyelinated, are more susceptible to local anes-

thetic action than the larger neurons. Usually, a definite order of blockade by local anesthetics on sensory functions can be observed with the sensation of pain first affected, followed by the sensations of cold, warmth, touch, and deep pressure. Recovery usually evolves in the reverse order.

EFFECT OF pH

Local anesthetics for therapeutic use are usually prepared in the form of a water-soluble salt since the free base is difficult to solubilize and is unstable. Most local anesthetics are secondary or tertiary amines and, as a consequence, can exist as either the uncharged base or as the positively charged substituted ammonium cation. The relative percentages of such forms are dependent on the dissociation constant (pK_a) and pH of the solution.

This chemical rearrangement can be illustrated in the following equation:

$$R:N + HOH \rightleftharpoons R:NH^+ + OH^-$$
Base   Cation

Since the pK_a of most local anesthetics is between 8.0 and 9.0, only about 2 to 20 percent of the agent will usually be found in the free-base form at the pH of most tissues. The penetration of a local anesthetic to its site of action is largely dependent upon its ability to cross lipid membranes. The free-base form has a high oil/water distribution coefficient and can therefore penetrate such membranes easily. Cationic forms, because of their charge, are unable to penetrate such barriers quickly. The limiting factors with respect to local anesthetic distribution and penetration through nerve sheaths are, therefore, its rate of conversion to the base form and the lipophilic character of the base.

EFFECTS ON ORGAN SYSTEMS

Local anesthetics influence all neurons, as well as a variety of other tissues, with which they come in contact. Such systems include sensory fibers, motor fibers, ganglia, portions of the central nervous system, and various muscular tissue. As a consequence, the therapeutic reference to the so-called "local" actions of such agents is merely a manifestation of dose, site, method of administration, dimensions of the nerve fiber, and the physical properties of the agent employed. It is obvious that systemic absorption of such compounds may initiate many unintentional pharmacologic actions. Clinically, the most serious effects are related to the central nervous, cardiovascular, and respiratory systems.

Central Nervous System

Most local anesthetics, if absorbed in sufficient amounts, will produce central nervous system stimulation. The extent of such effects, as previously noted, depends primarily upon the specific agent, and the concentration, method, and rate of administration of the drug. High blood levels of such agents may produce excitement, apprehension, disorientation, confusion, tremors, and clonic convulsions. Central nervous system stimulation of this type is almost always followed by depression and exhaustion. Death may ensue due to respiratory failure as a result of medullary depression. The peculiar effects of nitrogenous local anesthetics on the central nervous system are based on the lipophilic nature of such compounds. Because of the basic form engendered by the pH of the plasma, these agents readily pass the blood-brain barrier and produce a direct and rapid action on the brain. Such systemic effects are likely to be more prominent with cocaine than with other members of the group and may possibly be responsible, in some manner, for the addicting qualities of this agent. In addition, the facility of such agents for penetrating the blood-brain barrier may also explain why even rapidly hydrolyzable drugs, such as procaine, produce distinct central nervous system effects when sufficient concentrations are absorbed into the bloodstream.

Cardiovascular Effects

Most local anesthetics, with the exception of cocaine, will produce arteriolar dilatation, primarily due to a direct action on the smooth muscle wall, probably by interference with the excitation-contraction coupling action of calcium. Cocaine possesses the unique intrinsic characteristic of blocking the uptake of norepinephrine at sympathetic nerve terminals, thus prolonging adrenergic action and fostering vasoconstriction. Clinically, small systemic amounts of local anesthetics have little appreciable effect on blood vessels. Excessive absorption or administration of such agents into the bloodstream, however, may produce a generalized vasodilatation leading to sustained hypotension and cardiovascular collapse. Usually combined with this action on blood vessels is a direct depressive effect on the myocardium. The action of local anesthetics, in sufficient concentrations, on the heart usually involves a reduction in myocardial excitability and contractility with bradycardia frequently observed. Cardiac output diminishes and may progress rapidly to a cardiac standstill. This ability of local anesthetics, such as procainamide and lidocaine, to depress cardiac tissue by increasing the effective refractory period, elevating the threshold for stimulation, and prolonging conduction time has considerable therapeutic usefulness in various arrhythmias.

ABSORPTION, DISTRIBUTION, AND METABOLISM

The effect of pH on local anesthetic penetration through tissue has been mentioned previously, as well as the need for a basic, uncharged form of optimal diffusion. An optimal combination between a satisfactory oil/water distribution coefficient coupled with an effective hydrophilic group, to allow adequate water solubility, is essential to provide good diffusion capability for a local anesthetic.

Local anesthetics manifest little penetration through intact skin. However, with the exception of a number of esters such as procaine and the insoluble local anesthetics, fairly rapid absorption is obtained through various mucous membranes. Upon injection and subsequent absorption, most local anesthetics have little difficulty penetrating membrane barriers including the placenta.

As with all drugs, rates of metabolic transformation play an important role in determining the duration of action and toxicity of a compound. Biotransformation mechanisms associated with these agents are highly dependent on chemical structure, and local anesthetics containing an ester linkage, such as procaine, are inactivated by hydrolysis. Procaine is metabolized primarily in the plasma by the enzyme serum cholinesterase. Lidocaine, an amide, is primarily metabolized in the liver by microsomal enzymes. Several pathways occur in the inactivation of this compound. The primary route of inactivation involves the removal of one of the ethyl groups on the terminal tertiary amine of lidocaine, followed by hydrolysis of the amide linkage to form xylidine and monoethylglycine. Oxidation may then occur prior to sulfate conjugation. Both free and conjugated forms are excreted in the urine of humans, with 3 to 11 percent of the total administered dose found in an unchanged form.

VASOCONSTRICTORS

Vasoconstrictors, such as epinephrine hydrochloride, are very frequently combined with local anesthetic solutions to prevent their vasodilatating effects and rapid removal from the site of injection. Typical exceptions to the use of vasoconstrictors are procedures where the circulation may be compromised, as in anesthesia involving the toes, fingers, and penis. A distinct disadvantage of vaso-constrictors is the possibility of systemic toxicity following the administration of high concentrations of a drug such as epinephrine. Reactions far too frequently seen in dental and medical practice include anxiety, tachycardia, palpitation, and elevated blood pressure. It is therefore necessary to adhere strictly to dosage requirements when local anesthetics are combined with vasoconstrictors. Local anesthetics such as lidocaine and mepivacaine require smaller concentrations of such vasoconstrictors because of their potency and diminished vasodilatating effect.

TOXICITY

The serious manifestations associated with rapid local anesthetic absorption have been discussed earlier in this chapter and involve central nervous system stimulation followed by depression, respiratory depression, cardiac dysfunction, and generalized vasodilatation. As with most drugs, toxic symptoms may be elicited in conditions where hepatic or renal disease is present. The clinical entity associated with the presence of atypical cholinesterases in some individuals may also present a potential hazard when ester anesthetics are administered.

Hypersensitivity to local anesthetics is rare. The syndrome consists of an allergic dermatitis or asthmatic attack or, in some cases, evolves into a full-blown anaphylactoid reaction. Such sensitivity is usually encountered with procaine-like local anesthetics which may exhibit cross-sensitivity to other members of the para-aminobenzoate family. Skin and patch tests currently available are ineffective in predicting these reactions. However, lidocaine and other amides do not exhibit this cross-sensitivity and can be utilized in these cases. Prolonged or frequent contact with a number of local anesthetics may produce dermatologic reactions, and these are often observed in practitioners who continually handle such agents.

METHODS OF ADMINISTRATION

Surface Anesthesia

This method refers to the topical application of local anesthetic agents to induce surface anesthesia in the eye; in various mucous membranes including the nose, throat, and trachea; and in the skin. As has been mentioned previously, local anesthetics will penetrate through intact skin to some extent. However, local anesthetics, with the notable exception of the insoluble compounds, will be rapidly absorbed through mucous membranes.

Local anesthetics may be used for a variety of ocular operations or to produce surface anesthesia of the cornea in simple procedures such as tonometry. Agents used for surface ophthalmic anesthesia include tetracaine, lidocaine, and dibucaine.

Agents such as lidocaine or tetracaine are frequently applied to the throat, larynx, or trachea in an aerosol spray or by a swab. Water-soluble jellies are also utilized in such cases. Burns and surface pain on the skin, as well as less sensitive mucous membranes, are often treated with preparations such as cyclomethycaine, benzocaine, lidocaine, and tetracaine. Abraded or ulcerated areas are much more susceptible to systemic absorption than is intact skin, and as a consequence, indiscriminate application of local anesthetic agents to these areas may produce adverse reactions.

Infiltration Anesthesia

This method of administration is commonly used in a number of minor surgical procedures, particularly the injection of an anesthetic agent intradermally or subcutaneously at or around the area to be anesthetized. Low concentrations are usually required in this procedure for anesthetizing small peripheral nerve endings. A "ring" or "triangle" method is commonly employed in which small wheals are formed around the operative area and subsequently connected by infiltration with the local anesthetic agent, usually procaine or lidocaine solution.

Nerve Block Anesthesia

Blockade of this type involves a variety of anatomically diverse nerve trunks or spinal routes. It may refer to regional blockade of the cervical plexus or to direct injection into the spinal cord. All such procedures necessarily require a high degree of specialization and experience and should not be attempted by the untrained.

Spinal Anesthesia Spinal anesthesia is also referred to as *intrathecal* or *subarachnoid block*. It offers the distinct advantage of muscular relaxation for operations in the lower part of the body, without the attendant trepidation associated with the loss of consciousness. Injection of a local anesthetic into the subarachnoid space of the lumbar area almost immediately initiates the onset of anesthesia. Diffusion or spread of local anesthetic in the spinal cord is primarily dependent on the concentration and physical characteristics of the agent employed. Anesthetic localization at a specific level of the spinal cord can be facilitated by using solutions which exhibit varying specific gravities. Solutions registering a specific gravity greater than that of spinal fluid are referred to as *hyperbaric*; those manifesting specific gravities lower than spinal fluid are called *hypobaric*. A solution of equivalent density to that of cerebral spinal fluid is called *isobaric*. Utilization of a solution of proper specific gravity combined with careful positioning of the patient permits diffusion of the agent to the desired level of contact in the spinal cord.

Typical average durations of action of some of the commonly used agents are procaine, 1 to 1.5 h; lidocaine, 2.5 to 3 h; tetracaine, 3 to 5 h; and dibucaine, 4 to 6 h.

Continuous Spinal Anesthesia By placing a catheter within the spinal subarachnoid space, intermittent injections of an anesthetic can be given to produce continuous anesthesia for unlimited periods of time. In this way, the level of anesthesia can be maintained and regulated accurately for long durations. Procaine and tetracaine are frequently utilized in such procedures.

Epidural Anesthesia Epidural or peridural anesthesia is produced by injection of a local anesthetic into the space surrounding the dura mater, within the spinal canal. This procedure essentially accomplishes most of the objectives desired with spinal anesthesia, except that the subarachnoid space is not entered and many of the complications of this action are avoided. The principle of epidural anesthesia is based on the diffusion of the agent through tissue surrounding the dura mater.

One of the most serious disadvantages of this technique, beyond the skill required, is the relatively large volume of local anesthetic solution needed to produce anesthesia. This may result in a high incidence of systemic reactions; moreover, chance placement of the needle in the subarachnoid space may prove fatal. Lidocaine and mepivacaine are commonly utilized in these procedures because of their good diffusion capabilities through tissue.

Epidural anesthesia, induced by administering the anesthetic solution into the sacral canal through the sacral hiatus, is referred to as *caudal anesthesia* and is often used in obstetrics.

PREPARATIONS AND DOSES

Amides

Lidocaine Hydrochloride (Xylocaine)

$$\text{CH}_3 \quad \text{O}$$

—NHC—CH$_2$N(CH$_2$CH$_3$)$_2$·HCl

$$\text{CH}_3$$

Lidocaine hydrochloride, 2-diethylamino-2',6'-acetoxylidide hydrochloride, was introduced into general medical practice in 1948. The compound represented a distinct departure from the classic procaine structure because of the substitution of an amide for an ester linkage, and because lidocaine is not a derivative of benzoic acid. Lidocaine is an unusually stable compound. Investigations have determined the potency to be approximately 2 to 3 times that of procaine. Clinically it produces a more rapid, longer lasting, and more extensive anesthesia than procaine (Table 7-1). Unlike procaine, lidocaine does exhibit a surface anesthetic action and can be applied topically to mucous membranes. It is compatible with epinephrine, but manifests an

intrinsic property which permits it to leave the site of injection at a slower rate than procaine. Consequently, in procedures where small volumes are utilized, lidocaine can be injected without epinephrine. These desirable properties have allowed lidocaine to virtually supplant procaine as the local anesthetic of choice in a variety of procedures.

Lidocaine and other amides may induce drowsiness instead of stimulation as an indication of toxicity. In instances of slow absorption of high concentrations of the drug, the toxic symptoms usually associated are drowsiness, dizziness, blurred vision, nausea, tremors, convulsions, and respiratory arrest. The most serious toxicity is related to rapid onset of action. Here, rapid action of lidocaine produces, with little warning, unconsciousness, respiratory depression, cardiovascular dysfunction, and cardiac arrest.

Lidocaine is used extensively for infiltration, nerve block, and epidural anesthesia, as well as for topical application. Preparations for infiltration anesthesia are available in concentrations from 0.5 to 1 percent. A wide variety of solutions from 1 to 2 percent are available with and without epinephrine for regional blockade. This agent is also used in the management of cardiac arrhythmias.

Mepivacaine Hydrochloride (Carbocaine)
Mepivacaine hydrochloride, 1-methyl-2',6'-pipecoloxylidide hydrochloride,

$$\text{CH}_3 \quad \text{O}$$

—NHC— ...·HCl

$$\text{CH}_3 \qquad \text{CH}_3$$

possesses an amide linkage and is similar in chemical structure and pharmacologic activity to lidocaine. Both lidocaine and mepivacaine exhibit approximately equivalent actions with respect to potency and toxicity (Table 7-1). The duration of action is slightly longer with mepivacaine, and the need for vasoconstrictor assistance in absorption and prolongation of effect is consequently decreased. In many instances, therefore, mepivacaine may be utilized without epinephrine.

The toxic actions of mepivacaine are similar to those discussed above with lidocaine. Mepivacaine

Table 7-1 Comparative Properties of Local Anesthetics

Anesthetic	Potency	Toxicity	Duration of action, h
Dibucaine	15	15	3+
Tetracaine	10	10	2+
Lidocaine	2	2	2+
Mepivacaine	2	1–2	2+
Procaine	1	1	1

is rapidly absorbed from the epidural space into the maternal bloodstream and readily crosses the placenta. This diffusion may induce toxic effects in the mother and depression of the infant at birth. Although certain advantages can be claimed for mepivacaine, it should by no means be considered an advancement comparable to that achieved by lidocaine over procaine.

Dibucaine Hydrochloride (Nupercaine) Dibucaine hydrochloride, 2-butoxy-*N*-(2-diethylaminoethyl) cinchoninamide hydrochloride,

$$\cdot HCl$$

is another example of a local anesthetic with an amide linkage. Dibucaine is one of the most potent local anesthetics, registering a potency and toxicity approximately 15 times as great as procaine (Table 7-1). Associated with this action is increased latency and duration of action. Dibucaine is usually combined with epinephrine to diminish absorption and lessen toxicity. It is infrequently used in infiltration and nerve block anesthesia; however, the compound finds substantial use in topical and spinal anesthesia. The progression of adverse effects is similar to that discussed for other amide local anesthetics, with the added caution regarding the high toxicity of this compound.

Esters

Procaine Hydrochloride (Novocain) Procaine hydrochloride, 2-diethylaminoethyl-*p*-aminobenzoate hydrochloride,

$$\left[H_2N - \bigcirc - \overset{O}{\underset{\|}{C}} - OCH_2CH_2\overset{H}{\underset{+}{N}}(C_2H_5)_2 \right] Cl^-$$

is poorly absorbed from mucous membranes and therefore produces anesthesia only upon injection. In contrast to cocaine, procaine produces not vasoconstriction but vasodilatation, and consequently is rapidly carried away by the bloodstream from the site of injection. Thus, a vasoconstrictor drug, such

as epinephrine, is usually administered with it. Procaine is one of the least toxic of the commonly used anesthetics for infiltration, producing prompt and adequate anesthesia. The duration of action is short unless administered with a vasoconstrictor.

Low toxicity is primarily the result of rapid inactivation by plasma cholinesterase. Central nervous and cardiovascular adverse reactions are less frequently observed with procaine than with many of the other local anesthetics due to its low toxicity, although in higher doses the same general spectrum of reactions will be manifested as with lidocaine (Table 7-1). Some patients are extremely susceptible to even small doses of procaine and may react with flushing of the skin and a sensation of warmth. Other patients may evidence dermatitis or other reaction due to prior sensitization with procaine, either as a local anesthetic or as a procaine penicillin preparation. One of the metabolic products of procaine is *p*-aminobenzoic acid, and increased concentrations of this metabolite will antagonize the therapeutic action of sulfonamides. In conditions where sulfonamides are therapeutically administered, procaine should not be utilized.

The use of procaine in the treatment of cardiac arrhythmias was limited by the rapid hydrolysis of the compound. Removal of one oxygen atom from procaine and replacement by an —NH— group resulted in the compound *procainamide*, which is resistant to plasma hydrolysis. This agent is used exclusively in the management of cardiac irregularities.

Tetracaine Hydrochloride (Pontocaine) Tetracaine hydrochloride, 2-dimethylaminoethyl *p*-butylaminobenzoate hydrochloride,

$$\left[H_9C_4 - \overset{H}{\underset{|}{N}} - \bigcirc - \overset{O}{\underset{\|}{C}} - OCH_2CH_2\overset{H}{\underset{+}{N}}(CH_3)_2 \right] Cl^-$$

is a local anesthetic which is at least 10 times as potent as procaine (Table 7-1). The drug is effective when applied to mucous membranes and is used as a surface anesthetic for the eye, nose, and throat. Tetracaine produces a marked and sustained anesthesia. The compound has a significant latency of action, in many cases as long as 15 min. When used in ophthalmology, tetracaine does not produce paralysis of accommodation, corneal ulceration, or increased intraocular pressure, nor does it dilate the pupil as does cocaine. Substantially utilized in spinal anesthesia, tetracaine is infrequently employed in infiltration and field block anesthesia.

Cocaine, Cocaine Hydrochloride   Cocaine is an alkaloid obtained from the plant *Erythroxylon coca* or is semisynthetically produced from ecgonine.

Natives of Peru and other countries adjacent to the Andes still indulge in the ancient practice of chewing the coca leaf for the stimulatory properties and the relief from fatigue that the drug temporarily offers. This practice is widespread and constitutes an integral part of the culture of these tribes. Cocaine has substantial historical importance, as well as significant use as an experimental pharmacologic tool. Although the drug still retains a number of zealous advocates for its topical use, there is little reason for its therapeutic administration as a practical local anesthetic when so many more desirable synthetic local anesthetics are available. The unpredictability and resultant toxicity, as well as the addictive nature of cocaine, long ago limited the use of this drug to topical application primarily in ophthalmology. The compound is regulated by federal narcotic laws. Cocaine, when applied to the cornea, constricts the conjunctival vessels, blanches the sclera, and produces mydriasis. Corneal clouding and pitting leading to ulceration of the eye are frequently associated with cocaine administration.

Acute cocaine poisoning is very similar in its progression to the other local anesthetics previously discussed. The primary and most serious consequences are related to the central nervous and cardiovascular systems. Cocaine provokes a powerful and rapid stimulation of the central nervous system, followed by symptoms of depression. Such symptoms as excitement, confusion, nausea, sweating, and tachycardia may occur. Features peculiar to cocaine intoxication include dilation of the pupils and exophthalmos. In addition, one may observe Cheyne-Stokes respiration and the usual local anesthetic symptoms of intoxication, that is, convul-

sions and unconsciousness, leading to death due to cardiovascular depression without the appearance of central nervous system effects. Cocaine is slowly metabolized in the liver, and this may contribute to the overall toxicity of the compound. The problem of chronic cocaine addiction represents an entirely different area of involvement and is discussed elsewhere in this text.

Surface Anesthetics

Many of the compounds described above possess the ability to produce good surface anesthesia when applied topically, as well as local anesthetic action upon injection. However, a number of compounds, because of poor solubility or other chemical properties which limit their diffusion capabilities, are valueless upon injection, but demonstrate excellent therapeutic qualities when applied to the skin or mucous membranes. It should be noted that most of the compounds in this classification do not conform to the structure previously described for classic local anesthetics. The following drugs are representative of those utilized as surface anesthetics.

Cyclomethycaine Sulfate (Surfacaine)   Cyclomethycaine sulfate, 3-(2-methylpiperidino)propyl-*p*-cyclohexyloxybenzoate sulfate,

is used for topical application only. The compound induces sustained anesthesia when applied to the mucous membranes of the rectum, vagina, urethra, and urinary bladder, but exhibits little effect upon the mucous membranes of the bronchi, trachea, nose, and eye. As with most poorly soluble local anesthetics, it can be applied to the skin whether abraded or intact. Cyclomethycaine is utilized for the relief of surface irritation and itching due to pruritus, insect bites, minor burns, and hemorrhoids, and is also used for urethral instillation prior to urologic examination. The drug is available in a variety of lotions (0.5 percent) and ointments (1 percent); a jelly (0.75 percent) for cystoscopic examination; and an aerosol spray (0.25 percent).

Benzocaine (Ethyl Aminobenzoate) The compound benzocaine and its close relative, butyl aminobenzoate (Butesin), are esters of para-aminobenzoic acid, yet differ from the parent procaine-type esters in that they do not contain the terminal hydrophilic amine group.

$$H_2N\!-\!\!\bigcirc\!\!-\!\!\overset{\overset{\displaystyle O}{\|}}{C}\!-\!OC_2H_5$$

Benzocaine is, therefore, very slightly soluble in water and is slowly absorbed, with a prolonged duration of action. Sensitization may occur with these compounds when in contact with susceptible patients, when applied over extensive areas, and when utilized repeatedly. Benzocaine produces a sustained and effective local anesthetic action when applied to abraded skin. These drugs are employed as topical anesthetics on intact or abraded skin, as antipruritics, and for various dermatologic conditions. Ethyl aminobenzoate is available in a 5 or 20 percent ointment and is also supplied in suppository form. Butyl aminobenzoate is combined chemically with trinitrophenol to form the compound Butesin Picrate. As an ointment, Butesin Picrate is widely used in the treatment of minor burns.

Miscellaneous

Ethyl Chloride Ethyl chloride is a highly flammable and volatile liquid which is used in the form of a spray on surface areas to obtain brief periods of local anesthesia. Its anesthetic action is based on the principle of rapid evaporation which produces localized freezing of the tissue, promoting loss of peripheral sensory function. (Freon, because of similar physical properties, also exhibits this action.) Ethyl chloride is useful for the temporary relief of pain in inflamed areas and for muscle spasms. The compound is available in spray bottles.

Part Three

Central Nervous System Drugs

Chapter 8

Sedatives and Hypnotics

In the treatment of organic and emotional disorders, drugs are frequently required to provide adequate relaxation and sleep. The substances employed for this kind of therapy are classified as hypnotics and sedatives. *Hypnotics* (also called *soporifics* or *somnifacients*) are used to induce sleep. *Sedatives* are directed toward a milder degree of central nervous system depression. Their purpose is to decrease excitement and allay anxiety without causing marked drowsiness or inefficiency. With only a few exceptions the same drugs can be utilized for sedation and hypnosis. The differences in effects are dependent on the dose.

BARBITURATES

The barbiturates used as hypnotics and sedatives have the following structure:

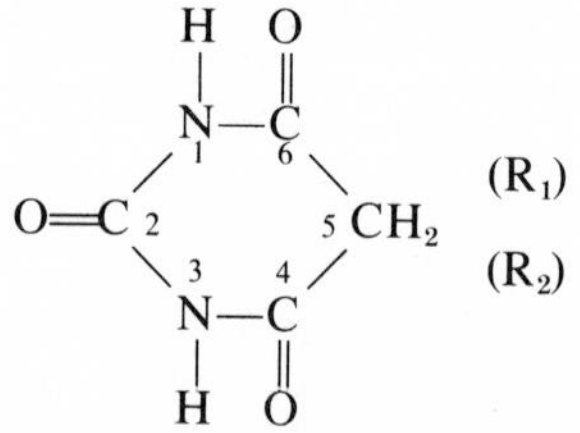

Barbituric acid

The parent compound, barbituric acid or malonylurea ($R_1 = R_2 = H$), is formed by the condensation of malonic acid ($HOOCCH_2COOH$) with urea (NH_2CONH_2). The formulas of some barbiturates available commercially in the United States are shown in Table 8-1.

A number of factors, both physicochemical and physiologic, influence the hypnotic or anesthetic potency of barbiturates. Some of these are water solubility, ionization, distribution between water and lipids, rate of entry into the brain compared with other tissues, volume of distribution in the body, and the rates of metabolism and excretion. On theoretical grounds it might be predicted that the most potent barbiturates would be characterized by a low, but definite, solubility in water, weak ionization, a high lipid/water partition coefficient, rapid entry into the brain, a volume of distribution not greatly exceeding that of total body water, and rates of metabolism and excretion slow enough so that the drug escapes appreciable destruction and elimination before reaching its site of action. However, some of these factors are interrelated in such a way that no drug fulfills all of the above conditions.

Barbituric acid and derivatives possessing only one substituent are devoid of central depressant activity. The 5,5-dimethyl and the 5-ethyl-5-methyl derivatives have some hypnotic activity, but this is too feeble to be of practical interest. The 5,5-diethyl derivative (barbital) is a clinically useful soporific. Barbiturates with an ethyl group and a longer chain are more potent than barbital, but when the chain length exceeds four or five carbon atoms, activity begins to decrease again. Increasing the length of the second ethyl group causes some increase in potency, but when the sum of the carbon atoms in both chains exceeds eight, toxicity generally increases more rapidly than clinical efficacy.

A barbiturate with a branched chain usually has greater hypnotic activity than the corresponding drug with a straight chain. Those containing a phenyl group in the 5 position are less potent somnifacients than their aliphatic or alicyclic analogues, but they have enhanced anticonvulsant and antiepileptic activity. Replacement of the oxygen in the 2 position by sulfur causes a marked increase in the lipid/water partition coefficients of 5,5-disubstituted barbiturates. The resulting drugs have greater hypnotic potency than their oxygen analogues when given intravenously, but their instability and their localization in depot fat make them unsuitable for oral administration as somnifacients. Their greatest usefulness is as intravenous anesthetics.

Mechanism of Action

Actions on the central nervous system of sedative and hypnotic doses of the barbiturates are expressed in many ways, ranging from subtle changes in mood to more profound effects such as sleep or ataxia. The physiology of such effects remains unknown at present, however.

From a chemical point of view, it seems clear that the barbiturates act in an unmetabolized form rather than as metabolites of the drugs. The fact that barbiturates are partially ionized at biologic pH's poses the question of whether the active form is the free acid or the anion or both. Available evidence indicates that the free acid alone is responsible for the depressant effects. Moreover, the drugs cross cellular membranes only in the form of the undissociated molecules. Data indicating that the

Table 8-1 Names, Chemical Structures, and Hypnotic Doses of Some Clinically Useful 5,5-Disubstituted Barbiturates

Barbiturate	Trade name	R_1	R_2	Hypnotic dose
Amobarbital	Amytal	Ethyl	Isoamyl	0.1–0.3
Barbital	Veronal	Ethyl	Ethyl	0.3–0.5
Butabarbital	Butisol	Ethyl	1-Methylpropyl	0.1–0.2
Pentobarbital	Nembutal	Ethyl	1-Methylbutyl	0.05–0.2
Phenobarbital	Luminal	Ethyl	Phenyl	0.1–0.2
Secobarbital	Seconal	Allyl	1-Methylbutyl	0.1–0.2

barbiturates are uniformly distributed within the central nervous system appear to eliminate the possibility that the selective actions can be attributed to localization of the drug at particular sites.

Effect on Organ Systems

Central Nervous System The central depressant actions of the barbiturates resemble those of the gaseous anesthetics, alcohol, and most of the hypnotic drugs discussed in subsequent sections. Depending on the dose administered, all the clinically useful drugs produce a broad range of effects extending from mild sedation to deep coma or anesthesia. The effects of the sedative-hypnotic barbiturates depend upon the nature of the subject and the situation in which the drug is administered.

Sedation and Hypnosis Although the doses employed for hypnosis are larger than those for sedation, the therapeutic goal is the same: to reduce awareness of external stimuli and, in appropriate circumstances, to promote sleep. The barbiturates most favored for daytime sedation are those which have a long or intermediate duration of action, for example, phenobarbital or butabarbital.

In general, barbiturates with a short or intermediate duration of action, such as secobarbital or amobarbital, are employed as hypnotic agents. The hypnotic action is sometimes apparent as early as 15 min after ingestion of the drug, but usually 30 to 60 min are needed. Sleep is usually maintained uninterrupted for 5 to 6 h. The incidence of rapid eye movement (REM) sleep and dreams is reduced. In REM sleep, also called "paradoxical" sleep, periods of rapid eye movements under closed eyelids alternate with periods of quiescence during physiologic sleep. Episodes of rapid eye movement have been correlated and associated with dreaming. Prolonged deprivation of REM sleep will generally result in reversible gross behavioral effects. The barbiturates reduce REM sleep somewhat but do not obliterate it totally, and therefore do not generally alter the personality behavior of the individual.

Anesthesia In sufficiently large doses, all the barbiturate hypnotics are capable of producing surgical anesthesia. However, only ultra-short-acting barbiturates are useful anesthetics. The ultra-short action of useful intravenous anesthetics, such as thiopental and methohexital, depends upon re-

distribution of the drugs from the brain (which is entered rapidly) to the other tissues (which are entered more slowly). Pentobarbital does not enter the brain as rapidly as thiopental or methohexital, and redistribution plays a relatively small role compared with metabolism in determining its duration of effects. Although barbiturates of the sedative-hypnotic type are no longer given to humans in doses sufficient to cause anesthesia, pentobarbital and secobarbital are sometimes administered intravenously in doses ranging from 0.2 to 0.8 g in conjunction with nitrous oxide anesthesia for moderately long operations.

Anticonvulsant Effects All the hypnotic-sedative barbiturates are effective antidotes to convulsant drugs, and in large doses they suppress the convulsions of tetanus and status epilepticus. Phenobarbital, however, differs from the other barbiturates in possessing a selective action which is utilized to prevent epileptic seizures, particularly of the grand mal type. The basic mechanisms involved in the antiepileptic action of phenobarbital are unknown. Apart from phenobarbital, the only barbiturates which have proved useful in the treatment of epilepsy are metharbital (N-methylbarbital) and mephobarbital (N-methylphenobarbital). The pharmacology of antiepileptic drugs is discussed in Chap. 12.

Analgesia The barbiturates differ from narcotic and antipyretic analgesics in lacking significant ability to obtund pain in doses not impairing consciousness. The remarkable effectiveness of the ordinary analgesic drugs precludes using barbiturates routinely for relief of pain. However, increased comfort is often achieved by combining barbiturates with aspirin or small doses of narcotics.

Respiratory System Sleep induced by hypnotic doses of barbiturates involves no more depression of the respiratory system than occurs in normal sleep. Progressively larger doses cause progressive reduction of the minute volume; the rate may be increased or decreased. The respiratory-stimulating action of 5 to 10 percent carbon dioxide becomes weaker and weaker and finally disappears. Death from barbiturate poisoning can usually be attributed to respiratory failure. With overwhelming doses the mechanism appears to be direct paralysis of the medullary respiratory center. However, in barbiturate poisoning generally, pulmonary edema or hypostatic pneumonia often plays a role in embarrassing the respiration. Laryngospasm appears to be a rare complication of ordinary barbiturate poisoning but is of considerable importance in connection with the intravenous administration of the ultra-short-acting barbiturates.

Circulatory System The circulation is not significantly affected by sedative or hypnotic doses of barbiturates. Greater effects on the blood pressure are observed in hypertensive patients; the decreases in both systolic and diastolic pressure are attributable to inhibition of the central neurogenic component of the hypertension. Doses large enough to cause coma or anesthesia generally produce a sustained decrease in the mean arterial pressure and pulse pressure, although the effects may be small.

Liver The barbiturates are metabolized primarily in the liver, but the evidence is entirely negative that these drugs have any direct toxic effect on the organ. In normal subjects, hypnotic doses do not alter the results of any of the usual clinical tests of hepatic function. Even in patients with severe liver disease the tests reveal no changes suggestive of deleterious effects of the drugs.

Barbiturates in the liver may cause a striking enhancement of the activity of enzymes involved in the metabolism of a variety of drugs and certain normal body constituents, particularly steroids. The mechanism of this effect is not fully understood but appears to involve increased synthesis of enzymes in the cytoplasmic reticulum. Barbiturates have a definite effect on the drug microsomal metabolizing system which may be of clinical significance (see Chap. 4). For example, a few therapeutic doses of phenobarbital may increase the rate of metabolism of the coumarin anticoagulants sufficiently to necessitate increased doses to achieve the desired reductions in clotting time. Moreover, withdrawal of the barbiturates without an adjustment in the dose of the anticoagulant may result in hemorrhage.

Routes of Administration

Barbiturates are administered orally, rectally, intramuscularly, or intravenously. The oral route should be employed whenever possible. In infants or in patients who are vomiting, the drugs may be given rectally in the form of a suppository or retention enema. When rapid onset of action is needed, as in patients with convulsions, the drugs may be injected intramuscularly or intravenously.

Absorption, Distribution, and Fate

The barbiturates are readily absorbed from the stomach, small intestine, rectum, and intramuscular sites. The mechanism of absorption from the gastrointestinal tract is nonionic diffusion (see Chap. 3). Following absorption, the drugs are present in all tissues and fluids of the body. Furthermore, barbiturates cross the placental barrier and become widely distributed in the fetal tissues. The drugs differ considerably in their binding to plasma albumin: For instance, thiopental is bound to the extent of about 65 percent; pentobarbital is approximately 40 percent bound; secobarbital, 45 percent; and phenobarbital, about 20 percent. Binding to tissue proteins parallels the binding to plasma proteins. Therefore, the drugs are rather uniformly distributed throughout the body. Ultra-short-acting barbiturates attain much higher concentrations in depot fat than in other tissues of the body.

Barbiturate hypnotics are metabolized primarily in the liver by oxidation of the substituents in the 5 position. Hydrolysis of the barbituric acid ring is generally only a minor reaction. Ethyl groups are quite resistant to oxidation. Therefore, barbital, which contains two ethyl groups, is excreted almost completely unchanged. Longer alkyl chains are oxidized to form secondary alcohols, ketones, or carboxylic acid derivatives; the latter are sometimes subjected to beta oxidation to form carboxylic acids with two fewer carbon atoms. The phenyl group in phenobarbital is hydroxylated in the *para* position. Phenolic as well as alcoholic metabolites are conjugated with glucuronic acid to varying extents. The allyl ($CH_2\!\!=\!\!CHCH_2$) group present in a number of barbiturates usually escapes metabolic alteration, but in secobarbital it is converted in part to a 2,3-dihydroxypropyl ($CH_2OHCHOHCH_2$) group.

Excretion

The barbiturates and their metabolites are eliminated primarily by renal excretion, involving glomerular filtration and tubular back diffusion of the free-acid forms of the drugs. Alkalinization of the urine does little to expedite the elimination of most barbiturate hypnotics, but has a marked effect on the excretion of phenobarbital. The basis for this difference is that phenobarbital has a lower pK_a (7.2) than do the other barbiturates. Therefore, increasing pH in the physiologic range converts a greater fraction of phenobarbital to the anionic form, to which tubules are impermeable.

Toxicity

Acute Poisoning The wide use of the barbiturate hypnotics provides ample opportunities for accidental intoxication and suicide attempts. Most cases of barbiturate poisoning stem from attempted suicide, but some are accidental, and a few may result from what has been called *automatism*. This is a state of drug-induced confusion in which the patient forgets having taken the medication and ingests more of it. The fairly wide difference between the usual hypnotic dose and toxic dose of barbiturates casts doubt on the plausibility of automatism as a common source of serious poisoning except possibly in addicts. Furthermore, the concept undoubtedly provides a convenient device for protecting patients and their families from the social stigma of suicide. Nevertheless, many clinicians are persuaded that automatism is a genuine phenomenon of considerable importance.

The diagnosis of barbiturate intoxication is based on the history, physical examination, and detection or determination of drugs in the blood, urine, or gastric contents. Poisoning by barbiturates seldom can be distinguished on purely clinical grounds from that caused by other hypnotic drugs. The cardinal signs are stupor or coma and respiratory depression. The respiration is affected early in the course of intoxication. The minute respiratory volume is decreased, sometimes sufficiently to cause cyanosis. The rhythm may be slow or rapid or may have a Cheyne-Stokes pattern. Ordinarily the blood pressure falls appreciably only in the presence of marked respiratory depression. Undoubtedly, hypoxia plays an important role in causing the hypotension, since merely providing adequate ventilation often restores blood pressure to normal. However, severely poisoned patients may develop circulatory shock.

The treatment of barbiturate poisoning includes removing any unabsorbed drug from the stomach, supporting the respiration and circulation, expediting elimination of drug which has been absorbed, and preventing complications. It should always be kept in mind that acute intoxication may be superimposed upon chronic intoxication. After emerging from coma every patient poisoned by barbiturates should be questioned about chronic use of the drugs and treated accordingly.

Chronic Toxicity The clinical picture of chronic barbiturate intoxication resembles that of mild acute barbiturate or alcohol intoxication. Barbiturate addicts differ from alcoholics in that they usually maintain a good state of nutrition. The signs and symptoms vary considerably in different individuals and in the same subject at different times. The effects are greatest when the drug is taken on an empty stomach. They are least marked upon arising and increase during the day as successive doses are consumed. The mental changes include impairment of intellectual ability, defective judgment, loss of emotional control, and accentuation of pathologic features of the personality. Most addicts prefer pentobarbital, secobarbital, or amobarbital to phenobarbital. The drugs are usually taken by mouth, although some narcotic addicts inject them intravenously.

The severity of the abstinence syndrome depends on the individual patient as well as on the daily dose and the duration of the intoxication. Abrupt withdrawal of barbiturates from chronically intoxicated individuals is absolutely contraindicated. The patient should be hospitalized and stabilized on the smallest amount of the drug which maintains a continuous state of mild intoxication. A period of 2 to 3 weeks is usually required to withdraw barbiturates safely. Rehabilitation and psychotherapeutic treatment of recovered barbiturate addicts is the same as that for alcoholics or narcotic addicts.

Therapeutic Uses

Hypnosis Barbiturates are extremely useful in inducing sleep in ordinary insomnia, but should not be regarded as a substitute for a concerted effort to discover and treat the basic causes of the disorder. Patients should be urged to provide an environment maximally conducive to sleep and to seek methods of relaxing at bedtime. As has been mentioned, pentobarbital and secobarbital in 0.1 to 0.2 g doses have become almost the standard hypnotic in the United States, and their efficacy has been proved in many kinds of patients. In recommending drugs to be administered during the night, it is advisable that the dose to be consumed is isolated from the main supply to guard against accidental ingestion of an excessive amount. Continuous use of barbiturates in recommended doses may result in dependence (see Chap. 15). The patient should be told that the first night after discontinuing the drug may be less restful than usual.

Sedation Some of the common conditions in which barbiturate sedation is used are anxiety-tension states, neurasthenia, hyperthyroidism, essential hypertension, coronary vascular accidents, cardiac failure, peptic ulcer, and colitis. The drugs relieve the anxiety associated with these disorders without noticeable impairment of mental performance.

Anticonvulsant Uses The barbiturates are superior to other hypnotic-sedative drugs for the treatment of acute convulsions arising from various disease processes or from the ingestion of poisons. Thus they are employed in the therapy of status epilepticus, eclampsia, and cerebral hemorrhage. The therapeutic use of phenobarbital and mephobarbital in the treatment of epilepsy is discussed in Chap. 12.

Specialized Uses
Preanesthetic Medication Pentobarbital and secobarbital are widely employed as preanesthetic medication. In the absence of pain, they are the only central depressants needed to provide the serenity desired before anesthesia.

Obstetric Amnesia The barbiturates are commonly used during labor, either alone or in combination with scopolamine, to produce amnesia by means of ''twilight sleep.'' The objective is to render the patient sufficiently drowsy that she will sleep between pains and not remember the ordeal but remain able to assist in the delivery. The barbiturates most often employed are secobarbital and pentobarbital.

Idiosyncrasy and Contraindications

Idiosyncrasy Abnormal reactions to the barbiturates may be encountered in certain patients who have not had prior experience with the drugs (*natural idiosyncrasy*). In some individuals hypnotic doses of the barbiturates consistently produce excitement and inebriation. Others respond with headache, nausea, and vomiting or diarrhea. Occasionally the drugs appear to be responsible for myalgia, neuralgia, or arthralgia, which may persist for several days after discontinuation of medication.

Hypersensitivity reactions to the barbiturates most commonly involve the skin, although the blood and blood-forming organs may also be affected. Phenobarbital occasionally causes exfoliative dermatitis, which may be accompanied by parenchymatous hepatitis. A few cases of agranulocytosis and thrombocytopenic purpura have also been attributed to this drug.

Contraindications The barbiturates are definitely contraindicated in patients who have become sensitized to them. Severe pulmonary insufficiency constitutes a contraindication, since patients with disorders such as chronic emphysema are often extremely sensitive to the respiratory depressant action of ordinary hypnotic doses. The drugs should be avoided in individuals with acute intermittent porphyria because they may precipitate an acute attack. Barbiturates which depend upon the kidney for their elimination should be avoided or used guardedly in patients with renal insufficiency. Hepatic disease, unless extremely severe, is not a contraindication for barbiturates metabolized by the liver. Great caution must be exercised in prescribing barbiturates for the individual with a suicidal tendency or a predilection to abuse them.

Preparations and Doses *Amobarbital* sedative dose is 20 to 40 mg, two or three times daily; hypnotic dose, 0.1 to 0.3 g. It is available as a powder, and tablets of 8, 15, 30, 50, or 100 mg.

Sodium amobarbital doses are the same as for the free acid. It is available as a powder in pulvules or capsules containing 60 to 200 mg; suppositories of 200 mg; and ampuls containing 65, 125, 250, 500, or 1,000 mg of sterile powder.

Sodium pentobarbital hypnotic dose is 0.1 g. It is available as a powder in capsules of 30, 50, or 100 mg; suppositories of 30, 60, 120, or 200 mg; and sterile injection solutions containing 50 mg/ml.

Phenobarbital sedative dose is 15 to 30 mg, three or four times daily; hypnotic dose, 0.1 to 0.2 g. It is available as a powder; an elixir containing 4 mg/ml; and tablets of 15, 30, 60, or 100 mg.

Sodium phenobarbital doses are the same as for the free acid. It is available as a powder; sterile injection solutions containing 75 or 150 mg/ml; ampuls containing 120 or 300 mg of sterile powder; and tablets of 30 or 100 mg.

Sodium secobarbital hypnotic dose is 0.1 to 0.2 g. It is available as a powder; pulvules or capsules of 30, 50, or 100 mg; ampuls containing 250 mg of sterile powder; suppositories of 30, 60, 120, or 200 mg; an elixir containing 4 mg/ml; and a sterile solution containing 50 mg/ml.

NONBARBITURATES

Chloral Hydrate

Chloral hydrate $(CCl_3CH(OH)_2)$ is an aldehyde hydrate which has a pungent odor and somewhat caustic taste. Chloral hydrate is usually taken by mouth but is sometimes given rectally. Its irritant action precludes subcutaneous or intramuscular injection. Intravenous administration of solution in sterile saline is feasible but should be reserved for emergencies.

Mechanism of Action   Part of the hypnotic action of chloral hydrate can be attributed to trichloroethanol formed by the chemical reduction of the drug in tissues.

Little is known about the mechanisms by which chloral hydrate or trichloroethanol causes sedation or sleep. Most studies on the neurologic effects of hypnotics have involved the use of barbiturates rather than chloral hydrate. It may be presumed that the actions of chloral hydrate and trichloroethanol are the same as those of the barbiturates.

Effects on Organ Systems   The central depressant actions of chloral hydrate resemble those of alcohol, the barbiturates, and the gaseous anesthetics. In small doses the principal effect is sedation. Somewhat larger doses taken under appropriate circumstances induce sleep. In ambulatory individuals, the drug may produce the signs and symp-

toms of drunkenness. Larger doses lead to coma or anesthesia. However, the drug is not used for intravenous anesthesia because the margin of safety is too narrow.

Controlled clinical studies have proved the effectiveness of the usual hypnotic dose (0.5 to 1 g) of chloral hydrate in inducing and maintaining sleep. In most individuals sleep occurs within 1 h after swallowing the drug and continues for 5 h or longer. At any time during the hypnotic response, the patient can be readily aroused. The duration of action of chloral hydrate is short enough so that the incidence of aftereffects (hangover) is insignificant.

Doses of chloral hydrate larger than the therapeutic cause deeper and longer sleep and increase incidence of hangover. Pain is obtunded, and the body temperature may fall. Loss of all reflexes and depression of the medullary respiratory and vasomotor centers occur after doses in the lethal range.

Therapeutic doses of chloral hydrate ordinarily cause no changes in the respiration, blood pressure, or heart rate beyond those occurring in normal sleep. However, extremely large doses may cause myocardial depression or arrhythmias, in which central vagal stimulation appears to be involved. Chloral hydrate has an irritant action on the gastric mucosa and therefore should be taken well diluted, or it may cause nausea and vomiting. Like many other hypnotics, chloral hydrate has the ability to enhance hepatic microsomal drug-metabolizing activity.

Absorption, Fate, and Excretion   Chloral hydrate is efficiently absorbed from the gastrointestinal tract including the rectum. The drug and its metabolites appear to be widely distributed throughout the body. In humans chloral hydrate is partly oxidized to trichloroacetic acid and partly reduced to trichloroethanol. Trichloroethanol is responsible for many of the hypnotic effects of chloral hydrate, while trichloroacetic acid is devoid of hypnotic action. Conjugated products appear in the urine.

Preparations and Doses   Chloral hydrate is available in solutions of various strengths and in 0.25 and 0.5 g capsules. The usual adult hypnotic dose of chloral hydrate is 0.5 to 1 g. Larger amounts may be employed in the treatment of delirium or maniacal states, but should be given cautiously.

Toxicity

Acute Poisoning The signs of poisoning by chloral hydrate resemble those from alcohol or the barbiturates. The usual features are coma, depressed respiration, hypotension, and hypothermia. The ingestion of large doses may cause death almost immediately. If the patient survives for several hours, the prognosis is generally good, although transient jaundice or albuminuria may be present during recovery. The average *lethal* dose has been estimated to be about 10 g. In the past many cases of poisoning occurred from chloral hydrate added illicitly to alcoholic beverages ("knockout drops," "Mickey Finn"); however, the belief that the activity of chloral hydrate is enhanced by a chemical reaction with alcohol is erroneous. The metabolism of ethanol is not appreciably altered by chloral hydrate. However, blood trichloroethanol reaches earlier and higher peak levels when chloral hydrate is administered with ethanol, an effect attributed to decreased oxidation of the halogenated drug to trichloroacetic acid.

Trichloroacetic acid binds strongly to plasma albumin. Thus it may interact with other drugs which bind to this serum protein by displacing them and causing a sudden rise in blood level of the free drug.

Treatment of acute poisoning consists of gastric lavage, support of respiration and circulation, and maintenance of normal body temperature.

Chronic Poisoning Chloral hydrate is very similar to alcohol, the barbiturates, and other hypnotics in respect to habituation, tolerance, and addiction. Addiction to chloral hydrate is uncommon and protocols for treatment have not been formulated in detail, although experience with barbiturate addiction suggests that gradual reduction of the daily dose would be preferable to abrupt withdrawal of the drug. Delirium, mania, or convulsions occurring during withdrawal should receive the same treatment as that given for alcohol or barbiturate abstinence.

Therapeutic Use Chloral hydrate is used primarily in the treatment of insomnia. Its rapid onset of action and short duration of effect make it particularly suitable for individuals whose main difficulty is falling asleep. For patients whose trouble is maintaining sleep, the drug can be prescribed to be taken during the night at the time of awakening.

However, for this condition most physicians prefer longer-acting drugs (e.g., pentobarbital) to be taken at bedtime.

Contraindications The drug should be used cautiously in the presence of severe hepatic, renal, or cardiac disease. Oral administration is wisely avoided in patients with esophagitis, gastritis, or gastric or duodenal ulcers. Continued administration of chloral hydrate may increase the activity of the drug-metabolizing enzymes of the hepatic endoplasmic reticulum. This effect is of particular importance in patients receiving coumarin anticoagulants, because withdrawal of the somnifacient may decrease the rate of biotransformation of the anticoagulant and thereby increase bleeding tendency.

Paraldehyde

Paraldehyde, a trimer of acetaldehyde, has the following structure:

$$CH_3$$
$$|$$
$$CH$$
$$O \diagup \quad \diagdown O$$
$$CH_3{-}CH \quad CH{-}CH_3$$
$$\diagdown O \diagup$$

It is a colorless liquid with a characteristic penetrating odor and a disagreeable burning taste. Over a prolonged period of time, the combined action of air and sunlight convert it almost entirely to acetic acid. The drug is dispensed in amber-colored 1-oz bottles to protect it from sunlight and air.

Mechanism of Action It appears likely that the central depressant actions of paraldehyde can be attributed to the drug rather than to one of its metabolites. Most studies on the mechanism of action of hypnotics have involved the barbiturates rather than paraldehyde, but it may be assumed that the mechanism of action of paraldehyde is the same as that of barbiturates.

Effect on Organ Systems The hypnotic and sedative actions of paraldehyde are indistinguishable from those of chloral hydrate, alcohol, or the barbiturates. The usual hypnotic doses of paraldehyde taken orally probably induce sleep somewhat more rapidly than equally depressant doses of chloral hydrate or barbiturates. The duration of the hypnotic action is brief, and the incidence of depressant aftereffects is low.

Paraldehyde undoubtedly possesses some ability to decrease pain, but it is used as an analgesic only in obstetrics. Paraldehyde is seldom employed to prevent seizures, but is of definite value in treating status epilepticus.

Therapeutic or somewhat larger doses of paraldehyde do not significantly depress respiration or circulation. Lethal doses taken orally or rectally usually cause death by paralysis of the medullary respiratory center. However, a few fatalities have been attributed to pulmonary edema and right-sided heart failure. Paraldehyde is irritating to the gastric and rectal mucosa and therefore should always be administered adequately diluted.

Absorption, Fate, and Excretion Paraldehyde is absorbed rapidly from the gastrointestinal tract including the rectum. The drug is extensively metabolized in the body; 11 to 28 percent is excreted unchanged through the lungs and 0.1 to 2.5 percent through the kidneys. The fate of the remaining drug appears to involve conversion to acetaldehyde and subsequent oxidation via the tricarboxylic acid cycle to carbon dioxide and water.

The liver seems to be the principal organ involved in the metabolism of paraldehyde. In some patients with severe hepatic disease, the drug is detoxified at an abnormally slow rate, and the hypnotic effects are prolonged. The abstinence syndrome resembles delirium tremens.

Preparations and Doses Paraldehyde is dispensed as the pure liquid; 1 g capsules and 2, 5, and 10 ml ampuls are also commercially available. The usual oral doses for hypnosis range from 3 to 8 ml; however, in delirium tremens and other psychotic conditions characterized by excitement, it may be necessary to administer 15 or 30 ml, or even more. When large doses are needed, or when the oral route is contraindicated, the drug may be administered rectally combined with two parts of olive oil.

Toxicity Paraldehyde is quite similar to chloral hydrate, alcohol, and the barbiturates in regard to tolerance, habituation, and addiction. However,

habituation and addiction to paraldehyde are relatively uncommon because of esthetic considerations. The usual features of acute poisoning are coma, depressed respiration, and hypotension. After intravenous administration, signs of pulmonary edema and right-sided heart failure may also be present. The use of decomposed paraldehyde has been responsible for several cases of serious corrosion of the stomach and rectum.

The treatment of acute poisoning by paraldehyde consists of gastric or rectal lavage to remove unabsorbed drug, maintenance of body temperature, and support of respiration and circulation. The patient may remain in coma for many hours, since the rate of metabolism of paraldehyde is not rapid. Paraldehyde addiction is probably more common than chloral hydrate addiction but less common than barbiturate addiction. Gradual reduction of the dose constitutes better treatment than abrupt withdrawal of the drug. Chronic ingestion of large quantities of paraldehyde may lead to severe metabolic acidosis. The mechanisms involved have not been elucidated.

Therapeutic Uses The odor it imparts to the breath restricts the use of paraldehyde for most ambulatory patients, but the drug may be utilized as a hypnotic in bedridden or other individuals with limited social contact. It is also employed in the treatment of delirium tremens and other psychotic conditions characterized by extreme excitement. It may be given to severely burned patients. Administered intravenously, it is useful for the emergency treatment of tetanus, eclampsia, status epilepticus, or convulsions induced by poisons, although barbiturates are usually favored. Administered rectally, paraldehyde has also been employed for basal anesthesia and obstetric analgesia.

Contraindications Because of its irritant action, oral administration of paraldehyde is contraindicated in esophagitis, gastritis, or gastric or duodenal ulcers, and rectal administration should be avoided in the presence of inflammatory conditions of the anus or lower bowel. Some physicians consider the drug contraindicated in patients with asthma or other bronchopulmonary diseases. Paraldehyde is also contraindicated in patients taking disulfiram.

Ethchlorvynol

Ethchlorvynol is an effective hypnotic, but in the recommended doses its actions are less profound than those produced by chloral hydrate or the barbiturates. Ethchlorvynol is a synthetic organic compound with the following structure:

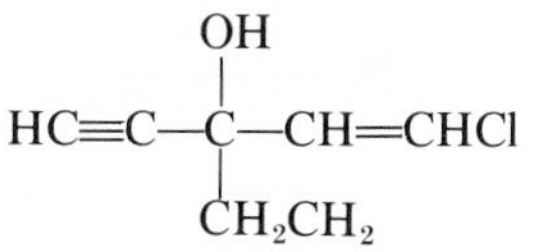

$$HC{\equiv}C{-}\underset{\underset{CH_2CH_2}{|}}{\overset{\overset{OH}{|}}{C}}{-}CH{=}CHCl$$

Effect on Organ Systems Ethchlorvynol has approximately the same potency and toxicity as phenobarbital, but its hypnotic effects are achieved more rapidly and disappear more quickly. The drug has anticonvulsant activity and is occasionally useful in the treatment of epilepsy. It is not effective as an analgesic. Therapeutic doses of ethchlorvynol have no important actions on organ systems other than the central nervous system. However, some patients taking the drug complain of an unpleasant aftertaste. Ethchlorvynol appears to lack the ability to induce hepatic drug-metabolizing enzymes.

Preparations and Doses Ethchlorvynol (Placidyl) is available in 0.1, 0.2, and 0.5 g capsules for oral administration. The recommended adult hypnotic dose is 0.5 g, although 1.0 g doses are employed rather frequently. The doses recommended for daytime sedation range from 0.1 g twice daily to 0.2 g three times a day.

Toxicity Ethchlorvynol taken in quantities substantially larger than the therapeutic dose produces an array of signs and symptoms indistinguishable from those caused by other hypnotics. Chronic intoxication with ethchlorvynol resembles chronic poisoning by alcohol or the barbiturates. Patients may exhibit ataxia, confusion, disorientation, and occasionally visual or auditory hallucinations. A daily dose of 2 g appears sufficient to cause physical dependence. Withdrawal of the drug may result in grand mal seizures or psychotic behavior.

Reversible toxic amblyopia has been seen in connection with continued use of ethchlorvynol. Apparently extremely rare, this effect may be related to idiosyncrasy.

Therapeutic Uses Ethchlorvynol may be employed as a hypnotic in patients with uncomplicated insomnia. It can also be used as a daytime sedative for persons with organic or functional disorders characterized by anxiety or tension.

Contraindications Since ethchlorvynol was reported to have precipitated an attack of porphyria, the drug is not recommended for patients with this condition. Exaggerated side effects and delirium have been reported in patients receiving tranquilizers, monoamine oxidase inhibitors (MAOI), or tricyclic antidepressants. The underlying mechanisms are unknown.

Ethinamate

Ethinamate is somewhat more potent a somnifacient than ethchlorvynol and in the recommended dose is a reliable hypnotic with brief duration of action. Ethinamate is a synthetic organic compound with the following structure:

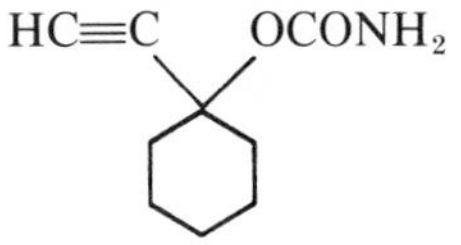

Effect on Organ Systems The central depressant effects of ethinamate closely resemble those produced by such barbiturates as pentobarbital or secobarbital. Also, the therapeutic index (lethal dose/hypnotic dose) is about the same as that of the barbiturates.

No important actions on organ systems other than the central nervous system have been reported. Intravenous injection of the drug may cause transient hypotension and bradycardia. However, hypnotic doses given orally cause little change in the pulse, blood pressure, or respiration. The drug is considered nonirritating, but in an occasional patient causes a burning sensation in the epigastrium. Thrombocytopenic purpura and drug fever have been reported.

Absorption, Fate, and Excretion Ethinamate is rapidly absorbed from the gastrointestinal tract. Most of the drug is hydroxylated in the *para* position of the cyclohexane ring. About half of the 4-hydroxyethinamate is excreted as such; the remainder is excreted as a glucuronide conjugate. Since the hydroxylation of other drugs is achieved almost entirely by hepatic microsomes, it may be presumed that the liver is the most important organ in the detoxification of ethinamate.

Preparations and Doses Ethinamate (Valmid) is available in 0.5 g tablets for oral administration. The minimal effective hypnotic dose for adults is 0.5 g. Many patients require 1.0 g and some as much as 2.0 g.

Toxicity Many cases of attempted suicide with ethinamate have been reported, but fatalities have been relatively few, and these have often involved complicating factors. Death is usually attributed to respiratory failure, although circulatory collapse has also been observed. Treatment of ethinamate poisoning consists of maintaining body temperature and supporting the respiration and circulation; gastric lavage is useful if the patient is seen shortly after taking the drug. Extracorporeal hemodialysis is effective in eliminating the drug but is probably less useful than in treatment of poisoning from hypnotics with a longer duration of action.

Addiction to ethinamate has been reported. The clinical picture resembles that of chronic barbiturate intoxication. Ethinamate addicts ingest as much as 15 g of the drug daily, and hallucinations and convulsions may occur during abstinence.

Therapeutic Uses Ethinamate may be used to advantage in situations indicating a hypnotic with a short duration of action. It is particularly suitable for patients who have trouble falling asleep but not staying asleep. It may also be recommended for individuals who are unusually susceptible to hangover from drugs which act for longer periods of time. The drug may be given to patients who have become hypersensitive to barbiturates. Ethinamate is unsatisfactory for daytime sedation and offers no definite advantages for preanesthetic medication.

Glutethimide

Glutethimide is a very satisfactory hypnotic and sedative. Its extensive abuse, both in the United States and abroad, has led to many cases of addiction and acute poisoning. Glutethimide has the following structure:

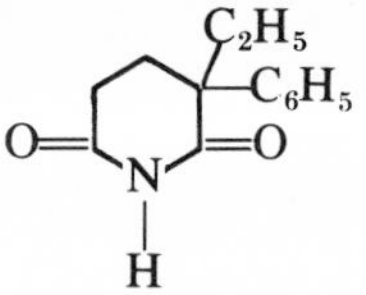

Effect on Organ Systems In humans the hypnotic effects of 500 to 700 mg glutethimide are about the same as those of 100 to 150 mg, respectively, of pentobarbital. Controlled studies have also indicated that glutethimide in a dose of 125 mg three or four times daily is a satisfactory daytime sedative. Ordinary hypnotic doses do not produce reliable analgesic, antipyretic, anticonvulsant, antiepileptic, antiemetic, or antitussive actions. However, sedative doses confer some protection against seasickness. Therapeutic doses of glutethimide have no important actions on organ systems other than the central nervous system. Like the barbiturates, glutethimide enhances the ability of the hepatic microsomes to metabolize drugs other than itself. This effect may be of considerable clinical importance in patients receiving coumarin anticoagulants.

Absorption, Fate, and Excretion Studies indicate that glutethimide is adequately absorbed from the gastrointestinal tract. Marked cyclical changes in the depth of coma in patients taking large amounts of glutethimide with suicidal intent have raised the question of whether considerable quantities of the drug pass into the intestines and remain there undissolved for variable lengths of time prior to absorption. After absorption the drug is widely distributed and reaches somewhat higher concentrations in fat than in other tissues. Glutethimide is almost completely metabolized during its sojourn in the body. Less than 0.2 percent of a therapeutic dose appears unchanged in the urine. Some of the metabolites are excreted into the bile but are reabsorbed and ultimately excreted in the urine. Fecal excretion amounts to only 1 to 2 percent of the dose in the form of metabolites.

Preparations and Doses Glutethimide (Doriden) is available as 125, 250, and 500 mg tablets for oral administration. The usual hypnotic dose is 500 mg, but 750 mg or 1 g is needed for the more severe cases of insomnia. For daytime sedation, doses of 125 or 250 mg are given three times daily, usually after meals.

Toxicity The clinical picture of glutethimide poisoning consists of prolonged coma, with more hypotension and less respiratory depression than are usually encountered in barbiturate intoxication. Many patients exhibit markedly dilated and fixed pupils plus facial twitching or hyperreflexia or intermittent spasticity of the extremities. Paralytic ileus, atony of the urinary bladder, and hyperthermia (less often, hypothermia) may also occur. The urine often contains an unexpectedly large number of casts. Prolonged coma leads to a high incidence of pulmonary complications. Careful attention must be given to maintaining a clean airway, and infections must be treated aggressively with antibiotics. Extracorporeal hemodialysis is of definite value in eliminating glutethimide from the body. Sudden and unexpected death is a common feature of severe glutethimide poisoning; this has sometimes been attributed to laryngospasm or cardiac arrest for want of a better explanation. The usual postmortem findings in glutethimide intoxication are cerebral edema, pulmonary edema, pneumonia, and visceral hemorrhages. Chronic ingestion of glutethimide in doses exceeding the therapeutic may lead to the development of addiction. Supplementary signs and symptoms consist of mydriasis, suffusion of the conjunctiva, and dryness of mouth. Glutethimide addicts consume from 2.5 to 12 g of the drug daily, but the average daily dose is about 5 g. Withdrawal of the drug may provoke excitement, hallucinations, or grand mal seizures. As is true of addiction to all other hypnotics including alcohol, absolute abstinence is not necessary for the appearance of withdrawal phenomena; a marked reduction in the daily dose is sufficient. The treatment of glutethimide addiction consists of gradual withdrawal of the drug over a period of about 2 weeks.

Therapeutic Uses Glutethimide may be prescribed for the treatment of insomnia in individuals who cannot tolerate barbiturates. In therapeutic doses its effectiveness appears to be about equal to that of pentobarbital or secobarbital. In doses of 125 mg taken three or four times daily, glutethimide has proved to be a satisfactory daytime sedative; however, butabarbital, which is cheaper, appears to be superior in most patients. Owing to its propensities for causing serious poisoning and addiction in individuals who abuse it, the drug should be prescribed with the same vigilance exercised with the barbiturates.

Methyprylon

The hypnotic potency of methyprylon is greater than that of any of the drugs discussed above and is exceeded only by some of the barbiturates. Numerous clinical trials and wide clinical use have established its value as a somnifacient. Methyprylon has the following structure:

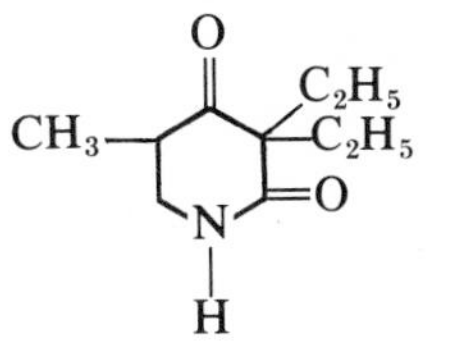

Effect on Organ Systems Therapeutic doses of methyprylon have little effect on any of the organs of the body except the central nervous system. Like all other hypnotics, the drug occasionally causes nausea and vomiting. Instances of neutropenia and thrombocytopenia have been observed clinically. However, it is not certain if methyprylon or its metabolites are responsible for these reactions.

Absorption, Fate, and Excretion Methyprylon is adequately absorbed from the gastrointestinal tract. The metabolism of methyprylon involves the formation of a double bond between the fifth and sixth carbon atoms of the piperidine ring.

Preparations and Doses Methyprylon (Noludar) is available in tablets of 50 and 200 mg, and in capsules of 300 mg. The usual hypnotic dose for adults is 200 to 400 mg by mouth at bedtime. Doses of 50 to 100 mg three or four times daily have been used for daytime sedation.

Toxicity Large doses of methyprylon cause coma which may be accompanied by respiratory depression or hypotension or both. Excitation and convulsions have been observed occasionally in patients during recovery from a toxic dose of methyprylon. These effects have usually been treated by the cautious administration of a barbiturate with a short duration of action.

It is clear that chronic abuse of methyprylon results in the development of tolerance and physical dependence. Abrupt withdrawal of methyprylon is accompanied by marked nervousness, generalized hyperreflexia, auditory hallucinations, and convulsions.

Therapeutic Uses Methyprylon closely resembles pentobarbital and secobarbital, and may be prescribed as a hypnotic for patients who cannot tolerate these barbiturates.

Methaqualone

Methaqualone is a synthetic organic chemical unrelated to the piperidinediones or any of the other groups of soporifics discussed above. It does not appear to offer any advantages over the better-known somifacients. It has the following structure:

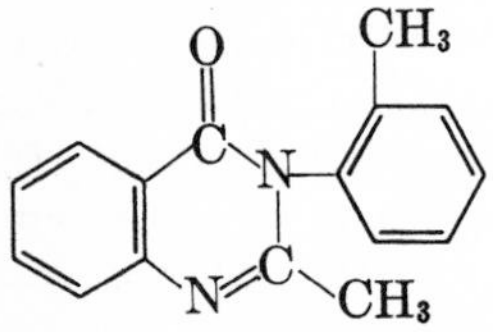

Effect on Organ Systems This drug may resemble mephenesin more than the barbiturates or the hypnotics discussed above. Large doses of methaqualone exert a selective depressant effect on polysynaptic spinal reflexes. Methaqualone appears to lack significant analgesic activity, but it enhances the effect of codeine. Side effects of a mild and transient nature have been encountered in about 5 percent of all patients receiving hypnotic doses. These include headache, drowsiness, dizziness, anorexia, nausea and vomiting, dryness of the mouth, epigastric discomfort, diarrhea, tachycardia, diaphoresis, and skin rashes. Paresthesias preceding the onset of sleep have been mentioned by a few patients.

Absorption, Fate, and Excretion Methaqualone appears to be adequately absorbed from the gastrointestinal tract. It is almost entirely degraded during its sojourn in the body. A large number of products are formed by the oxidation of the methyl groups and the hydroxylation of the aromatic rings. The alcoholic and phenolic metabolites are then conjugated with glucuronic acid. Some of the metabolites of methaqualone appear to be secreted into the bile and reabsorbed through the intestine prior to excretion in the urine.

Preparations and Doses Methaqualone (Quaalude, Sopor, Somnafac, Parest) is available as scored 150 and 300 mg tablets and 200 mg capsules. The usual hypnotic dose is 150 to 300 mg at bedtime. Doses of 75 mg after each meal have been used for daytime sedation.

Toxicity Large doses of methaqualone cause coma which may be accompanied by thrashing movements or tonic convulsions or both. Pulmonary and cutaneous edema is a common finding, regardless of the therapy employed or its results. Gastric and nasal hemorrhages are also encountered frequently. Therapy is focused on controlling seizures and maintaining adequate respiration and circulation. The continued ingestion of methaqualone in doses exceeding the therapeutic dose may lead to severe psychologic or physical dependence. Some patients have been known to consume as much as 7.5 g of the drug daily.

Therapeutic Uses Methaqualone might be considered for patients who have had unsatisfactory results with other hypnotics. However, there are no grounds for anticipating benefits not shared by more established drugs.

Flurazepam

Flurazepam hydrochloride, a useful hypnotic agent, is a benzodiazepine derivative (see Chap. 10). Satisfactory hypnotic effects begin within 20 to 45 min after oral administration and last for 7 to 8 h. The exact site and mode of action of flurazepam are unknown. Flurazepam, like chloral hydrate and methaqualone, does not decrease dream time as measured by the number of REM. Clinical studies have not been performed utilizing this agent in reduced dosage as a daytime sedative.

Adverse Reactions The incidence and type of untoward effects caused by flurazepam hydrochloride are similar to those produced by other agents in this class. The possible development of psychic and physical dependence on the drug should be considered.

Dosage and Preparations The usual hypnotic dose is 15 to 30 mg before retiring. Flurazepam (Dalmane) is available in 15 and 30 mg capsules for oral use.

Nonprescription Hypnotics

American citizens spend millions of dollars annually to treat themselves with hundreds of different products advertised to produce safe and restful sleep or to relieve nervous tension. Most of these remedies contain a 25-mg dose of an antihistaminic drug, usually methapyrilene hydrochloride but sometimes pyrilamine maleate. Some also contain scopolamine amine oxide, 0.15 mg per capsule. These drugs have been promoted as hypnotics because of the drowsiness observed in connection with their use in treating allergic disorders and preventing motion sickness. Their efficacy in inducing and maintaining sleep has not been fully established. One controlled study indicated that the hypnotic effects of 50 mg methapyrilene were approximately equivalent to those of 100 mg phenobarbital. The safety of these drugs compared with the recognized hypnotics is also uncertain. At least two fatalities from the accidental or intentional ingestion of methapyrilene have been reported, but the available data do not permit an estimate of the lethal dose. Scopolamine amine oxide in a dose of 1 mg three times a day within 24 to 36 h produces a high incidence of blurred vision and dry mouth. Double this dose leads to nightmares, hallucinations, and mania. Although abuse of antihistaminic drugs by individuals predisposed to drug addiction is not unknown, fortunately it does not appear to be a common occurrence.

ALCOHOL

Ethyl Alcohol

The ethyl alcohol in all alcoholic beverages results from the fermentation of sugar by yeast. If a cereal is the raw material for the beverage, it must first be malted to convert the starch to maltose, since yeast will not ferment starch. For wines and distilled liquors, the bottle label must state the percentage of alcohol expressed by volume or as a number followed by the word "proof." In this country the proof number is twice the percentage of alcohol by volume. The term *proof* originated in an old English custom of testing the alcohol content of whisky.

The whisky was poured over gunpowder and a flame applied to it. If the gunpowder exploded, the whisky was said to be of "proof strength." For whisky to ignite, it must contain at least 50 percent alcohol by volume.

Effect on Organ Systems Alcohol evaporates readily from the skin, producing a cooling effect. It lowers surface tension and is also a good solvent for many substances found there. Alcoholic sponge baths, therefore, are useful both for cleansing and as an aid in reducing fevers. As an antiseptic, 70 percent by weight is generally considered the optimum concentration for penetration and denaturation of bacterial proteins, although 50 to 95 percent solutions are effective. Ingestion of moderate quantities causes dilatation of skin blood vessels, with flushing of the face, neck, and upper trunk area. This effect prevents normal cutaneous vasoconstriction on exposure to cold, so that intoxication hastens the fatal outcome in "freezing to death." Central vasomotor depression probably plays a major role in the production of this peripheral vasodilatation.

Since, during active absorption of alcohol, high concentrations of alcohol reach the liver via the portal vein, and since the liver bears the brunt of oxidizing alcohol to acetaldehyde, it is conceivable that alcohol may have a direct hepatotoxic action. However, in chronic alcoholics, it is generally believed that hepatic cirrhosis is due not to prolonged high intake of ethyl alcohol but rather to the associated dietary deficiencies.

Although ethyl alcohol exerts the above pharmacologic actions, its main effect is on the central nervous system. The effect is always a depression, beginning with the higher functions and later extending to the more vegetative mechanisms as the percentage of alcohol in the central nervous system increases. The common idea that alcohol is a stimulant is due to its power to lessen inhibitions, thus causing impulsive behavior. The more important effects of alcohol on the central nervous system are:

1 *Impairment of vision* Alcohol reduces visual acuity. The alcohol in two or three cocktails may cause a reduction in visual acuity of more than 50 percent. Diplopia may occur if the blood alcohol concentration reaches 0.2 to 0.3 percent.

2 *Muscular incoordination* Small doses of alcohol impair the ability of the brain to coordinate muscular activity. With high concentrations of alcohol in the body, the manifestations of muscular incoordination are slurred speech and staggering gait, then complete loss of the power of speech and locomotion, and finally coma and surgical anesthesia.

3 *Lengthened reaction time* The mean normal reaction time is around 0.29 s to light and 0.19 s to sound. Blood alcohol concentrations below 0.1 percent have very little effect on reaction time. Levels between 0.1 and 0.2 percent usually lengthen the reaction time from 10 to 50 percent.

4 *Euphoria* The drinker sees the world and himself through rose-colored glasses. The desire to secure this effect is the chief reason for the popularity of alcoholic beverages, except for those who use these beverages sparingly as a condiment. Euphoria usually begins at levels of blood alcohol below those causing definite muscular incoordination.

5 *Removal of inhibitions* Alcohol, even in rather small amounts, causes loss of inhibitions, and the individual responds to many impulses which are ordinarily repressed. The resultant behavior may consist of silly speech and harmless antics, but sometimes becomes vicious and antisocial.

Blood Alcohol Level and Impairment There is a direct correlation of the concentration of alcohol in the blood with pharmacologic effects leading to impairment. One type of impairment, frank intoxication, exhibits the common signs of drunkenness, including slurred speech, difficulty of locomotion, and obvious loss of inhibitions. The results of several studies have been summarized as follows: For six zones of blood alcohol concentration (expressed in milligrams per 100 milliliter), the average percentage of subjects adjudged to be intoxicated were 0 to 50, 10 percent; 51 to 100, 34 percent; 101 to 150, 64 percent; 151 to 200, 86 percent; 201 to 250, 96 percent; and 251 to 300, 99 percent. These studies agree that almost all subjects with blood alcohol levels above 200 mg/100 ml (0.20 percent) were definitely *drunk*.

Fate of Alcohol in the Body After absorption, over 90 percent of ethyl alcohol is metabolized. The remainder is eliminated unchanged. For man the average rate at which this occurs is 100 mg/kg/h

and it is reflected as a corresponding fall in blood alcohol in the body. In other words, a 150-lb person can rid himself of 7 g (9 ml) of absolute alcohol or about ⅔ oz of 100-proof whisky every hour. For each gram of alcohol metabolized, 7 kcal is made available to the body.

The metabolism of alcohol may be divided into three stages, which take place concurrently.

Stage I During this stage alcohol is oxidized to acetaldehyde by alcohol dehydrogenase with diphosphopyridine nucleotide (NAD, coenzyme I) acting as the immediate hydrogen acceptor:

$$CH_3\text{---}CH_2OH + NAD \xrightarrow[\text{dehydrogenase}]{\text{alcohol}}$$

$$CH_3\text{---}CHO + NADH + H^+$$

Stage I occurs almost exclusively in the liver. Kidney tissue shows some activity, but most other tissues cannot oxidize alcohol. The rate at which alcohol is changed to acetaldehyde is constant and is the prime factor that determines the rate of disappearance of alcohol from the body.

Stage II In this step the acetaldehyde is oxidized to acetic acid, and the latter buffered to form acetate. Since there is still some question regarding the enzyme and the hydrogen acceptor involved in the reaction, we will simply write the equation:

$$CH_3CHO + H_2O \longrightarrow CH_3\text{---}COOH + (2H)$$

Stage II is a very rapid reaction, so that only small traces of acetaldehyde appear in the blood, even after excessive consumption of alcohol. However, after the administration of certain drugs, notably disulfiram (Antabuse), the enzyme in stage II is inhibited and pronounced acetaldehydemia results, even following rather low doses of alcohol.

Stage III The acetate formed in stage II increases the body's pool of acetate, which is finally oxidized to CO_2 and H_2O. The overall reaction can be written:

$$CH_3\text{---}COOH + 4(O) \longrightarrow 2CO_2 + 2H_2O$$

The actual reaction is much more complicated, and most of the acetate probably goes through the Krebs cycle. The CO_2 formed then enters the body's pool of bicarbonate, almost all of which finally exists as pulmonary CO_2.

Therapeutic Uses Alcohol and hydroalcoholic solutions are excellent solvents and preservatives for many drugs. As pointed out previously, sponging large areas of the body with rubbing alcohol (isopropyl alcohol), is sometimes useful in reducing fevers. Ethyl alcohol is an effective antiseptic in concentrations from 50 to 95 percent, depending on how and when used. However, 70 percent is a very satisfactory concentration because it is strongly germicidal, wets the skin well, spreads smoothly, and is less irritating than 95 percent ethyl alcohol. However, isopropyl alcohol is probably a better antibacterial agent than ethyl alcohol.

The use of alcohol to dilatate coronary vessels and for treating peripheral vascular diseases is unreliable. However, alcoholic drinks may be of benefit to patients with cardiac disease in that the mild sedation permits rest and relaxation.

Alcoholism, Acute and Chronic

The symptoms of severe, acute alcoholism are much like those of an overdose of ether, with shallow respiration and some impairment of circulation. The face and body surface are pale, and the extremities are cold. Death is due to respiratory failure. Chief postmortem findings are hyperemia of the stomach mucosa and edema at the base of the brain.

No specific treatment for severe acute alcoholism has been found. Treatment is symptomatic. If the patient can be kept alive and hypoxia avoided, he will usually recover as the absorbed alcohol is metabolized.

Chronic alcoholism presents a serious medical, social, and economic problem. At present there is no scientific explanation for the fact that some persons continue excessive drinking to the point where their lives become "utterly unmanageable," to quote a phrase from Alcoholics Anonymous.

The chronic alcoholic cannot refrain from excessive drinking, and he is distressed and upset without the euphoria produced by alcohol in his system. Some chronic alcoholics often do not drink to the point of marked intoxication; others are quite drunk most of the time. The outstanding symptom is an intense craving for alcohol, the desire to drink being about the only interest in life. There are, of course, varying gradations of the affliction.

About 15 percent of chronic alcoholics develop various psychoses, including delirium tremens, Korsakoff's syndrome, and chronic alcoholic deterioration. *Delirium tremens* usually occurs as a sequel to heavy, excessive drinking over a period of 2 to 6 weeks. The initial symptoms are restlessness, insomnia, tremor, fear, perspiration, and headache. This is followed by the second stage, which is characterized by hallucinations and delirium. The hallucinations are predominantly visual but may be tactile and auditory; they generally involve great fear. Alcoholics call the first stage the "shakes" and the second stage the "horrors." Convulsions sometimes occur. The delirium usually lasts 3 or 4 days, disappearing after a terminal sleep. The reported mortality in delirium tremens varies from 1 to 37 percent.

The *Korsakoff syndrome* appears in a few alcoholics, the incidence of this disorder being about one-tenth that of delirium tremens. The chief signs of the Korsakoff syndrome are impairment of memory of recent events, lessened learning ability, disorientation in space and time, and polyneuritis involving pain in the extremities and partial or total paralysis of the arms and legs. The polyneuritis appears to be due to a marked deficiency of vitamin B_1 (thiamine). Treatment consists of fairly high dosage of thiamine (some investigators have recommended the addition of nicotinic acid), together with a well-balanced diet.

A third type of alcoholic psychosis is called *chronic alcoholic deterioration*. Some of the signs are dilatation of the facial capillaries, a "bloated" look, flabby muscles, fine tremors, and impaired physical capacity and stamina. There is a marked diminution of will power, and the memory is impaired. The emotions are very labile, depending on surroundings. Treatment is difficult, if not impossible in advanced cases.

Some cases of chronic alcoholism, both psychotic and nonpsychotic, terminate fatally in a few months or years. However, many chronic alcoholics have a fairly normal life expectancy, aside from being bad safety risks. Chronic alcoholics are sick persons and should be treated as such.

Many physicians refer their alcoholic patients to Alcoholics Anonymous. However, sometimes disulfiram (Antabuse) is employed to bolster sobriety by the production of unpleasant symptoms. When taken by itself in small doses, disulfiram produces no apparent pharmacologic effects. If, however, after several days of such medication, small amounts of alcohol are imbibed, a toxic reaction follows which persists as long as the alcohol is being metabolized. Roughly in order of their appearance, the symptoms and signs are a cutaneous sensation of heat, flushing, vasodilatation, hypotension, palpitation, increased heart rate, dizziness, vomiting, unconsciousness, and collapse. The magnitude of these symptoms is subject to individual variation and is proportional to the dosage of both disulfiram and alcohol. In some patients only discomfort has been observed; in a few instances death has occurred. Disulfiram should be used only to bolster the determination of the patient not to drink and should be accompanied by good psychiatric and medical treatment.

Chapter 9

Psychotomimetic Drugs

Psychotomimetic drugs are chemical substances capable of inducing psychic and behavioral patterns characteristic of psychosis. These drugs are most commonly known as *hallucinogens*. They also, however, produce delusions, disturbances in thinking, and behavioral changes that resemble psychosis—a state characterized by maladaptive behavior to an individual's environment.

CLASSIFICATION OF PSYCHOTOMIMETIC SUBSTANCES

Most psychotomimetic substances have strong effects on the peripheral autonomic nervous system as well as on the central nervous system. Since the neurohumors of the peripheral autonomic nervous system are moderately well understood, many investigators have made conclusions about the neuropharmacologic modes of action of psychotomimetic

agents on the basis of peripheral mechanisms. Consequently, many psychotomimetic agents can be placed into three broad classes: (1) agents demonstrating peripheral adrenergic activity, (2) drugs eliciting anticholinergic actions, and (3) agents exhibiting miscellaneous actions. The main psychotomimetics belonging to the adrenergic class are LSD, mescaline, phencyclidine, and the amphetamines. The anticholinergic class includes scopolamine and atropine, while the miscellaneous group includes marihuana.

ADRENERGIC PSYCHOTOMIMETIC COMPOUNDS

The prototype of this group is LSD (lysergic acid diethylamide); therefore, it will be discussed in detail, and the others will be described only in relation to it. The structure of LSD is as follows, the broken line indicating the tryptamine structure within the LSD molecule.

LSD

Pharmacodynamics of LSD

LSD is a very potent stimulant of the central nervous system. Human beings remain sleepless for many hours after ingesting it. The earliest and longest lasting effect, occurring even with very small doses, is pupillary dilation. Pupillary inequality (anisocoria) is common in human subjects, as is hippus, a rhythmic dilation and contraction of the pupils, often synchronous with respiration. Hyperreflexia, also occurring uniformly, is another evidence of overstimulation of the nervous system. This may progress to spontaneous clonus of the antigravity muscles, especially the quadriceps group. Masseter hyperreflexia causes feelings of tightness of the jaw which, however, does not progress to actual trismus. Waves of piloerection often occur. The pupillary and hyperreflexic effects are inversely correlated with age, being greater in young adults and less in older subjects. Increases in body temperature are sometimes encountered in human beings but are not very great. Even without fever, the subjects feel hot and look flushed.

Sialorrhea, nausea, and vomiting are common gastrointestinal effects. Subjects may feel unusually hungry but be unable to eat much. Hypermotility of the gut is frequently present.

Cardiovascular effects include tachycardia and a moderate increase in blood pressure. These may be secondary to the general state of excitement rather than direct effects of the compound. LSD does not affect cerebral circulation significantly.

LSD increases contractility in uterine muscle, but is less active than ergonovine in this respect.

Sensory and Subjective Effects of LSD Along with the overexcitation and hyperreflexia described above, sensory distortions occur regularly. A sense of variation in lighting progresses to vivid visual illusions, pseudohallucinations, and after sufficiently large doses, true hallucinations. Typically, the visual images are of vividly colored geometric patterns, often moving kaleidoscopically, or of halos or rainbows around lights. Often, any moving object seems to be followed by a stream of color. True auditory hallucinations are extremely rare, although illusions, distortions, and synesthesias occur. Bizarre paresthesias and distorted proprioception are frequent, ranging from formications to sensations of walking on a pebbly or hot surface.

Distortions in perceptions of size and distance and other spatial distortions are very common and are often associated with distortions of body image. Feelings of separation of part of the body, or loss of a part, or failure to recognize a part as one's own are also common. Sometimes a subject may feel quite small, and cower in the middle of a bed, terrified of falling off and being killed. In others, perceptions of other people may be altered so that they look horrid and threatening.

Emotional Effects of LSD Although enthusiasts have extolled the euphoria produced by LSD, dysphoria is at least as frequent. Typically, there is alternation or the two supposedly opposite poles actually seem mixed. Feelings of anxiety and tension are almost always present. This may often progress to irrational terror which may alternate chaotically with hilarity. A less common occurrence is catatonia, in which the subject may stand and gaze at a cigarette and match in his hands for several minutes without lighting them.

Tolerance of LSD Although tolerance develops to some of the effects of LSD with daily usage, dilated pupils and some degree of hyperreflexia persists. The tolerance is not accompanied by physical dependence, and abrupt discontinuance does not precipitate any withdrawal symptoms.

Mechanism of Action of LSD Whatever the biochemical mechanism, the pharmacodynamic action responsible for the psychotomimetic effects of LSD probably is associated with the overstimulation it produces. This may operate to disrupt the ordinary flow of cerebral activity and thus produce the disorganized psychophysiologic picture described above.

Distribution and Metabolism Given intravenously, LSD is quickly bound to plasma proteins. It disappears rapidly from the bloodstream, having a half-life of 175 min. It tends to concentrate in the liver and to lesser extents in the spleen, kidneys, and adrenals. The amount reaching the brain is tiny, about 0.01 percent of the given dose. Although the compound encounters no special hindrance at the blood-brain barrier, neither has it any special affinity for the brain. Since we assume its significant actions take place in the brain, this makes its potency all the more impressive.

LSD is metabolized entirely in the liver, conjugated mostly to glucuronide and excreted mainly in bile (about 80 percent) and to some extent in urine (about 8 percent), the latter possibly depending on pH.

Antagonism of LSD Effects Research on the antagonistic substances of psychotomimetic compounds is of interest for three reasons: (1) It may promote greater understanding of the biochemical or physiologic modes of action of psychotomimetics. (2) Antidotes for any drug under study are always desirable. (3) A new compound antagonistic to a psychotomimetic compound could have some therapeutic effect against clinical mental illness.

Several compounds have been reported to be effective against LSD. Some steroids, including progesterone, are antagonistic to it, as are the phenothiazine derivatives and diazepam.

Tryptamine Derivatives

A number of substituted tryptamine compounds have been obtained from natural sources or prepared by chemical modifications. All have actions very similar to those of LSD. They differ in respect to potency, time of onset and duration of action, and the degree to which they produce cardiovascular or gastrointestinal effects. With some of the

compounds, the latter effects may submerge the LSD-like actions. These tryptamine derivatives are of interest mainly from two viewpoints: (1) the identification of active principles in natural products with psychotomimetic activity and (2) structure-activity relationships, with the goal of trying to uncover pharmacodynamic modes of action basic to the psychotomimetic effect of these drugs.

The most ubiquitous of these tryptamine derivatives in natural sources are N,N-dimethyltryptamine (DMT) and bufotenin, occurring in many plants with wide geographic distribution. The isomer of bufotenin, 4-hydroxy-N,N-dimethyltryptamine, is psilocin, one of the active principles of the *Psilocybe* mushrooms. Psilocybin is its phosphoryl ester. The phosphate is rapidly hydrolyzed off in the body, so that both psilocin and psilocybin amount to the same compound. They are very potent compared with other compounds in this group, a dose somewhat less than 0.1 mg/kg producing a full-blown, long-lasting LSD-like reaction.

β-Phenylethylamine Derivatives

Mescaline The oldest β-phenylethylamine is mescaline, or 3,4,5-trimethoxyphenylethylamine, obtained originally from peyote. Mescaline is among the least potent of the compounds ordinarily classified as psychotomimetic. The most consistent effect is nausea and vomiting, which tends to occur early after administration and subsides as the psychotomimetic effects begin. These are much like the effects of LSD, but perhaps not so long lasting, depending on the amounts taken.

Humans excrete about 58 percent of a dose of mescaline unchanged. The metabolic fate of the remainder is oxidation of the side chain to form 3,4,5-trimethoxyphenylacetic acid, which is inactive. A small amount of the intermediate 3,4,5-trimethoxyphenylacetaldehyde can also be detected.

Mescaline-Amphetamine Intermediaries A drug related to mescaline which has attracted some notice is 4-methyl-2,5-dimethoxyphenylisopropylamine, known as DOM or STP. There has been a flurry of abuse of this compound. However, careful laboratory study has shown its effects to be comparable to those of mescaline, although it is more potent. It may be longer acting, but once again there is the problem of determining equivalent doses, since duration of action of these compounds varies with dose.

Amphetamines   Amphetamine was introduced as a stimulant drug and has also been employed as a nasal decongestant, an antiobesity agent, and in the treatment of hyperkinesia in children. Amphetamine, methamphetamine, and others have been serious problems from the standpoint of misuse. Although these ordinarily had not been classified as psychotomimetic, all these compounds are such if sufficient doses are taken. Methamphetamine (Methedrine, deoxyephedrine, Desoxyn, "speed"), the most potent member, has been particularly misused.

The basic pharmacology of amphetamines in ordinary doses is given in Chap. 17. People who misuse amphetamines tend to escalate their doses rapidly for a combination of reasons. Tolerance to amphetamine occurs rapidly so that with steady intake, larger doses must be taken for a given intensity of effect. Also, these people often take the drug not for the usual reasons of simple mood elevation, etc., but for more intense drug effects. With very large oral doses, up to 500 mg/day, the user experiences time distortion, flight of ideas and fantasies, and overexcitability or irritability. The effects of large oral doses tend to subside rather rapidly, and the user may then become intolerably depressed or sleepy unless he takes more drug. After a number of hours of very sound sleep, he may awaken with no apparent adverse effects.

Intravenous injection of methamphetamine has become a significant problem. The choice of methamphetamine may have been determined in part by the fact that in the early 1960s this was the only amphetamine available in a form for parenteral injection. With sharply increased restrictions on supplies from legitimate manufacturers, illicit laboratories began manufacturing methamphetamine, which is a fairly simple molecule. Their product is preferred now because addicts have begun to inject such large doses that the legitimate commercial product is too dilute for them. These persons ordinarily inject 200 to 300 mg intravenously as often as every 2 h around the clock for a total daily dose of 2.4 to 3.6 g. Daily doses as large as 15 g have been reported. To accomplish this, users inject very concentrated, syrupy solutions. They keep this up

for several days, during which time they often eat little or nothing because of the anorexigenic effect of the drug. It is during these sustained high-dosage bouts that the psychotomimetic effect of the drug appears.

Initially, the user may become bustling and busy. He may actually accomplish some things early in the course, but very soon his performance deteriorates. Activity may continue but is usually of a pointless, highly stereotyped sort. The user gets "hung up" doing one thing over and over again, sometimes for hours. At about this time the psychosis becomes apparent. It is paranoid in character, with marked ideas of reference, usually having to do with possible detection by the authorities. Although the taker may say he feels elated, he appears glum, depressed, and withdrawn. Visual hallucinations do not occur as with LSD, although distortions and illusions may. Auditory hallucinations also probably do not occur, but hyperacusis does, often related to the paranoia.

After discontinuance of the drug, profound sleep follows, often for 12 to 18 h. Upon awakening, the user may feel depressed and want to resume drug taking immediately. No actual withdrawal syndrome occurs, but some persons experience disagreeable depressed feelings ("crash") with discontinuance of these large-dose bouts.

Sudden death sometimes occurs with this kind of drug abuse. This may be due to cardiac arrhythmia or to cerebral damage secondary to circulatory derangement.

Cross-Tolerance among Adrenergic Psychotomimetic Compounds

A clue to whether any two compounds act by the same biochemical pharmacologic mechanism occurs when they share cross-tolerance. By this criterion LSD, psilocybin, and mescaline belong together, while amphetamine does not. This fits with the behavioral effects, since the psychosis caused by amphetamine is different as well.

Phencyclidine

Phencyclidine

Phencyclidine (PCP) was investigated for use as a general anesthetic in humans. However, because of the high incidence of emergence delirium, it was dropped from further consideration for this purpose, and a derivative was introduced, namely ketamine. PCP is still utilized in veterinary practice to immobilize primates. Because of the psychotomimetic effect of PCP, the drug has gained wide popularity as a drug of abuse, especially for replacing LSD as a hallucinogen. PCP has not been found to be teratogenic or to produce "flashbacks" with repeated use. The psychotomimetic effects last longer than do those of LSD and appear to be less intense. The dose of PCP as a hallucinogen is high (in the milligram range) compared to the dose of LSD (in the microgram range). During the psychotomimetic effect of PCP, the sympathetic nervous system appears to be stimulated, as evidenced by an elevation in arterial blood pressure and pulse rate, and by dilation of the pupils and dry mouth. Recent animal studies indicate that PCP potentiates the adrenergic nervous system by blocking the "re-uptake" of norepinephrine and by a localized adrenergic receptor effect. The toxic effects in chronic users may be expressed as increased sympathetic nervous system activity as reviewed above.

The psychotomimetic effect of PCP, however, has been explored more fully because this drug is chemically different from all of the other compounds and because the character of its effects is also different. Some investigators have concluded that the effects of phencyclidine mimic schizophrenia much more accurately than do those of other psychotomimetic compounds. One interesting finding is that the effects of phencyclidine are mitigated by sensory deprivation, as are the symptoms of schizophrenia.

Cocaine

Cocaine in large doses is psychotomimetic. Apparently the effects and the mechanism are similar to those of the amphetamines. Cocaine takers become severely paranoid and may attack murderously as a result of their delusions. The attack may be directed toward their visual hallucinations rather than at an actual person, but this cannot be relied on. Cocaine is discussed more fully in Chap. 7.

ANTICHOLINERGIC PSYCHOTOMIMETIC COMPOUNDS

The prototypes of this group are atropine and scopolamine. Their basic pharmacology is given in Chap. 19. At present, the most plausible explanation for the actions of these compounds is that by blocking cholinergic mechanisms in the brain, they allow predominance of adrenergic and possibly dopaminergic mechanisms.

The peripheral effects of anticholinergic psychotomimetics resemble those of the parent compound atropine and include dilated pupils; dry, hot, flushed skin; dry mouth; and tachycardia. Blood pressure changes are those of postural hypotension and are usually unimpressive except in severe toxicity when hypotension occurs because of ganglionic blockage. The nausea and emesis seen with use of the adrenergic compounds do not occur. Instead, dry throat may be severely painful. The muscle cramps and paresthesias associated with adrenergic compounds are absent, but tremors, rigidity, and mass muscle movements of hyperkinesis may be observed. Clonus of antigravity muscles may occur soon after administration but then disappears as the other effects develop.

The most marked subjective effects are confusion and disorientation. Attention span is reduced almost to the vanishing point. Visual hallucinations of a highly structured, concrete sort occur regularly. The individual becomes preoccupied with these and disregards everything else.

Restlessness and overactivity continue for many hours. Because of this and the disregard of environment, the person may injure himself by stumbling over unnoticed objects or by falling. Exhaustion, with dehydration and electrolyte depletion, can result from sustained activity and refusal of food and drink. In advanced toxicity, pyrexia is uniform and is the lethal factor in fatalities due to these compounds.

Antagonism of the atropine-like psychotomimetic compounds would seem to require a drug with muscarinic or anticholinesterase activity. Accordingly, physostigmine, a "reversible" cholinesterase inhibitor, has been shown to be effective. Physostigmine has a short duration of action compared with that of the anticholinergics, an advantage because the patient can then be titered for the proper amount of antagonism. Careful continual monitoring of the patient is very important so that he gets enough but not too much physostigmine.

MISCELLANEOUS PSYCHOTOMIMETIC COMPOUNDS

Marihuana

There is only one species of hemp, *Cannabis sativa* (κάννᾰβις meaning hemp, *sativa* meaning cultivated), from which marihuana is obtained. Other names such as *indica* merely describe the country of origin, in this case India. The same plant is grown for rope fibers, although today this has been largely displaced by synthetics such as nylon and polyesters.

The marihuana plant is dioecious, and the top of the female flowering plant is rich in a sticky resin in which the active psychotropic principles are concentrated. Their activity has been known for many centuries and in many cultures. The history of marihuana is reflected in the many names given to different preparations by different peoples: bhang, kif, dagga, charas, majun, ganja, marihuana, marijuana, Mary Jane, hashish, hash, tea, pot, grass, muggles, reefers, and so on. Generally speaking, in the United States, marihuana and related names refer to chopped dried plant preparations intended for smoking, while hashish refers to resinous extracts intended for swallowing or, more commonly, for mixing with tobacco for smoking. Because of the crudeness of the preparations, injection has not been practiced.

Chemistry of Marihuana   The pharmacologically active substances in marihuana are nitrogen-free tricyclic compounds referred to as *cannabinoids*. Several occur in the natural resin, and hundreds of isomers and related compounds have been prepared and studied. The active natural compound is *l*-Δ^9-*trans*-tetrahydrocannabinol. The Δ^8 isomer also is active.

l-Δ^9-*trans*-Tetrahydrocannabinol

Pharmacologic Effects of Marihuana   The effects of marihuana vary greatly, depending on whether administration is by ingestion or by smoking. Smoking results in rapid absorption of small amounts of active substances. The effects are therefore fleeting, and the intensity can be regulated by the rate of smoking. Swallowing leads to slower absorption of usually larger amounts of substances. The effects, therefore, are slower in onset, much more intense, and much more lasting.

A constant effect of marihuana preparations is peripheral vasodilatation. This is most obvious in the conjunctivae, so that bloodshot eyes are among the most frequent signs of marihuana intoxication. Marihuana does not cause pupillary dilation. Some of the compounds have marked effects on standing blood pressure and can cause significant orthostatic hypotension. Ordinarily this would occur only with oral administration. Increased pulse rate seems to be a common effect.

Persons using marihuana often report a craving for sweets. However, marihuana does not affect blood sugar, at least when smoked. The mechanism of this effect, whether psychologic or pharmacologic, therefore remains unexplained.

The most immediate effects of small doses of marihuana, such as from smoking, are shortened attention span and distortion of time sense. Large doses lead to marked impairment of abstract thinking and inappropriate affect. Stimulus bondage also is quite common. This is the basis for the claim that users can concentrate better on music, for example; in fact, they are unable to attend to or deal with a diversity of stimuli. Unsteadiness, staggering, wide-base gait, and slurred speech also are common with large doses, such as after swallowing. Even with smoking, naïve subjects exhibit some degree of psychomotor impairment; however, practiced subjects are able to overcome or compensate for this.

In smaller doses, marihuana is not psychotomimetic. As the dose increases, distortions, illusions, and hallucinations occur. These are again predominantly visual, and often vividly colored. Distortions of auditory stimuli occur, but true auditory hallucinations are doubtful. However, as with LSD and other such compounds, synesthesias are often described. Thus as with the other substances described in this chapter, the effect seems to be that of a nonspecific toxic state of the brain, although the character of the subjective experience is different from that of LSD. This may occur because marihuana is basically sedative, whereas LSD is stimulatory.

Although the effects from smoking are fleeting, the effects after swallowing marihuana preparations are quite long lasting. These more intense effects tend to be biphasic. Following an initial lag of 30 to 60 min, the subject enters a phase of euphoria. In this phase, his behavior is not unlike that of a person intoxicated with alcohol, and the eyes are markedly bloodshot. After 3 to 4 h, depending on the dose, this phase passes, and fatigue ensues. Hallucinosis, if present, passes away at this point. The individual then continues for many hours in a worn-out, physiologically depressed state. This biphasic aspect is not unlike that of ethanol qualitatively, but differs in being much more protracted in time. Persons who drink large amounts of alcohol have an initial euphoria which can be accompanied by transient delirium or hallucinosis, which is not the same as delirium tremens. This phase is succeeded by depression, sleep, or even coma. Thus there are strong similarities in the actions of alcohol and marihuana, although they differ quantitatively.

Tolerance to Marihuana and Its Metabolic Fate
Increasing tolerance to marihuana apparently does not occur. Indeed, rather the opposite is probably the case, so that with succeeding doses the user becomes more susceptible to the effects and perhaps more likely to have spontaneous recurrence of effects, sometimes called "flashbacks." Naïve users are often disappointed in the effects of their first dose. Several exposures are sometimes neces-

sary for the taker to decide that he is experiencing what others have described. This can be explained as a sort of learning or "sensitization." An alternative explanation can be found in the apparently long duration of action of marihuana substances which may, in turn, be related to long half-life in the body.

Nutmeg

Nutmeg is the dried kernel of the seed of an evergreen tree, *Myristica fragrans*. The active compound is myristicin, the structure of which follows:

Myristicin

The psychotomimetic effect of nutmeg has been known for a long time. Poisoning with powdered nutmeg was common in Great Britain early in this century when it was used for attempted abortion. Intoxication with nutmeg is long lasting and has features somewhat similar to those of the anticholinergic compounds, i.e., dry mouth, tachycardia, sensations of hot skin, plus typical visual hallucinations, and so on. Difficulties with urination and defecation are common. The pupils of the eye are constricted rather than dilated, however. Characteristically, intoxication with nutmeg is followed by a hangover consisting of severe influenza-like aching all over the body.

Chapter 10

Antipsychotic and Antianxiety Agents

ANTIPSYCHOTICS

Drugs which produce tranquilization or "peace of mind" are classified by pharmacologists and psychiatrists as antipsychotic and antianxiety agents. The antipsychotics such as chlorpromazine produce emotional calmness and mental relaxation and are, therefore, highly effective in controlling the symptoms of acutely and chronically disturbed psychotic patients. These agents also cause reversible extrapyramidal symptoms in susceptible patients and have little or no tendency to produce physical dependence or habituation. Use of such drugs is therefore indicated in excited, delusional, or other psychotic states.

In contrast, the antianxiety drugs produce calmness and relaxation, but not of the same "quality" as that induced by the antipsychotic drugs. Hence, such drugs are particularly effective in common psychoneurotic states but are ineffective in severely disturbed psychotic patients. These drugs do not produce extrapyramidal symptoms and have a relatively low incidence of unwanted effects, although some physical dependence may occur, depending on the dose and length of time used. The antianxiety drugs are employed in common mental disorders such as nervous tension and psychosomatic reactions.

Phenothiazine Derivatives

The phenothiazines are extremely complex pharmacologically, with effects on both central and peripheral nervous systems, and have important metabolic effects as well. Each compound differs quantitatively and qualitatively in the extent to which it produces each of these pharmacologic effects. All of them act on the central nervous system to produce (1) mild sedation, in which afferent stimuli can easily arouse the patient; (2) antiemetic effects; (3) alteration of temperature regulation which may result in either hypothermia or hyperthermia, depending upon environmental temperature; (4) alteration of skeletal muscle tone which may relieve, as well as produce, extrapyramidal symptoms; (5) an antipruritic effect; (6) rarely analgesic effects; and (7) endocrine alterations including a "pseudopregnancy." These drugs also act on the autonomic nervous system, producing (1) α-adrenergic blockade; (2) antiadrenergic uptake, adrenergic potentiation, and prevention of retention of adrenergic amines; (3) serotonergic blockade; (4) antihistaminic effects; (5) cholinergic blocking effects at both nicotinic ganglionic and muscarinic receptor sites; (6) inhibition as well as activation of cholinesterase; (7) potentiation of d-tubocurarine; and (8) local anesthetic effects.

Chemical Structure The phenothiazines are classified according to their chemical structure. This is based on the type of substitution in the 10 position of the phenothiazine ring which contains a tertiary nitrogen (see Table 10-1).

Comparative Pharmacologic Activities It is difficult to make valid generalizations regarding structure-activity relationships. However, a few principles have emerged which summarize some of the known facts about phenothiazines (Table 10-2). Although most phenothiazines exhibit to some degree the various effects listed in Table 10-2, the predominant pharmacologic effect is usually deter-

Table 10-1 Some Therapeutically Useful Phenothiazines

Subgroup	Trade name	R_1	R_2
1 Propylamino			
Promazine	Sparine	$CH_2-CH_2-CH_2-N(CH_3)_2$	H
Chlorpromazine	Thorazine	$CH_2-CH_2-CH_2-N(CH_3)_2$	Cl
Triflupromazine	Vesprin	$CH_2-CH_2-CH_2-N(CH_3)_2$	CF_3
2 Propylpiperazine			
Prochlorperazine	Compazine	$CH_2-CH_2-CH_2-N\diagdown N-CH_3$	Cl
Trifluoperazine	Stelazine	$CH_2-CH_2-CH_2-N\diagdown N-CH_3$	CF_3
Fluphenazine	Permitil, Prolixin	$CH_2-CH_2-CH_2-N\diagdown N-CH_2-CH_2OH$	CF_3
3 Ethylpiperidyl			
Thioridazine	Mellaril	$(CH_2)_2-$ (N-piperidyl, CH_3)	SCH_3
4 Ethyldimethylamino			
Promethazine	Phenergan	$CH_2-CH-N(CH_3)_2$ with CH_3	H

Table 10-2 Comparative Pharmacologic Activities of Phenothiazine Derivatives

Phenothiazine derivatives	Anti-histaminic effects	Anti-psychotic effects	Adrenergic blocking effects	Extra-pyramidal symptoms	Cholinergic blocking effects	Antiemetic effects
Promethazine	High	Low	Moderate	Low	Moderate	Moderate
Promazine	Moderate	Moderate	High	Moderate	Moderate	Moderate
Chlorpromazine	Moderate	High	Moderate	Moderate	Moderate	Moderate
Triflupromazine	Moderate	Highest	Low	Highest	Moderate	High
Thioridazine	Moderate	High	Moderate	Low	High	Low

mined by the chemical substitution on the phenothiazine nucleus.

Actions on the Central Nervous System

Behavioral Effects The administration of chlorpromazine and related phenothiazines primarily produces depression of the central nervous system. Generally the individual may become sedated but behavioral arousal occurs quite easily. After being given chlorpromazine, psychotic patients appear less severely disturbed and have fewer hallucinations and delusions. This antipsychotic effect is more often seen with long term rather than emergency administration. Administration of the drug for acute conditions does produce a quieting effect in grossly agitated and disturbed patients. Interestingly, after long-term administration of phenothiazines, tolerance to the antipsychotic effects does not develop although tolerance does develop to the drowsiness and orthostatic hypotension. In general, chlorpromazine markedly reduces motor activity.

Antiemetic Actions In addition to a vomiting center in the medulla, there is a bilateral area on the floor of the fourth ventricle which can be stimulated by chemical agents such as apomorphine to cause emesis. This area is called the *chemoreceptor trigger zone*. Hence bilateral destruction of the chemoreceptor trigger zone prevents apomorphine-induced vomiting. However, reflex vomiting due to irritants such as copper sulfate in the stomach still occurs. Apomorphine-induced vomiting is blocked by very small doses of chlorpromazine, although reflex vomiting still occurs. The blocking action of chlorpromazine and related phenothiazines directly involves the chemoreceptor trigger zone. However, large doses of chlorpromazine may depress the vomiting center directly.

Effects on Central Skeletal Motor Mechanisms Usually following chronic, but occasionally after acute, administration of some phenothiazines, extrapyramidal side effects may develop. Some sex differences have been demonstrated in that akathisia (motor restlessness) and extrapyramidal reactions occurred twice as often in women as in men. In men dyskinesia (dystonic reactions) is twice as common as in women. Generally drugs like benztropine or diphenhydramine easily control the extrapyramidal symptoms induced by these phenothiazines. It is interesting that those substituted phenothiazines which have the greatest antihistaminic and anticholinergic properties produce the fewest extrapyramidal symptoms, as exemplified by thioridazine.

Alteration of Temperature Regulation The phenothiazines depress temperature-regulating mechanisms. They may produce hypothermia or hyperthermia, depending on the environmental temperature. In climates where the temperature is high, patients on phenothiazine medication may suffer a hyperthermic episode because of failure to lose body heat. Normally phenothiazines lower body temperature, a hypothermic effect.

Sites of Action in the Central Nervous System The central sites of action of chlorpromazine and related phenothiazines are multiple. These compounds do not produce significant cortical depression but act primarily subcortically. Chlorpromazine produces mild depression of some neurons in the brainstem reticular formation. It has been demonstrated that the reticular formation has an important role in regulating sensory function. One of the actions of chlorpromazine is to enhance reticular inhibition of sensory input. It has been suggested that chlorpromazine increases the filtering mechanisms of the brainstem activating system and thereby reduces afferent input. The actions of chlorpromazine on the limbic system are complex and involve both inhibitory and excitatory effects.

Although phenothiazines have a wide variety of biochemical effects, only one correlates with their clinical antipsychotic potency. This correlation concerns the influence upon certain catecholamines in the brain, especially dopamine. Dopamine is an established brain neurohumor present in high concentrations in the substantia nigra and terminals of the corpus striatum. In these areas dopamine action has been associated with various behavior effects and central muscular activity. Phenothiazines block the dopamine receptors in the brain and this blockade appears to be closely related to their therapeutic action as antipsychotic drugs.

Endocrine Actions The endocrine effects of the phenothiazines are due primarily to their action on the brain including the hypothalamus. The hypothalamus inhibits the production of lactogenic hormone in the anterior pituitary. Depression of the hypothalamus releases lactogenic hormone, which induces lactation. Thus, some patients complain of increased lactation following chronic use of chlorpromazine and other drugs which depress hypothalamic function. The phenothiazines which are especially likely to cause abnormal lactation include chlorpromazine, thioridazine, trifluoperazine, and fluphenazine.

The phenothiazines release melanocyte-stimulating hormone from the pituitary which results in abnormal pigmentation. There is a correlation between the effectiveness of various phenothiazines in releasing melanocyte-stimulating hormone and their antipsychotic potency.

The effects of the phenothiazines on ovulation and menstruation depend on the dose and duration of treatment. Therapeutic doses delay ovulation, as judged by biopsy, basal body temperatures, and menstruation. It has been shown that some phenothiazines, especially in high dosage, produce amenorrhea.

Peripheral Nervous System Effects The pheno-thiazines have multiple peripheral nervous system actions. These compounds produce α-adrenergic blocking and adrenergic potentiating effects, depending on the dose and duration of therapy. With a single small dose, especially with chlorpromazine, the α-adrenergic blockade is more consistent. Although most of the phenothiazines produce α-adrenergic blockade, their actions on norepinephrine are not so consistent as might be expected from classic α-adrenergic blocking agents such as phenoxybenzamine. This is because the phenothiazines are also adrenergic potentiators. Particularly with chronic administration, one can easily demonstrate that the phenothiazines potentiate the blood pressure responses of norepinephrine. This is due to an inhibition of the uptake mechanism for amines or to prevention of their retention. This phenomenon readily occurs peripherally but not in the central nervous system. The phenothiazines also block the nicotinic and muscarinic actions of acetylcholine. Generally these actions are weak and are seen primarily as side effects. However, some phenothiazines such as thioridazine are effective anticholinergics. The phenothiazines also vary widely in antihistaminic action, promethazine being more antihistaminic than chlorpromazine.

Potentiation of the Action of Various Drugs The phenothiazines are known to enhance the actions of various drugs such as the barbiturates and narcotics. This effect is dose-dependent. An interesting dissociation between potentiation of the miotic and sedative effects of morphine, but not respiratory minute volume, by chlorpromazine has been reported. Chlorpromazine has been shown to depress the level of alcohol dehydrogenase. As would be expected, this increases the blood levels of ingested ethyl alcohol. Patients should be warned about this effect because phenothiazines and even moderate amounts of alcohol are a potent combination which can result in a "dead drunk."

Administration, Distribution, and Metabolic Fate Many of the phenothiazines can be given intravenously, subcutaneously, intramuscularly, and orally. They must be given very slowly intravenously because of local irritation and possible severe hypotension due to central vasomotor depression and α-adrenergic blockade. Following absorption, they are distributed diffusely in the body but disappear from the blood very rapidly. Significant blood levels are present only 2 to 3 h after injection.

The most common pathway in the metabolism of chlorpromazine and similar phenothiazines is by hydroxylation (see below) and subsequent conjugation with glucuronic acid. The second most common pathway is by the formation of the sulfoxides (see below) occurring in the liver by the drug microsomal metabolizing system. In addition, demethylation and side chain oxidation can also occur in the liver.

Hydroxylation

Sulfoxide formation

With chlorpromazine, the percentage of metabolites appearing in the urine varies considerably, depending on the species. In man, at least five metabolites of chlorpromazine are found: chlorpromazine sulfoxide, desdimethylchlorpromazine sulfoxide, glucuronides, hydroxyl derivatives, and chlorpromazine itself. Chlorpromazine is also dechlorinated to promazine.

Although the metabolic excretion pattern of chlorpromazine and related phenothiazines may last for many weeks, the duration of action of these drugs is relatively short, especially on single-dose administration. Compounds such as chlorpromazine have a duration of action of approximately 6 h; it is necessary to administer the medication three to four times a day to maintain an adequate blood level. In the case of some phenothiazines, such as trifluoperazine, drug administration twice a day is sufficient.

Untoward Effects and Toxicity The phenothiazines produce numerous undesirable effects. These include lethargy, drowsiness, tachycardia, hypothermia, dryness of the mouth, orthostatic hypotension, lactation, and extrapyramidal symptoms. It is interesting that the potency of the substituted phenothiazines correlates best with the extrapyramidal reactions and inversely with sedation, undesirable autonomic effects, seizures, dermatitis, jaundice, and agranulocytosis. The autonomic nervous system effects are most prevalent with weaker drugs such as promazine. Autonomic side effects are less frequent with the potent agents such as trifluoperazine and fluphenazine.

Allergic reactions to the phenothiazines usually occur in the first few months of treatment. These include various forms of dermatitis, jaundice, agranulocytosis, and photosensitivity. Most blood dyscrasias occur within the first few weeks of therapy. Agranulocytosis, although rare, is more prevalent with chlorpromazine and promazine than with the other more potent phenothiazines. If it is recognized and the drug stopped, the patient will recover completely.

Extrapyramidal symptoms induced by the phenothiazines are frequently dramatic. Akathisia (motor restlessness) occurred in approximately 21 percent, tremors in 15 percent, and dyskinesia (dystonic reactions) in 2 percent of the cases in one study. A correlation has been found between the percentage of occurrence of such reactions and the milligram potency of the drugs. Some interesting sex differences have been observed. Akathisia and tremors occurred twice as often in women as in men. In men, dyskinesia occurred earliest (90 percent within 4½ days), akathisia next, and tremors last. Dyskinetic symptoms included bizarre neuromuscular manifestations which could be mistaken for seizures, tetanus, meningitis, encephalitis, and poliomyelitis. The induced extrapyramidal symptoms are completely reversible upon discontinuation or reduced dosage of the phenothiazine.

There is also a tardive dyskinesia which occurs, usually in older patients and more commonly in women, after administration of large doses of phenothiazines for long periods of time. The onset is insidious and the movements are rhythmic and coordinated rather than spasmodic. The tongue, lips, face, and jaws are most commonly involved. The late dyskinesia is not only irreversible, but it is usually intensified when the phenothiazine is withdrawn. This state may be suppressed with high doses of phenothiazines. Estimates of the incidence of this toxic effect vary.

Thioridazine appears to produce significantly fewer untoward side effects, such as extrapyramidal symptoms, lethargy, drowsiness, orthostatic hypotension, convulsions, and photosensitivity, compared with other phenothiazines. However, this compound has its own side effects, including atropine-like actions and, when given in massive doses, pigmentary retinopathy. Temporary failure of ejaculation has also been described following this medication.

Three types of pathologic liver conditions are associated with phenothiazine medication. The most frequent type is a diffuse inflammatory change associated with biliary stasis. The clinical picture is that of obstructive jaundice with a moderate elevation of alkaline phosphatase level. The next type of liver-induced ailment resembles acute hepatitis with evidence of parenchymal liver damage as indicated by elevated thymol turbidity and prothrombin deficiency. In the third and least common type of reaction, early cirrhosis is observed.

The most common adverse effects in children are extrapyramidal symptoms, which may be confused with encephalitis or other neurologic syndromes. The less common complications of phenothiazine therapy in children include jaundice, granulocytopenia, cutaneous eruptions, and hyperpyrexia.

Patients who take an excessive amount of phenothiazines present two different clinical pictures. The first is related to extreme somnolence; with prodding, the patient can be aroused but promptly falls back into a deep sleep. The second is hypotension. There may be a mild-to-moderate drop in blood pressure; the patient may or may not be conscious. The skin may be markedly gray but warm and dry. The nailbeds are usually still pink and the pulse is strong but more rapid than normal. Respiration usually is slow and regular. Hypotension may be severe, in which case the patient may present symptoms of shock, including weakness, cyanosis, perspiration, and a rapid thready pulse.

Therapeutic Uses   The phenothiazines are used widely as antipsychotics. Although these agents are not curative, they do reduce psychiatric symptoms sufficiently to allow the mentally disturbed patient to have better contact with reality and to be discharged to a home and family environment. Owing

to these drugs, community psychiatric treatment is a reasonable possibility. They are also used occasionally to relieve very severe anxiety and especially panic reactions induced by amphetamine and LSD. The phenothiazines have been used as antiemetics and antihistaminics and to potentiate the actions of narcotics and other agents.

Tolerance and Withdrawal   Tolerance occurs to phenothiazine-induced drowsiness and orthostatic hypotension. Interestingly, tolerance does not occur to the antipsychotic effects of these drugs. There is no typical withdrawal syndrome as is characteristic of barbiturates and narcotics.

Thioxanthene Derivatives

Chlorprothixene, the first clinically successful thioxanthene, and thiothixene are very similar in pharmacology to their corresponding phenothiazine derivatives. All the known side effects of the phenothiazines have been observed with the thioxanthenes, although some researchers claim that the incidence of certain side effects is less. Structurally they differ in that they have a carbon in place of a nitrogen in the center ring (Table 10-3).

Butyrophenone Derivatives

Although the butyrophenone derivatives have pharmacologic properties very similar to those of the phenothiazines and thioxanthenes, they are chemically quite different. Two butyrophenones, haloperidol and droperidol, are now in clinical use. Haloperidol has the following structure:

Like the phenothiazines, haloperidol produces extrapyramidal reactions. This, in fact, is its major shortcoming, although it can usually be avoided by careful control of dosages. It is an effective antipsychotic and antiemetic, has antidopaminergic actions, especially in the basal ganglia, and produces peripheral α-adrenergic blockade.

Haloperidol is widely used as a long-acting and very effective antipsychotic. It has a long plasma half-life so that a cumulative effect readily occurs.

Table 10-3 Therapeutically Useful Thioxanthenes

Generic name	Trade name	R_1	R_2
Chlorprothixene	Taractan	$=CH-CH_2-CH_2-N(CH_3)_2$	Cl
Thiothixene	Navane	$=CH-CH_2-CH_2-N\bigcirc N-CH_3$	$\overset{O}{\underset{O}{\overset{\uparrow}{\underset{\downarrow}{S}}}}-N(CH_3)_2$

It is advisable to give small doses to titrate the patient to the proper antipsychotic level, thus keeping objectionable extrapyramidal symptoms minimal. Haloperidol is effective in treating Gilles de la Tourette disease.

Although haloperidol produces a high incidence of extrapyramidal symptoms, it produces little sedation and perhaps fewer autonomic side effects, such as severe hypotension, than do the phenothiazines. Haloperidol has also induced tardive dyskinesia after prolonged use. When used in combination with lithium carbonate for the treatment of acute mania there have been reports of severe encephalopathy. If haloperidol is taken during the first trimester of pregnancy, limb malformations in the fetus may occur.

Droperidol (Inapsine) was designed as a more easily biotransformed butyrophenone with an action of less than 24 h. It has been used as a neuroleptic in combination with a very potent synthetic meperidine derivative, fentanyl, to produce a state called *neuroleptanalgesia*. This very interesting combination is known by the trade name *Innovar*.

Other Antipsychotics

The *Rauwolfia* alkaloid reserpine was first used in psychiatry in the mid-1950s primarily for its sedative effect. However, since the introduction of the phenothiazines, the use of reserpine has decreased considerably in psychiatry. The major reasons for this are that the phenothiazines have been found to be more effective as antipsychotic agents and their activity is easier to control than that of reserpine.

In addition, reserpine may cause a dose-dependent marked mental depression with chronic use. The only indication for reserpine in psychiatric disorders is in patients who cannot tolerate phenothiazines. Consequently, further discussion of this drug will be deferred to Chap. 18.

Selected Preparations and Doses

Phenothiazine Derivatives *Chlorpromazine* and its hydrochloride (Thorazine, Thorazine Hydrochloride) are available in tablets, 10, 25, 50, 100, and 200 mg; suppositories, 25 and 100 mg; sustained-release capsules, 30, 75, 150, 200, and 300 mg; solutions (oral use), 30 mg in 1 ml; injection, 25 mg in 1 ml, 50 mg in 2 ml, and 250 mg in 10 ml; syrup, 2 mg/ml. Dosage varies widely, depending upon child, adult, outpatient, inpatient, etc.; usually in adults 200 to 1,000 mg total per day in divided doses, three or four times a day.

Fluphenazine hydrochloride (Permitil, Prolixin) is available in tablets, 0.25, 1, 2.5, and 5 mg; extended-action tablets, 1 mg; elixir, 0.5 mg/ml; solution (injection), 25 mg in 10 ml; dosage: 2.5 mg initial oral dose for major psychoses.

Prochlorperazine and its ethanedisulfonate and maleate (Compazine) are available in tablets, 5, 10, and 25 mg; solution (injection), 10 mg in 2 ml, and 50 mg in 10 ml; syrup, 1 mg/ml; suppositories, 2.5, 5, and 25 mg; dosage: 30 to 40 mg divided daily oral doses for severe psychotic patients.

Promazine hydrochloride (Sparine hydrochloride) is available in tablets, 10, 25, 50, 100, and 200 mg; solution (injection), 50 mg in 1 ml, 50 mg in

1, 2, and 10 ml, and 250 and 500 mg in 10 ml; syrup, 2 mg/ml; dosage: 25 to 300 mg orally in divided daily doses.

Thioridazine hydrochloride (Mellaril) is available in tablets, 10, 25, 100, 150, 200 mg; dosage: 300 mg orally in divided doses.

Trifluoperazine hydrochloride (Stelazine hydrochloride) is available in tablets, 1, 2, 5, and 10 mg; solution (injection), 20 mg in 10 ml; dosage: 1 to 4 mg orally per day.

Triflupromazine hydrochloride (Vesprin) is available in tablets, 10, 25, and 50 mg; solution (injection), 3, 10, and 20 mg in 1 ml; suppositories, 35 and 70 mg; dosage: 50 mg orally in divided daily doses.

Thioxanthene Derivatives *Chlorprothixene* (Taractan) is available in tablets, 10, 25, 50 mg; solution (injection), 25 mg in 2 ml; dosage: 10 mg orally three or four times daily, individualized for particular patient; much higher doses in hospitalized patients.

Thiothixene (Navane) is available in capsules, 1, 2, 5, 10 mg; dosage: individually adjusted from 1 to 20 mg/day total; usually given twice or once daily because of prolonged half-life.

Butyrophenone Derivatives *Haloperidol* (Haldol) is available in tablets, 0.5, 1.0, and 2.0 mg; oral concentrate, 2.0 mg/ml; dosage: individually adjusted; total daily dose, 1 to 15 mg, usually divided twice a day.

Rauwolfia Alkaloids *Reserpine* (Rauloydin, Raurine, Rau-Sed, Reserpoid, Sandril, Serpasil, Serpate) is available in tablets, 0.1, 0.2, 0.25, 0.5, 1, 2, 4, and 5 mg; solution (injections), 5 mg in 2 ml and 25 and 50 mg in 10 ml. Also available as elixirs and capsules; dosage: 0.25 to 1 mg orally daily for mild anxiety and mild hypertension. Much higher doses may be used in severe cases.

Lithium

When the term *lithium* is used in conjunction with psychopharmacology it refers to the lithium ion or lithium salt. Lithium is administered in the form of lithium carbonate for the treatment of mania.

Mechanism of Action The exact mechanism whereby lithium exerts its antimanic effect has not yet been identified; however, it may be related to incomplete ion substitution for other extracellular and intracellular cations such as sodium and potassium. Its action would then be localized at the cell membrane.

Absorption, Distribution, and Excretion The lithium ion is rapidly and almost completely absorbed from the gastrointestinal tract and passes directly from the blood to the tissues. It is not bound to protein. After absorption and distribution, an equilibrium is established between lithium in the tissues and plasma. Since this equilibrium is dynamic, the concentration of lithium in the serum reflects the amount of lithium in the body. Thus, serum lithium concentration [measured in milliequivalents per liter (meq/l) of blood] provides an objective monitor for lithium treatment. Lithium is eliminated almost entirely by renal excretion. About 80 percent of the lithium in the glomerular filtrate is reabsorbed by the tubules. It has a half-life of approximately 24 h.

Adverse Reactions

Acute Undesirable reactions associated with relatively low serum lithium levels are more of an inconvenience than a danger and include such symptoms and signs as anorexia, transient gastric discomfort, vomiting, diarrhea, excessive thirst, polyuria, and tremor (Table 10-4). Another type of adverse effect is associated with the rapid attainment of high plasma lithium levels. This type of effect includes reactions seen in cases of overdosage or poisoning which may occur in suicide attempts with lithium. When it is used in combination with haloperidol for the treatment of acute mania, there have been reports of severe encephalopathy.

Symptoms of toxicity often coincide with serum lithium peaks and may be related more to the rapidity of the rise of lithium levels than to the absolute levels attained. These toxic effects may disappear or diminish without reduction in dosage or may respond to a rescheduling of the dosage over a 24-h period. Some effects, such as polyuria and tremor, may persist.

Toxic reactions seen at blood levels above 1.5 meq/l are more serious and include muscle fasciculation and twitching, hyperactive deep tendon reflexes, somnolence, confusion, and sometimes epileptiform seizures. There is no specific antidote for severe lithium intoxication. Treatment consists

Table 10-4   Adverse Reactions to Lithium

Gastrointestinal
1 Anorexia
2 Nausea
3 Vomiting
4 Diarrhea
5 Thirst
6 Xerostomia
7 Weight loss

Neuromuscular
1 Muscle weakness
2 Ataxia
3 Tremor
4 Muscle hyperirritability
   a Fasciculation
   b Twitching
   c Clonic movements of whole limbs
5 Choreoathetotic movements
6 Hyperactive deep tendon reflexes

Central nervous system
1 Anesthesia of skin
2 Incontinence of urine and feces
3 Slurred speech
4 Blurring of vision
5 Dizziness
6 Giddiness
7 Epileptiform seizures
8 Blackout spells

Mental
1 Psychomotor disturbances
2 Somnolence
3 Confusion
4 Restlessness
5 Stupor
6 Coma

Cardiovascular
1 Hypotension
2 Electrocardiographic changes
3 Peripheral circulatory collapse
4 Cardiac arrhythmias

Miscellaneous
1 Polyuria
2 Glycosuria
3 Fatigue
4 Lethargy
5 Dehydration
6 Tinnitus

of cessation of lithium and general measures to correct the effects of water and electrolyte imbalance.

Chronic   In general, prolonged use of lithium has been singularly free from harmful effects. A syndrome resembling diabetes insipidus is a fairly rare effect. Thyroid enlargement during prolonged lithium therapy has now been well documented, although the incidence is low, about 1 to 2 percent of the patients. Most patients are euthyroid, although some may exhibit hypothyroid symptoms. Withholding lithium usually leads to a return to normal thyroid function. One other area of toxicity that has not been clearly resolved is the potential for teratogenic effects. As a general principle, it is considered best not to give lithium to pregnant patients.

Therapeutic Use   The main indication for lithium carbonate is the manic phase of manic-depressive illness. Lithium carbonate maintenance therapy prevents or diminishes the intensity of subsequent episodes in those manic-depressive patients with a history of mania. Lithium does not appear to be effective in acute depression.

Preparations and Dosage   Lithium carbonate (Eskalith, Lithane, Lithoxate, Lithotabs) is available in tablets and capsules of 300 mg. Optimal patient response can usually be established at the outset with 600 mg three times a day. Such doses will usually produce the desired serum lithium level, ranging between 0.5 to 1.5 meq/l. It is important, however, to reduce the dosage rapidly to maintenance levels (0.5 to 1.0 meq/l) when the acute mania subsides, to avoid excessive serum concentrations and resultant toxic reactions. The recommended dosage to maintain this level is 300 mg three times a day.

ANTIANXIETY DRUGS

The critical factor determining whether a drug is used clinically as a mild antianxiety agent or as a sedative-hypnotic is the slope of the dose-response curve for central nervous system depression. Sedatives with relatively shallow dose-response curves tend to be used primarily as antianxiety drugs because a wide dose range is available which produces calming or ataraxia without objectionable side effects, such as drowsiness, sleep, ataxia, or slurred speech. On the other hand, sedatives with steeper dose-response curves are used primarily as soporifics to promote sleep.

Pharmacologically, the antianxiety drugs differ from the antipsychotic drugs in the following ways: (1) Antianxiety drugs produce a lower incidence of toxic and side effects; (2) they do not cause extrapyramidal signs; (3) they possess central skeletal muscle relaxing properties; and (4) they produce a higher incidence of habituation and possible physical dependence. This is particularly true of meprobamate.

Propyl Alcohol Derivatives

Meprobamate Meprobamate's chemical structure may be represented as follows:

$$
\begin{array}{c}
O \\
\parallel \\
H_2C\!-\!OCNH_2 \\
| \\
CH_3\!-\!C\!-\!CH_2CH_2CH_3 \\
| \\
H_2C\!-\!OCNH_2 \\
\parallel \\
O
\end{array}
$$

The principal pharmacologic action of meprobamate is depression of the central nervous system. It has a mild sedative effect.

Sedative and Hypnotic Effects Meprobamate is somewhat similar to the barbiturates, particularly phenobarbital, but is shorter acting. It promotes sleep in persons with insomnia. However, like the barbiturates, it decreases that portion of sleep associated with dreaming and REM. The compound also causes skeletal muscle relaxation. The critical question of whether this effect is due to a specific central skeletal muscle–relaxant action or is secondary to a sedative effect has never been adequately answered. Meprobamate is about as effective as most centrally acting skeletal muscle relaxants now available.

Absorption and Metabolic Fate Administered orally meprobamate is readily absorbed into the bloodstream. Peak blood concentrations occur 1 to 2 h after administration. The levels then decline for 10 h or more. The major metabolite of meprobamate has recently been established to be 2-methyl-2-(β-hydroxypropyl)-1,3-propanediol dicarbamate.

Pharmacologically this compound is relatively inert.

Physical Dependence It is now well known that meprobamate produces physical dependence if taken in sufficient dosage. Several studies have been made on the effects of meprobamate with regard to physical dependence and withdrawal symptoms in man. It has been shown that 2,400 mg or less of meprobamate per day does not lead to withdrawal symptoms in the majority of patients. On the other hand, doses of 3.2 to 6.4 g of meprobamate and more per day over a prolonged period cause definite physical dependence and withdrawal symptoms. The typical syndrome of meprobamate withdrawal consists of insomnia, vomiting, tremors, muscle twitching, anxiety, anorexia, and ataxia.

Untoward Effects and Toxicity Considering its widespread use, meprobamate taken in usual therapeutic doses produces relatively few adverse side effects. Serious effects, such as thrombocytopenic purpura, leukemia, and aplastic anemia, have been reported but are rare. Allergic symptoms also have been observed. These usually occur after a few doses of the drug. The incidence of reactions is not related to a previous history of allergy. Mild reactions consist of an urticarial or erythematous maculopapular rash which may be confined to the groin or may be generalized. Acute nonthrombocytopenic purpura with fever and edema also has been noted. Serious reactions include high fever, fainting spells, angioneurotic edema, and bronchospasms.

Ingestion of large amounts of meprobamate, particularly in cases of overdosage with suicidal intent, may result in coma, cardiovascular shock, respiratory collapse, and death. Drowsiness, lethargy, stupor, and coma in adults have occurred with doses of 4 to 9.6 g. Accidental meprobamate overdosage in children occurs but not so often as might be expected, perhaps in part because of the bitter taste of the drug. The clinical picture of overdosage in children resembles that in adults.

Derivatives of Meprobamate The commercial success of meprobamate prompted the synthesis of analogues which would have somewhat more selective pharmacologic actions. Tybamate (Tybatran) has pharmacologic actions similar to those of meprobamate except that its plasma half-life is approximately one-half that of meprobamate. This has clinical importance in that the drug is shorter acting. Furthermore, the tissues of the body apparently are not exposed to high and prolonged blood levels so that physical dependence and withdrawal symptoms have not been observed following even rather large doses.

Carisoprodol (Rela, Soma), like meprobamate, is a central nervous system depressant, but it is thought to be more selective as a skeletal muscle relaxant. Its principal side effect is drowsiness, suggesting that it is not unlike meprobamate in pharmacologic properties, although there is some evidence of increased potency as a skeletal muscle relaxant.

Another analogue of meprobamate, mebutamate (Capla), is a mild central nervous system depressant in which a vasomotor depressant action is said to predominate and to have negligible muscle relaxant effects. Chemically this drug is very similar to meprobamate. Its action to depress blood pressure is central; it has no direct action on autonomic ganglia or blood vessels.

Benzodiazepines

Several benzodiazepines are available to the medical practitioner. Chlordiazepoxide, diazepam, flurazepam and oxazepam are the principal derivatives. Their structural formulas are as follows:

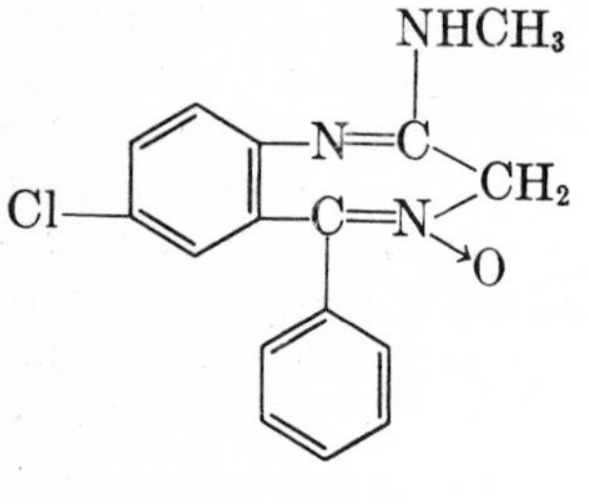

Diazepam

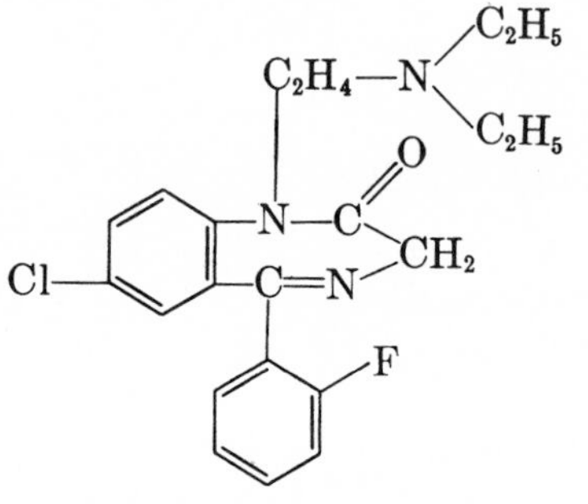

Flurazepam

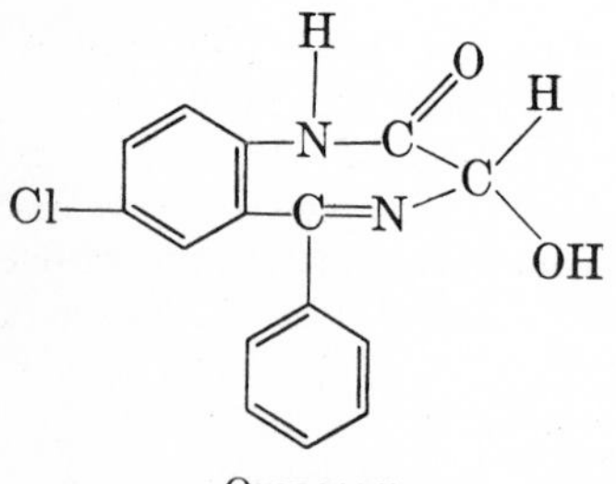

Chlordiazepoxide

Oxazepam

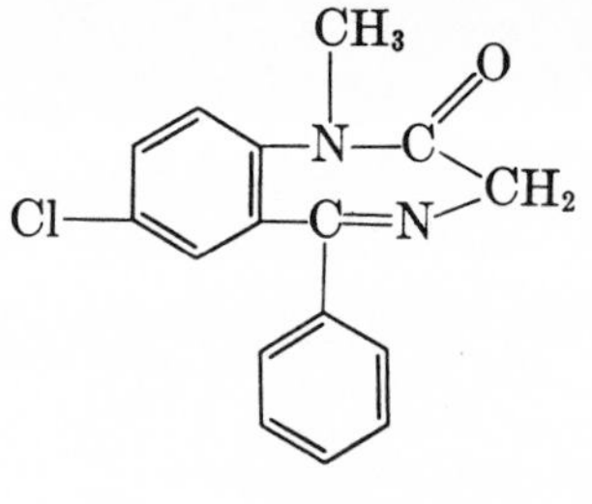

Oxazepam is a natural metabolite of diazepam in the body. It differs from diazepam by hydroxylation and demethylation in the diazepine ring as illustrated. The compound; flurazepam, is presently utilized primarily as a hypnotic and not as an anti-anxiety agent. The other benzodiazepines have sedative, anticonvulsant, and skeletal muscle-relaxant properties, but weak hypnotic effects. They appear pharmacologically related more to meprobamate than to other derivativies, but have distinct differences from it. Single or repeated doses do not affect arterial blood pressure, responses to epinephrine, or respiration. These compounds are effective in relieving anxiety and its accompanying somatic reactions. Elderly patients have been found to be very prone to central nervous system depression following even small doses. Chlordiazepoxide tends to exhibit a cumulative effect. On the basis of determining plasma levels in man, chlordiazepoxide has been shown to have a half-life of approximately 48 h following extremely large daily doses of 300 to 600 mg. It should be noted that these are about 10 times the usual therapeutic dose. Chlordiazepoxide has the longest duration of action, diazepam a shorter, and oxazepam the shortest.

Oxazepam is more poorly absorbed than diazepam and so requires larger dosage orally.

As an anticonvulsant and a muscle relaxant, diazepam is a more potent, shorter-acting analogue of chlordiazepoxide. Like chlordiazepoxide, diazepam has negligible cardiovascular depressant effects.

Absorption, Distribution, and Excretion The drug appears in the blood a few minutes after oral administration, and peak levels are obtained about 2 h later. Chlordiazepoxide is rapidly absorbed from the intestine. Part of the drug is secreted into the stomach and reabsorbed, while part is excreted into the feces. These effects persist for about 48 h. After very large daily doses of chlordiazepoxide to psychiatric patients, it has been estimated that the plasma half-life is approximately 48 h.

Physical Dependence There is no evidence that the chronic ingestion of chlordiazepoxide or diazepam in usual therapeutic doses recommended by the manufacturer leads to physical dependence. However, enormous doses of chlordiazepoxide (300 to 600 mg) and diazepam (80 to 100 mg) daily, given to psychiatric patients for several months, produce physical dependence. Depression, agitation, insomnia, loss of appetite, nausea, aggravation of psychoses, and grand mal seizures may be noted following abrupt withdrawal of the drug.

Untoward Effects and Toxicity The most frequent side effects of the benzodiazepines are drowsiness, ataxia, and lethargy. Syncope following large doses of chlordiazepoxide has been observed in aged and debilitated patients. Skin rashes, nausea, altered libido, menstrual and ovulatory irregularities, agranulocytosis, and increased sensitivity to alcohol also have been observed. Chlordiazepoxide causes paradoxical rage, excitement, hostility, confusion, or depersonalization in some severely ill schizophrenic patients. In patients who ingested chlordiazepoxide with suicidal intent, using single doses up to 2,250 mg, sedation, ataxia, dysarthria, and occasionally sleep and coma have been observed. It has been repeatedly observed in many patients who attempted suicide with chlordiazepoxide that although they fell asleep, they could easily be aroused and were able to talk, eat, and drink.

Several suicide attempts with diazepam have been made. The maximum single dose taken has been reported to be between 300 and 400 mg. This is a massive dose compared with the average therapeutic dose. Following such a massive dose, the patient became ataxic and drowsy.

Heterogenous Chemicals

Hydroxyzine Hydroxyzine has antihistaminic, antiemetic, and sedative actions. It has been used in the symptomatic treatment of anxiety and tension in neuroses, but is of little value in psychoses. The most common side effect of hydroxyzine is drowsiness, which is seen in about 25 percent of the patients. Headache, jitteriness, nausea, and xerostomia also have been noted. The toxicity of hydroxyzine appears to be low. Hydroxyzine enhances the depressant effects of opiates and barbiturates.

Chlormezanone Chlormezanone produces mild central nervous system depression and skeletal muscle relaxation similar to the effects of meprobamate, although the compounds are chemically unrelated. The drug is rapidly absorbed from the gastrointestinal tract. The duration of action is approximately 4 to 6 h. Its metabolic fate is unknown.

Clinical studies with this drug suggest that it has weak sedative effects; its muscle-relaxant actions are probably related to sedation rather than to any specific effect on spasticity or rigidity. Its side effects are mild and relatively infrequent. Drowsiness, lethargy, dizziness, flushing, dryness of the mouth, and skin rashes have been observed.

Preparations and Dosage *Chlordiazepoxide hydrochloride* (Librium) can be given orally and parenterally. There is wide variation in the effective dose. The usual daily oral dose is 15 to 40 mg in most adults. Preparations: capsules, 5, 10, and 25 mg; powder and solvent for parenteral injection, 100 mg.

Chlormezanone (Trancopal) is given orally. The adult dose is 300 to 800 mg/day. Preparations: tablets, 100 and 200 mg.

Diazepam (Valium) is administered orally and parenterally. There is wide variation in dosage, depending on the patient. The usual dose is 2 to 10 mg two, three, or four times a day. Preparations: scored tablets, 2, 5, and 10 mg; injectable preparation as 2 ml containing 5 mg/ml; 5 to 10 mg may be given intramuscularly or intravenously.

Hydroxyzine hydrochloride or pamoate (Atarax, Vistaril) may be given as the hydrochloride salt orally, intramuscularly, or intravenously. Usual oral dose for adults is 25 to 100 mg/day. The pamoate salt appears to offer no more sustained effect orally (it is converted to the HCl form in the stomach) than does the HCl salt. Preparations: hydroxyzine HCl solution for injection, 50 and 100 mg in 2 ml, and 250 mg in 10 ml; syrup, 2 mg/ml; tablets, 10, 25, and 100 mg. Hydroxyzine pamoate capsules, 25, 50, and 100 mg; suspension for oral use, 5 mg/ml.

Meprobamate (Equanil, Miltown) is administered orally. The usual dose for adults is 400 mg three or four times daily. Preparations: capsules (sustained-release), 200 and 400 mg; oral suspension, 40 mg/ml; tablets, 200 and 400 mg.

Oxazepam (Serax) is administered orally. Dosage varies from 10 to 30 mg three or four times a day, depending on severity of symptoms. Preparation: capsules, 10, 15, and 30 mg.

Chapter 11

Antidepressant Drugs

Two distinct classes of antidepressant drugs are therapeutically useful, the tricyclic antidepressants and the monoamine oxidase inhibitor (MAOI) antidepressants, although nonspecific central nervous system stimulants such as dextroamphetamine and methylphenidate are occasionally used in the symptomatic treatment of mild depressive reactions.

TRICYCLIC ANTIDEPRESSANT DERIVATIVES

The tricyclic derivatives imipramine, desipramine, amitriptyline, nortriptyline, protriptyline, and doxepin constitute the most widely used group of drugs currently available for the medical treatment of depression. There is general agreement that in comparison to the MAOI (described below), the tricyclic compounds are consistently more effective and potentially less toxic. Either advantage alone would warrant preference over the MAOI.

Chemistry

The basic chemical structure (Fig. 11-1) and the pharmacologic and toxicologic actions of the tricyclic compounds resemble those of the phenothiazine and thioxanthene derivatives. Structurally there are three series of tricyclic antidepressants: dibenzazepine, dibenzocycloheptadiene, and dibenzoxepin derivatives.

Imipramine, the first tricyclic antidepressant compound introduced, is a dibenzazepine derivative and differs structurally from the phenothiazine antipsychotic drug promazine only in that the sulfur atom is replaced by an ethylene group, thus forming a seven-membered iminodibenzyl ring system. The N-desmonomethyl metabolite of imipramine possesses antidepressant activities similar to those of the parent molecule and is available as desipramine.

The structural relationship of amitriptyline, a

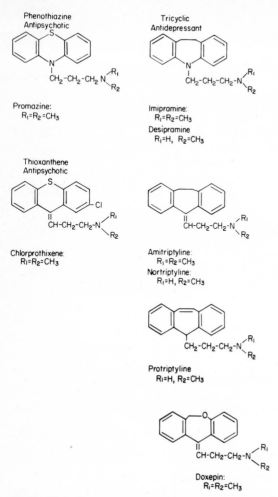

Figure 11-1 Comparison of phenothiazine and thioxanthene antipsychotic and tricyclic antidepressant structures.

dibenzocycloheptadiene derivative, to the thioxanthene antipsychotic drug chlorprothixene is comparable to that of imipramine to promazine. However, amitriptyline does not have a chlorine atom. The biologically active *N*-desmonomethyl metabolite of amitriptyline is available as nortriptyline. A shift in the position of a double bond in the nortriptyline molecule yields the antidepressant analogue protriptyline.

Doxepin is a dibenzoxepin derivative differing from amitriptyline in having an oxygen in place of a carbon atom in the center ring of the molecule.

Mechanism of Action

The Catecholamine Hypothesis   Soon after reserpine came into clinical use both as an antipsychotic and antihypertensive agent, it was noted that some patients became depressed during treatment. The depressive reactions from reserpine were often indistinguishable from those which occurred spontaneously. Many persisted for considerable periods after the drug was withdrawn, requiring electroconvulsive therapy to bring them under control, and some led to suicide. These reactions suggested that the reserpine-induced depressive reaction provided a good model for naturally occurring depressions. The discovery that reserpine depleted stores of serotonin and norepinephrine in the nervous system led to the proposal that naturally occurring depressions might be associated with decreased availability of norepinephrine at the central adrenergic synapses. It also focused attention on the levels of these biogenic amines in the nervous system to explain the actions of centrally acting drugs. Presumably, if depletion of amines were associated with sedation, an increase in brain amines should be associated with stimulation.

The tricyclic antidepressant imipramine, with structural and pharmacologic resemblances to chlorpromazine, at first seemed to be an exception to the rule. Its unexpected efficacy as an antidepressant and lack of efficacy as an antipsychotic were not readily explained. The crucial difference in action between imipramine and chlorpromazine, it turned out, was that the former led to potentiation of sympathetic responses, while the latter blocked them. One of the ways in which imipramine and other tricyclic compounds augment sympathetic responses is by blocking the uptake of norepinephrine after it has been released by the presynaptic neuron. Chlorpromazine and its congeners are believed to act by preventing the release of norepinephrine from the nerve ending into the synaptic cleft. Both drugs are known to stabilize cell membranes, but it would seem at first sight that one must construct a procrustean bed to explain how one drug does it one way and the other another. Still, it should be remembered that the spatial characteristics of imipramine and chlorpromazine may be more dissimilar than they appear. Furthermore, membrane theory is still rudimentary, and it is quite possible that membranes are not spatially symmetric on both sides. If so, it is conceivable that one drug could find suitable receptors on one side of a membrane, and another drug on the other side of the same membrane.

The present model of the central adrenergic synapse is as follows: When a nerve impulse or drug activates the sympathetic fiber, norepinephrine is released from storage granules located at the ends of the fiber close to the synaptic cleft. After the brief period of synaptic transmission, most of the norepinephrine is taken back into the neuron for further storage. The norepinephrine that is not reabsorbed is catabolized by the enzyme catechol-O-methyltransferase, the end product being normetanephrine. Within the neuron, synthesis and degradation of norepinephrine are in a state of dynamic equilibrium, some norepinephrine being constantly catabolized by MAO. The end products of this intraneuronal pathway are deaminated metabolites: first, 3,4-dihydroxymandelic acid, and second, 3-methoxy-4-hydroxymandelic acid (vanillylmandelic acid, VMA). It is believed that the major portion of VMA comes from the process of endogenous turnover, so that its excretion can be used as a marker for this process. On the other hand, only norepinephrine released at the synapse results in the production of normetanephrine, the excretion of which is used as a marker for physiologically active norepinephrine.

Despite some reservations, the catecholamine hypothesis has been the product of considerable efforts to elucidate the biochemical substrates of depressive reactions and explain the actions of antidepressant drugs.

The tricyclics also have sedative properties. Indeed, doses of 25 mg of amitriptyline were about equivalent to 100 mg of secobarbital sodium when given to preoperative patients as a hypnotic. Although marked sedative or hypnotic effects are less often seen in depressed patients treated with tricyclics, drugs with direct stimulant effects, such as tranylcypromine, amphetamines, and MAOI, are generally considered less effective antidepressants.

Rather than one mechanism being totally responsible for the antidepressant effects of a drug, it may be that a combination of effects may be needed. Drugs such as the tricyclics, which combine the effects of potentiation of norepinephrine, central anticholinergic action, and sedation, not only illustrate the adage that few drugs have only single

effects but raise the possibility that a combination of effects may be desirable for maximum therapeutic efficacy.

Effects on Organ Systems

Central Nervous System Most nondepressed subjects given tricyclics experience sleepiness or fatigue. In depressed patients, sedative effects are most apparent from amitriptyline and least from the monodesmethylated derivatives, such as desipramine or nortriptyline. The dissociation between antidepressant efficacy and customary stimulation is quite apparent. Perceptual changes induced by these drugs appear to be nonspecific and of little value in predicting utility or clinical responses in patients. Both imipramine and amitriptyline evoke epileptiform seizures. Intravenous doses of amitriptyline may evoke or enhance paroxysmal activity in epileptics. Only nonspecific changes similar to those produced by chlorpromazine and imipramine are noted in depressed nonepileptic patients.

Cardiovascular System The cardiovascular effects of the tricyclic antidepressants are similar to those of the phenothiazines; tachycardia and orthostatic hypotension are common. At usual therapeutic doses, both imipramine and amitriptyline may cause flattened T waves, prolonged Q-T intervals, and depressed S-T segments in the electrocardiogram. Toxic doses of these drugs cause multiple cardiac arrhythmias, including first-degree atrioventricular block, which indicates that these drugs may interfere with atrioventricular conduction.

Absorption, Fate, and Excretion

The tricyclic antidepressants are adequately absorbed after oral administration. The plasma half-life is more than 12 h following a single dose.

The metabolic routes of inactivation of the tricyclic antidepressants are somewhat similar to those of the phenothiazines. Hydroxylation and N-demethylation are the principal metabolic pathways of the tricyclics. Hydroxylation may occur at either the 2 or 10 position; 10-hydroxylated compounds of imipramine, desmethylimipramine, and didesmethylimipramine are excreted in urine. 10-Hydroxyiminodibenzyl may occur, as well as the corresponding glucuronides of these compounds;

imipramine *N*-oxide accounts for only 2 percent of the dose of imipramine excreted in urine. Amitriptyline is metabolized in a similar fashion to imipramine.

Wide variations in plasma levels of desipramine have been described in patients under steady-state conditions, the variations being at least eightfold probably because of individual variation in the rate of hydroxylation. While it is still questionable whether these are important considerations in therapeutic effects, they seem reasonable conclusions concerning side effects related to extensions of pharmacologic actions.

Adverse Reactions

Although the incidence of minor side effects is relatively high, the tricyclic compounds produce fewer serious toxic disturbances than do the MAO inhibitors. Adverse reactions encountered with the tricyclic antidepressants are in many respects similar to those of the phenothiazine and thioxanthene antipsychotics (Table 11-1).

Central and peripheral neurologic disturbances have been produced by the tricyclic compounds. Older patients may develop ataxia and incoordination, resulting in serious injury from falls. Unilateral and bilateral peroneal palsies have followed the use of both imipramine and amitriptyline. Both imipramine and amitriptyline evoke epileptiform seizures.

The tricyclics are directly anticholinergic both peripherally and centrally. Urinary retention and paralytic ileus are the most important adverse consequences. The cardiovascular effects of the tricyclic antidepressants are similar to those of the phenothiazines. As mentioned previously, toxic doses of these drugs may cause multiple cardiac arrhythmias.

Imipramine may cause cholestatic jaundice resembling jaundice from phenothiazines in every respect. As with the latter drugs, it is now a rare complication. Instances of agranulocytosis due to tricyclics, also resembling those due to the phenothiazines, continue to occur sporadically.

Tricyclic antidepressants should be used with caution—if at all—in the presence of glaucoma because of their anticholinergic effects. Their role in the genesis of seizures is uncertain, so caution is recommended during the early phases of treatment in epileptics.

Table 11-1   Incidence of Adverse Reactions to Tricyclic Antidepressant Drugs

Adverse reaction	Incidence*
Autonomic and cardiovascular disturbances	
Xerostomia	4
Constipation	3
Urinary retention	2
Disturbed vision	3
Sweating	4
Palpitations	2
Dizziness	3
Central and peripheral neurologic disturbances	
Drowsiness	2
Tremor or twitching	2
Confusion	2
Hyperactivity	2
Hematologic, Dermatologic, and Hepatic Disorders	
Leukopenia	1
Agranulocytosis	1
Skin rash	1
Pruritus	1
Photosensitization	1
Cholestatic jaundice	1

* 4, High; 3, moderate; 2, low; 1, rare.

The acute toxicity of the tricyclic antidepressants appears to be more serious than that of the phenothiazines and other antipsychotics. The major distinguishing feature of intoxication with the tricyclic antidepressants are disturbances of all types in cardiac rhythm and conduction.

Therapeutic Uses

The tricyclic antidepressants should be considered the drugs of choice for retarded or endogenous depressions. Patients must be kept on the drug for a period of at least four weeks, since therapeutic improvement may not be seen until that time. Comparisons of the tricyclic antidepressants suggest that the drugs are at least equal in overall therapeutic efficiency. Amitriptyline is approximately equal to imipramine in therapeutic effectiveness and may possibly be better in the older, more psychotic, depressed patient. The monodesmethyl derivatives of imipramine and amitriptyline have been shown to be less sedating than their parent compounds. Protriptyline is the least sedating, however. Although the desmethylated analogues are said to act more rapidly, this has never been adequately documented. Doxepin appears to be of value in treating mild depression where anxiety is prominent.

MONOAMINE OXIDASE INHIBITOR ANTIDEPRESSANTS

This designation refers to a group of psychotropic agents classified on the basis of their presumed biochemical mode of action, that is, inhibition of the enzyme MAO. The MAOI were introduced as the first antidepressants.

Chemistry

The MAOI are of two chemical types, hydrazides and nonhydrazides (Fig. 11-2). Hydrazide derivatives include isocarboxazid and phenelzine. Iproniazid was the first hydrazide, but it has been withdrawn from the market because of hepatotoxicity. Since part of the toxicity of iproniazid was thought to be the result of formation of free hydrazine, later variants of this group tended toward structures which protected the hydrazide moiety, as in the case of isocarboxazid. The nonhydrazide MAOI, tranylcypromine, chemically resembles dextroamphetamine in having a cyclopropyl rather than an isopropyl chain, and is the only clinically useful antidepressant of the nonhydrazide series. This chemical difference significantly enhances its ability to inhibit MAO as compared to dextroamphetamine. However, tranylcypromine retains some of the sympathomimetic actions of dextroamphetamine.

Mechanism of Action

Clinically available MAOI produce an irreversible inactivation of MAO by forming stable complexes with the enzyme. MAO normally limits intracellular levels of biologically active amines. Consequently, MAOI increase the amounts of endogenous amines such as norepinephrine, epinephrine,

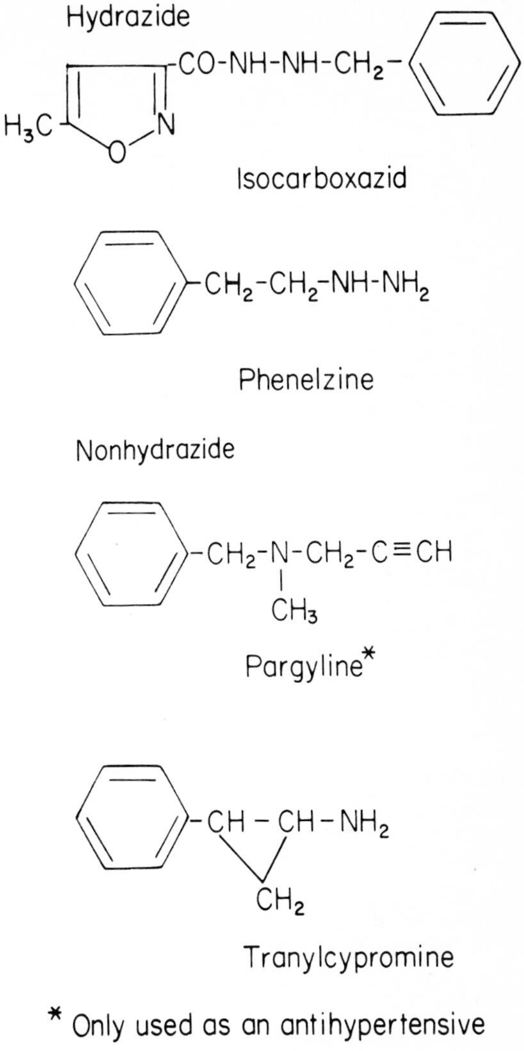

Figure 11-2 Monoamine oxidase inhibitor antidepressants.

dopamine, and serotonin in various tissues including brain, heart, intestines, and blood.

There are several amine oxidases of which MAO is only one. The clinically useful MAOI are not entirely specific for MAO since they also inhibit the metabolism and inactivation of certain drugs such as meperidine by other pathways.

As stated previously, a decreased availability of biogenic amines at central adrenergic synapses may be associated with naturally occurring depressions. The MAOI increase the availability of endogenous amines by inhibiting intracellular deamination of these amines, and their antidepressant effect might result from this inhibitory action.

Tranylcypromine possesses two modes of action. The first is due to its potent inhibition of MAO and the second is the result of an amphetaminelike action. The latter effect has been attributed to the release of norepinephrine from central neurons and also possibly to a reduction in the neuronal reuptake of norepinephrine. The rapid onset of action of tranylcypromine is a consequence of its amphetaminelike action, and its sustained antidepressant effects are related to the inhibition of MAO. This nonhydrazide derivative has sometimes been referred to as a *bimodal* antidepressant.

Effects on Organ Systems

Central Nervous System   All the MAOI produce low-voltage, fast activity changes in the EEG. They do not seem to alter thresholds at which stimulation of the reticular formation evokes EEG arousal. These drugs produce the same type of central motor stimulation and antagonize the sedative effect of reserpine when given prior to the depressant drug.

Cardiovascular System   Drugs in this group are likely to produce a greater incidence of postural hypotension than of hypertension. Pharmacologically, this effect may be due partly to an inhibition of transmission in sympathetic ganglia. This inhibition of ganglionic transmission is transient and weak, however. Another and perhaps more important mechanism of the hypotensive effect is a blockade of the release of adrenergic transmitters in certain organ systems by the MAOI.

Of far greater importance are the serious *acute* hypertensive reactions which may occur following the interactions of MAOI with a variety of pressor drugs, or food substances which have a high tyramine content, such as cheese, liver, and beer.

Liver   Enhancement of drug action can be attributed to an inhibition of the oxidative enzyme systems in the liver by MAOI.

The effects of a number of anesthetic agents, ganglionic blockers, atropine, morphine, meperidine, and other narcotic agents, and antimalarials such as chloroquine, are markedly enhanced by all hydrazide MAOI.

Absorption, Fate, and Excretion

The currently available MAOI are readily absorbed when given by mouth. The rate at which they produce inhibition of MAO is not known. It is postulated that these agents are present in the body for only a short time, but that they produce long-lasting effects by irreversible inactivation of the enzyme. The termination of drug effect depends upon enzyme regeneration, a process which takes weeks.

The hydrazide MAOI are thought to be cleaved, with resultant liberation of active products. On the other hand, the nonhydrazide MAOI apparently combine directly with the enzyme.

Adverse Reactions

Reported effects of acute overdosage with MAOI include agitation, hallucinations, hyperpyrexia, and both hypotension and hypertension. Among the most serious toxicities are those involving the liver, brain, and cardiovascular system. All stimulant drugs can detrimentally alter behavior by increasing tension, producing insomnia, aggravating psychoses, and possibly converting a retarded depression into an agitated one. Excitatory reactions are more likely with MAOI than with tricyclic antidepressants, since the latter have intrinsic sedative effect.

The occurrence of acute hypertensive crisis with fatal subarachnoid or intracranial hemorrhage led to the sharply curtailed use of tranylcypromine. While it is a unique drug in that the direct sympathomimetic effects may ultimately be potentiated by the slower-developing inhibition of MAO, all MAOI have been associated with such reactions.

Tremors, twitches, hyperreflexia, convulsions, and other neurologic signs have been produced by some MAOI. The appearance of hyperreflexia may be used to signify the upper dosage level of hydrazide derivatives, and thus more disabling neuromuscular disturbances may be avoided by reducing dosage. Peripheral neuropathy associated with the hydrazide drugs presumably has the same basis as that associated with isoniazid, i.e., is related to pyridoxine deficiency (see Chap. 37).

The numerous autonomic effects of the hydrazides are somewhat perplexing. Inhibition of MAO might be expected to increase tissue concentration of catecholamines with resultant sympathomimetic effects, but some symptoms, such as orthostatic hypotension, are inconsistent. The latter paradoxic symptom is believed to result from the formation of a false adrenergic transmitter, octopamine. One of the MAOI, pargyline (Eutonyl), is used exclusively as an antihypertensive.

The hydrazides produce hepatocellular jaundice, which had a high fatality rate in the case of iproniazid, but seems to be both milder and less common with the currently marketed hydrazide derivatives.

By blocking the catabolism of amines, MAOI may potentiate the actions of numerous drugs: amphetamines, barbiturates, meperidine, methyldopa, and possibly others. Even certain foods and beverages, such as cheeses, herring, beer, and wines, may contain enough tyramine or other related pressor amine materials to cause dangerous hypertensive episodes in the presence of a MAOI. Patients on these drugs should be warned explicitly about these hazards.

The MAOI should be employed with caution in conjunction with alcohol, ether, barbiturates, procaine, chlorothiazide, and phenylephrine, since there is potentiation of the effects of these agents. Tranylcypromine should not be administered with sympathomimetics, such as levodopa and dopamine.

Therapeutic Use

MAO inhibition takes place approximately 2 to 3 weeks after the onset of treatment, a period which corresponds to the time of therapeutic improvement. Numerous reports documenting relatively low clinical effectiveness coupled with high toxicity have markedly reduced the enthusiasm for MAOI as antidepressants suitable only for patients refractory to other forms of antidepressant therapy. Most studies indicate that phenelzine and tranylcypromine are the most useful available drugs of this class. Phenelzine is the preferred agent, since it does not seem to be associated with as high an incidence of hypertensive crisis.

The effects of a MAOI inhibitor may persist for a substantial period after discontinuation of the drug, and this should be borne in mind when another drug is prescribed following a MAOI. MAOI therapy should be terminated at least 14 days prior to initiation of therapy with another agent.

CENTRAL NERVOUS SYSTEM STIMULANTS

Chemistry

The older sympathomimetic stimulants, exemplified by dextroamphetamine, are phenylalkylamines. Newer members of this group are characterized by having a piperidine ring in a structure resembling the diphenylmethanes, such as methylphenidate.

Amphetamine   Methylphenidate

Mechanism of Action

The primary action of dextroamphetamine and methylphenidate in depression is to release norepinephrine at synapses, thus increasing the availability of the amine at central adrenergic synapses (see Chap. 17).

Absorption, Fate, and Excretion

Dextroamphetamine and methylphenidate are effective after oral administration, and their effects last for several hours. Substantial amounts of dextroamphetamine are excreted unchanged in the urine. The rate of excretion of this basic compound is highly pH-dependent, being considerably faster when the urine is acid than when it is alkaline. Most of the metabolites are parahydroxylated compounds.

Adverse Reactions

The acute toxic effects of dextroamphetamine and methylphenidate are usually extensions of their therapeutic actions, and as a rule result from overdosage. Although the stimulating effect of amphetamines is considered almost axiomatic, clinical effects are often paradoxic. The type of patient who experiences mood elevation and stimulation may be one whose personality is that of a "thinker," while the one who experiences paradoxic tranquilization may have the personality of a "doer." The interplay between personality and drug action is only beginning to be appreciated, not only for sympathomimetic stimulants but for most other types of psychotherapeutic drugs. Fatigue and depression usually follow the central stimulation. As might be expected with a sympathomimetic drug, there is an increase in both pulse rate and blood pressure.

Chronic intoxication can cause symptoms similar to those of acute overdosage, but abnormal mental conditions are more common. In addition, tolerance to and dependence on psychomotor stimulants often occur.

Therapeutic Use

Dextroamphetamine and methylphenidate, which should meet the requirements as antidepressants according to their presumed action on norepinephrine, are clearly effective stimulants but are not usually considered effective for severe depression. Some patients, especially those with reactive depression following some loss or physical illness, may respond to the euphoriant effects of central nervous system stimulants. Generally, such use of these drugs should be limited in duration since the development of tolerance to or dependence on these drugs may occur.

SUMMARY

The drugs available for treating depressions are listed in Table 11-2. Although some individuals have doubted the efficacy of both the tricyclic

Table 11-2   Current Antidepressant Drugs

Generic and trade names*	Total daily dosage, mg	
	Outpatient range	Hospital range
Tricyclics		
Amitriptyline (Elavil)	50–150	75–225
Desipramine (Norpramin, Pertofrane)	75–150	75–200
Doxepin (Adapin, Sinequan)	75–150	150–300
Imipramine (Tofranil, Presamine)	50–150	75–225
Nortriptyline (Aventyl)	20–100	40–100
Protriptyline (Vivactil)	10–20	15–60
MAOI		
Isocarboxazid (Marplan)	10–30	10–50
Phenelzine (Nardil)	15–30	15–75
Tranylcypromine (Parnate)	None	20–30
Stimulants		
Dextroamphetamine (Dexedrine)	15–30	30–60
Methylphenidate (Ritalin)	10–30	30–60

* Trade name is in parentheses following generic name.

drugs and MAOI, the tricyclic compounds definitely appear to have a place in the treatment of moderate, and perhaps even severe, depression.

Chapter 12

Antiepileptic and Antiparkinsonian Drugs

ANTIEPILEPTIC AGENTS

Convulsions of greater or lesser complexity constitute one of the common medical emergencies requiring suppressive therapy. Included in the category of convulsive disorders are certain syndromes so characteristic they have been named since ancient times. Epilepsy, the "sacred disease," in its various forms has been estimated to affect from 0.5 to 1.5 percent of the population. The essential requirement of antiepileptic drug therapy is that it control the syndrome without undue sedation and change in behavior so that the individual may remain a useful member of society.

Epileptiform Syndromes

Grand Mal The grand mal attack is one of the most dramatic and frequently encountered seizure types. The attack has its onset with or without premonitory signs (the aura) and consists of loss of consciousness followed by tonic and clonic spasms

of the musculature. Cessation of respiration, tongue biting, and urinary and fecal incontinence occur during the convulsive phase. As the tonic aspects of the seizure develop and respirations are suspended, the individual becomes deeply cyanotic, but as this gives way to the onset of clonic movement, irregular and stertorous breathing ensues. As the movements gradually subside, the patient relaxes, respiration becomes normal, and the patient regains consciousness. Typical postseizure phenomena include sleep, confusion, headaches, and gastric disturbance.

Petit Mal Petit mal attacks are primarily encountered in childhood, having their onset early in the first decade of life and rarely persisting beyond twenty years of age. The attacks are characterized by a sudden brief lapse in consciousness with or without minor motor movements of the eyes, head, or extremities. Falling does not occur, but there may be staggering, drooping of the head, and on

115

rare occasions, urinary incontinence. The attack is brief, lasting 5 to 30 s, following which the patient is immediately alert and able to resume normal activity. Petit mal seizures can be induced in most cases by 1 to 3 min of hyperventilation. In contrast to most other seizures, petit mal occurs with great frequency. Attacks rarely occur in such close succession as to impair consciousness for long periods of time.

Psychomotor Psychomotor attacks are manifested as episodes of alteration in behavior, perception, or affect. In most instances clouding of consciousness, automatic patterned movements, and total amnesia for the episode occur. The patient is completely out of contact with his or her environment but does not fall. The movements may be simple and brief, such as slapping the hands or smacking the lips, but may also take the form of a sequence of behavioral activity, such as getting out of a chair and walking across a room and performing a seemingly purposeful activity. On occasion, aimless running, fugal states, and sudden alteration in mood are encountered. Aggressive behavior is sometimes demonstrated, but rarely are violent acts committed.

Focal A focal seizure is one in which the clinical manifestations can be intimately correlated with the site of cerebral origin of the attack. Such seizures are most frequently encountered in symptomatic seizure disorders, and they usually imply a macroscopic or microscopic lesion of the cortex. When the attack remains limited to one segment or function of the cerebral cortex, the term *focal* is applied. However, if the attack begins in a segment and spreads in marchlike fashion following the homologue of the cerebral cortex, it is referred to as a *Jacksonian seizure*. In a classic example of such a seizure, convulsive movements start in the distal portion of an extremity, such as the finger, and progress to involve the rest of the hand, the arm, and the foot of the homolateral leg. Consciousness is retained unless the attack spreads to the opposite side of the body. If this kind of spread occurs, consciousness is lost, and generalized grand mal seizure may ensue.

Minor Motor Seizures in this group have in common brief duration, frequent occurrence, and

lack of postseizure abnormalities. They are often associated with other seizure types as well as with diffuse brain damage.

Drugs Useful in Grand Mal

Barbiturates All barbiturates are useful in convulsive states but only some appear to be particularly selective in epilepsy because they are effective in doses below those needed for marked sedation.

Phenobarbital Phenobarbital is the prototype barbiturate antiepileptic. It and other barbiturates designed for this purpose, as well as primidone, a closely related drug, are shown in Table 12-1.
Central Nervous System Effects Phenobarbital raises the threshold for electroshock seizures in experimental animals, tending to abolish the tonic phase of the convulsion in doses which do not cause obvious sedation. In humans also, the dose necessary for antiepileptic activity has only a minimal sedative effect.
Toxicity The toxicity of phenobarbital when used in epilepsy is the same as that when it is given

Table 12-1 Barbiturates and Related Compounds Effective in Grand Mal Epilepsy

Compound	R₁	R₂	R₃
Phenobarbital	(phenyl)	—C_2H_5	—H
Mephobarbital	(phenyl)	—C_2H_5	—CH_3
Metharbital	—C_2H_5	—C_2H_5	—CH_3
Primidone*	(phenyl)	—C_2H_5	—H

* Not a barbiturate: replacement of C=O at position 2 by CH_2 changes ring to pyrimidine.

as a general sedative and hypnotic. However, in epilepsy the drug is used for long periods of time (months and years); thus certain toxicities are more likely to develop. Skin rashes may eventually occur even after the drug has been used for years. This requires withdrawal of the drug, for there is always the possibility of exfoliative dermatitis. A certain degree of tolerance and dependence on the drug occurs, for sudden withdrawal in epileptic patients may precipitate seizures and occasionally leads to status epilepticus (repeated seizures without rest periods). For this reason barbiturates should be withdrawn slowly and replaced by other drugs to prevent this complication. Rarely do the usual doses employed in epileptic therapy lead to dependence or barbiturate "inebriation."

Mephobarbital The structure of mephobarbital (Table 12-1) is closely related to that of phenobarbital. In fact, it is phenobarbital methylated in the 3 position of the ring structure. This change makes the compound more fat-soluble and less water-soluble, a characteristic of many antiepilepsy drugs.

The potency of mephobarbital is somewhat less than that of phenobarbital, but since its sedative effects are also less, the therapeutic index is close to that of its parent structure. In all respects its actions on the central nervous system are quite similar to those of phenobarbital.

Gastrointestinal absorption of mephobarbital is less complete than that of phenobarbital. In the liver, demethylation occurs. About 75 percent of a given oral dose will be converted to phenobarbital in 24 h. Chronic administration of the drug leads to accumulation of phenobarbital, rather than mephobarbital, in the plasma. Thus it is difficult to establish whether mephobarbital, or its metabolite, phenobarbital, is the active ingredient in long-term use.

Mephobarbital (Mebaral) is available in tablets of 30, 100, and 200 mg. The usual dosage varies from 0.2 to 0.8 g in adults and from 0.03 to 0.3 g in children.

Metharbital Metharbital is the 3-methyl derivative of barbital (Table 12-1). It thus bears the same relationship to barbital that mephobarbital bears to phenobarbital. Like the former drug, it is demethylated in the liver, although the process of conversion is slower than that of mephobarbital. Metharbital

(Gemonil) is available in tablets containing 0.1 g. Usual dosage is 0.2 to 0.8 g per day. The toxicity of metharbital is similar to that of barbital and phenobarbital.

Primidone The chemical structure of primidone is shown in Table 12-1. It does not have a barbituric acid ring structure, yet it bears a close resemblance to the barbiturates. It will be noted that the only difference lies in the replacement of the $C=O$ group in position 2 by CH_2. Primidone is oxidized in the liver to phenobarbital. It is also metabolized to phenylethylmalonamide which possesses anticonvulsant activity. Side effects such as ataxia and sedation are quite marked, even in minimal anticonvulsant doses. Because of the high incidence of drowsiness it can seldom be used alone. The somnolence tends to decrease as the drug is continued. Other side reactions common to barbiturates, such as skin rashes, also occur. Rare instances of megaloblastic anemia have been reported. Primidone (Mysoline) is available in 0.25 g tablets and a 5 percent suspension for children. The usual adult daily dose is 0.25 to 2 g.

Hydantoin Derivatives The chemical structure of two antiepileptic hydantoins is shown in Table 12-2. It will be noted that they have a five-membered ring structure, in contrast to the six-membered barbiturates, and also that the point of difference lies in the absence of a $C=O$ group. All the hydantoins are highly fat-soluble and insoluble in water.

Table 12-2 Drugs Mainly Effective in Grand Mal Epilepsy

Drug	R_1	R_2	R_3
Diphenylhydantoin	phenyl	phenyl	—H
Mephenytoin	phenyl	$—C_2H_5$	$—CH_3$

Phenytoin (Diphenylhydantoin) In its overall effects on the central nervous system this drug comes close to being an ideal antiepileptic drug, since in full anticonvulsive doses it has only minor sedative effects. Even in large doses it does not cause hypnosis.

Mechanism of Action Certain aspects of the effect of diphenylhydantoin on suppression of seizure spread have now been clarified to some extent. One current theory concerns the function of the PTP (posttetanic potential) in the spread of excitation throughout the cerebral cortex. At a focal point in the cerebral cortex where there is a rapid negative firing and rapid discharge of impulses (as in an epileptic focus), the spread of such excitation requires the formation of the PTP, which results in an enhancement of synaptic transmission. The PTP is an important mechanism in developing high-frequency trains of impulses for excitatory feedback circuits and in spreading impulses to other areas of the cortex. It is believed that diphenylhydantoin promotes the extrusion of sodium from neural fibers in the cortex. The alteration in ionic concentration inhibits the formation of the PTP and consequently retards significant spread of excitation throughout the brain.

To some extent diphenylhydantoin is a folic acid antagonist. Particularly with chronic use the brain level of folate falls, and this has been used by some authorities to explain the mechanism of action of diphenylhydantoin. Additional support for this theory stems from the fact that large doses of folate will cause the return of convulsions in epileptics well controlled by diphenylhydantoin.

Absorption, Fate, and Excretion Diphenylhydantoin is readily absorbed from the gastrointestinal tract, reaching highest concentrations in the liver and central nervous system. Because of its long plasma half-life (approximately 22 h), plateau levels of diphenylhydantoin in plasma can be attained in 7 to 8 days; these levels can usually be maintained with 200 mg daily by mouth. Moreover, there is no significant difference at any time between plasma levels attained by giving a single daily dose and those attained by giving the same dose in three divided portions several hours apart.

Diphenylhydantoin is metabolized by hydroxylating microsomal enzymes in the liver. Its metabolism can be increased and its pharmacologic effect decreased by drugs such as phenobarbital, which induce increased activity of hepatic microsomal enzymes. Drugs which appear to decrease diphenylhydantoin metabolism include bishydroxycoumarin and isonicotinic acid hydrazide.

One of the major metabolic pathways for disposition of diphenylhydantoin is parahydroxylation of one of the phenyl groups, with subsequent glucuronic acid conjugation and elimination. The urinary output of this compound may account for 50 to 70 percent of the total amount of drug given, with unmetabolized drug accounting for less than 5 percent. Some patients have developed toxicity on ordinary doses of the drug as a result of a defect in parahydroxylation or because of drug interactions.

Preparations and Doses Diphenylhydantoin sodium (Dilantin, phenytoin sodium): capsules of 30, 50, and 100 mg; oral suspension of 30 and 125 mg per 5 ml; injection of 50 mg/ml. The usual adult dose is 0.2 to 0.6 g.

Toxicity In human use most side effects begin at a dose level of 0.5 g/day. Most subjects complain of ataxia, lack of coordination, tremors, nystagmus, and diplopia. Usually there is a tendency for increased irritability, but some subjects experience drowsiness. Reduction of the dose below 0.5 g generally clears up these symptoms.

Nausea and vomiting caused by the alkalinity of the drug are best combatted by ingestion of large quantities of water, and by taking the drug only during or after a meal. A skin rash is uncommon, and when it occurs it is not considered a contraindication to continuation of the drug. Long-continued use of the drug leads to hyperplasia of the gums, especially in the young. The connective tissue and the capillaries proliferate, with no evidence of pain or inflammation. Often the subject is unaware that hyperplasia is occurring. The mechanism is unknown, but fortunately it regresses as the drug is withdrawn. Hirsutism is another troublesome symptom which occasionally is seen with these drugs. Fortunately, diphenylhydantoin has rarely caused serious blood dyscrasias other than a transient eosinophilia.

A rare complication of therapy with diphenylhydantoin is lymphadenopathy, a syndrome that closely mimics malignant lymphoma and is termed *pseudolymphoma*. All signs disappear with cessation of therapy. Other rare toxic reactions are the lupus erythematosus cell (and syndrome) and erythema multiforme exudativum. Both may represent hypersensitivity reactions.

The most notable signs of toxicity with intravenous use of diphenylhydantoin are cardiovascular collapse and/or central nervous system depression. Cardiac arrhythmias, including atrial and ventricular conduction depression and ventricular fibrillation or arrest, may also occur. Parenteral diphenylhydantoin sometimes causes drowsiness, nystagmus, circumoral tingling, vertigo, nausea, and, rarely, vomiting.

Therapeutic Uses   The two major clinical uses of diphenylhydantoin are in the treatment of grand mal epilepsy, and in cardiac arrhythmias, which is discussed in Chap. 22 under Antiarrhythmic Agents.

Clinical response determines the dosage of antiepileptic medication. However, drug blood level determinations are helpful in the management of some patients, particularly those who do not respond to average or maximal doses or who manifest signs or symptoms of toxicity while receiving small or conventional doses of anticonvulsant agents. The usual therapeutic and tolerable blood-serum levels of diphenylhydantoin are, respectively, 10 to 20 μg/ml. In some patients, levels of 20 μg/ml provoke nystagmus ataxia and diplopia. In excess of 30 μg/ml, drowsiness and lethargy are encountered. With levels greater than 50 μg/ml, extreme lethargy and sometimes coma are observed.

Mephenytoin   As seen in Table 12-2, mephenytoin differs in two respects from diphenylhydantoin. At position 5 an ethyl group is substituted for one of the phenyl rings; at the 3 position a methyl group is added. These changes, while retaining the fundamental characteristics of diphenylhydantoin, make mephenytoin more potent and more toxic and add a sedative action.

Mephenytoin is well absorbed in the gut. The liver demethylates the drug to 5-phenyl-5-ethylhydantoin. This metabolite is inactive and is excreted conjugated with glucuronic acid.

Mephenytoin (Mesantoin) is available in 0.1-g tablets. The average adult daily dose is 0.2 to 0.6 g.

Toxicity   The toxicities of mephenytoin are similar to those of diphenylhydantoin, except there is more sedation. In addition, mephenytoin depresses the bone marrow sufficiently often to cate-

gorize it as a hazardous drug. Patients on mephenytoin must have frequent blood counts, especially in the first months of therapy. Hyperplasia of the gums does not occur, but the drug does cause pigmentation of the face in susceptible patients.

Ethotoin   The most recent of the hydantoin derivatives is ethotoin. It is less potent than diphenlhydantoin and also less toxic. It is a satisfactory drug but has few or no advantages over diphenylhydantoin. Ethotoin (Peganone) is available in 250-mg tablets. The usual adult daily maintenance dose is 2 to 3 g.

Tricyclics

Carbamazepine   Carbamazepine (Tegretol) is an iminostilbene derivative.

Carbamazepine

It is metabolized in the liver and its serum half-life is between 14 and 29 h. Because its use involves performing frequent laboratory tests and because of potential serious side effects, carbamazepine is indicated only in patients who have not responded satisfactorily to treatment with other antiepileptic drugs. The conditions responding to carbamazepine are grand mal, psychomotor, temporal-lobe, and mixed seizures. The major toxicities include: aplastic anemia, cholestatic and hepatocellular jaundice, acute urinary retention, oliguria, elevated blood pressure, impotence, dizziness, drowsiness, blurred vision, disturbances of coordination, erythematous rashes, congestive heart failure, thrombophlebitis, and cataract formation. Other anticholinergic symptoms may also develop.

The initial adult dose of carbamazepine is 200 mg twice a day, which is then gradually increased; dosage should not exceed 1,200 mg daily. The minimum effective dose is 800 to 1,200 mg daily.

Drugs Useful in Petit Mal

Oxazolidines   There are two drugs in this group which are closely related. They are trimethadione and paramethadione, and their use is restricted to the therapy of petit mal epilepsy.

Trimethadione

Chemistry　The five-membered ring structure is identical to that of the hydantoins except that oxygen replaces nitrogen in the 1 position. As the name implies, trimethadione has 3,5,5-methyl substitutions.

Trimethadione

Central Nervous System Effects　Trimethadione has little sedative or hypnotic action; it is, however, analgesic. Few other effects of the drug are notable.

Absorption in the gastrointestinal tract is efficient and rapid. The methyl group on the nitrogen atom is removed in the liver. The demethylated product is excreted slowly and, in patients on continuous therapy, tends to accumulate. It may be that the protection afforded by trimethadione is the result of its metabolite rather than of the parent structure.

Preparations and Dose　Trimethadione (Tridione) is available in capsules containing 0.3 g, in tablets of 0.15 g, and as a solution containing 40.6 mg/ml. The usual oral daily dose is 1 to 2 g.

Toxicity　Considering that the anticonvulsive dose of trimethadione is 10 times that of phenobarbital and causes only mild analgesia yet still affords several times the protection against convulsions, its superiority for its stated purposes is realized. Extremely large doses do cause ataxia, sedation, coma, and respiratory failure. There are instances of bone marrow depression when the drug is used experimentally in large doses for long periods of time. This is reversible on withdrawal of the drug.

Patients are not aware of the analgesic effects. The most common complaints are skin rashes, photosensitivity, and gastric irritation. In the higher dosage ranges (over 1 g daily), ataxia and drowsiness are likely to occur. About one-quarter of the

subjects complain of seeing "snow." This is caused by *hemeralopia*, a visual aberration in which visual acuity is diminished and objects appear whitish and sometimes dazzling. The symptom disappears gradually on withdrawal of the drug. No optic nerve damage has been documented. Although aplastic anemia and severe agranulocytosis are rare, it is advisable to perform frequent blood examinations when using this drug. Another rare toxicity is the precipitation of a nephroticlike syndrome which may be fatal. The urine should be repeatedly examined for cells and protein. In fact, as with all antiepileptic drugs, careful and continual supervision of the patient is essential.

Paramethadione　Paramethadione (Paradione), the other oxazolidine antiepileptic, offers no clinical advantage over trimethadione and its use is limited.

Phenylsuccinimides　Another group of five-membered ring structures effective in petit mal epilepsy are the succinimides. The most important drug in this category is ethosuximide.

Ethosuximide

Preparation and Dose　Ethosuximide (Zarontin) is available in capsules of 250 mg. The daily dose is 0.75 to 1.5 g.

Ethosuximide

Toxicity　In large doses the succinimides cause sedation and drowsiness. Ethosuximide causes the least sedation of the succinimides. Minor side reactions are nausea and vomiting, dizziness, headache, dreamlike state, and skin rashes. Severe blood dyscrasias have occurred with ethosuximide, and the blood count must be watched. More recently there have been reports of hepatic and renal dysfunction associated with this drug. Fatal bone marrow aplasia has also been reported with ethosuximide. Ethosuximide is of value only in petit mal and minor motor epilepsies.

Other Phenylsuccinimides Two other drugs in this category are phensuximide and methsuximide, but they exhibit no major clinical advantages over ethosuximide. It is of interest that methsuximide is also useful in psychomotor epilepsy.

Phensuximide (Milontin) is available in capsules of 0.5 g in a suspension of 62.5 mg/ml. The daily dose is 1.5 g.

Methsuximide (Celontin) is available in capsules of 0.3 g. The daily dose is 0.6 to 1.2 g.

Other Antiepileptic Drugs

Phenacemide

Chemistry Phenacemide (phenylacetylurea) is structurally a hydantoin ring between positions 1 and 5.

Phenacemide

Although often drawn in the projected ring form of hydantoin, it is doubtful that in the natural state the steric forces in the molecule would ever hold it in that shape.

Absorption and Fate Like other antiepileptic drugs which have a low water solubility, it is very well absorbed from the gastrointestinal tract. Metabolism is probably complete in the liver, since metabolites have not been identified nor does the drug appear in the urine. The action of phenylacetylurea is markedly prolonged in the presence of liver injury.

Central Nervous System Side Effects and Toxicity In spite of the large dose required, it causes little sedation or other undesirable neurologic effects. Unfortunately, in clinical use phenacemide has proved to be extremely toxic. Aside from minor side effects such as ataxia, anorexia, weakness, and headache, there are three areas of severe toxicity: hepatotoxicity, bone marrow depression, and toxic psychosis.

Preparation and Dose Phenacemide (Phenurone) is available in 0.5-g tablets. The daily dose may vary from 0.75 to 3.5 g.

Acetazolamide The carbonic anhydrase inhibitor, acetazolamide, has been found clinically useful in all types of epilepsy. However, the therapeutic effect is seldom complete, and it is best used in conjunction with other drugs. Often the beneficial effects are not sustained even with increased dosage.

Preparation and Dose Acetazolamide (Diamox) is available in 0.25-g tablets. The usual adult dose is 0.5 to 1.0 g daily.

Toxicity Drowsiness, anorexia, and paresthesias of the hands and feet are occasional side reactions. Skin rashes, drug fever, and blood dyscrasias have been very rarely reported.

Benzodiazepines These drugs, represented by chlordiazepoxide and diazepam in clinical practice, are used mainly as antianxiety agents. They have mild sedative effects along with anticonvulsant and muscle-relaxing properties. They are used extensively in status epilepticus and other convulsive seizures. The precise pharmacophysiologic mechanism by which these agents produce their anticonvulsant effects has not been fully defined.

ANTIPARKINSONIAN AGENTS

Although the clinical features are distinctive, parkinsonism is a syndrome of diverse etiology. The chief manifestations are rigidity, akinesia, resting tremor, and a characteristic flexed posture and shuffling gait. Iatrogenic parkinsonism due to antipsychotic drugs also accounts for a large number of cases, seen mostly in psychiatric practice. Parkinsonian features may be among the symptoms of brain tumor, cerebral vascular disease, and other degenerations of the central nervous system.

For over a century, the treatment of parkinsonism has rested primarily on the use of centrally active anticholinergic agents. Initially, various preparations of the belladonna alkaloids were used, including stramonium, atropine, and hyoscine. Recognition of the role of acetylcholine in nervous function, and particularly its probable role in the central nervous system, led to the suggestion that the clinical efficacy of atropine and scopolamine in parkinsonism might be due to their antagonism of acetylcholine.

An appreciable body of evidence has accumulated to show parkinsonism as a pathophysiologic state resulting from disease or dysfunction of a dopaminergic neuronal system arising in the midbrain chiefly in the substantia nigra and projecting to the corpus striatum. Physiologic studies indicate that dopamine exerts an inhibitory influence on the striatum. Thus in parkinsonism, the striatum would appear to be released from an inhibitory dopaminergic influence. The observation that centrally active cholinergic agents such as physostigmine exacerbate the parkinsonian state, whereas centrally active anticholinergic agents reduce its intensity, suggests that the symptomatology reflects the disinhibited activity of striatal cholinergic systems. According to this hypothesis a beneficial action could be exerted in parkinsonism either by blocking the excessive stimulation of the cholinergic system or restoring the normal function of the inhibitory dopaminergic system by restoration of its deficient neurohumor.

Levodopa

Of the several methods attempted to correct dopamine deficiency in the parkinsonian brain, administration of the immediate precursor of dopamine, levodopa, is the logical therapy because dopamine does not cross the blood-brain barrier. It is believed that the therapeutic effect of levodopa reflects the restoration of striatal dopamine toward normal. The diseased dopaminergic neuron which normally must synthesize dopamine from tyrosine (Fig. 12-1) can presumably do so more easily starting from dopa.

Preparations and Dosage Levodopa (Bendopa, Dopar, Larodopa) is available in oral tablets and capsules of 100, 250, and 500 mg. Therapy is started with small doses and increased every 2 to 3 days according to the patient's tolerance of side effects. The average dose thus achieved is 5.5 g daily.

Toxicity Anorexia, nausea, and vomiting are the chief dose-limiting side effects in the initial period of treatment. Others include tachycardia, palpitations, orthostatic hypotensive episodes, insomnia, agitation, and, rarely, more severe mental disturbances with delusions and hallucinations. Cardiac arrhythmias can be quite severe. These effects diminish with time or on lowering of the daily dose. They are less frequent if individual doses of levodopa are taken only after meals. Choreiform involuntary movements develop in a large proportion of patients receiving long-term treatment. Usually these do not appear until the third month of treatment; in some cases they do not

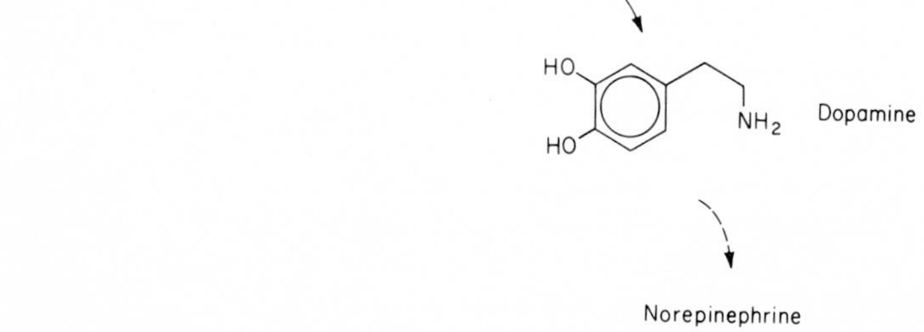

Figure 12-1 Schematic pathway of synthesis of dopamine from tyrosine in dopaminergic neurons. Presumably, increasing the supply of dioxyphenylalanine (DOPA) would increase the production of dopamine.

appear until the fifth or sixth month of treatment. If the movements are severe or if they interfere with function, the dose should be decreased until a satisfactory compromise is achieved.

Drug Interactions Many patients benefit from the combination of levodopa with one of the anticholinergic agents. The dosage requirement of levodopa can be reduced without altering clinical effectiveness by combining it with the decarboxylase inhibitor α-methyldopahydrazine. This compound does not penetrate the blood-brain barrier to inhibit central decarboxylase. This results in more levodopa entering the brain, thus permitting the dosage to be reduced without reducing the striatal dopamine effect. Pyridoxine markedly reduces or completely annuls the beneficial effect of levodopa administration. Pyridoxine appears to accelerate the metabolism of the drug in extracerebral tissues, thereby preventing it from gaining access to the central nervous system. Phenothiazines such as chlorpromazine antagonize the effect of levodopa and are best avoided.

Anticholinergic Agents

Today the belladonna alkaloids have been replaced in the treatment of parkinsonism by the synthetic anticholinergic antiparkinsonian agents listed in Table 12-3. Although less potent than the natural alkaloids, these synthetic agents possess similar pharmacologic properties and are strongly anticholinergic. The wide distribution of cholinergic neurons in the central nervous system makes it difficult to identify the specific structure involved in the beneficial effect of the anticholinergic drugs.

Therapy There is little reason for preferring one of the anticholinergic antiparkinsonian drugs over another. In general, treatment is begun with small doses which may be increased gradually until further increases yield no benefit or side effects are encountered. The benefits obtained are limited to a partial and often unsatisfactory reduction in the intensity of the parkinsonian state. A decrease in muscular resistance to passive movement, i.e., rigidity, is the most striking effect observed. There is also a general improvement in motor function and posture. Tremor may be reduced but is rarely

Table 12-3 Preparations and Doses of Anticholinergic Antiparkinsonian Agents

Drug	Availability	Usual daily dosage, mg
Trihexyphenidyl	Tablets, 2 and 5 mg	
Procyclidine	Tablets, 2 and 5 mg	1-15
Biperiden	Tablets, 2 mg Ampuls, 5 mg	
Benztropine	Tablets, 0.5, 1, and 2 mg Ampuls, 2 mg	1-6
Diphenhydramine	Capsules, 25 and 50 mg	
Orphenadrine	Tablets, 100 mg Ampuls, 60 mg	50-200

abolished and is generally the least responsive feature of the parkinsonian syndrome.

Toxicity Side effects attributable to the anticholinergic activity of these drugs are encountered in nearly all patients, and usually some compromise must be made in adjusting the dosage between therapeutic effects and the side effects common to all anticholinergic drugs.

Amantadine

The antiviral agent *amantadine* was accidentally discovered to relieve parkinsonism when used prophylactically against viral infection. The antiparkinsonian action of amantadine is probably related to stimulation of dopaminergic receptors.

Amantadine has a unique chemical structure consisting of four fused cyclohexane rings substituted with a single amine group.

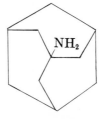

Amantadine

It is well absorbed from the gastrointestinal tract. The side effects suggest action on transmission in the central nervous system. Among the numerous reactions are hyperexcitability, tremors, ataxia, slurred speech, psychic depression, insomnia, lethargy, and, in high doses, convulsions. Other side effects probably not related to the central nervous system are dry mouth, gastrointestinal symptoms, skin eruptions, polyuria, and nocturia.

It is difficult to evaluate the pure therapeutic potency of this drug because in the clinical studies, amantadine was given to patients who were already receiving conventional therapy. Nevertheless, a marked improvement in clinical signs, symptoms, and functional disability was noted after the addition of amantadine.

The treatment of parkinsonism by combining levodopa, anticholinergic agents, and amantadine has produced better results than are seen with any of these drugs alone. This combined therapeutic program is of particular importance in those individuals who cannot tolerate higher dosages of levodopa because of toxic side effects.

Chapter 13

Narcotic Analgesics

OPIUM ALKALOIDS

Morphine

Narcotic analgesics obtund severe pain in the conscious state and produce some degree of central nervous system depression. Despite interesting new prospects, morphine, the oldest narcotic analgesic, is the best understood and remains the standard with which all others are compared. Therefore, morphine is discussed most completely and serves as the reference for other compounds described below.

Source and Chemistry Morphine is obtained from opium, which comes from the unripe seed capsules of *Papaver somniferum*. Opium contains two series of alkaloids. The phenanthrene series, of which morphine is a member, also includes codeine, which constitutes 0.7 to 2.5 percent, and thebaine, 0.3 to 1.5 percent. The benzylisoquinoline

series includes papaverine, 0.8 to 1.0 percent, noscapine (narcotine), 3 to 10 percent, and other alkaloids. The latter series has no narcotic activity.

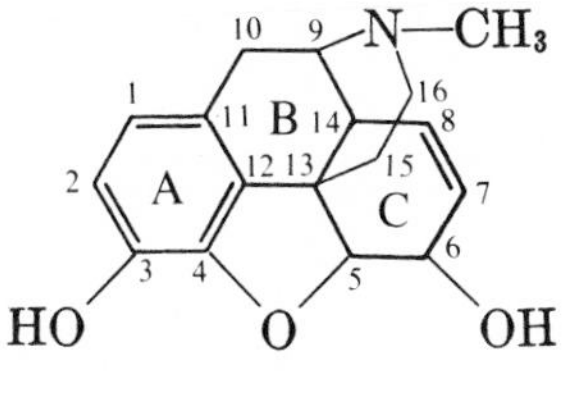

Morphine

The three rings of the phenanthrene nucleus, which are composed of C-1 to C-14, are designated A, B, and C, respectively. The fourth ring, composed of C-9 and C-13 to C-16 and the tertiary amine nitrogen, amounts to a piperidine ring, a structure present in most narcotic analgesics. The two hydroxyl groups, on C-3 and C-6 of the

125

phenanthrene nucleus, are phenolic and alcoholic hydroxyl, respectively. The 6-hydroxyl group forms ethers with difficulty but acetylates readily. This ester is more resistant to hydrolysis than a 3-ester. Any change in the substituents of the 3- and 6-hydroxyl groups alters the pharmacologic activity of morphine. Changes in the substituent on the nitrogen also lead to profound changes in activity.

Mechanisms of Action   The mechanisms of action by which morphine produces analgesia are enigmatic. Morphine can be shown to increase pain thresholds by a variety of methods, but the relationship of this fact to clinical relief of pain is indefinite. Most of the "analgesic" action of morphine probably derives from its power to exert a calming, soothing, fear-relieving effect. Although this effect is generally assumed to occur in the cerebral cortex, the neurophysiologic mechanisms are entirely unknown. Most, if not all, of the known diverse effects of morphine on various organ systems are probably irrelevant to the production of analgesia.

Effects on Organ Systems

Central Nervous System   Morphine has both stimulant and depressant effects on the CNS, and there are great variations in the degree to which either of these is more prominent. Cats are usually wildly excited by it; in contrast, the usual effect of morphine on humans is sedative. However, some humans are made excited, even maniacal, by morphine. Typically, a level of sedation is produced which is not so deep as that of a hypnotic agent such as a barbiturate: the patient may doze but can be readily aroused. Morphine is often described as producing a sense of euphoria. This is not always true. Some persons are made euphoric by morphine; others, dysphoric. The foggy, "other world" sensation is regarded as pleasant by some persons and unpleasant by others. Accompanying the sedation and mood effect, morphine produces feelings of dizziness, warmth, itching, and frequently nausea. The nausea produced by morphine is probably due to a combination of two factors: (1) morphine stimulates the chemoreceptor trigger zone of the medulla oblongata, and (2) morphine can cause some degree of orthostatic hypotension. Therefore, subjects given morphine who sit up or walk about

are more prone to nausea than are those who lie quietly in bed. The chemoreceptor trigger zone activates the nearby emetic center of the medulla. Antagonistic to the effect of stimulating the trigger zone, morphine depresses the emetic center. Morphine also possesses antitussive activity. The effects of morphine on spinal cord reflexes are very complex. Spinal cord stimulation is always present but is often masked by central nervous system depression.

Autonomic Nervous System   Morphine inhibits the release of acetylcholine in postganglionic structures of the gut, presumably by making them less excitable. Morphine also indirectly stimulates the postsynaptic elements of the adrenal medulla, causing release of epinephrine and norepinephrine and partial depletion of adrenal medullary catecholamine stores.

Respiratory System   Morphine is a powerful respiratory depressant, acting by medullary depression which in turn reduces carbon dioxide drive. Alveolar and serum P_{CO_2} both increase after morphine administration, and this may occur before any reduction in respiratory rate or tidal volume is noted.

Cardiovascular System   Morphine causes orthostatic hypotension in some patients because of depression of the vasomotor center of the medulla or possibly because of histamine release. Sufficiently large doses of morphine can cause hypotension even in the horizontal position; very large doses cause bradycardia.

Gastrointestinal System   The emesis following oral morphine administration is caused by a direct effect on the upper portion of the gastrointestinal tract which produces vigorous contractions and spasms of the smooth muscles of gut walls and sphincters. This results in hypertonic delay of peristalsis, with delayed gastric emptying time, and in constipation, which can become very severe, alternating with waves of overactivity. Tolerance does not develop to this effect of opiates, the mechanism of which remains unknown.

Hepatic System   The drug has no significant effect on the liver, even in large chronic doses. The action of morphine on the gallbladder, bile ducts, and sphincters is the same as that on the gut; as a result, morphine produces greatly increased cholecystic and choledochal pressures.

Skin Morphine occasionally causes urticaria, and some cases of contact dermatitis have been reported. Morphine causes an increase in sweating as well as histamine release, which in turn accounts for the reddened eyes and itching skin.

Genitourinary System Morphine decreases the volume of urine, probably because of release of antidiuretic hormone from the neurohypophysis. As in the gut, morphine causes spasm of the smooth muscles of the urinary tract, so that the detrusor and sphincter are spastic. The result of all these effects is oliguria, which may become clinically significant. Morphine also depresses sexual activity. Chronic dosage in humans causes absence of libido; addicts are reportedly able to maintain erection, but ejaculation is delayed or absent. In women, chronic morphinism causes oligomenorrhea or amenorrhea. Involution of the female genitalia may eventuate. These effects are due to suppression by morphine of hypophyseal gonadotropins. Despite these profound effects, sterility does not necessarily ensue. Morphine has no significant direct effect upon contractions of the uterus in labor, but it mitigates the concomitant, involuntary ("bearing down") contractions of the abdominal musculature and thus can delay labor. Infants born to addict mothers exhibit a physical dependence on morphine.

Miscellaneous Systems Morphine inhibits thyroid hormone release, probably by interfering with the central pathways which permit release of thyroid-stimulating hormone (TSH) from the adenohypophysis. It also produces hyperglycemia. This effect results from the peripheral sympathetic discharge mentioned above and can be blocked by adrenergic blockade.

Morphine causes marked constriction of the pupil in those species in which the drug is sedative. This effect is apparently accomplished by an excitatory action on the visceral nuclei of the oculomotor nuclear complex. The effect can be blocked by atropine. Tolerance does not develop to this miosis, and the effect is so uniform in humans that it has been used for evaluating analgesic drugs.

Absorption, Fate, and Metabolism Because of its pK_a (7.92) and the relative aqueous and lipid solubilities of the ionized and nonionized forms, morphine is rather poorly absorbed from the gastro-intestinal tract. It is more readily and reliably administered by the parenteral route. After entering the bloodstream, morphine is rapidly distributed throughout the body. The basicity of morphine also ensures that it moves promptly to intracellular sites. As with many other agents which have potent mental effects, morphine shows no special affinity for the CNS, and only minute amounts are needed in the brain to elicit the typical pharmacologic effects. Metabolic transformation occurs mainly, though not entirely, in the liver. Morphine is partly converted to normorphine. Excretion products include free and conjugated forms of morphine and normorphine; a small amount of codeine may be formed as well. The principal excretion product is morphine 3-monoglucuronide. Some secondary conjugation may occur on the alcohol hydroxyl group to yield the 3,6-diglucuronide.

Excretion of morphine and its metabolic products occurs mainly via the kidney. Up to 90 percent has been accounted for by this route, mostly as the glucuronide.

Toxicity The cardinal acute toxic effect of narcotics is respiratory depression. This far outweighs all other adverse effects. Long-term chronic dosage leads to physical dependence, which might be regarded as a kind of toxicity, but no other direct untoward effects occur.

Acute oral toxicity occurs mostly in children, from overdosage with paregoric (Camphorated Opium Tincture). Acute parenteral toxicity most often occurs because of self-administered overdosage in addicts. This is not uncommon, due to unreliability of supplies and overestimation by addicts of their own tolerance.

Pinpoint pupils are among the most constant findings in addiction, but in terminal narcosis, the pupils become dilated. Early in narcosis the skin is clammy and pale; later it becomes cyanotic. Respirations are slow, shallow, and irregular; occasionally, periodic (Cheyne-Stokes) respiration is seen. The heart rate is slow, and blood pressure is somewhat low, although shock is usually only a terminal event.

Therapeutic Uses, Hazards, and Contraindications These potent agents, with their formidable liabilities of respiratory depression and physical dependence, should never be used when less potent measures will suffice. The rule of *primum est non nocere* is never more cogent than with narcotics. However, there are a few instances in which lesser measures are often inadequate and utilization of narcotic agents is generally accepted. Once again, morphine is the prototype.

In myocardial infarction, when not only pain but apprehensiveness is often intense, morphine is of great value. It relieves the pain and at the same time calms the patient. Morphine may also decrease cardiac work in this crucial time, since even though it causes some catecholamine release, its central depressant property may yield a marked reduction in the physiologic release of catecholamines caused by pain and fear.

Morphine is invaluable in treating acute pulmonary edema. Of all unpleasant sensations, air hunger is one of the worst; morphine acts very powerfully to relieve this. In addition, morphine actually appears to aid in the disappearance of edema fluid from bronchioles and alveoli. This is true even though morphine is a potent bronchoconstrictor, which would seem to impede outflow and eventual removal of the fluid by coughing. This action would also seem to impair respiratory exchange, even though the patient becomes indifferent to the latter effect. For these reasons, aminophylline is often given at the same time for its bronchodilator action.

Another very common use for narcotics is as part of premedication for surgery. Proper use of narcotic agents can reduce the apprehension of the patient before induction of general anesthesia as well as reduce the amount of anesthetic drug necessary. Narcotics can also make spinal or local anesthesia tolerable. Again, the principal undesirable effect is respiratory depression; secondarily, hypotension may occur. These effects are also drawbacks to the so-called "lytic cocktail" as premedication for surgery. This procedure consists of inducing narcosis with an opiate and chlorpromazine. However, these agents have additive respiratory depressant effects, and hypotension is frequent. More recently, meperidine derivatives and butyrophenone congeners have been used in much the same way.

Use of morphine and similar drugs is contraindicated in biliary colic. In the past, use of atropine with morphine was recommended to overcome the intense constriction of the gallbladder, bile ducts,

and sphincters, but atropine is not sufficiently potent, and rupture of diseased tissue may still occur. Nitrites and aminophylline are more potent in this respect and by themselves can provide temporary relief from the pain by relaxing the spasm of the biliary tract. Similarly, morphine is contraindicated in acute pancreatitis when at least part of the cause may lie in spasm of the sphincter of Oddi or general contraction of the biliary or pancreatic ducts. Also, this is a relapsing disease, and addiction proneness tends to be extreme in these patients.

In chronic pain, opiates should be withheld if the reasonable life expectancy is more than 3 to 6 months, because in that interval tolerance will vitiate their usefulness. When opiates are given for chronic pain, they should be employed at irregular intervals and given only when absolutely necessary. As tolerance develops, dosage should be advanced only to the point of pain relief, not to the point of frank hypnosis. These measures will delay the progress of tolerance. Since cross-tolerance exists among all of these agents, switching drugs is of no help in avoiding or delaying tolerance.

Semisynthetic Derivatives of Morphine

The drugs discussed in this section have qualitatively the same actions and uses as morphine. They differ only in potency, speed, and duration of action.

Heroin Heroin, presently prepared by acetylating morphine, is considered the drug of first choice by "street addicts." Because of this and because heroin is more potent on a weight basis, greater profits can be obtained from it on the illicit market. It serves no therapeutic purpose that cannot be achieved by other drugs, and heroin is now legally banned in the United States and elsewhere. The

Heroin

drug enters the brain mainly as 6-monoacetylmorphine along with significant amounts of morphine. The onset of action of heroin is faster and the duration of action is shorter than with morphine.

Hydromorphone (Dihydromorphinone) Hydromorphone is formed by the catalytic transhydrogenation of morphine, which converts the 6-hydroxyl group to a ketone oxygen and saturates the neighboring double bond. Hydromorphone is approximately 8 times more potent than morphine on a milligram for milligram basis and sustains physical dependence at a dose roughly one-eighth that of morphine. Its absorption following oral administration is better than that of morphine and its onset of action is faster, while the duration of action is briefer. Hydromorphone is somewhat more sedative and less euphoriant than morphine.

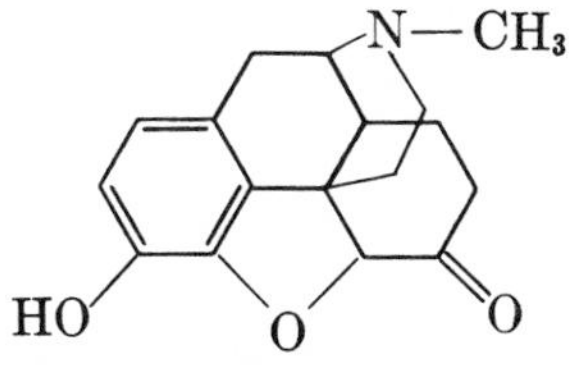

Hydromorphone

Oxymorphone Oxymorphone is the same as hydromorphone structurally except that it has a hydroxyl group on C-14. Oxymorphone is about 10 times as potent as morphine and causes more euphoria and more nausea and vomiting than do otherwise equivalent doses of morphine. The time-action curve of oxymorphone is about the same as that of morphine. Oxymorphone is a powerful respiratory depressant but is not very active as an antitussive. The addiction liability of oxymorphone is greater than that of morphine.

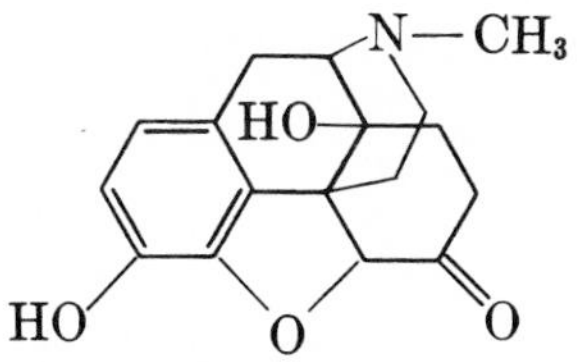

Oxymorphone

Codeine Codeine, the 3-methyl ether of morphine, is a natural alkaloid obtained from opium or synthesized by methylation of morphine. In analgesic effect, codeine is much less potent on a weight basis than morphine. Codeine produces little sedation; the stimulant component of its action is much less opposed by a sedative component, and hence it may produce excitement. Toxic doses in children may produce seizures. Codeine is much less potent as a respiratory depressant and also has much less effect on the gastrointestinal tract than does morphine in otherwise equivalent doses. Codeine is an effective antitussive.

In the body, codeine is demethylated; the 3-methyl and the *N*-methyl group are each removed to form morphine and norcodeine, respectively. Codeine in large doses can produce tolerance and dependence. Cross-tolerance occurs between codeine and other narcotic analgesics.

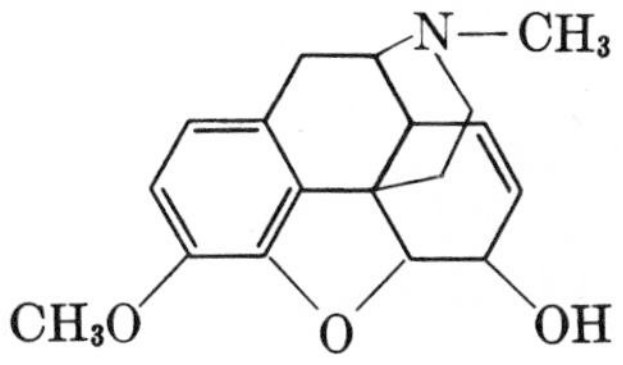

Codeine

Antagonism of Morphine and Morphine-like Actions

Nalorphine, or *N*-allylnormorphine, is remarkable because, when given alone, it has many of the actions of morphine, but when given in conjunction with morphine, it antagonizes many of these actions.

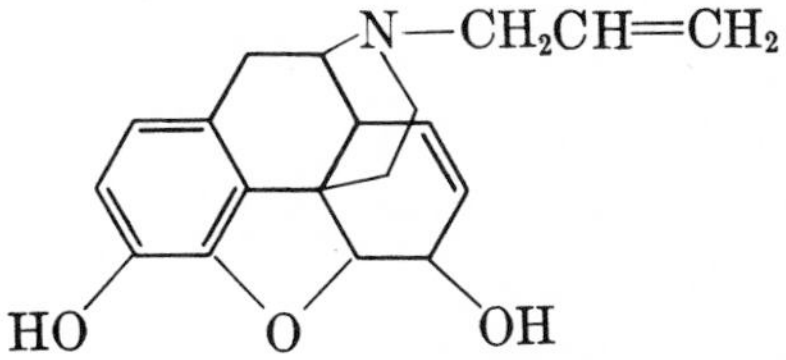

Nalorphine

Nalorphine is a powerful analgesic. Although tolerance and physical dependency occur on chronic dosage with nalorphine, it is relatively nonaddicting, and this should have made it invaluable. However, doses large enough to produce analgesia also produce a range of unpleasant mental effects, including malaise, dysphoria, confusion, disorientation, and visual hallucinations. These effects occur often enough and are severe enough to make nalorphine valueless as an analgesic.

Given in conjunction with narcotics, nalorphine acts rapidly as a highly specific antagonist against many of the actions of the narcotic. Individuals heavily sedated by morphine are very soon awake after administration of nalorphine. Since nalorphine antagonizes the hypoactivity and respiratory depression of morphine, the duration of action of nalorphine is shorter than that of morphine, and as the effect of the former disappears, the depressant and other effects of the latter appear.

Since nalorphine is a respiratory depressant by itself, it adds to the respiratory depressant effect of barbiturates, and in cases of respiratory acidosis, the compound is dangerous, as are the other opiates.

Nalorphine is used to treat acute morphine intoxication. A related use is in neonatal narcosis which eventuates from administration of analgesics to the parturient mother. Nalorphine is also employed in screening drugs for addiction liability and for diagnosing addiction.

Nalorphine antagonizes other narcotic analgesics as well as morphine. The dose of antagonist necessary to reduce a given level of effect of any narcotic by a given proportion is generally constant, but nalorphine is less effective against large doses of meperidine than against other commonly used narcotics.

Several other *N*-allyl congeners of narcotic analgesics have been prepared and studied. *N*-allyl-noroxymorphone, or naloxone,

Naloxone

is rated 6 times as potent an antagonist of the analgesic effects of morphine as levallorphan (see below) and 30 times as potent as nalorphine. This compound is atypical in several respects: it has

little or no subjective effects and does not cause miosis, a hallmark of narcotic effect. Tolerance and physical dependence do not occur. Naloxone is about 7 times as potent as nalorphine in precipitating the abstinence syndrome and retains this ability even with chronic dosage. It antagonizes other narcotic analgesic antagonists, including nalorphine, levallorphan, and pentazocine.

Naloxone is superior to nalorphine as a narcotic antagonist because it does not possess any morphine-like effects and consequently does not produce respiratory depression by itself. Thus it can be used in acute narcotic poisoning without the additional respiratory depression observed with nalorphine.

In the treatment of narcotic addiction, naloxone has been extensively used to prevent the euphoric effect associated with narcotic abuse. On a voluntary basis, the addict undergoes withdrawal and is then given daily doses of naloxone. Two of the major disadvantages to the use of naloxone are its short duration of action and its poor oral absorption. Presently, a new antagonist, naltrexone, is being clinically investigated for drug addiction programs.

Naltrexone

The advantages of this drug over naloxone are that it has a long duration of action and can be orally administered. The effectiveness of such a therapeutic approach with narcotic antagonists has not been fully evaluated and will require extensive clinical trials to determine its efficacy in the treatment of drug addiction.

SYNTHETIC ANALGESICS

Synthetic analgesics all have about the same pharmacologic actions as morphine, and with a few exceptions differ from it only quantitatively. Therefore, they will be discussed in reference to morphine, and the principal emphasis will be on the differences.

Phenylpiperidine Series

Meperidine The analgesic property of meperidine, the first entirely synthetic analgesic, was discovered after it was synthesized in the course of a program for developing synthetic atropinelike antispasmodic compounds. The effects of meperidine on the central nervous system are about the same as those of morphine.

Meperidine

Meperidine is a bronchoconstrictor and respiratory depressant. It has a greater respiratory depressant effect than do large doses of morphine. Although some antihistaminic and anticholinergic properties can be demonstrated, meperidine nevertheless also causes both histamine release and spasm of smooth muscle. Like morphine, therefore, meperidine causes biliary spasm. However, like codeine, it does appear to be less constipating than morphine. Unlike both morphine and codeine, meperidine is not an effective antitussive. Meperidine does not cause miosis but, rather, tends to cause mydriasis, which is one of the ways in which it is more like atropine than morphine. The effect of meperidine on heart rate is variable. As with morphine, meperidine causes postural hypotension.

Meperidine is addictive but will substitute only partially for morphine or heroin in addicts. Physical dependence caused by meperidine is more resistant to "unmasking" by nalorphine. Meperidine is probably the narcotic most frequently abused by physicians and nurses, and is also the most common agent in iatrogenic addictions.

The toxic effects of meperidine resemble those of atropine or scopolamine: mydriasis, dry mouth, tachycardia, and excitement which progresses to delirium with disorientation and hallucinations. The acute toxic effects of meperidine are not so favorably counteracted by nalorphine as are the effects of morphine.

Unlike morphine, meperidine is well absorbed by the oral route. Excretion is mainly in the urine. In general, meperidine more closely resembles codeine than morphine. It differs from codeine in being slightly more potent, in having a shorter time-action curve, and in having some undependable anticholinergic effects.

Diphenoxylate Diphenoxylate is effective in reducing gut motility in small oral doses. For this reason, it has gained wide popularity as an antidiarrheal drug in combination with atropine (Lomotil). Larger doses have effects similar to those of codeine, and the compound therefore is not devoid of addiction liability. Indeed, it has been employed successfully to prevent withdrawal effects in addicts. Although dependence to diphenoxylate is theoretically possible, at very low doses the incidence of physical dependence is extremely low. Nevertheless, caution should be exercised when giving this preparation to patients receiving addicting drugs or to individuals who are addiction-prone.

Other drugs in the phenylpiperidine series include alphaprodine, anileridine, ethoheptazine, fentanyl, and piminodine.

Diphenylheptane Derivatives and Analogues

Methadone The pharmacologic activity of methadone is very similar to that of morphine. However, methadone is well absorbed orally and is longer acting than morphine. By the parenteral route, methadone is about equal to or slightly more potent than morphine in producing analgesia. Methadone can substitute completely for morphine in addicts at about one-fourth the dose. Controlled withdrawal utilizing methadone is milder and less acute than with morphine; this is one of the most important current uses of methadone.

Methadone

Another important use for the drug is in methadone maintenance programs for narcotic dependence. Since methadone can be administered orally, it is used as substitute therapy for heroin or other narcotic analgesics. The narcotic addict is placed on daily doses of methadone sufficient to prevent withdrawal symptoms. While on methadone, the addict is physically dependent on it and precaution must be taken to avoid sudden withdrawal of the drug.

Propoxyphene Propoxyphene is structurally very similar to methadone. Its analgesic potency is less than that of codeine. In large doses, propoxyphene has some opiatelike effects. In general, propoxyphene's pharmacologic effects are similar to the opiate group; however, it does not compare with this group in analgesic potency. Propoxyphene can produce drug dependence which may be characterized as psychic as well as physical dependence.

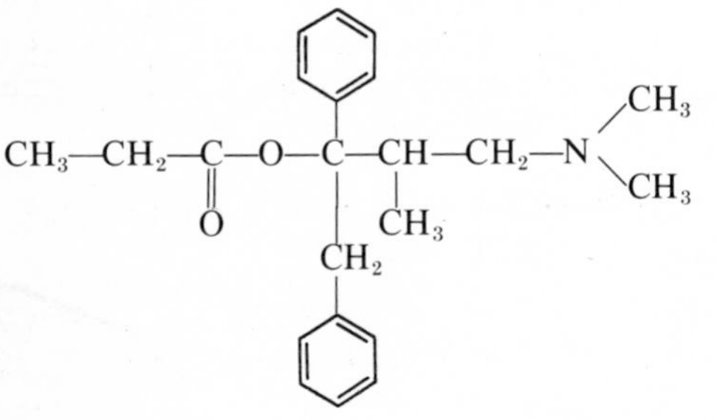

Propoxyphene

Morphinan Series

Removal of the ether oxygen, the hydroxyl groups, and the N-methyl group from morphine results in morphinan. Compounds of the morphinan series are chemically intermediate between opiate analgesics and the other synthetic analgesics. They contain the phenanthrene nucleus of morphine but are manufactured by synthesis rather than by chemical modification of morphine.

Methorphan The levorotatory isomer levomethorphan produces intense opiatelike effects; it can be substituted for morphine, and it is fully addictive. The dextro isomer, dextromethorphan, is not analgesic, will not substitute for morphine, and is not addicting. Dextromethorphan, however, has useful antitussive activity.

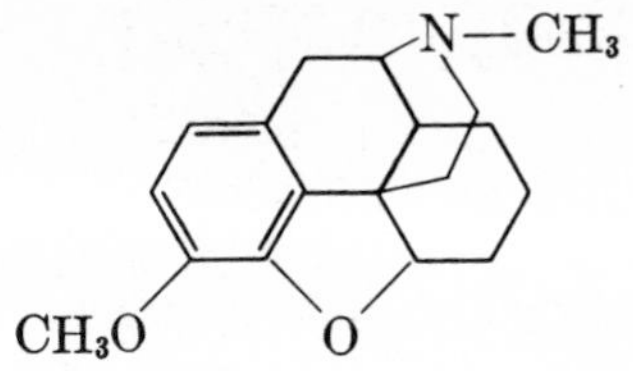

Methorphan

Levorphan Levorphan, or levorphanol, is the most potent of the morphinan derivatives. It is more potent than morphine and at least as addictive. The duration of action is about the same. The only advantage levorphan offers over morphine is that of reliable oral absorption.

Levallorphan The N-allyl congener of levorphan, like the N-allyl congener of morphine, is a potent narcotic antagonist. Again, the levorotatory isomer is active while the dextro form is not. Levallorphan is more potent than nalorphine but probably has no greater therapeutic ratio.

Benzomorphan Derivatives

Benzomorphan derivatives are structurally another step further removed from morphine than the morphinan series. One ring of the phenanthrene nucleus has withered to two alkyl groups, usually methyl, as in pentazocine. However, the piperidine ring containing the tertiary nitrogen still remains, as does the hydroxyl group in a position analogous to the 3-hydroxyl group of morphine.

Pentazocine

Pentazocine is a weak antagonist of morphine but by itself has strong analgesic effect. Respiratory depression is by far the most serious drawback. Pentazocine is about one-third to one-fourth as active orally as parenterally. When administered parenterally, pentazocine is about one-half as potent as morphine in producing respiratory depression, but only about one-fourth as potent in causing analgesia. When administered orally its analgesic potency is about equal to that of codeine. Untoward effects which are fairly common are dizziness, sweating, nausea, and vomiting. Tachycardia and hypertension occur only with large doses. The respiratory depression can be antidoted with naloxone. Psychic and physical dependence on pentazocine have been reported.

Pentazocine

PREPARATIONS AND DOSES

Morphine Sulfate Available in tablets of 5, 8, 10, 15, and 30 mg. These can be given orally or dissolved in water for parenteral use. Official solutions for injection are also available. Morphine hydrochloride is also available; this salt does not differ importantly from the sulfate. The usual analgesic dose range by the subcutaneous route is 8 to 15 mg. From 8 to 20 mg may be given orally.

Paregoric Formerly called Camphorated Opium Tincture, still widely used in treatment of diarrhea. Paregoric contains 2.0 mg morphine, the only active ingredient, in 5 ml (about a teaspoonful).

Hydromorphone Hydrochloride Available as follows: ampuls for injection containing 1 to 4 mg/ml; rectal suppositories containing 3 mg; tablets containing 1 to 4 mg. Multiple-dose vials are also marketed containing 10 or 20 ml, with 2 mg/ml. The usual dosage range is 1 to 4 mg orally, subcutaneously, or intravenously.

Oxymorphone hydrochloride Available as follows: solutions for injection containing 1 mg/ml; tablets of 10 mg for oral use; and suppositories of 2 or 5 mg. Usual doses are 1.5 mg subcutaneously or intramuscularly, 0.75 mg intravenously, 5 to 10 mg orally, or 2 to 5 mg rectally.

Codeine Phosphate Available in 15-, 30-, and 60-mg tablets for oral or hypodermic use. The usual dose range of codeine phosphate is 15 to 60 mg, either orally or subcutaneously.

Meperidine Hydrochloride Available in the following solutions for injection: 25, 50, 75, or 100 mg/ml. Meperidine is also available in tablets of 50 or 100 mg, and an elixir containing 10 mg/ml. The usual dose range is 50 to 100 mg intramuscularly or orally.

Methadone Hydrochloride Available in solutions of 10 mg. Also available in tablets of 2.5, 5, 7.5, and 10 ml, and a syrup which contains 0.33 mg/ml. The usual oral dose range is 2.5 to 10 mg. The usual parenteral dose is 7.5 mg; this may be repeated after 4 h. The usual oral maintenance dose for treating narcotic addiction ranges between 10 and 80 mg daily in the methadone maintenance programs.

Propoxyphene Hydrochloride Available in capsules of 32 and 65 mg for oral use. The usual dosage is 32 or 65 mg 3 or 4 times a day.

Propoxyphene Napsylate Available as 100-mg tablets and as a suspension containing 50 mg/5 ml. The usual oral dose is 100 mg.

Levorphan Tartrate Available in solutions containing 2 mg/ml. Tablets containing 2 mg are also available. The usual dose is 2 to 3 mg subcutaneously or orally.

Pentazocine Hydrochloride Available as 50-mg tablets. The usual oral dose is 50 mg.

Pentazocine Lactate Available in solutions containing 30 mg base/ml. The recommended adult dose is 30 mg subcutaneously, intramuscularly, or intravenously.

Nalorphine Hydrochloride Available in ampuls for injection containing 0.2 mg/ml, 5 mg/ml, and a multiple-dose vial containing 50 mg/10 ml. Usual dose range is 2 to 20 mg in divided doses. Doses may be repeated at 10- or 15-min intervals to a maximum of three doses. For asphyxia neonatorum due to opiates given the mother, the dose is 0.2 mg into the umbilical vein or alternatively by the intramuscular or subcutaneous route. This may be repeated at 2-min intervals to a maximum cumulative dose of 0.5 mg.

Naloxone Hydrochloride Available in ampuls for injection containing 0.4 mg/ml. Usual dose for improvement of respiratory function is 0.4 mg which may be repeated at 2- or 3-min intervals for a total of three doses.

Levallorphan Tartrate Available in solutions of 1 mg/ml. The usual dosage for narcotic antagonism is 1 mg intravenously initially with one or two additional doses, if necessary, of 0.5 mg at 3-min intervals.

Chapter 14

Nonnarcotic Analgesics and Antipyretics

SALICYLATES

Aspirin is probably used more widely and in larger quantity than any other therapeutic agent today. The first pharmacologic data on aspirin appeared in 1899; in 1967, nearly one-half billion dollars was spent on the purchase of nonprescription salicylate preparations. Approximately 12,000 tons of aspirin are consumed in the United States each year—more than 150 tablets for each inhabitant. Salicylates are most commonly used as antipyretic and analgesic agents in the relief of headaches and minor aches and pains. Probably the most important use of salicylates is in the treatment of arthritis and rheumatic fever. The mechanism of action of the salicylates in these conditions is discussed later in this chapter.

Sources, Chemical and Physical Properties

The chemical structures of the principal salicylates are given below. All of them are now prepared exclusively by synthesis.

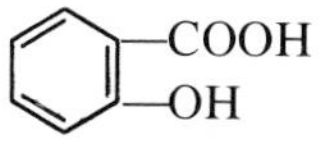

Salicylic acid

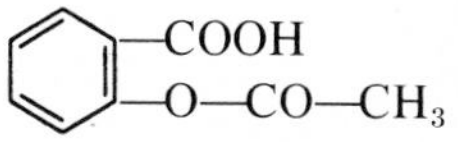

Acetylsalicylic acid

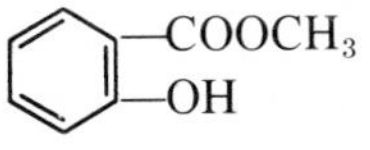

Methyl salicylate

Salicylic Acid Salicylic acid forms white crystals, usually in fine needles or as a fluffy white crystalline powder.

Sodium salicylate, the most widely used salt, forms white microcrystals.

Acetylsalicylic Acid (Aspirin) Acetylsalicylic acid (aspirin) forms white crystals. It is stable in dry air but gradually hydrolyzes in moist air to salicylic and acetic acids. It usually has a slight acetic acid odor which may be pronounced if tablets have remained in a warm place for prolonged periods.

Methyl Salicylate Methyl salicylate, or oil of wintergreen, is a colorless or slightly yellowish liquid having the characteristic odor and taste of wintergreen.

Effects on Organ Systems or Physiologic Function

Antipyretic Action One action of salicylates is that of *antipyresis*, or the reduction of an elevated body temperature. At therapeutic doses, the drugs usually are without effect on normal body temperature and affect only the patient with fever. This action is believed to be centrally mediated through the hypothalamus. In contrast, in toxic doses they act as pyretic agents, probably by a peripheral metabolic action.

Antipyretic drugs produce a fall in elevated body temperature by virtue of increased heat loss. The action is nonspecific in that it is not related to the elimination of the infection or underlying cause, and thus the definition does not ordinarily apply to chemotherapeutic agents. The antipyretic drugs appear to exert little effect on heat production in therapeutic doses. Their principal action seems to be through a marked dilation of the small vessels of the skin, possibly mediated through a central effect on the hypothalamus.

Analgesic Action Many pharmacologists have contended that the ability of salicylates to relieve painful sensation is centrally mediated, largely because antipyretic and analgesic coordination occurs in the same areas of the hypothalamus. In contrast, other investigators feel that salicylate action is peripheral and quite unlike that of the centrally acting narcotic analgesics such as morphine. Much of the controversy may lie in the variability and inadequacy of analgesic assays, with the possibility that they are evaluating a multitude of complex factors other than relief of pain.

Central Nervous System Depression Limited experiments suggest that salicylates have some slight tranquilizing action. Like tranquilizers, aspirin can have synergistic action upon the hypnotic effect of

barbiturates. Central nervous system disturbances, such as delirium and occasionally psychoses, may develop in patients after high doses of salicylate. In their mild forms such symptoms are so common that the term *salicylism* is generally applied to them (see Toxicity).

Respiratory System The average analgesic dose of acetylsalicylic acid (0.3 g) does not affect respiration. However, it is increased in both rate and depth after large doses of aspirin or other salicylates. This is largely the result of a direct stimulating action of the drug, although it has been suggested that peripheral metabolic stimulation and overproduction of carbon dioxide might contribute to the effect.

In most reported cases of salicylate poisoning, respiration is deep and rapid and the rate may be as high as 38 per minute. Occasionally, the hyperpnea of the Kussmaul type is difficult to distinguish from that found in diabetic acidosis. Most of the recent evidence supports the view that there is first a primary hyperventilation due to central stimulation, which then leads to a carbon dioxide–deficit type of alkalosis with an alkaline urine and a low blood-bicarbonate level. Later a ketosis develops, with a bicarbonate-deficit type of acidosis.

Acid-Base Balance Acid-base balance changes and disturbances in electrolyte pattern probably are related to both respiratory stimulation and metabolic effects. The respiratory stimulation tends to lead to respiratory alkalosis; the altered metabolism produces more acidic intermediary metabolites, which, together with the ingestion of the acidic drug, result in metabolic acidosis.

In advanced salicylate intoxication, particularly in children, serum sodium, serum–carbon dioxide content, and pH may be decreased, but this effect is usually preceded by ketosis and follows an initial period of hyperventilation and uncompensated respiratory alkalosis.

Gastrointestinal Tract Nausea and vomiting probably are produced by central stimulation. In rheumatic fever patients in whom high plasma levels of salicylate are maintained, nausea is common as a side effect, but nausea is almost as frequent after intravenous as after oral administration of the drug and occurs even when the gastric contents contain no salicylate.

Direct gastrointestinal irritation may occur after large doses of salicylates. In some cases of intoxication the gastrointestinal tract shows hemorrhage and other alterations, but in other cases signs of gastrointestinal involvement are absent. In dogs it is possible to produce petechial hemorrhages of the gastric mucosa by intravenous administration of large doses of sodium salicylate, oral ingestion of large doses of aspirin, or the subcutaneous administration of methyl salicylate. Gastric ulceration in rats can be produced by the oral administration of large doses of aspirin for 10 days and by subcutaneous administration of the drug.

Blood   Several reports have appeared which show that high dosages of salicylates may produce hypoprothrombinemia. Ingestion of 85 mg/kg for 6 days increased the prothrombin time in 8 of 10 human subjects, but there was no effect on bleeding time, platelet count, or prothrombin consumption. The prothrombin levels have been reported to be 10 to 60 percent below normal in acute rheumatic fever at salicylate levels of 35 mg/100 ml, but the prothrombin time returned to normal despite continued salicylate therapy. In another study, children with rheumatic fever who were on salicylate therapy developed hypoprothrombinemia without hemorrhage.

A number of recent reports deal with the effect of salicylate upon platelet aggregation. Platelet aggregation by epinephrine and the release of serotonin is blocked by aspirin. The possible relationship of both to aspirin-induced gastric hemorrhage and to the treatment of thromboembolic disease is obvious. Aspirin as well as corticoids dramatically prevented platelet clumping in over 1,000 pulmonary infarction patients at doses from 4 to 6 g daily.

Changes in the sedimentation rate are common after salicylate administration. The plasma fibrinogen may be reduced proportionally to the total dose given rather than to the plasma-salicylate level. Sedimentation rates are inversely related to the fibrinogen concentration in both normal subjects and rheumatic fever patients. The alteration of the fibrinogen content of the plasma by salicylates is attributed to a direct action on the plasma and on liver function.

Anti-inflammatory and Antirheumatic Actions
Probably the most important indications for the use of salicylates are in the treatment of rheumatic fever and rheumatoid arthritis. Salicylates alter inflammation induced by a variety of experimental methods. Whether they act at the mediator phase (prostaglandins) or elsewhere in the complex reactions leading to inflammation remains unknown and is an interesting area for investigation.

Uric Acid Excretion   Drugs which tend to enhance the excretion of uric acid are termed *uricosuric agents.*

There seems to be no doubt that salicylates can lower the renal threshold for uric acid and the urate level in the blood. However, it has long been recognized that salicylate may produce a paradoxical effect, depending on the dose administered. At doses in the range of 5 g/day salicylate may increase urate excretion by 40 percent; given with sodium bicarbonate, it may increase excretion up to 80 percent. However, at low doses such as 1 g/day, it will decrease urate excretion by 20 percent. Furthermore, even at high doses, it will antagonize the uricosuric effect of probenecid, phenylbutazone, and sulfinpyrazone.

It is believed that uric acid is filtered in the glomeruli but is then actively reabsorbed to the extent of 90 to 95 percent in the proximal tubules. Most of the urate in the urine results from distal secretion. At low tubular salicylate concentrations this secretion is depressed, leading to higher blood levels of uric acid. At high tubular salicylate concentration, both the urate reabsorption and secretion are blocked, the net result being uricosuria. Alkali administration enhances this effect by increasing tubular salicylate concentration. In confirmation, uricosuric doses of salicylates also inhibit renal transport of amino acids and of *p*-aminohippurate.

Skin   Skin irritation is readily produced by free salicylic acid and by methyl salicylate. Topical application of salicylic acid produces a slow and painless destruction of the epithelium. It may be used for this purpose to remove corns and warts. While it may have some direct action against certain fungi, it is more likely that its effectiveness in this area is due chiefly to keratolytic action.

Routes of Administration

Under ordinary circumstances absorption of salicylates in the gastrointestinal tract is so rapid that there is seldom need for parenteral administration. There is, however, convincing evidence that the relief afforded by salicylates, particularly in rheumatic fever, is proportional to the plasma level, and it may be difficult because of gastrointestinal irritation to give salicylates orally at a rate sufficient to attain high plasma levels in less than 2 days. For this reason some have advocated the intravenous administration of sodium salicylate. There is no doubt that high plasma levels are obtained rapidly in this manner, but the attendant dangers associated with the administration of large doses of salicylate by this route are ordinarily considered to outweigh the advantages.

Salicylates may be given rectally in doses of up to 3 to 6 g 3 to 4 times daily, with each dose dissolved in about 120 ml of plain water. Doses for children are proportionately smaller. A recent report stresses that in dogs rectal suppositories can produce mucosal irritation ranging from hyperemia to ulceration and perforation.

Absorption

The salicylates are among the most rapidly absorbed drugs by most routes of administration. Although the rate of absorption depends somewhat on the pH, it is nevertheless rapid at all hydrogen-ion concentrations within the physiologic range.

Absorption of the free acid, salts, and esters of salicylates occurs readily after cutaneous application. Methyl salicylate, which frequently is applied to the skin by rubbing, is absorbed so rapidly that traces may be detected in the urine within 15 min. Absorption is increased by dissolving the ester in alcohol, in liquid petrolatum, or in anhydrous lanolin. Normal human subjects to whom 0.2 g is applied locally excrete about one-quarter of the methyl salicylate in the urine. Poisoning has been reported in children following the application of salicylate ointments to a large area of the skin.

When salicylates are given orally to human subjects, the rate of absorption depends to an appreciable extent on the emptying time of the stomach in addition to stomach contents. When the drug is in solution, absorption is primarily dependent on the pH of the solution, since it is the nonionized form of the drug that is absorbed.

While the half-life for absorption of aspirin is less than ½ h in a fasting stomach, in nonfasting subjects the half-life is more than doubled. Effervescent drug mixtures decrease the emptying time of the stomach, owing partly to the weak alkalinity of the solution and probably to the carbon dioxide produced.

The administration of an alkali salt exerts an additional effect by modifying solubility of the salicylate preparation. Mildly buffered tablets of aspirin presumably lead to temporary dissolution of the drug in the stomach, but in the acid environment the drug will slowly reprecipitate in microcrystalline form, leading to greater absorption than would be expected from the administration of the unbuffered drug.

The salicylate concentration is usually greater in the serum than in whole blood. It appears that the red cell membrane is readily permeable to salicylate and that the drug is not bound by the proteins of the erythrocytes.

Conjugation and Degradation of Salicylates

Conjugation of a fraction of the administered salicylic acid with glycine to form salicyluric acid, the o-hydroxy analogue of hippuric acid, has been known for a long time. Salicyluric acid has no therapeutic effect in rheumatic fever patients and is excreted unchanged. Thorough studies in children leave no doubt that this conjugation product is a major metabolite. Little salicylurate is found in plasma and, of the tissues, only the kidney contains significant amounts.

When salicylates or aspirin are administered to human patients, two glucuronides are formed in roughly equal parts, an ester glucuronide and an ether glucuronide. Glucuronides may be synthesized by several organs, but the liver is presumably the major site of formation. Because of the more rapid renal clearance of glucuronides compared with that of salicylate, plasma levels in humans never exceed 1 percent of the salicylate level.

Excretion

Administered salicylate is excreted primarily in the urine. From 80 to 95 percent of the total dose administered is excreted in human patients in the form of compounds containing a salicyl group. Rate of excretion during the first day may be reduced by as much as 15 percent in rheumatic fever as well as in other pathologic conditions including nephritis, tuberculosis, and alcoholism.

It has long been known that patients tolerate salicylates better when sodium bicarbonate is given simultaneously, since the latter lessens the tendency to nausea and vomiting. This beneficial effect of sodium bicarbonate has often been attributed to reduction of a local irritating effect on the gastrointestinal tract, but many observations show that the main effect of sodium bicarbonate is to increase free salicylate excretion, thus lowering serum-salicylate levels. Sodium bicarbonate increases the urinary excretion of salicylate in children to such an extent that the blood levels 4 h after its administration may be only half those attained without sodium bicarbonate. Similar results are obtained during aspirin administration. Potassium citrate produces an increase in salicylate excretion analogous to the action of sodium bicarbonate.

Tolerance

Tolerance to the therapeutic effects of salicylates probably does not occur, although some patients may be under almost constant therapy for long periods of time. Occasionally the dose of salicylate required to control pain becomes somewhat greater, but this increase may coincide with the progression of the disease.

Idiosyncrasy

Idiosyncrasy, usually manifested as bronchoconstriction, urticaria, angioneurotic edema, or anaphylactic shock, may develop from the administration of relatively small amounts of salicylate. An asthmatic patient who took 0.3 g aspirin died within 10 min. She had previously experienced two severe reactions to the drug and had known that she was hypersensitive to it. In another asthmatic patient, known to be hypersensitive to the drug, death occurred after ingestion of 0.6 g aspirin. Hypersensitivity to aspirin as manifested by an angina pectoris syndrome has been described in two patients, one of whom also developed urticaria. A small "granule" of aspirin applied to the tongue produced a violent attack of coughing, asthma, and itching within 1 min in persons hypersensitive to the drug.

Preparations and Doses

Acetylsalicylic Acid (Aspirin)   Thus drug is used as 0.3- and 0.6-g compressed tablets or capsules, which is the usual adult dose. Tablets containing 0.3 g of aspirin plus an effervescent base are commonly available. Candylike tablets of aspirin containing 80 mg per tablet are available for children but have obvious dangers. Suppositories up to 0.9 g are available.

Sodium Salicylate   This drug may be obtained as 0.3- and 0.6-g tablets or in sterile solution for injection. The average dose of sodium salicylate is 1 g.

Salicylic Acid   Salicylic acid is most commonly used in ointment form in the treatment of epidermophytoses. Whitfield's ointment is Benzoic and Salicylic Acid Ointment, which contains 6 percent salicylic acid and 12 percent benzoic acid in a wool-fat and petrolatum base.

Methyl Salicylate (Oil of Wintergreen)   For external use only.

Toxicity

Despite their relatively low toxicity, the various forms of salicylate are responsible for more accidental fatal poisonings than any substances other than the barbiturates, alcohol, and carbon monoxide, and rank high on the list of causes of suicide by poisoning.

Apparently, there is no clear evidence of chronic toxicity; arthritic patients take up to 10 g a day for many years without apparent harmful effects. It is quite possible, however, that the kidney damage often referred to as *phenacetin nephritis* may in part be related to chronic consumption of salicylates (see Acetophenetidin and Acetaminophen Toxicity below).

Salicylates are also responsible for a high percentage of childhood poisonings due to all causes. Most of the cases in infants may be due to overzealous therapeutic use; in older children and adults they are due to accidental ingestion. Methyl salicylate is a fairly frequent offender because of its pleasant odor, the general impression of its being innocuous, and the ease with which toxic doses of the liquid are ingested. Fatalities in children have resulted from 4 ml of oil of wintergreen.

Fatalities result from salicylate toxicity in children with greater frequency than in adults, apparently because of lessened ability to withstand acid-base changes and dehydration. Initially the effects of salicylate overdose are those of respiratory stimulation, both in depth and rate, with resultant hypocapnia and respiratory alkalosis. Accompanying these may be irritability, dizziness, tinnitus, hallucinations, fever, nausea, and vomiting.

In early stages, the pH of the blood is usually high, ranging up to 7.6, but after several hours, particularly in children, both the serum–carbon dioxide content and the pH are frequently distinctly decreased. The causes of this metabolic acidosis may include the following contributory factors. Ketosis, with its acidic metabolites, is a frequent finding and has been shown to result from simple hyperventilation. Furthermore, the concentration of salicylate itself in plasma may be appreciable, namely 40 to 80 mg/100 ml, representing several milliequivalents per liter of acid. Finally, unidentified anions may accumulate in the blood and may amount to 8 to 18 meq/liter. These may be acidic intermediates, such as ketone bodies and lactic acid resulting from incomplete carbohydrate and lipid metabolism. The metabolic effects already mentioned might well account for such findings.

The net result of these effects is a disturbance which may be either respiratory alkalosis or metabolic acidosis or a combination of both. Blood pH rather than urinary pH is a better measure of the acid-base imbalance. Some of the interrelationships are illustrated in Fig. 14-1. The picture of hyperpnea, hyperglycemia, ketosis, acidosis, polyuria, and dehydration may be similar to that seen in diabetic acidosis. It can usually be distinguished by a history of salicylate ingestion and the presence of tinnitus, muscle irritability, and petechiae. Other disturbances associated with acute salicylate intoxication may be vomiting and diuresis occurring during the early phases of intoxication. Accompanying these are electrolyte disturbances, including hyponatremia and hypokalemia. Tetany and changes in

the ECG have been reported. Delirium, coma, and oliguria may follow, and death has resulted after 2 h to several days.

Treatment of acute poisoning may be aimed at preventing absorption; at treatment of the fluid, acid-base, and other electrolyte problems; or at promoting elimination of the drug. Activated charcoal may be of considerable value in reducing absorption even several hours after drug ingestion. In rats, blood levels only reached 40 percent of the expected level when charcoal was given 30 min after the salicylate.

Salicylism   A series of reactions called *salicylism* frequently occurs when the therapeutic dose of salicylate is high, as in rheumatic fever and gout. These symptoms, which may be manifested at plasma levels in excess of 25 mg/100 ml, consist of nausea and vomiting, tinnitus, deafness, severe headache, mental dullness and confusion, quickened pulse, and increased respiration. The condition, resembling cinchonism, may be troublesome,

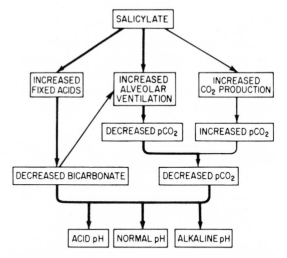

Figure 14-1   Summary of the pathogenesis of mixed disturbances of acid-base equilibrium in salicylate intoxication. From above downward are depicted the basic actions of salicylate, the separate effects of these actions on acid-base equilibrium, and the interaction of these effects in dictating the final pH. The line connecting "decreased bicarbonate" and "increased alveolar ventilation" is meant to imply that low blood pH may augment the primary effect of the drug upon respiration.

but the effects are usually without danger and disappear promptly when the drug is discontinued. In long-term therapy, there is some evidence that tolerance may develop to high doses and symptoms of toxicity may diminish. The aural manifestations are usually reversible.

Gastrointestinal Bleeding   A large number of reports indicate that human subjects may bleed acutely after aspirin ingestion. In upward of 70 percent of normal subjects ingesting even low doses of the drug, the fecal blood levels are increased. A high correlation between exacerbation of ulcers and recent ingestion of aspirin has also been observed.

Therapeutic Uses

Analgesia   Analgesia constitutes the major use of salicylates. The lay public employs aspirin particularly in the treatment of simple headache or neuralgic pain in doses of 0.3 to 0.6 g. Other salicylates are probably less effective. Probably relatively little of the total amount consumed in the United States is prescribed by a physician. The drug is especially useful in pain of low intensity, either when circumscribed or widespread in origin. The intense pain associated with coronary occlusion, although it emanates from a very limited area, is little alleviated by aspirin. On the other hand, the widespread joint pain of rheumatic fever is dramatically abolished.

Pain with Accompanying Inflammation   This is also extensively treated with the salicylates. A major application is rheumatoid arthritis. At a low dose of aspirin, perhaps 2.6 g/day, relief of pain alone is seen; at a high dose (greater than 5 g/day) objective changes are seen as well, such as changes in joint size, grip strength, etc.

Rheumatic Fever   Acute rheumatic fever is an inflammatory disease which follows infection with β-hemolytic streptococci. Significant features of the disease include arthritis, carditis, chorea, and a well-defined rash. Large doses of salicylates not only are of value in the symptomatic therapy of the disease, but may also affect the progressive valvular deformity which is often associated with continuation and/or recurrence of the rheumatic process. Salicylates are of no value in preventing later attacks of rheumatic fever, which may be prevented by the long-term administration of penicillin.

Antipyresis   Antipyresis has long been recognized as a nonspecific action of the salicylates, and they are commonly used for this purpose. Patients with fever are often restless and extremely uncomfortable, and there is no reason to believe that judicious administration of antipyretics to such patients is not desirable. Obviously, if specific chemotherapeutic agents are available, they will be used, but salicylates are of value as adjunctive therapy.

Gout   An acute attack of gout is caused by the precipitation of uric acid crystals in a joint. Hyperuricemia refers to an increase over the normal level of urate in the blood. It may be caused by an increased production or decreased excretion by the kidney. It may be idiopathic or secondary (such as in acute leukemia or renal failure). Since urate is relatively insoluble, it may precipitate, giving rise to tophi. When this occurs in the kidney, permanent damage may result. Not all cases of hyperuricemia need be treated, but when it must be, several drugs are available to lower the level of urate in the body. In a comparative study, it was observed that administration of salicylates resulted in lower serum–uric acid levels than did the administration of probenecid. However, uricosuric doses in adults usually consist of 5 g or more of sodium salicylate or aspirin daily, and this dosage is likely to produce salicylism. Lower doses of salicylate may increase the level of uric acid in the blood. As a result, salicylates have been replaced by other agents for the treatment of hyperuricemia.

NONSALICYLATES AND DRUGS USEFUL IN GOUT

During the latter half of the last century many drugs were synthesized and introduced for their antipyretic action. Many are now of greater interest as nonnarcotic analgesics. Of considerable importance, in addition to the salicylates, are acetophenetidin and acetaminophen. Some drugs, such as phenylbutazone and indomethacin, have valuable anti-inflammatory properties and are useful in the therapy of rheumatic diseases. Other drugs, such as colchicine, probenecid, and allopurinol are not analgesic or anti-inflammatory drugs but are of importance in the treatment of gout. Table 14-1 summarizes the pharmacologic effects of some nonnarcotic analgesic drugs and drugs useful in gout.

Acetophenetidin and Acetaminophen

Acetaminophen and acetophenetidin are employed for much the same purpose as are the salicylates, although their primary use is for the relief of ordinary aches and pains. In contrast to the salicylates, however, they are devoid of anti-inflammatory or antirheumatic properties and are not specifically employed in the treatment of rheumatic fever, rheumatoid arthritis, or gout.

NH—CO—CH$_3$ NH—CO—CH$_3$

OH   OC$_2$H$_5$

Acetaminophen   Acetophenetidin

Mechanism of Action   The antipyretic action of acetophenetidin and acetaminophen may be cen-

tral. Heat loss is increased by dilation of the cutaneous vessels and increased sweating. Although the drugs have little influence on normal temperature, the antipyretic response occurs also when the temperature is only slightly elevated. Their primary action may be in the hypothalamus and thalamus at the central endings of the nerves carrying painful stimuli. The antipyretic center is known to reside in the hypothalamus, and it has been suggested that the center of analgesic action may be located in approximately the same position. However, the peripheral action of these drugs may be a more important mechanism than their central action, as discussed under Salicylates.

Effect on Organ Systems   Aside from the depressant effect of acetophenetidin on the central nervous system, an action not shared by acetaminophen, these drugs are without major effect on other organ systems, with the exception of the blood and perhaps the kidney. These effects will be discussed under Toxicity, below.

Routes of Administration   Acetophenetidin and acetaminophen are given orally. There is no reason under ordinary circumstances for any other method of administration.

Absorption, Distribution, and Fate   Acetophenetidin and acetaminophen are absorbed rapidly after

Table 14-1   Summary of Pharmacologic Effects of Nonnarcotic Analgesic Drugs and Drugs Useful in Gout*

Drug	Analgesic	Antipyretic	Anti-inflammatory	Uricosuric	Relief in acute gout	Toxic
Salicylate	3+	3+	3+	2+ (high doses)	−	±
Acetophenetidin	3+	3+	−	−	−	+
Acetaminophen	3+	3+	−	−	−	±
Phenylbutazone	3+	3+	3+	+	2+	3+
Oxyphenbutazone	3+	3+	3+	+	2+	3+
Sulfinpyrazone	±	±	±	4+	−	+
Indomethacin	3+	3+	3+	−	2+	2+
Probenecid	−	−	−	3+	−	+
Allopurinol	−	−	−	−	−	±
Colchicine	−	−	−	−	3+	2+

* Effects range from −, or none, to 4+, or marked

oral administration despite their limited solubility in water.

Tolerance Tolerance probably does not exist for the drugs. Idiosyncrasy to these drugs occurs only rarely and may involve skin rashes, hemolytic anemia, thrombocytopenia purpura, and possibly agranulocytosis. This is in contrast to the salicylates to which sensitivity has been reported more frequently.

Preparations and Doses
Acetophenetidin (Phenacetin) Available as a powder. The usual dose is 0.3 g.

Acetaminophen (N-Acetyl-p-Aminophenol) Available as tablets of 0.3 g and as various elixirs.

The use of acetophenetidin with aspirin or salicylate and usually with caffeine, as in the APC (aspirin, phenacetin, caffeine) combination, has been popular for many years, although clinical superiority over aspirin alone has not been demonstrated. The mixture allows a decrease in the dose of the two analgesics, resulting theoretically in a decrease in possible adverse effects, whereas the analgesic activities are additive. Caffeine reduces cerebral blood flow, and it may counteract the dilation or excessive pulsation of cerebral blood vessels implicated in headache pain. Its therapeutic contribution is most questionable, however. For the occasional user of analgesic agents, aspirin produces such minimal risk of side effects that this drug alone probably is preferable.

Toxicity
Blood The most frequent manifestation of acute toxicity of large doses is cyanosis, which is due to the formation of *methemoglobin*. After chronic administration of the drugs to humans, cumulation of methemoglobin is unlikely because of the ready disappearance of the altered pigment from the system.

Acetaminophen has been reported to produce less methemoglobin in man than an equimolar amount of acetophenetidin, probably because there is less likelihood of the formation of a toxic metabolite.

There is considerable variation among individuals in the tendency to form methemoglobin. Children are more susceptible than adults.

Acetophenetidin, especially on long-continued administration of large doses, may give rise to a small amount of altered blood pigment other than methemoglobin. Although it is commonly referred to in the literature as *sulfhemoglobin*, it is not a well-characterized pigment and does not occur in normal blood. Acetaminophen is less apt to produce this abnormal pigment.

A mild *hemolytic anemia* has been reported in many cases with chronic drug ingestion. The deposition of hemosiderin and other iron-associated pigments in the spleen, liver, and kidney following acetophenetidin probably represents hemolyzed erythrocytes.

Kidney Although renal injury has been claimed infrequently during the first 60 years of use of acetophenetidin, clinical investigators reported in 1953 that many persons with chronic renal diseases had been consuming large amounts of analgesic mixtures over many years. Reports, mainly from Switzerland, Scandinavia, Australia, and occasionally the United States, soon followed, associating analgesic abuse with an increasing incidence of interstitial nephritis, tubular and papillary necrosis, and chronic pyelonephritis.

The toxicity has been termed *phenacetin nephritis,* but the pathologic criteria have not been clearly and uniformly defined, and the evidence linking the responses specifically to acetophenetidin rather than to aspirin is very inconclusive. There is little question that the syndrome is associated with analgesic abuse. There is not yet sufficient experience with acetaminophen to evaluate its potential nephrotoxic effect.

Therapeutic Uses These drugs are active antipyretic agents in febrile states. Like the salicylates, their principal use at present is to relieve ordinary aches and pains. They are most effective in pain of moderate intensity, such as headache, osteoarthritis, and dysmenorrhea, and are useful in patients who cannot tolerate salicylates. Gastric bleeding, which has been reported following salicylate administration, is not seen with these drugs.

Acetaminophen is probably the best substitute for aspirin as an antipyretic or analgesic drug, but not as an anti-inflammatory compound. Acetophenetidin and acetaminophen are relatively ineffective for intense or visceral pain.

Phenylbutazone

Phenylbutazone (Fig. 14-2) has been used to a considerable extent in acute gout, rheumatoid arthritis, and other conditions, where it produces a prolonged action. Its similarity in action to cortisone was soon noticed, and, being appreciably less expensive, it was rapidly accepted as a therapeutic substitute in certain conditions. It is not usually employed as an ordinary analgesic for headache and other mild to moderate pain because of its frequent toxicity.

Effect on Organ Systems As far as is known, phenylbutazone acts as an antipyretic and analgesic in much the same way as do salicylates. Its similarity in action to cortisone probably cannot be attributed to stimulation of the pituitary, since large doses in experimental animals do not deplete the adrenals of ascorbic acid. Large doses do not reduce liver glycogen content in experimental animals, as do the salicylates. At high drug concentrations the drug demonstrates some uricosuric actions; that is, it furthers the excretion of uric acid by blocking its tubular reabsorption, thus lowering serum–uric acid levels.

Routes of Administration Generally phenylbutazone is given orally. Intramuscularly there is some pain at the site of injection. Thrombosis of the veins occurs frequently after intravenous administration.

Absorption, Distribution, and Fate Comparison of plasma levels following oral and intramuscular administration indicates that phenylbutazone is absorbed completely from the gastrointestinal tract. Oral administration of the drug results in peak plasma levels within 2 h.

Phenylbutazone is bound to a large extent to the nondiffusible constituents of the plasma. At plasma levels of 50 to 150 mg/liter, which are within the range of therapeutic concentrations, approximately 98 percent of the drug is bound to plasma proteins.

A number of acidic drugs and normal substrates compete with phenylbutazone for binding sites on serum proteins. For example, the anticoagulant warfarin competes for the same binding site on human albumin; and tolbutamide, other sulfonylureas, sulfonamides, and indomethacin apparently behave similarly. Since displacement of a drug from its binding site by phenylbutazone would lead to an increase in the concentration of the freed drug, an increased pharmacologic action of that drug would be expected, such as increased therapeutic or toxic effects. Indeed, clinically phenylbutazone potentiates the anticoagulant effect of warfarin and has produced hemorrhagic complications; it has increased the hypoglycemia following tolbutamide and even insulin.

Experiments with phenylbutazone and other drugs have revealed a remarkable adaptive phenomenon in drug-metabolizing enzymes. Chronic

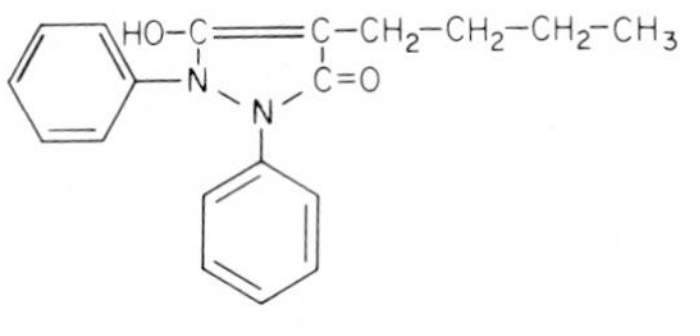

Phenylbutazone

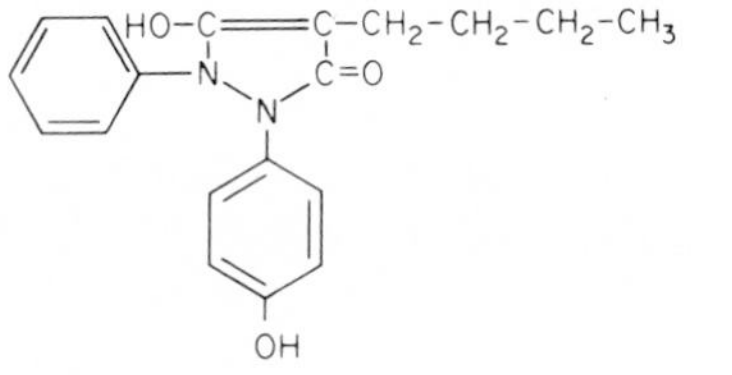

Oxyphenbutazone

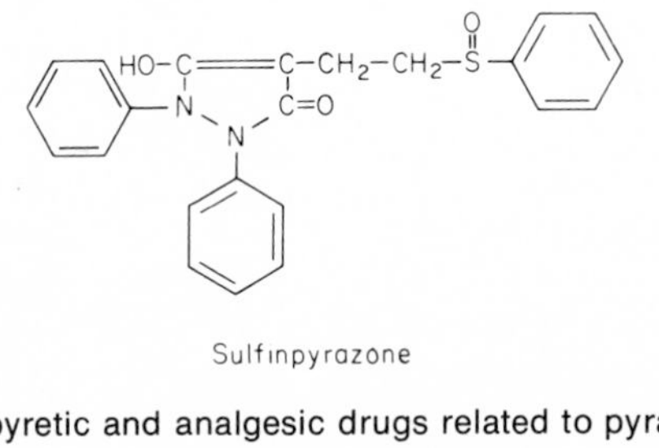

Sulfinpyrazone

Figure 14-2 Antipyretic and analgesic drugs related to pyrazoline.

pretreatment of animals, and apparently of human beings also, with phenylbutazone produces a sharp increase in the rate of drug metabolism by induction of liver microsomal enzyme synthesis.

When phenylbutazone is given to human subjects, virtually all of it undergoes metabolic transformation. The products include several metabolites. One such product has been identified as the *p*-hydroxy derivative of phenylbutazone, oxyphenbutazone. This compound possesses the potent antirheumatic and sodium-retaining properties of the parent drug and is described separately below.

Preparations and Doses Phenylbutazone (Butazolidin) is available as 100-mg tablets. It is also available as a buffered preparation and with steroids. It is usually administered orally at an initial dosage of 300 to 600 mg daily, divided into three or four doses and given with milk or meals to diminish gastric intolerance. This dosage may be continued for 1 week and, if improvement occurs, is followed by maintenance doses gradually reduced to 100 to 200 mg daily. Drug treatment should cease with a reduction in the formed elements of the blood. On restoration of the normal blood picture, treatment with low doses of phenylbutazone may sometimes be resumed, but with great caution.

Toxicity Blood changes are the most common serious toxic effects resulting from the administration of phenylbutazone. The most serious effect is agranulocytosis, which may appear at any time following administration. This blood dyscrasia may have a very rapid onset and does not appear to be associated with high doses of the drug. Some workers point out that the agranulocytosis observed is not an ordinary toxic reaction but a hypersensitivity which takes some time to develop.

The appearance or reactivation of peptic ulceration following phenylbutazone administration has been noted even in the absence of previous history or symptoms of such ulcers. Cases of gastric ulcer and duodenal ulcer perforation during or immediately following phenylbutazone therapy have been described. The ulcers healed on discontinuation of the drug. Some nausea and vomiting have been reported after drug treatment. The effect on gastric mucosa is not a direct one, since it is not abolished when the drug is administered parenterally. Apparently the drug decreases the secretion of mucus by the gastric antrum.

Liver function tests and histologic studies show evidence of *toxic hepatitis* in some patients and a cholangiolitic change in others. Jaundice and increased prothrombin time with purpura have been observed, and toxic cirrhosis has led to death.

Kidney damage has involved hematuria, anuria, and uremia with severe destruction of the convoluted tubules.

Sodium retention due to increased reabsorption of sodium has been observed regularly, associated with retention of water and chloride, and edema formation. Presumably the effect occurs without impairment of general renal function.

Skin irritation in the form of drug rash with an occasional fatal exfoliative dermatitis is not uncommon after the administration of the drug. The skin rash frequently precedes the agranulocytosis by several days or weeks.

Therapeutic Uses The drug has been found to be effective in acute gout, rheumatoid arthritis, osteoarthritis, rheumatoid spondylitis, and related diseases. In acute gout, the response is frequently dramatic, with an initial relief of pain and gradual resolution of other signs such as joint inflammation. Colchicine is probably preferred unless the patient cannot tolerate its gastrointestinal effects or derives no benefit from it. If phenylbutazone is used, it should be employed only for 2 or 3 days.

If phenylbutazone is indicated, the patient should be under the close supervision of a physician and should receive frequent blood checks, including white cell and differential counts, even though this procedure will not always predict incipient toxicity. Patients with a history of peptic ulcer, drug allergy, blood dyscrasia, or hepatic or renal disease or those who may be subject to edema or congestive heart failure should not receive the drug. A diet low in sodium is helpful in view of the sodium retention produced by drug treatment. Fever, lesions of the mouth, and sore throat associated with phenylbutazone therapy may be symptoms of agranulocytosis, and drug therapy should be terminated upon appearance of these symptoms. Blood dyscrasias or allergic reactions, rash, symptoms of peptic ulcer, gastrointestinal bleeding, or hepatic dysfunctions are also contraindications for continued treatment. In general, the drug should be used for short periods of 1 week. An exception to this rule is the case of ankylosing spondylitis which is unresponsive to other medications.

Oxyphenbutazone

Oxyphenbutazone (Tandearil) (Fig. 14-2) was isolated during studies on the metabolic products of phenylbutazone. It differs from the parent drug in bearing a hydroxyl group on one of the benzene rings and possesses the potent antirheumatic and sodium retention properties of phenylbutazone. When administered, the metabolite is said to produce somewhat less gastrointestinal distress than the parent drug and may be preferred for this reason.

It is readily absorbed from the gastrointestinal tract, has a biological half-life in humans of about 12 h, is highly bound to serum albumin, and is excreted in metabolized form which includes a glucuronide.

Like phenylbutazone, the drug has anti-inflammatory, antipyretic, and analgesic properties. The drug decreases swelling and stiffness in joints in various rheumatic diseases and may be useful, like phenylbutazone, in the treatment of acute gout, active rheumatoid arthritis, and related diseases when used for short periods of time.

The use of oxyphenbutazone is like that of phenylbutazone. Dosage is described under Phenylbutazone. Maintenance doses of 400 mg/day are considered maximal.

Because of the high incidence and possible severity of adverse reactions to the drug, it should be used only when safer medication is ineffective. Adverse reactions and contraindications are the same as those described earlier in this chapter under Phenylbutazone.

Sulfinpyrazone

Pharmacologic evaluation of various analogues of phenylbutazone for antirheumatic and uricosuric properties revealed that the 4-phenylthioethyl derivative had marked uricosuric activity. Subsequently it was observed that this compound is metabolically altered to the sulfoxide, one of the most potent of uricosuric compounds. The latter drug is currently available as sulfinpyrazone (Anturane) (Fig. 14-2).

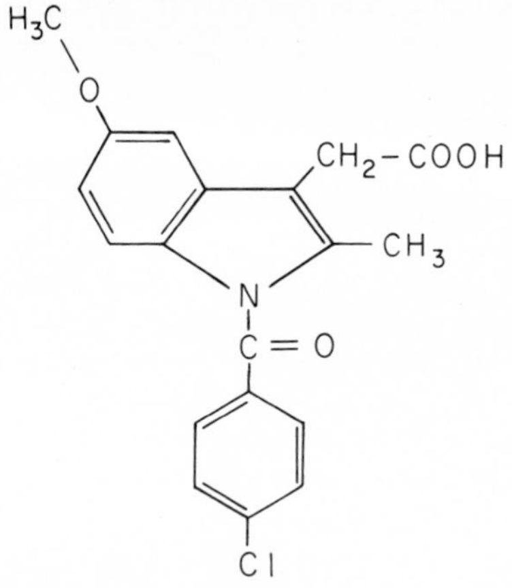

Figure 14-3 Indomethacin.

Indomethacin

Indomethacin (Indocin) (Fig. 14-3) is an anti-inflammatory agent used in joint diseases such as osteoarthritis and ankylosing spondylitis. It also possesses antipyretic and analgesic properties similar to those of phenylbutazone. It has been postulated that the drug inhibits leukocyte motility in the treatment of acute gout. Like many other anti-inflammatory drugs, it uncouples oxidative phosphorylation.

Absorption, Distribution, and Fate Indomethacin is absorbed promptly after oral administration, and peak plasma levels are reached within 2 to 4 h. About 90 percent of the drug in the plasma is bound to protein. About 90 percent of a single dose is excreted in 1 to 2 days, the mean half-life being about 10 h. In the urine the compound exists entirely as the glucuronide. Tubular secretion of indomethacin is inhibited by probenecid. The drug crosses the placental barrier.

Preparation and Dose Regular therapy should be initiated with small doses (25 mg twice daily) to minimize adverse reactions. Doses may be increased gradually until an effective level has been reached. Doses larger than 200 mg are not recommended. Upon control of the acute phases of rheumatoid arthritis, the dose should be reduced to a satisfactory maintenance level.

Toxicity The untoward effects of this drug are such that about 15 percent of patients discontinue therapy. About 20 to 30 percent of patients receiving indomethacin complain of headache, a smaller percentage of vertigo and mental confusion. These toxicities may disappear with continued use but warrant care with performance tasks such as driving. These symptoms may be alleviated by lowering the dose or giving it in divided amounts. Nausea, epigastric burning, stomatitis, and diarrhea also occur in 25 percent of patients. The gastrointestinal symptoms may be diminished by taking the drug after meals and with milk, but may also force discontinuation of therapy. Indomethacin is ulcerogenic and produces gastrointestinal bleeding and anemia. Aplastic anemia has apparently resulted from the drug. Hemoglobin determinations and other hematologic examinations are therefore indicated. Edema, blurred vision, tinnitus, and skin rashes may follow drug therapy. Epilepsy, parkinsonism, and emotional problems may be aggravated. Children may be particularly sensitive to this drug, and several deaths have been reported.

Therapeutic Use Indomethacin is of limited use in the treatment of rheumatoid arthritis. Certain cases derive benefit from it when it is added to the basic salicylate treatment program.

Indomethacin is very effective in acute gout and is considered by some clinicians to be the drug of choice. Indomethacin may be used together with probenecid in the treatment of gout since it does not block the uricosuric action of the latter.

Probenecid

As with salicylates and other uricosuric drugs, it is possible to show that very low doses of probenecid (Benemid), Fig. 14-4, block tubular secretion of urate; at conventional doses, however, inhibition of reabsorption of urate predominates.

Mechanism of Action Probenecid competitively inhibits the carrier system of renal tubular uric acid reabsorption in man.

Absorption, Fate, and Excretion Probenecid is absorbed readily from the gastrointestinal tract. The free acid or its soluble salts are equally well absorbed, reaching optimal plasma levels in about

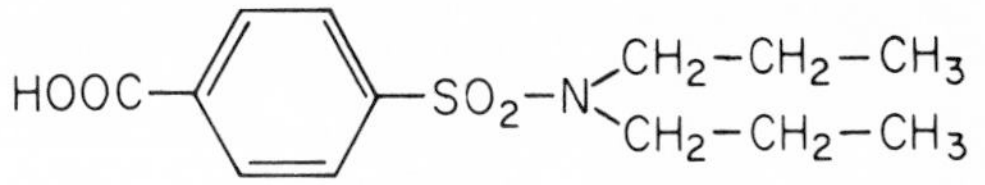

Figure 14-4 Probenecid.

2 to 4 h. More than three-fourths of the probenecid is bound to plasma albumin. The drug is excreted slowly, largely in the form of metabolites and a small amount of the unchanged compound.

Toxicity Although probenecid is well tolerated and the incidence of untoward effects is low at the usual dose, occasionally patients may experience nausea. The incidence of nausea can be reduced by taking the drug with food or an antacid or by reducing daily dosage. Skin rashes may appear in about 5 percent of the patients, and hypersensitivity reactions in 0.3 percent. Serious anaphylactoid reactions are extremely rare. These include massive necrosis of the liver and the nephrotic syndrome.

In patients receiving sulfonamides and oral hypoglycemic drugs concurrently with probenecid, blood levels of these drugs should be watched, since competition for excretion by the kidney may produce cumulative toxicity. In about 10 percent of patients receiving probenecid the rapid elimination of urate may precipitate an acute attack of gout.

Therapy of Gout Probenecid produces a large negative balance of uric acid when first administered, particularly at a time when the uric acid concentration in the plasma is high. It may be combined with sulfinpyrazone for enhanced uricosuric action. A uricosuric agent, like probenecid, is of no value in relieving the pain and inflammation in acute bouts of the disease and may actually aggravate the condition unless administered with colchicine. In refractory cases, allopurinol may also be combined with probenecid.

Salicylate even at uricosuric doses should not be administered with probenecid, since the actions of the two drugs are antagonistic; if an analgesic agent is needed, acetaminophen may be used. The use of chlorothiazide, hydrochlorothiazide, and related drugs in hypertension often results in urate retention because of depression of urate tubular secretion. Probenecid is effective in furthering the excretion of uric acid without altering the diuretic effects of these drugs.

Allopurinol

Allopurinol (Zyloprim) is a different type of agent for the treatment of gout and other hyperuricemias.

Mechanism of Action Allopurinol inhibits xanthine oxidase and thus reduces the conversion of body purines to uric acid.

Effect on Organ Systems In animals allopurinol produces no particular effect on the kidney except at very high doses, when xanthine may deposit. No evidence of significant action on hematopoietic, gastrointestinal, hepatic, vascular, or central nervous systems has been detected.

Route of Administration The drug is normally given orally.

Tolerance No appreciable difference in drug action has been found between acute and chronic administration, and xanthine oxidase levels were not induced or depressed by long-term drug treatment.

Preparation and Dose Allopurinol is available in tablets of 100 and 300 mg. Usually, sufficient drug is given to lower serum urate to normal levels. The usual dose is 200 to 300 mg/day in divided doses for mild gout, and 400 to 600 mg/day for moderately severe tophaceous gout. For the prevention of nephropathy during cancer chemotherapy, when considerable destruction of nucleic acids takes place, daily treatment up to 800 mg is recommended for 2 to 3 days. Fluid intake to assure urinary output of 2 liters/day, preferably slightly alkaline, is desirable. If mercaptopurine is also administered, the dose of this carcinostatic drug should be reduced, since its catabolism is prevented.

Toxicity Maculopapular skin rashes have been reported in about 3 percent of patients; occasionally exfoliative urticarial and purpuric lesions accompanied by fever may result, especially at higher doses. The development of pruritus should signal discontinuance of therapy with the drug. The onset of these rashes may be slow. Some gastrointestinal upset, drowsiness, hepatotoxicity, bone marrow re-

actions, and symptoms of idiosyncrasy have been observed. A few cases of a diffuse vasculitis have been reported. Children and nursing mothers normally should not receive the drug. Toxicity probably is limited because xanthine oxidase deficiency in xanthinuric patients apparently is not serious, and levels of hypoxanthine and xanthine are well within limits of solubility and clearance.

Therapeutic Uses Allopurinol is used in primary hyperuricemia, as in gout, and in secondary hyperuricemia resulting from malignancies, psoriasis, the use of thiazide diuretics, or the treatment of neoplastic diseases. The drug is especially useful in severe gouty arthritis or in individuals who form renal urate stones. It also effectively prevents recurrence of uric acid nephrolithiasis.

Allopurinol is probably preferred to uricosuric drugs when stones are already present in the urinary tract. Once begun, therapy is usually continued indefinitely.

Colchicine

Source and Chemistry Colchicine is an alkaloid found in the meadow saffron, or autumn crocus. Aside from its use in the therapy of acute gouty arthritis for about 1,500 years, colchicine is of considerable biologic interest because of its remarkable ability to arrest cell division in metaphase.

Mechanism of Action The way in which this drug relieves attacks of gout is not well understood. Colchicine has no effect on the urinary excretion of uric acid, its biosynthesis, or its plasma levels. There seems to be little evidence that it acts primarily as an analgesic, and it is usually ineffective in other arthralgias.

Toxicity Gastrointestinal symptoms after colchicine are common. They begin with nausea and abdominal discomfort, followed by violent and uncontrollable vomiting and diarrhea, spasm of the bladder, and great prostration. With somewhat higher doses, bone marrow depression, peripheral neuritis, myopathy, anuria, and alopecia have occasionally been reported.

Therapeutic Uses Administration of the drug should begin at the earliest possible moment after the appearance of one or more symptoms suggestive of acute articular distress. An acute attack of gout requires the ingestion of one tablet every hour until there is an unmistakable subsidence of articular symptoms or until the development of gastrointestinal distress, whichever subjective reaction is first observed. Usually the total amount of drug required is between 6 and 8 mg, but it depends on the severity of the attack. Should a second full course be indicated, it should not be given for at least 48 h following the termination of the first course. If the drug is given intravenously for a more rapid response, no more than 5 mg should be given, with no oral supplements of drug. In case of renal impairment, the dosage of colchicine should be reduced.

Chapter 15

Drug Dependence

TERMS CONCERNED WITH DRUG DEPENDENCE AND ABUSE

The terminology of drug dependence essentially derived from the concept of drug enslavement and designated different degrees of enslavement or compulsion to seek and take drugs. *Habituation* refers to the pattern of repeatedly taking a drug when the need is small, the dose is not increased, and no physical dependence on the drug is produced. *Psychologic dependence* generally means that the effect of the drug satisfies some psychologic need and is gratifying to the individual. Although habituation has frequently been equated with psychologic dependence, the latter term alludes to a mechanism underlying drug-taking behavior, while the former designates the pattern of drug-taking behavior. *Addiction* refers to a pattern of repeated drug-taking behavior where the need or compulsion is much stronger than it is in habituation. This definition of addiction has been formalized and extended to include, in addition to

a strong compulsion, the tendency to increase dose and the production of physical dependence (see below).

Both the Expert Committee on Addiction-producing Drugs of the World Health Organization and the Committee on Problems of Drug Dependence of the National Academy of Sciences have recommended that the general term *drug dependence* be substituted for the terms *addiction* and *habituation*, and that this general term be modified by the particular drug or groups of drugs abused (for example, drug dependence of the morphine type, drug dependence of the barbiturate type, etc.).

The term *drug abuse* is now frequently used to designate the inappropriate as well as excessive use of drugs. Drug abuse also implies that harm is done to the individual user and/or to society in general.

Perhaps one of the most effective ways of limiting drug abuse and dependence has been to determine the abuse potentiality of drugs, both new and old, and subject the agents to appropriate controls according to their potentiality for abuse. Further, *physicians should be clearly aware of the abuse potential of drugs in order that they practice knowledgeable and intelligent prescribing patterns*. Three major factors determine the abuse potential of drugs: (1) their capacity to induce compulsive drug-seeking behavior; (2) their toxicity; and (3) the social consequences of abusing drugs as well as the attitude of society toward drug abuse.

TOLERANCE AND DEPENDENCE

Drugs which induce tolerance and physical dependence seem to produce strong compulsive drug-seeking behavior which is characterized by frequent relapse following withdrawal or detoxification.

Tolerance

Tolerance to the actions of a drug may refer to several types of phenomena. When tolerance develops very rapidly, following either a single dose or a few doses given over a short period of time, it is called *acute tolerance*. When the drug must be administered over a long period of time to induce tolerance, it is called *chronic tolerance*. *Cross-tolerance* exists when tolerance to one drug confers tolerance to another. With some drugs under certain conditions, although the initial response is diminished, tolerance can be attained by increasing the dose. This type of tolerance is seen with barbiturates. With other types of drugs, partial or total refractoriness to the effects of the drugs may develop. Still another type of tolerance is when the initial response diminishes and is replaced by another response. An example of this type of tolerance is the changing of the euphoria produced initially by morphine or heroin to the lethargic feeling experienced when the drug is administered chronically. Another type of tolerance is seen when the action persists during chronic administration of stabilization doses, although additional large doses of the drug do not produce any additional changes. This type of tolerance develops in response to the respiratory depressant and miotic effects of morphine.

Physical Dependence

Physical dependence is a state of drug-induced physiologic change which becomes manifest as an abstinence syndrome when the effective dose of the drug is diminished by either withdrawing the agent or by administering appropriate antagonists which displace it from its site of action. When physical dependence develops at a very rapid rate over a matter of hours, it is called *acute physical dependence*. When it is produced by prolonged treatment with a drug, it is called *chronic physical dependence*. The abstinence syndrome that results from termination of the drug is termed *withdrawal abstinence*. In contradistinction, abstinence produced by administering a competitive antagonist such as nalorphine or naloxone to a subject physically dependent on morphine is called *precipitated abstinence* (sometimes referred to as acute abstinence).

Thus far, there have been four groups of drugs which have been unequivocally shown to produce tolerance and physical dependence: (1) the narcotic analgesics such as morphine, (2) narcotic antagonists with agonistic actions such as nalorphine, (3) sedative-hypnotic agents such as barbiturates, and (4) alcohol.

Physical dependence is closely associated with the phenomenon of tolerance. In determining the type of physical dependence an agent produces, both cross-tolerance and cross-dependence have been utilized. As an example, subjects tolerant to and physically dependent on morphine will be cross-tolerant to other narcotic analgesics such as methadone. Furthermore, other narcotic analgesics can be substituted, and if administered in sufficient doses, will completely suppress abstinence signs and symptoms in morphine-dependent subjects. It is a general rule that drugs of one type will suppress abstinence syndromes of drugs of the same type, but will not suppress abstinence of drugs producing different types of dependence. Actually, only certain types of cross-suppression have been studied, so it is only for these types that we are absolutely certain about the presence or absence of cross-suppression.

DEPENDENCE OF THE MORPHINE TYPE

The Bureau of Narcotics, on the basis of criminal records, estimated that there were approximately 100,000 active narcotic addicts in the United States in 1974. Most of these addicts lived in slum areas of large metropolitan cities, with the majority belonging to minority groups. Conditions in these areas are a powerful determinant for, and certainly predisposes individuals to, narcotic experimentation and abuse.

One of the drugs most frequently used by addicts in the United States is heroin. Over the past several years, heroin abuse has become more widespread, and its incidence is increasing. It has been estimated that there are over 375,000 heroin abusers in the United States alone. The drug has a somewhat more rapid onset of action than morphine when administered subcutaneously and intravenously, but is probably converted rapidly to morphine in the body. Heroin is 2 to 3 times more potent than morphine, which may be an important consideration for those engaged in the illegal importation of narcotics. Other minor differences between morphine and heroin have been reported, such as the greater capacity of morphine to produce the sensation of pins and needles and itching.

Narcotic analgesics produce a number of effects such as nausea, vomiting, profuse sweating, itching, and feelings of lethargy and sedation, some of which may be quite unpleasant to a naive subject; however, these agents also produce euphoria, tranquility, and somnolence, which to other individuals are very desirable effects.

The subjective changes produced by narcotic analgesics in nontolerant subjects closely resemble those produced by amphetamine and include feelings of relaxation, contentment, well-being, cheerfulness, and increased energy. These feelings may be associated with purposive or nonpurposive motor activity. In some individuals, or at other times, narcotic analgesics produce sedation. This may take the form of an apathetic detachment sometimes called "coasting" or may involve transient episodes of sleep spontaneously interrupted by waking, which is termed being "on the nod."

With continued use of narcotics, some effects are diminished (tolerance); and some effects are changed. Thus, with continued use the analgesic effect is diminished. Pupillary constriction and constipation persist throughout a period of chronic intoxication with an agent such as morphine, but are not increased even when very large additional doses of the narcotic are administered. Euphoria and feelings of well-being produced by morphine are replaced by feelings of lethargy and apathy during chronic administration.

The Narcotic Abstinence Syndrome

Both the precipitated and withdrawal abstinence syndromes in subjects chronically physically dependent on most narcotic analgesics show essentially the same spectrum of signs and symptoms and differ only with regard to their time course. Precipitated abstinence becomes manifest within a few minutes following the administration of an antagonist such as nalorphine or naloxone. The evolution of the abstinence syndrome following abrupt withdrawal is much slower but does vary with the drug of addiction. In a subject addicted to morphine, the initial abstinence symptoms emerge 6 to 12 h after the last dose and consist of an awareness of the impending illness and feelings of restlessness, tiredness, and weakness. After 12 h, certain signs of abstinence such as yawning, lacrimation, rhinorrhea, and perspiration emerge, and the patient may enter into a fitful sleep called "yen sleep." After 24 h, the patient becomes increasingly restless, twitching of various muscle groups appears, and the patient complains of back and leg pains and hot and cold flashes as well as chills. At the same time, other signs of disordered function of the autonomic nervous system become apparent, including fever, increase in both rate and depth of respiration, elevation of blood pressure and increased pulse rate, and dilation of previously constricted pupils. By 48 h the abstinence syndrome is nearing its peak, and the patient is nauseated, retches, vomits, has diarrhea, eats and drinks very little, and loses weight rapidly. The patient may lie in a fetal position, twitching and turning and covering him or herself with blankets even in hot weather. After 72 h the abstinence syndrome begins to subside slowly. Approximately 1 to 2 months after the drug has been withdrawn, autonomic signs return to normal or preaddiction level. At about this time a new syndrome emerges which has been called *protracted or secondary abstinence*. In humans, this syndrome is characterized by a slight lowering of blood pressure, pulse rate, and body temperature, decreased responsivity of the respiratory center to carbon dioxide, and a small degree of constriction of the pupils. This state persists for at least 4 to 6 months. During protracted abstinence, there is hyperresponsivity of the autonomic nervous system to nociceptive stimuli and an increased excretion of epinephrine in the urine.

Potential Hazards

There are several medical diseases and problems associated with narcotic addiction which are usually consequences of using unsterile techniques in administration of drugs. These include abscesses, hepatitis, subacute bacterial endocarditis, and tetanus. In past years, malaria has been another such illness. At the present time, there is evidence that an anicteric viral hepatitis is endemic among narcotic addicts, and special care should be taken when obtaining blood from patients suspected of being addicts.

Treatment

Treatment of narcotic addicts poses many practical problems. Under optimum conditions, the addict should be hospitalized on a ward in which there is a very close control of all drugs, including narcotics, preferably in a hospital specializing in the treatment of drug addiction. After the patient has been thoroughly examined and his or her physical condition assessed, the patient should be detoxified. This can be done with little discomfort by substituting methadone for the narcotic the addict has been taking. Methadone has two advantages: (1) it can be administered orally, and (2) it has a much longer duration of action than has morphine. A dose of 1 mg methadone will substitute for approximately 4 mg morphine sulfate in the dependent subject. When the patient is stabilized on methadone the dose can be reduced approximately 50 percent every other day, and methadone can be stopped in most patients by the sixth to tenth day. For several weeks after withdrawal, the patient may be quite restless and unable to sleep at night. Barbiturates, meprobamate, chlordiazepoxide, and phenothiazine tranquilizers have been employed to alleviate these late-coming minimal symptoms of primary abstinence.

During the past several years, a number of new treatment procedures have been proposed for the management of addicts after detoxification. Addicts may be encouraged to participate in *self-help* groups such as Alcoholics Anonymous, Addicts

Anonymous, and Narcotics Anonymous. The success of these organizations in helping dependent individuals depends on the patient's personal commitment to remain abstinent and upon peer group support. Several *addict communities*, such as Synanon and Day-top Lodge, have become widely known. In these communities, which have a strong leadership hierarchy and a very authoritarian structure, an attempt is made to indoctrinate, in a meaningful way, a body of community-oriented values through leadership, self-help, and group help. *Halfway houses* provide a transitional state for addicts in their evolution from a closely controlled prison environment into the greater freedom of society at large.

Two chemotherapeutic approaches to treating narcotic-dependent subjects have been introduced and are undergoing clinical trial. In the *methadone maintenance program*, in which patients are made dependent upon very large doses (approximately 100 mg/day orally) of the narcotic analgesic, methadone, a high level of cross-tolerance to morphine, heroin, and other narcotic analgesics is produced. As long as patients are maintained or maintain themselves on methadone, they are largely refractory to the subjective changes and effects produced by "street" heroin or other narcotic analgesics. While on methadone, patients appear to have better social adjustment (for example, better rates of employment and fewer arrests) than they had achieved prior to methadone treatment. The disadvantage of the methadone maintenance program is that patients thus have a high level of dependence on a narcotic analgesic.

A second chemotherapeutic approach proposed for the treatment of narcotic addiction is the use of a narcotic antagonist such as naloxone which antagonizes the effects of heroin and morphine, preventing the manifestation of the euphoric action and the development of physical dependence. Naloxone is administered at a dose of 0.8 mg/day intravenously after the patient has been detoxified with gradually decreasing doses of methadone. The patient does not receive supplemental doses of methadone while on narcotic antagonist therapy. The patient is rendered "drug free" except for the narcotic antagonist, which is nonaddicting. Patients on narcotic antagonists have thus been able to function without the disadvantages associated with methadone maintenance stated above. Recently, a newer narcotic antagonist, naltrexone, has been under investigation and appears to have properties similar to naloxone. However, naltrexone has a longer duration of action than does naloxone, and can be administered orally at a dose of 50 mg/day.

DEPENDENCE OF THE BARBITURATE TYPE

The abuse of barbiturates, sedative-hypnotics, alcohol, and minor tranquilizers continues to be a widespread phenomenon in the United States and Europe. These agents produce sleep, motor incoordination, and physical dependence. Four types of sedative-hypnotic abuse are common:

1 Sedative-hypnotics are used in excess to cope with anxiety feelings and distressing emotions.
2 Sedative hypnotics are used in excess to obtain a feeling of well-being, euphoria, or stimulation. Although the subjective effects of barbiturates can clearly be distinguished from those of narcotic analgesics, even narcotic addicts indicate a level of liking for barbiturates comparable to that obtained with highly euphorogenic doses of morphine. Some of the stimulatory changes induced by barbiturates have been interpreted as representing a release from inhibitory influences.
3 Barbiturates are used in combination with amphetamine or to counteract the stimulatory effects of amphetamine and to induce sleep.
4 Abusers of alcohol and narcotics may also abuse barbiturates and other sedative-hypnotic agents.

Chronic intoxication with barbiturates is similar to chronic alcohol intoxication and is characterized by signs of motor incoordination such as ataxia, dysarthria, dysmetria, and nystagmus, and difficulties in thinking, confusion, and emotional lability. Only partial and low-grade tolerance develops to the effects of barbiturates, with upper limits of intake ranging from 1.0 to 2.5 g/day orally. During the course of chronic intoxication, the most serious toxicologic effects are related to motor incoordination, which is responsible for self-inflicted injuries and involvement in accidents, and emotional lability, which results in quarrelsomeness and fights. Barbiturates, sedative-hypnotic drugs, minor tranquilizers, and alcohol may act synergistically or have additive effects which can result in severe, and at times fatal, intoxication.

The Barbiturate Abstinence Syndrome

If barbiturates are withdrawn from patients who are physically dependent on them, a serious abstinence syndrome emerges. During the period when the addict is becoming sober, many of the signs of chronic intoxication disappear, and the patient's improvement may give a false indication of recovery. From 12 to 24 h after the drug has been withdrawn, the patient addicted to the shorter-acting barbiturates complains of feelings of anxiety and weakness, loss of appetite, and insomnia, and exhibits coarse tremors. During the next 24 h, the abstinence syndrome increases in intensity and the following signs and symptoms may emerge if the level of dependence is sufficient: vomiting, hypotension, tachycardia, moderate or severe orthostatic hypotension, hyperactive deep tendon reflexes, fever, fasciculations, uncontrolled tremors, and grand mal convulsions. Seizures have been observed as late as 7 days after withdrawal. In addition, some patients may have psychotic episodes, either following seizures or without seizures, with visual and auditory hallucinations and delusions. The most serious consequences of barbiturate withdrawal are grand mal convulsions, delirium, and pyrexia, all of which may endanger life. During withdrawal, EEG abnormalities consist of random slow waves, spikes, paroxysmal spike and slow-wave discharges, and high-frequency high-voltage spikes, as well as susceptibility to photic stimulation.

Because of the serious nature of barbiturate abstinence, withdrawal should always be carried out in a hospital where drug use can be carefully controlled. Patients dependent on barbiturates should not be treated on an ambulatory basis. Pentobarbital or another barbiturate should be given until the patient is mildly intoxicated. When a stabilization dose has been established, the drug should be withdrawn slowly at a rate not exceeding 0.1 g/day. If convulsions have already occurred or delirium has developed, these should be controlled by giving 0.3 to 0.5 g pentobarbital or equivalent amounts of other barbiturates. The patient should then be given a mildly intoxicating stabilization dose every 4 to 6 h. Narcotic analgesics will not suppress the abstinence syndrome of patients physically dependent on barbiturates or other sedative-hypnotic agents.

A large number of agents, including ethyl alcohol, chloral hydrate, paraldehyde, meprobamate, glutethimide, ethinamate, ethchlorvynol, methyprylon, chlordiazepoxide, diazepam, and oxazepam, when taken chronically in sufficiently large doses, produce a type of physical dependence similar to that produced by barbiturates, if not indistinguishable from it. Dependence on these agents should be treated in the same manner and as cautiously as barbiturate dependence.

COCAINE AND AMPHETAMINE DEPENDENCE

Cocaine and amphetamine dependence are an important problem in the United States. Cocaine, amphetamines, and related drugs produce feelings of elation and, in so doing, alleviate fear and anxiety. Chewing of the coca leaf is practiced extensively by Indians in South America, particularly by laborers of the lower economic strata, to relieve feelings of fatigue and hunger. Cocaine is abused in this country primarily as a "spree" drug. The American addict usually takes the drug intravenously, although in the past snuffing of cocaine has enjoyed popularity. The latter practice can produce perforation of the nasal septum. Cocaine is commonly used with morphine and other opiates in a mixture called a *speedball*. Intravenous injection of cocaine produces a short-lived feeling of elation. The cocaine abuser may repeat the dose at frequent intervals to recapture these feelings and become acutely intoxicated. Acute intoxication is characterized by signs of autonomic stimulation including tachycardia, mydriasis, and hypertension, and by signs of central nervous system stimulation including hyperreflexia, tremors, muscle twitches, convulsions, delusions, and hallucinations. The patient suffering from cocaine paranoia may commit acts of violence.

The toxicologic effects of chronic cocaine abuse consist of emotional lability, loss of appetite, mental impairment, and the tendency to withdraw from social contacts. The excitant effects of cocaine, such as tremors, convulsions, delusions, and hallucinations, can readily be treated with barbiturates.

DEPENDENCE OF THE LSD TYPE

The use and abuse of LSD-like hallucinogens, like other abuse problems, has its roots in antiquity. Hallucinogens have been used in religious rites and as intoxicants for many centuries and in many societies; however, their use had been quite limited in most Western civilizations until the 1960s. The various LSD-like hallucinogens which are abused include LSD (lysergic acid diethylamide), mescaline and peyote, psilocin and psilocybin, dimethyltryptamine and STP (DOM or 2,5-dimethoxy-4-methylamphetamine). One of the reasons given for the use and abuse of these agents is that they increase insight, understanding, and enlightenment. There is no hard and objective evidence that LSD produces these effects, regardless of how LSD-induced changes are perceived and interpreted by the user.

Objective assessments of the effects of LSD and other LSD-like psychotogens show that the effects are dose-dependent. In most subjects, dose levels of 1 mg/kg or less may commonly produce euphoric and pleasurable subjective changes and feelings of relaxation. Larger doses tend to produce feelings of anxiety, perceptual distortion and hallucinations, and feelings of unreality which may be interpreted by many subjects as dysphoria. There is great individual susceptibility to the effects of the psychotogens. Of particular concern are several types of responses to LSD that have been reported.

1 Some subjects who take LSD have depressive reactions and attempt suicide. There have been several deaths reported following the use of LSD in which persons jumped from high places or walked into a flow of traffic. Whether these were intentional suicide attempts or the consequences of distorted judgment and perception is not known.

2 There have been several hundred cases of prolonged psychotic episodes or anxiety reactions reported following the use of LSD. The common type of psychotic reaction has been a schizophrenic state with paranoid delusions or hallucinations. Some of the patients exhibiting psychotic reactions have had previous histories of mental illness and psychosis, others have not. Psychotic episodes may last for several days to many months.

3 Some subjects have had spontaneous recurrence of delusions, hallucinations, perceptual distortion, or anxiety reactions many months after the last ingestion of LSD.

Part Four

Autonomic Nervous System

Chapter 16

Introduction to the Autonomic Nervous System

GENERAL CONSIDERATIONS

The autonomic nervous system provides one of the important means whereby organisms regulate the activities of the major organ systems so that the limits for survival are not surpassed. This system has been organized into two specialized subsystems, the parasympathetic and the sympathetic. In controlling bodily function under normal physiologic conditions the parasympathetic nervous system usually predominates, whereas the sympathetic nervous system generally directs the response of the organism to various environmental stresses. When mammals are confronted with danger, the heart beats more rapidly and more forcefully, the pupils dilate to permit more light to reach the retina, blood flow through skeletal muscles is enhanced, blood sugar is elevated, the sphincters of the alimentary tract close, and the mind becomes more alert. Each of these responses is brought about by the activation of the autonomic nervous system.

ANATOMIC CONSIDERATIONS

The pathways of each of the two major subdivisions of the autonomic nervous system consist of two neurons. The cell body of the first is found in the brain or spinal cord, and that of the second outside the CNS, either in discrete ganglia or within the innervated organ. In general, the preganglionic fiber is myelinated, and the postganglionic fiber is non-myelinated, but there are exceptions.

The *parasympathetic division* of the autonomic nervous system, with its preganglionic cell bodies in the brain steam (tectobulbar) and the sacral cord (S2–S4), is also called the *craniosacral division* (or tectobulbosacral division). The cells of origin of the postganglionic fibers of the parasympathetic division are near, on, or within the innervated organ. The cranial division of the parasympathetic system distributes fiber through the oculomotor (III), facial (VII), glossopharyngeal (IX), vagal (X), and bulbar accessory (XI) nerves to terminal ganglia which innervate structures of the head, neck, thoracic cavity, and abdominal viscera (with the exception of the descending colon and the pelvic viscera, which are innervated by the sacral division). The sacral division arises from the sacral cord (S2–S4) and forms the pelvic nerve (*nervus erigens*), which synapses in terminal ganglia near, on, or within the innervated organs. Only in the head are there found discrete parasympathetic ganglia separated from the innervated structure.

The *sympathetic division* of the autonomic nervous system, with its preganglionic cell bodies in the intermediomedial or intermediolateral column of the thoracic and upper lumbar (T1–L2 or L3, and more rarely C8, C7, or L4) spinal cord, is called the *thoracolumbar division*. Sympathetic preganglionic fibers pass out of the spinal cord with the ventral root and into the chain ganglia through the *white rami communicantes*. The cells of origin of the postganglionic sympathetic nerves are in autonomic ganglia of three types: (1) chain or paravertebral; (2) collateral or prevertebral; (3) terminal or peripheral. The synapses of sympathetic nerves occur in the first two ganglia, but occasional sympathetic nerves synapse in terminal ganglia.

When compared with other units of the nervous system, autonomic ganglia are regarded as relatively simple structures consisting of the small preganglionic nerve terminals, the ganglionic cells and their associated dendritic processes, and satellite or glial cells. There are, however, marked variations in the organizational patterns found among ganglia of the same species and between the same ganglia of different species. In mammalian sympathetic ganglia, the ratio of preganglionic fibers is of the order of 1:20. By contrast, mammalian parasympathetic ganglia usually have a ratio of 1:1 or 1:2 (for example, ciliary ganglion). The differences between sympathetic and parasympathetic ganglia, together with the widespread distribution of postganglionic sympathetic fibers as compared with postganglionic parasympathetic fibers, is often regarded as the anatomic basis for the different physiologic characteristics of the two divisions of the autonomic nervous system. While activation of the sympathetic division results in a generalized response of many organ systems, activation of the parasympathetic division results in a more localized and discrete response. The organization of para-

sympathetic innervation by the vagus nerve is a notable exception to this generalization. The ratio of preganglionic vagal fibers to postganglionic fibers in the plexuses of Auerbach and Meissner is about 1:8,000.

PHYSIOLOGIC CONSIDERATIONS

The actions of the various autonomic nerves of effector cells are summarized in Table 16-1 and require little additional comment. Many organs receive both sympathetic and parasympathetic fibers and are influenced in opposite ways by the two divisions of the autonomic nervous system. In some instances, for example, heart and intestine, the organs are endowed with inherent activity and require dual innervation with opposing actions in order to elevate or suppress inherent activity when appropriate. The cells of these organ systems are directly influenced by both sympathetic and parasympathetic nerves. In other instances, control of function is regulated by opposing actions on different effector cells. For example, pupillary constriction occurs following the activation of parasympathetic nerves to the circular muscles of the iris or following the inactivation of sympathetic nerves to the radial muscles of the iris. Conversely, pupillary dilation occurs following activation of sympathetic fibers to the radial muscles or the inactivation of parasympathetic fibers to the circular muscles. Stated in other terms, the circular muscles of the iris are under the control of parasympathetic nerves, and the radial muscles are under sympathetic control, with pupil size determined by the interplay between the sympathetic and parasympathetic nerves. Parallel action of sympathetic and parasympathetic innervation to effector cells is illustrated in a superficial way by the response of salivary glands to stimulation. The parallelism is incomplete because sympathetic activation of salivation results in a thick, viscid saliva and parasympathetic activation results in a copious, watery saliva. The increase in conduction rate in atrial fibers following either sympathetic or vagal stimulation is a second example of a parallel action of the two types of autonomic nerves. However, the increase in atrial conduction by vagal stimulation is not a constant finding.

It follows from these considerations that the activity of most organ systems reflects a balance of modulating influences between the sympathetic and parasympathetic nervous systems. Blockade of the sympathetic nervous system by drugs can be expected to result in an exaggeration of parasym-

pathetic activity. Conversely, blockade of parasympathetic activity results in the exaggeration of sympathetic activity. When both pathways are blocked, the effect on the organ system depends upon the status of organ activity prior to the blockade and on the pathway that normally dominates the organ system.

SYNAPTIC TRANSMISSION

The release of transmitter substances from the small, unmyelinated nerve endings is initiated by nerve action potentials (Fig. 16-1). Obviously, drugs or procedures modifying conduction of impulses in the nerve terminals can be expected to produce corresponding changes in the release of the synaptic transmitter. The presence of the vesicular organelles in nerve terminals is one of the most consistent ultrastructural features of junctional tissues. Depending upon the synapse examined, the vesicles vary in size and electron opacity. In cholinergic endings, the synaptic vesicles range in diameter from 200 to 400 Å; in electron micrographs, they appear as rings with centers of modest electron opacity. Adrenergic nerve endings and adrenal medullary cells contain vesicles that range in diameter from 400 to 1300 Å. The synaptic vesicles are believed to be the containers for transmitter substances that migrate toward the nerve terminal membrane during nervous stimulation to disgorge their contents into the synaptic cleft.

The neurotransmitter attaches reversibly with the receptor on the synaptic membrane at a rate rapid enough to cause changes in membrane activity. At many junctions the rate of dissociation of the transmitter and receptor must occur at a rapid rate for synaptic activity to remain responsive to succeeding incoming impulses. Equally important, mechanisms must be available for the elimination of the transmitter from the junctional region in order to prevent the accumulation within the synapse of concentrations of transmitter able to interfere with synaptic activity. Termination of transmitter activity can occur by a variety of means. After a dissociation of the transmitter from the postsynaptic receptor, the transmitter may diffuse away from the synapse, be converted to inactive degradation products by metabolic means, or be accumulated by the nerve terminals from the extra-

Table 16-1 Actions of the Autonomic Nerves on Various Effectors

Effector	Response to sympathetic nerves A, B*		Response to parasympathetic nerves
Eye			
Pupil		Dilation	Constriction
Iris			
Radial muscles	A	Contraction	
Circular muscles			Contraction
Accommodation			
Ciliary muscle	B	Relaxation	Contraction
Tarsal muscle	B	Contraction	
Orbital muscle			
Glands			
Sweat	A	Secretion†	
Salivary	A	Secretion	Secretion
Lacrimal			Secretion
Respiratory tract			Secretion
Gastrointestinal tract			Secretion
Piloerectors	A	Contraction	
Bronchioles	B	Relaxation	Contraction
Heart			
Sinus nodal rhythm	B	Acceleration	Slowing
AV node refractory period		Reduced	Increased
Atrial conduction rate	B	Increased	Increased
Atrial contraction force	B	Increased	Decreased
Ventricular contraction force	B	Increased	Decreased (?)
Blood vessels			
Muscle	A, B	Dilation	
Coronary	A, B	Dilation	Constriction
Skin	A	Constriction	
Viscera	A, B	Constriction	
Salivary gland	A	Constriction	Dilation
Erectile tissue	A	Constriction	Dilation
Gastrointestinal tract			
Muscle wall	A, B	Relaxation	Contraction
Sphincters	A	Contraction	Relaxation
Cardiac			Relaxation
Ileocecal	A	Contraction	
Spleen capsule	A	Contraction	
Urinary bladder			
Fundus	B	Relaxation	Contraction
Trigone and sphincter	A	Contraction	Relaxation
Uterus			
Nonpregnant	A, B	Contraction	
Pregnant	A, B	Contraction	
Liver	B	Glycogenolysis	

* Alpha, beta.

† Cholinergic fibers.

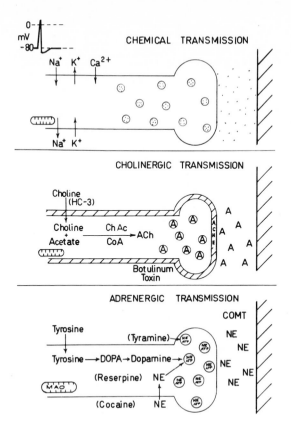

cellular space. At cholinergic junctions, a significant portion of the transmitter is eliminated by enzymatic means; at adrenergic junctions, reuptake of the transmitter by nerve endings accounts for the inactivation of the transmitter substance at that site.

CHOLINERGIC TRANSMISSION

The transmission of impulses at preganglionic nerve endings, postganglionic parasympathetic and some postganglionic sympathetic nerve endings, as well as somatic nerve endings, occurs by means of acetylcholine (ACh) liberated from storage granules within the nerve terminals.

The chemical processes involved in the formation of ACh within the nerves are complex and require at least two enzymatically controlled reactions. However, the major step in the synthetic process is the catalysis by choline acetylase of the acetylation of choline. This reaction requires the presence of CoA and the prior activation of acetate to its usable form, acetyl CoA. The sequence of reactions participating in the formation of ACh has been depicted as follows:

$$\text{``Activation'' of acetate} \longrightarrow \text{acetyl CoA}$$
$$\text{Acetyl CoA} + \text{choline} \underset{\text{acetylase}}{\overset{\text{choline}}{\rightleftharpoons}} \text{ACh} + \text{CoA}$$

Both organic and inorganic substances are known to affect the release of ACh. These substances are not selective for cholinergic nerve terminals. Among the inorganic ions present in nerve tissue, calcium appears to play a prominent role in the release mechanism. For example, in addition to the marked hyperirritability of neural structures associated with calcium deficiency, there is a profound reduction in the output of ACh from cholinergic nerves, resulting in turn in the failure of transmission. Conversely, an elevation in the concentration of calcium ions bathing the nerve terminals enhances the output of the transmitter.

Figure 16-1 Schematic representation of neurohumoral transmission at cholinergic and adrenergic junctions.

The *top* figure shows a general scheme for chemical transmisson. The conduction of the nerve action potential in the nerve ending is due to the movement of inorganic cations and is depicted by arrows showing the inward movement of Na^+ and Ca^{2+} and the outward movement of K^+. Restorative processes related to the extrusion of Na^+ and the accumulation of K^+ are depicted in a similar way on the bottom part of the diagram. The cellular inclusion bodies are indicated by the elongated oval (mitochondria) and spheres (synaptic vesicles containing transmitters). Dots in the junctional cleft indicate the diffusion of transmitter subsequent to release. The postjunctional membrane is indicated by the diagonal lines on the right side of the diagram.

The *middle* figure shows a conceptualized scheme for cholinergic transmission, and the details are presented in the text. The symbols are: HC-3 (hemicholinium), ChAc (choline acetylase), CoA (coenzyme A), ACh (acetylcholine), A (acetylcholine), AChE (acetylcholinesterase). The hatched lines on the nerve ending show the distribution of the enzyme acetylcholinesterase.

The *bottom* figure shows adrenergic transmission as described in the text. The symbols are NE (norepinephrine), ATP (adenosine triphosphate), MAO (monoamine oxidase), and COMT (catechol-O-methyltransferase).

Following its release from the nerve endings, ACh is subjected to a number of inactivation processes. These include diffusion from the site of release, dilution in extracellular fluids, binding to nonspecific sites, and enzymatic destruction. For most cholinergic junctions, the most important inactivation process is the enzymatic destruction of ACh to its hydrolysis products, acetic acid and choline. This reaction is catalyzed by the enzyme acetylcholinesterase and occurs at a rate sufficiently rapid to prevent the accumulation of ACh in the junction.

Acetylcholinesterase is one of a family of enzymes which catalyze the hydrolysis of ester linkages. In order to differentiate it from other esterases, it has also been named *true* or *specific* cholinesterase. Although this enzyme is associated primarily with neural structures, it is present also in such nonneural structures as the red blood cell and placenta. Another enzyme, closely related to acetylcholinesterase, which hydrolyzes ACh is called *nonspecific* or *pseudocholinesterase*. The nonspecific cholinesterase is found in the plasma, liver, and glial or satellite cells associated with nerve tissues.

ADRENERGIC TRANSMISSION

The transmission of impulses at sympathetic nerve endings occurs by means of *norepinephrine* liberated from storage granules within the nerve terminals. Norepinephrine is one of several naturally occurring biogenic catecholamines. Other important catecholamines are *epinephrine*, which is found in high concentrations in the adrenal medulla and other chromaffin cells, and *dopamine*, a precursor of both norepinephrine and epinephrine found in sympathetic nerve endings and in some areas of the CNS. The relationships of the three catecholamines are given in Fig. 16-2.

The synthetic pathway for norepinephrine in sympathetic nerve endings, appropriate cells of the CNS, and chromaffin tissues involves a complex series of enzymatic steps. In the first step of the series, the amino acid tyrosine undergoes hydroxylation to form dopa. The reaction is catalyzed by the enzyme tyrosine hydroxylase. When compared with other enzymes involved in the formation of catecholamines, the activity of tyrosine hydroxyl-

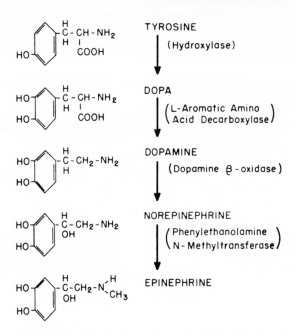

Figure 16-2 Metabolic pathway for the synthesis of norepinephrine and epinephrine from tyrosine.

ase is the lowest. Inhibition of this enzyme by analogues of tyrosine results in a depletion of catecholamine stores in the brain and adrenergic nerves. Indeed, the inhibitors of tyrosine hydroxylase are the most effective drugs for impairing the synthetic pathway for catecholamines. The hydroxylation of tyrosine is the primary rate-limiting step in the series of reactions. The second step in the pathway results in the conversion of dopa to dopamine by a decarboxylation reaction catalyzed by dopa decarboxylase (L-aromatic amino acid decarboxylase). The enzyme is not specific for dopa and will bring about the decarboxylation of histidine, tyrosine, and 5-hydroxytryptophan. In addition, the enzyme is present in most nonnervous tissues. The hydroxylation of the β carbon of dopamine to form norepinephrine takes place under the control of the enzyme dopamine-β-oxidase. This enzyme has been isolated from the chromaffin granules of the adrenal medulla and the synaptic vesicle of adrenergic nerves. The formation of epinephrine from norepinephrine is confined primarily to the adrenal medulla (and similar tissues), and the enzyme catalyzing the conversion is localized to those tissues. Except for the adrenal medulla, midbrain, and heart, very little phenylethanolamine-N-methyltransferase activity is present in most tissues.

There is some evidence to suggest that adrenergic nerve endings transport tyrosine from the extracellular fluid to the intraneuronal cytoplasm by metabolically dependent processes. However, relatively little is known about the chemistry of amino-acid transport in neural structures. After passing to the intracellular site, tyrosine is acted upon by the several enzymes to form norepinephrine, which is stored in the adrenergic nerve terminals in the form of vesicles. As mentioned before, the synaptic vesicles of adrenergic nerves have an electron-dense core and range in size from 400 to 1300 Å. In addition, the vesicles have dopamine-β-oxidase activity and contain a high concentration of norepinephrine. The vesicles also contain relatively high concentrations of ATP in a ratio of ATP to norepinephrine of 1:4. The granulated storage sites also have the capacity for concentrating norepinephrine and other catecholamines, such as epinephrine and dopamine, from the cytoplasm.

Calcium ions appear to be the required link between membrane excitation and the release of catecholamines from the nerve endings and adrenal medullary cells. At both sites calcium deprivation causes a failure of the release mechanism, and at both sites there is an influx of calcium ions during the release of the catecholamines. The mechanism whereby calcium brings about the release of norepinephrine is not known at present. In view of the intragranular binding between the catecholamines and ATP, calcium ions may participate in an enzymatic breakdown of the catecholamine-ATP complex. Some experiments have shown that calcium causes the release of both ATP and catecholamines from isolated synaptic vesicles.

By comparing the depletion of catecholamine stores produced by nerve stimulation, tyramine, and reserpine, it is apparent that the intraneuronal distribution, binding, and release of catecholamines is heterogeneous. As determined by isotopically labeled norepinephrine, there are two major neuronal compartments for the storage of catecholamines. The first compartment contains norepinephrine which undergoes rapid turnover (half-life of 2 h). The second compartment contains a storage form of norepinephrine with a slow turnover rate (about 24 h). Norepinephrine released from the first compartment is metabolized by the enzyme catechol-O-methyltransferase, and that released from the second compartment is metabolized by MAO.

When considering the various ways for terminating the actions of the catecholamines, distinction must be made between circulating and neuronal catecholamines. The term *circulating catecholamines* refers to catecholamines present in the blood as a consequence of sympathetic nerve activity, release from the adrenal medulla, or release from chromaffin tissues. The term *neuronal catecholamines* refers to the adrenergic nerve transmitter and its disposition within the adrenergic nerve ending. Insofar as neuronal catecholamines are concerned, distinction must also be made between the two principal compartments of intraneuronal catecholamines and the manner by which the catecholamines are released.

There are two major enzyme systems involved in the transformation of the catecholamines to inactive degradation products (Fig. 16-3). Oxidative deamination of epinephrine and norepinephrine is catalyzed by MAO. Adrenergic nerve endings contain large quantities of the enzyme so that tissues receiving sympathetic nerves also have large amounts of MAO. The enzyme is localized in the mitochondria. Apparently, because of its intraneuronal localization, MAO plays more of a role in the regulation of the intraneuronal disposition of catecholamines than the termination of circulating catecholamines. Inhibition of MAO leads to an increase in the tissue concentration of the catecholamines but has no appreciable effect on the responses to injected epinephrine or norepinephrine.

The second major enzyme involved in the metabolism of the catecholamines is catechol-O-methyltransferase. This enzyme is responsible for the inactivation of circulating catecholamines. Although the enzyme is widely distributed, it is concentrated in the liver and kidneys. Sympathetic nerves contain very little O-methyltransferase activity. The metabolic conversion by O-methyltransferase of the catecholamines to inactive forms is due to the transfer of a methyl group from "activated" methionine to the hydroxyl groups of the phenyl ring. Part of the norepinephrine released from adrenergic nerves during nerve stimulation is acted upon by O-methyltransferase. Similarly, circulating catecholamines are subjected to inactivation by O-methyltransferase activity.

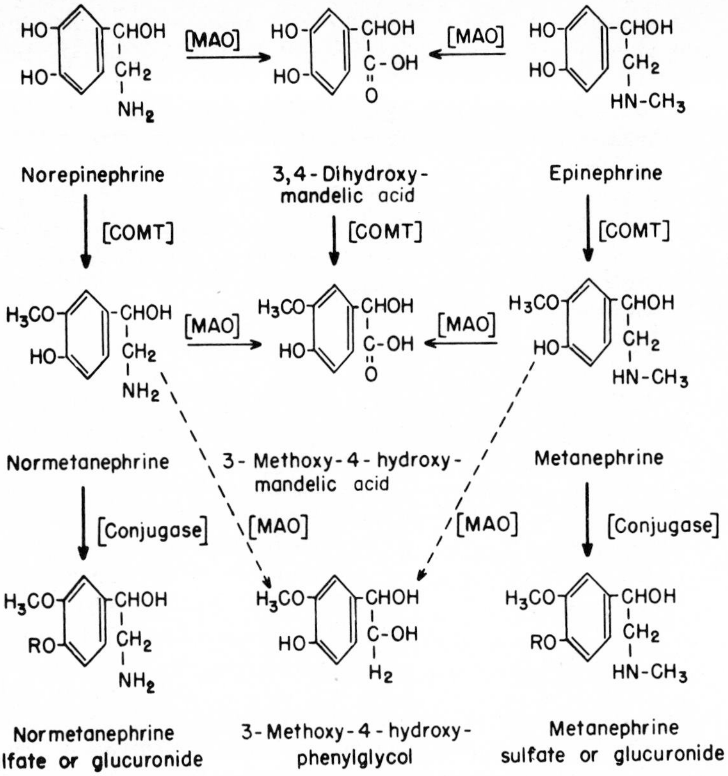

Figure 16-3 Metabolic pathways showing the inactivation of epinephrine and norepinephrine by various enzyme systems.

The uptake of catecholamines from the extracellular fluid by transport systems in adrenergic nerve endings probably accounts for the inactivation of a major portion of circulating catecholamines.

RECEPTORS

The demonstration that drugs such as epinephrine and ACh, which mimic the effects of activation of autonomic nerves, produce their characteristic effects on suitably denervated structures led to the proposal that the drugs act directly on the effector cell rather than on the nerve endings and that the drugs react with a special *receptive substance* on the cell.

In effector cells innervated by sympathetic and/or parasympathetic fibers, there are responses to the chemical mediator upon activation of the nerve fiber or to the administered mimetic agent. It is therefore postulated that responding cells possess receptors for ACh and other receptors for norepinephrine. These two general classes of receptors are often referred to as *cholinergic receptors* and *adrenergic receptors,* respectively.

Cholinergic Receptors

There are many peripheral efferent nerves which are cholinergic. It is convenient and, as we shall see, empirically useful to group them into three categories: (1) preganglionic fibers of the autonomic nervous system; (2) postganglionic fibers of the parasympathetic division and some postganglionic fibers of the sympathetic division; and (3) somatic motor nerves. Although each of these nerves transmits to a cell which contains receptors for ACh (cholinergic receptors, cholinoceptive sites), and each of these cells responds to properly applied exogenous ACh, the pharmacologic characteristics of the receptors at the three sites are different in significant ways. Drugs that mimic the effects of ACh at one cholinergic junction may have a markedly reduced effect at another. Similarly, drugs that block cholinergic transmission at one site may have no effect on cholinergic transmission at another site.

Earlier investigators clearly separated the *muscarine* actions and the *nicotine* actions of ACh. The alkaloid, muscarine, produces all the effects of postganglionic parasympathetic nerve stimulation and also induces sweating (a response produced by a cholinergic sympathetic postganglionic fiber). The effects of muscarine are readily suppressed by atropine, as are those of ACh on these same responses. On this basis, the receptors for ACh on effector cells innervated by postganglionic cholinergic fibers (all parasympathetic and certain sympathetic postganglionic fibers) may be called *muscarinic receptors* or *atropine-sensitive receptors*.

Drugs with the same pattern of activity as muscarine have been termed *muscarinic agents* or *parasympathomimetic drugs*. Muscarinic cholinoceptive sites are found also in some tissues that are not innervated by the parasympathetic division. Most arterioles do not receive parasympathetic innervation but are extremely sensitive to the actions of muscarine and muscarinelike drugs.

The receptors in autonomic ganglia and at the neuromuscular junction are responsive to low concentrations of nicotine and to ACh applied in adequate concentrations by an appropriate route of administration. The responses to ACh at these sites are called *nicotinic actions*, and the respective cholinoceptive sites *nicotinic receptors*. The nicotinic actions of ACh are subdivided into two groups, since there are some drugs which selectively interfere with transmission in autonomic ganglia and others that selectively interfere with neuromuscular transmission.

The three groups of cholinergic receptors all

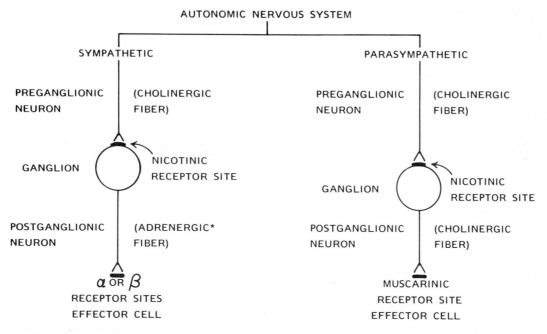

*EXCEPT POSTGANGLIONIC NEURONS TO SWEAT GLANDS AND PILOERECTOR MUSCLE AND THEIR RECEPTOR SITES, WHICH ARE MUSCARINIC RECEPTOR SITES.

Figure 16-4 Diagrammatic representation of the distribution of cholinoceptive and adrenoceptive sites in the peripheral autonomic nervous system.

respond to ACh; the differences among the receptors have been determined by using drugs which act like ACh or which antagonize the effects of ACh.

Adrenergic Receptors

The organs innervated by adrenergic nerves respond to epinephrine or norepinephrine in a manner which qualitatively mimics the effect of nerve stimulation. The primary reaction between norepinephrine or epinephrine and the effector cell is mediated by *adrenergic receptors (adrenoceptive sites)*.

A careful study of the relative potencies of several sympathomimetic amines for producing the characteristic sympathetic response in several tissues has suggested that adrenergic receptors could be grouped into two classes on the basis of the relative potencies of the sympathomimetic amines. It was found that in those noncardiac tissues showing excitatory responses to adrenergic stimulation, the relative order of potencies was first norepinephrine, then epinephrine, then isoproterenol. For the heart and those tissues inhibited by adrenergic stimulation, a different order of relative potencies

was found, that is, first isoproterenol, then epinephrine, then norepinephrine. The suggestion was made that the excitatory adrenergic receptors be called *alpha-adrenotropic receptors*, and that the receptors in inhibited cells and in the heart be called *beta-adrenotropic receptors*. This classification is now in general use.

The catecholamines cause striking changes in the metabolism of most organs. An increase in oxygen consumption, a breakdown of glycogen, an increase in the formation of lactic acid, and an increase in the mobilization of free fatty acids represent the major metabolic effects of the catecholamines. In mammals, the metabolic effects of epinephrine include hyperglycemia, the release of free fatty acids, and an increase in plasma lactic acid. There is a good probability that many of these effects of the catecholamines can be attributed to the increased formation of cyclic 3',5'-AMP by the adenyl cyclase enzyme system.

Figure 16-4 illustrates the distribution of cholinoceptive and adrenoceptive sites in the peripheral autonomic nervous system.

Chapter 17

Adrenergic Drugs

The sympathetic nervous system, in general, directs the response of an organism to various environmental stresses. Substances which evoke physiologic responses similar to those produced by the sympathetic adrenergic nerves are known as *sympathomimetic amines*.

Chemically, most of the adrenergic drugs are related to β-phenylethylamine; pharmacodynamically, epinephrine can be considered the prototype. Some of these agents occur in nature; all can be, and are, made synthetically.

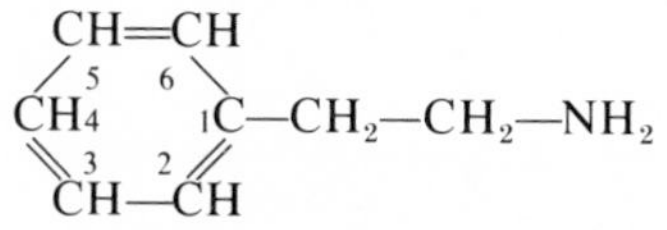

$$\underset{\text{β-Phenylethylamine}}{\overset{\displaystyle \overset{\text{CH}=\text{CH}}{\underset{\text{CH}-\text{CH}}{\text{CH}_4 \quad \text{C}-\text{CH}_2-\text{CH}_2-\text{NH}_2}}}{}}$$

The adrenergic agents can be classified into three general groups:

1 *Direct-acting* agents are those whose site of action is identical to that of the adrenergic neurotransmitter.
2 *Indirect-acting* agents are those whose site of action is on the postganglionic adrenergic nerve ending.
3 *Mixed-acting* agents are those whose action is both indirect and direct.

The first part of this chapter deals with the *direct-acting* catecholamines, which have been differentiated into alpha- or beta-adrenergic types. The rest of the chapter is devoted to a large number of sympathomimetic amines which are mostly mixed-acting.

DIRECT-ACTING SYMPATHOMIMETIC AMINES

Agents which have been shown to interact directly with adrenergic receptors are known as *direct-*

acting drugs. These include epinephrine, norepinephrine, isoproterenol, phenylephrine, and dopamine.

Epinephrine has been known and studied for about seventy years and is available from several sources under various trade names. The generic name, levarterenol, is most widely known by its German chemical names, noradrenaline or norepinephrine, in which the German derivation of the word *nor* stands for *N(itrogen) o(hne) R(adikal)*.

Epinephrine, Norepinephrine, and Isoproterenol

Source and Chemistry Norepinephrine and epinephrine are, respectively, the levorotatory isomers of 3,4-dihydroxyphenylethanolamine and 3,4-dihydroxyphenylethanolmethylamine. The dextrorotatory isomers, *d*-norepinephrine and *d*-epinephrine, are less active. The third catecholamine of importance is the synthetic amine isoproterenol, or 3,4-dihydroxyphenylethanolisopropylamine. The levorotatory isomer is more than a thousand times more active than the dextrorotatory isomer. Only the racemic mixture is commonly available, and unless otherwise specified this is the form used.

Epinephrine

Norepinephrine

Isoproterenol

Norepinephrine is the neurotransmitter produced and released in adrenergic synapses. Both epinephrine and norepinephrine occur naturally in the adrenal medulla. The proportions in which they are found in adrenal medullary extracts are variable. In most animals, including human beings, the proportion is approximately 85 percent epinephrine and 15 percent norepinephrine. In cases of pheochromocytoma the proportion of norepinephrine in the extract of the tumor may increase up to about 90 percent.

The biosynthesis of these amines and their metabolic fate has been the subject of much study. As discussed in the previous chapter, one scheme of formation is from tyrosine to norepinephrine and epinephrine. Other pathways are available, so the exact mode of synthesis is probably species-dependent and subject to other variable controlling factors. Some of the end products that have been identified in studies of the metabolism of epinephrine and norepinephrine are also shown in the previous chapter.

Mechanism of Action The proposed mechanism by which most of these agents exert their effects is by direct activation of adrenergic receptors.

Alpha and Beta Receptors Epinephrine and related compounds produce adrenergic effects that are both excitatory and inhibitory. Those responses attributed to *alpha*-receptor activation are primarily excitatory with the exception of intestinal relaxation. Those responses attributed to *beta*-receptor activation are primarily inhibitory, with the exception of the myocardial stimulant effects (see Table 17-1). Epinephrine is the most potent activator of the alpha receptor, being 2 to 10 times more active than norepinephrine and more than 100 times more potent than isoproterenol. Isoproterenol is the most potent activator of the beta receptor, being 2 to 10 times more active than epinephrine and 100 or more times more active than norepinephrine. However, these potency rankings are relative, and all these drugs have been shown to possess some activity at both alpha- and beta-receptor sites.

The concept which proposes the existence of two distinct receptors, alpha and beta, can be supported by the use of blocking agents which are specific for these sites. As described in the chapter on adre-

Table 17-1   Functions Associated with Each of the Adrenergic Receptors

Alpha receptor	Beta receptor
Vasoconstriction (cutaneous, renal, etc.)	Vasodilatation (skeletal muscle, etc.)
Splenic-capsule contraction	Cardioacceleration
Myometrial contraction (rabbit, dog, human being, etc.)	Myocardial augmentation
Iris-dilator contraction (mydriasis)	Myometrial relaxation (rat, pregnant cat, human being)
Nictitating-membrane contraction	Bronchial relaxation
Intestinal relaxation	Intestinal relaxation
Pilomotor contraction	Glycogenolysis
	Lipolysis
	Calorigenesis

nergic blockers, such agents as phenoxybenzamine, phentolamine, and tolazoline specifically block only those effects mediated by activation of alpha-receptor activators, i.e., norepinephrine and epinephrine. On the other hand, agents capable of activating beta receptors can be blocked by drugs such as propranolol. The fact that suitable antagonists do exist for both alpha and beta receptors substantiates the theory and has led to useful clinical applications.

Role of Cyclic 3′,5′-AMP   Unfortunately, the exact nature of the alpha-adrenergic receptor is unknown. However recent data strongly suggest that the beta-adrenergic receptor is adenylate cyclase. Adenylate cyclase catalyzes the conversion of ATP to cyclic 3′,5′-AMP. Cyclic 3′,5′-AMP is then broken down to 5′-AMP, and this reaction is catalyzed by a phosphodiesterase. Epinephrine is capable of producing a positive inotropic effect and increased cyclic AMP concentration in perfused rat hearts, and both of these responses are prevented by pretreatment with the beta-receptor blocking agent. Phosphodiesterase is inhibited by the methyl

xanthines and in particular by theophylline (see Fig. 17-1). Changes in the adenylate cyclase–cyclic AMP system occur following administration of catecholamines and concomitantly with the observed mechanical response. This is insufficient evidence to establish conclusively that adenylate cyclase is the beta receptor at the present time. However, at least in certain tissues, the main response to a beta agonist involves the cyclic 3′,5′-AMP system, and obviously if adenylate cyclase is not the direct receptor, it is certainly most intimately involved, perhaps by a coupling mechanism as yet unknown.

Effects on Organ Systems

Peripheral Vascular System   The most dominant and easily apparent effects of alpha- and beta-receptor agonists are on the vascular system (Table 17-2). It is obvious from the table that the various catecholamines have profoundly different effects on vascular networks in various organs. Also evident is that a beta-receptor agonist such as isoproterenol has an overall effect of decreasing peripheral resistance and increasing peripheral blood

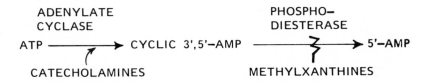

Figure 17-1   Effect of catecholamines and methylxanthines on the metabolism of cyclic 3′,5′-AMP.

Table 17-2   Effects of Alpha and Beta Agonists on the Peripheral Vascular System

Organ or variable	Alpha (norepinephrine)	Beta (isoproterenol)	Alpha and beta (epinephrine)
Resistance	Increased	Decreased	Small doses—decreased Large doses—increased
Blood flow	Reduced	Increased	Variable
Skin	Vasoconstriction	Negligible	Vasoconstriction
Mucous membranes	Vasoconstriction	Negligible	Generally vasodilation
Skeletal muscle	Generally vasoconstriction	Vasodilation	Generally vasodilation
Renal blood flow	Vasoconstriction	Slight vasoconstriction	Vasoconstriction
Hepatic Mesenteric Uterine Pulmonary	Vasoconstriction	Negligible	Vasoconstriction
Coronary	Dilation	Negligible	Vasodilation

flow. The effects of norepinephrine are exactly opposite, whereas those of epinephrine vary with dose and organ.

Myocardium and Cardiac Output Epinephrine evokes three distinct responses in the heart: (1) cardiac acceleration through the sinoatrial node (chronotropic effect); (2) increased force of contraction (inotropic effect); and (3) altered rhythmic function of the ventricle (ventricular extrasystoles, tachycardia, and potential fibrillation). These responses are usually accompanied by increased oxygen consumption and cellular metabolism.

In isolated heart preparations the cardioaccelerator effect is easily demonstrated. However, in intact animals, the vagal reflex triggered by the elevated arterial pressure usually averts any significant appearance of tachycardia.

The effect of epinephrine on cardiac output cannot be categorically stated. Both the inotropic and chronotropic actions would tend to increase the output. However, if the rate increases too much, the output may decrease because of insufficient ventricular filling time. In addition to reflecting the pumping action of the heart, cardiac output is dependent on the venous return and the resistance of the peripheral arterial system.

The effect of epinephrine on coronary blood flow has been extensively studied, but the final answer is not yet at hand. There can be no question that coronary flow per se is markedly increased by epinephrine in the intact animal. Whether the effective coronary flow, which may be defined as the flow necessary to supply the oxygen requirements of the myocardium, is increased, and whether epinephrine is a direct coronary dilator, is the troublesome question.

Arterial Pressure Recording the effect of epinephrine administered intravenously on the arterial pressure is a standard pharmacologic procedure. The result is often predictable and always spectacular.

In humans the responses to epinephrine and norepinephrine are strikingly different. With intravenous infusion of about 4 μg epinephrine per minute, the heart rate increases, systolic and mean pressure increase, and diastolic pressure usually decreases. The cardiac output is increased, and the total peripheral resistance declines. In contrast, with norepinephrine, while systolic, diastolic, and mean pressure increase, peripheral resistance increases, and the heart rate and cardiac output diminish. These results are interpreted by some as demonstrating that in man norepinephrine is a stronger vasoconstrictor than epinephrine.

The intense beta activation of epinephrine to produce tachycardia overcomes any vagal slowing due to the rise in blood pressure. Norepinephrine is less active than epinephrine in increasing heart rate, so that the usual response to norepinephrine is an increase in blood pressure and reflex vagal bradycardia. The cardiac output response reflects primarily the peripheral vascular effects; epinephrine increases cardiac output because of augmented venous return, and norepinephrine decreases output because of diminished return. In addition, myocardial stimulation contributes to the epinephrine pressor effect. It must be kept in mind also that the amount of the amine administered will alter the response. Although a small dose of epinephrine may act as an overall vasodilator and produce only tachycardia, large doses can increase peripheral resistance and mean arterial pressure and produce reflex bradycardia. The comparative effects of epinephrine and norepinephrine on various aspects of the cardiovascular system are summarized in Table 17-3.

Table 17-3 Comparative Effects of Epinephrine and Norepinephrine on the Human Cardiovascular System

Response	Epinephrine Minimal dose	Epinephrine Large dose, IV	Norepinephrine Minimal dose	Norepinephrine Large dose, IV
Blood pressure,				
Mean	0*	↑ ↑	↑	↑ ↑ ↑
Systolic	sl ↑	↑ ↑ ↑	↑	↑ ↑ ↑
Diastolic	sl ↓	↑	↑	↑ ↑ ↑
Cardiac output	↑	↑ ↑	0	0 or ↓
Pulse rate	0 or ↑	↑ ↑	0	0 or ↓
Peripheral resistance	↓	↑ ↑	↑	↑ ↑

*↑ = increase; ↓ = decrease; 0 = no change; sl = slight.

Effects on Other Systems

Bronchi The smooth muscle of the bronchi is relaxed by epinephrine. This muscle has beta-adrenergic receptors, since norepinephrine is less active than epinephrine and isoproterenol more active. The relaxant effects of isoproterenol and epinephrine are abolished by beta blocking agents. Relaxation of the bronchi has little noticeable effect on respiratory activity. It is only in the presence of bronchial constriction that relaxation produces an observable increase in tidal volume.

Eye Two groups of smooth muscle associated with the eye, the radial muscle of the iris and the smooth muscle of the orbit, respond to epinephrine. Both contract under the influence of epinephrine. Contraction of the radial muscle produces mydriasis; and that of the orbital muscle, an appearance of exophthalmos. When epinephrine is applied locally to the eye, little effect is noted unless a relatively high concentration is used.

Gastrointestinal Tract The usual effect of epinephrine, norepinephrine, and isoproterenol on the smooth muscle of the gastrointestinal tract is inhibitory. It would appear that the smooth muscle of the gastrointestinal tract has both alpha and beta receptors and that both receptors subserve relaxation or inhibition. If the intestinal adrenergic receptive mechanism consists of both types of receptors, it follows that all adrenergic agents should produce intestinal inhibition. This is true for nor-

epinephrine, ephedrine, amphetamine, metaraminol, methoxamine, and various related experimental compounds.

Uterus The response of the myometrium to epinephrine or sympathetic nerve stimulation varies in association with several factors. In addition to species variation, there is a variation in response observed with different phases of the estrous cycle and with pregnant and nonpregnant uteri.

Epinephrine usually inhibits the human uterus in vivo, but isolated segments of the human uterus are contracted. It is apparent, then, that both alpha and beta receptors are associated with the myometrium. The type of receptor differs in each species and varies with other conditions, presumably hormonal in nature.

Glands Most endocrine or exocrine glands are not affected to any great extent by epinephrine or the other adrenergic agents. Among the exocrine glands only the salivary glands respond significantly, producing a thick sparse secretion. The secretion rate of the other glands may be indirectly affected in that, if blood flow or pressure is increased, the glands become more active, and if vasoconstriction occurs, decreasing the local blood supply, the activity of the gland may decrease.

Metabolism Epinephrine produces a variety of metabolic effects. These include liver glycogenolysis, which results in hyperglycemia, and muscle glycogenolysis, which results in lactacidemia and hyperkalemia. In addition to this, epinephrine can produce an inhibition of glucose uptake by tissue, mobilization of fat involving an increase in plasma-free fatty acids, inhibition of cholesterol, and fatty acid synthesis. The metabolic effect that has received the most attention is the glycogenolysis resulting from activation of glycogen phosphorylase in liver. The overall increase in metabolic rate is a complex and probably indirect effect. Epinephrine has a generalized calorigenic action. The fundamental cause of this increase in respiratory metabolism, which occurs in all species, has not been fully determined.

Central Nervous System   Although epinephrine is not a central stimulant in the usual sense of the word, it does produce some effects that might be thus classified. The intravenous administration of epinephrine or norepinephrine produces opposite effects, which are best described as alerting effects. Anxiety and tremors appear as adverse reactions during the use of epinephrine and isoproterenol. In some instances the peripheral action of epinephrine may be manifested as an apparent central nervous system stimulation.

Routes of Administration   To obtain the systemic actions of epinephrine or norepinephrine, parenteral administration is required. When these drugs are administered orally, effectiveness is poor. Three probable reasons for the lack of response to oral administration of epinephrine or norepinephrine are: (1) inactivation by the digestive secretions; (2) local vasoconstriction, diminishing blood supply and absorptive ability of the mucous membranes; and (3) rapid enzymatic inactivation in the liver or intestinal wall. Epinephrine is usually administered subcutaneously or intramuscularly. In emergency it may be given intravenously, but cautiously and in reduced dosage. Norepinephrine is administered intravenously.

For local action, epinephrine is applied directly to mucous membranes or to cut surfaces to control capillary bleeding. When used with local anesthetics, it is injected intracutaneously or subcutaneously. In bronchial asthma, an epinephrine solution is nebulized in a suitable atomizer and the fine mist inhaled through the mouth. Some systemic effect can be observed occasionally with this method.

Metabolic Fate   It is obvious that the catecholamines are metabolized by a variety of biochemical processes; at least three such processes are implicated, including deamination, oxidation, and conjugation. Only a very small fraction of circulating epinephrine and norepinephrine is excreted unchanged in the urine. More detailed information on the metabolic fate of epinephrine and norepinephrine is found in the preceding chapter.

Termination of Catecholamine Activity   Despite the importance of enzymatic degradation of the catecholamines by the two enzyme systems MAO and catechol-*O*-methyltransferase, the biologic actions of the catecholamines are terminated principally by uptake by the sympathetic nerve ending processes. Inhibition of this uptake mechanism by agents such as cocaine produces a much greater potentiation of the mechanical effects of epinephrine or norepinephrine than does inhibition of either MAO or catechol-*O*-methyltransferase.

Selected Preparations and Doses

Epinephrine Injection and Epinephrine Solution These are aqueous solutions containing epinephrine hydrochloride equivalent to 0.1 percent epinephrine base. The only difference between these preparations is that the former must be sterile.

Epinephrine Inhalation   This is a 1 percent aqueous solution of epinephrine as the hydrochloride. To all aqueous solutions of epinephrine is added a reducing agent to prevent oxidation of the amine. Sodium bisulfite, 0.1 to 0.2 percent, or ascorbic acid can be used. The former, by local irritation, increases the rate of epinephrine absorption from subcutaneous or intramuscular injection.

Sterile Epinephrine Suspension   This is a sterile suspension of epinephrine base in a fixed oil suitable for intramuscular injection. The usual preparation contains 2 mg/ml.

The official dose of epinephrine in aqueous solution is 0.2 to 1 mg by any parenteral route other than intravenous. In the form of the oil suspension, the dose is 2 mg intramuscularly. These doses should be regarded as the maximal amounts to be given at one time. Several solutions for inhalation are available which contain synthetic, racemic epinephrine. These should contain about 2 percent of the amine in order to be equivalent in potency to the official inhalation.

Levarterenol (Norepineprhine) Bitartrate Injection
This is a sterile, aqueous solution usually containing 0.2 percent of the salt (equivalent to 0.1 percent of the free base), sodium chloride, and sodium bisulfite. It is available in ampuls of 4 ml under the trade name Solution Levophed Bitartrate.

Isoproterenol Hydrochloride Inhalation This is a solution of isoproterenol hydrochloride in an isotonic solution, usually available in concentrations of 1:100 or 1:200.

Isoproterenol Hydrochloride Injection This is a sterile solution of isoproterenol hydrochloride in water for injection. Injection usually available contains 0.2 mg in 1 ml or 1 mg in 5 ml.

Toxicity The usual therapeutic doses of epinephrine may produce what might be termed minor toxic effects. Anxiety, tremor, headache, fear, and palpitations are the usual symptoms. These are transient and not regarded as dangerous.

The toxic effects of overdosage or inadvertent intravenous injection are of three kinds. Elevated arterial pressure may result in cerebrovascular hemorrhage. Since this may occur readily in elderly patients, it should be emphasized again that, although small doses of epinephrine may produce a fall in peripheral resistance and only slight pressor effect, large doses produce an extremely high arterial pressure.

Because of the peripheral constriction and cardiac stimulation, pulmonary edema from pulmonary arterial hypertension may be a fatal toxic response to epinephrine. If epinephrine is used in the presence of excessive doses of digitalis or the mercurial diuretics, or in cyclopropane anesthesia, fatal ventribular fibrillation may follow.

No chronic toxicity of significance occurs with norepinephrine. Repeated local injections of epinephrine could result in necrosis at the site of injection due to excessive vasoconstriction. This might also be due to local inflammation produced by the preservative, sodium bisulfite.

Dopamine

Dopamine, 3,4-dihydroxyphenylethylamine, is one of the intermediate products in the synthesis of norepinephrine and is formed by the decarboxylation of dihydroxyphenylalanine. Dopamine has been found in sympathetic nerves and ganglia and in the CNS.

Dopamine

The peripheral actions of dopamine resemble those of a weak adrenergic activator. However certain differences between dopamine and norepinephrine have been reported. Dopamine in low doses caused a fall in arterial pressure, middle doses caused a biphasic pressor-depressor effect, and the larger doses produced a purely pressor response. The pressor effect of dopamine was reduced by phenoxybenzamine; the depressor effect was not reduced by dichloroisoproterenol. It is obvious that dopamine produces a vasodepressor effect that does not involve activation of the beta receptor, but rather a dopaminergic receptor. The positive inotropic and chronotropic effects elicited by dopamine are inhibited by beta-receptor blockade. Dopamine increases renal but not femoral flow. The renal effects of dopamine in humans also include an increased sodium excretion and glomerular filtration rate. Epinephrine and norepinephrine produce renal constriction. Dopamine produces little change in the peripheral resistance. Intra-arterial injection of dopamine reportedly had little effect on forearm blood flow, but a marked vasodilation occurred following phenoxybenzamine treatment. However, the exact physiologic role of dopamine is presently unknown. Because of its ability to increase renal blood flow, it has been suggested as an agent for the treatment of certain types of shock.

Phenylephrine Hydrochloride

Phenylephrine hydrochloride (Neo-Synephrine HCl), the levo isomer of 3-hydroxyphenylethanolmethylamine (the same as epinephrine but lacking the 4-hydroxyl group), is in action essentially similar to norepinephrine. It differs in only two ways: it is less potent and it has a longer duration of action. Parenteral administration in humans produces peripheral vasoconstriction, increased arterial pressure, and reflex bradycardia. It does not induce ventricular tachycardia or fibrillation in the presence of cyclopropane, nor does it produce central stimulation.

Phenylephrine

Phenylephrine, one of the most useful adrenergic agents, is employed as a pressor agent, decongestant, and mydriatic, and as an antiallergenic agent. Occasionally, phenylephrine will produce "rebound" congestion.

MIXED- AND INDIRECT-ACTING SYMPATHOMIMETIC AMINES

It has been suggested that the adrenergic agents (sympathomimetic amines) be classed into three categories: (1) those potentiated by denervation (direct-acting agents); (2) those not much affected by denervation (direct and indirect, or mixed-action, agents); and (3) those markedly less effective after denervation (indirect-acting agents). The prototypes for the three categories are norepinephrine (direct action), ephedrine (mixed action), and tyramine (indirect action). Although the classification of adrenergic agents into three categories is theoretically possible, it is more realistic to assume that all adrenergic agents except the catecholamines possess some degree of both direct and indirect effects to a greater or lesser extent.

The adrenergic responses to tyramine may be blocked by the appropriate adrenergic blocking agents. The indirect nature of this action of tyramine may be demonstrated by the following series of simple experiments utilizing various blocking agents. The pressor response in the anesthetized dog (an alpha effect) can be reduced by phenoxybenzamine (an alpha blocking agent). The inhibitory response to tyramine in the isolated rat uterus (a beta effect) can be blocked by dichloroisoproterenol (a beta blocking agent). The blockade produced by both blocking agents is specific and at the receptor level. Both responses to tyramine can be blocked by bretylium, an agent that acts to prevent the liberation of catecholamines by sympathetic nerves. This effect of bretylium is above the receptor level and is probably exerted at the endings. Although tyramine is of little clinical value, it is important as a laboratory tool.

It may thus be stated that the total action of adrenergic agents depends upon their ability to activate alpha and beta receptors by a direct action of the drug on the receptors or indirectly by triggering the release of catecholamines which will then activate both alpha and beta receptors.

Ephedrine

Source and Chemistry Ephedrine is an alkaloid which occurs in certain species of the genus *Ephedra*. Although available from plant sources, most of the ephedrine currently used is prepared by organic synthesis. Chemically, ephedrine is phenyl-isopropanolmethylamine.

Ephedrine

Effect on Organ Systems

Cardiovascular System Ephedrine is a mixed-acting sympathomimetic amine. The effect of ephedrine administered intravenously is similar to that of epinephrine. The arterial pressure—systolic, diastolic, and mean—rises and vagal slowing occurs. Compared with epinephrine, the pressor response to ephedrine occurs somewhat more slowly and lasts about 10 times longer. Furthermore, it requires more ephedrine than epinephrine to obtain an equivalent pressor response. It is commonly accepted that it requires about 250 times more ephedrine than epinephrine to achieve equipressor responses.

If a second dose of ephedrine is administered too soon, its pressor response proves weaker than that of the first dose. This phenomenon, known as *tachyphylaxis,* occurs with many adrenergic agents and is related to the duration of action of the drugs. The longer-acting the adrenergic agent, the more marked the tachyphylaxis. The shorter the time interval between doses, the smaller the pressor response to each subsequent dose. There are two explanations for tachyphylaxis. First, the initial dose of ephedrine may so deplete the norepinephrine stores of the nerve ending that very little norepinephrine is left to be released and subsequent doses of ephedrine exert only the direct component of its action. Second, one effect of ephedrine is to change the receptors so as to make them less responsive.

In humans, ephedrine increases the arterial pressure both by peripheral vasoconstriction and by cardiac stimulation. The heart rate is usually increased, as is pulse pressure, both suggesting increased cardiac output. The cardiovascular response to ephedrine is quite variable, however. In some cases the arterial pressure is not elevated, and in others bradycardia occurs at the height of the pressure rise; the peripheral resistance has been reported as increasing, decreasing, or remaining unchanged. Like epinephrine, ephedrine often produces a secondary congestive response.

Thus, based on the observed cardiovascular response, it can be stated that ephedrine directly and indirectly activates the same adrenergic receptors as does epinephrine but is less potent and has a longer duration of action.

Bronchi The smooth muscle of the bronchial tree is relaxed by ephedrine. Compared to epinephrine, the action of ephedrine is slow in onset, becoming complete only an hour or more after administration.

Eye Ephedrine produces mydriasis when applied locally to the conjunctiva, as well as after systemic absorption. In humans, there is a striking disparity between the mydriatic effects of ephedrine in Caucasians and Chinese or Negroes, being most active in the Caucasian, less active in the Chinese, and almost completely inactive in the Negro. The reason for this differential effect on irises of different races has not yet been completely explained.

Other Smooth Muscles In general, ephedrine produces qualitatively the same effects on smooth muscle as does epinephrine. Inhibition of the intact gastrointestinal musculature and contraction of the splenic capsule and of pilomotor muscles are produced. Ephedrine has the same myometrial and urinary bladder actions as does epinephrine.

Glands The effects of ephedrine are similar to those of epinephrine. However, ephedrine is much less potent, and with routes of administration other than intravenous, the glandular responses do not always occur. Ephedrine does produce hyperglycemia and eosinopenia.

Central Nervous System All the adrenergic agents possessing an unsubstituted phenyl ring and a methyl group on the α carbon atom are corticomedullary stimulants. Depending on the dose, the stimulant action in humans results in feelings of anxiety, tremor, insomnia and mental alertness, and increased respiration. When ephedrine is used as a central stimulant, the adrenergic effect becomes the side action. Ephedrine increases oxygen consumption and metabolic rate, presumably by central stimulation.

Routes of Administration Ephedrine can be administered by almost any route. Most frequently it is given orally, but is also injected subcutaneously, intramuscularly, or intravenously. For local action, as in the eye or on the nasal mucosa, ephedrine solutions are applied directly by drops, on a tampon, or as a spray.

Absorption, Fate, and Excretion Ephedrine is readily and completely absorbed after oral or parenteral administration. It does not produce enough local vasoconstriction to hinder absorption after subcutaneous or intramuscular injection. Ephedrine is resistant to MAO, but is deaminated to some extent in the liver, probably by the ascorbic-dehydroascorbic acid system. Conjugation also occurs. This is most apparent in the rat but probably occurs in other species. In addition, up to 40 percent of the ephedrine administered may be excreted unchanged in the urine. Inactivation and excretion are so slow that the action of ephedrine may persist for several hours.

Toxicity Most of the untoward actions of ephedrine are due to its effects on the CNS. These are nausea, vomiting, sweating, vertigo, tremor, nervousness, apprehension, and insomnia. Other effects, due probably to peripheral adrenergic action, are urinary retention and palpitation. None of these symptoms, which frequently appear with ordinary therapeutic doses, are dangerous, but they may preclude use of the drug in susceptible patients.

There are no chronic toxic effects of ephedrine; nor is there any evidence that true habituation or addiction occurs. Tolerance may develop with long-continued usage, but this may be only a reflection of the phenomenon of tachyphylaxis, and is therefore controllable by reducing the frequency of administration.

Therapeutic Uses Ephedrine is an orally effective long-acting sympathomimetic agent. Its clinical applications include bronchial asthma, allergic disorders, and nasal decongestion; it can be used as a pressor agent in spinal anesthesia, for mydriasis, and occasionally as a central nervous system stimulant. It should be used only with great caution in patients with organic heart disease, hypertension, and hyperthyroidism.

Amphetamines

This term is conventionally used to indicate racemic and dextrorotatory amphetamine and its N-methyl derivative, methamphetamine.

Amphetamine

In general amphetamines have the same adrenergic actions as ephedrine, producing mydriasis, inhibition of the gastrointestinal tract, and a pressor response by vasoconstriction. The action of these amines on the bronchial musculature is less potent than that of ephedrine, and bradycardia rather than tachycardia is the usual cardiac response. In addition, tachyphylaxis is very marked.

Therapeutic Uses The amphetamines are recommended for use in only a few selected conditions. These include narcolepsy and the management of children with the hyperkinetic syndrome. Adjunctively, amphetamine can be used as an anorexiant in the treatment of obesity, but only when combined with a program of caloric restriction, appropriate exercise, and psychologic support. Dextroamphetamine appears to be more useful than amphetamine as an anorexiant, since the dextrorotatory isomer is a more potent appetite suppressant. Dextroamphetamine generally should be used no longer than 2 weeks at a time, and new dietary habits should be developed so that decreased caloric intake continues after the drug is discontinued.

Tolerance to the effect of the amphetamines may occur within several weeks. In such instances, the anorexiants should no longer be regarded as acceptable adjuncts in the treatment program and should be discontinued.

Adverse Reactions The untoward effects produced by the amphetamines are related to their spectrum of pharmacologic actions. Adverse reactions affecting the CNS include psychic and even physical dependence in susceptible individuals, insomnia, restlessness, nervousness, dizziness, tremor, and dystonic movements of the head, neck, and extremities. If insomnia occurs, the last dose should be given in midafternoon. Serious depressive reactions which may sometimes be psychotic in nature have followed the intensive use of dextroamphetamine within a program of strenuous dieting in some individuals. Toxic psychoses have occurred with large dosage. Cardiovascular stimulation may cause increased pulse rate, as well as hypertension, headache, and palpitation. The drug should be discontinued promptly if chest pain or arrhythmias occur. Dryness of the mouth, mydriasis, nausea, diarrhea, and constipation have also been reported.

Acute overdosage results in accentuation of the usual pharmacologic effects: excitement, agitation, hypertension, tachycardia, mydriasis, slurred speech, ataxia, tremor, chills, hyperreflexia, tachypnea, fever, and toxic psychoses characterized by auditory and visual hallucinations and paranoid delusions. If these symptoms occur, the drug should be discontinued, sedatives prescribed, and custodial care and psychotherapy employed when needed. In severe cases, overdosage may cause acute circulatory failure and death.

The physician should be aware that susceptible patients may develop psychic dependence and even physical dependence from the use of amphetamines and amphetaminelike agents.

Although amphetamine, dextroamphetamine, and methamphetamine are available in sterile solutions for intravenous use, this dosage form is absolutely contraindicated for any condition. Individuals who abuse these amphetamines frequently inject the drug 4 to 6 times daily with total daily doses as large as several grams. Polyarteritis nodosa (necrotizing angiitis) has been associated with the intravenous administration of large doses of methamphetamine and dextroamphetamine in drug abusers.

Withdrawing amphetamines from abusers may unmask symptoms of chronic fatigue (mental depression, asthenia, tremors, and gastrointestinal disturbances), and in some individuals the fatigue may be followed by drowsiness and prolonged sleep.

Generally, amphetamines should not be prescribed for patients with hypertension, cardiovascular disease, and hyperthyroidism because their sympathomimetic effect may aggravate these conditions. They are contraindicated in those receiving MAOI and guanethidine and should be used with caution in patients who are overly sensitive to adrenergic agents. These drugs should not be given to individuals who are known drug abusers.

Methamphetamine Hydrochloride

Methamphetamine hydrochloride (Methedrine HCl, Desoxyn HCl, desoxyephedrine HCl), the dextrorotatory isomer of phenylisopropyl methylamine, may be regarded as a derivative of either amphetamine or ephedrine. Like both of these, it is a mixed-acting adrenergic activator depending on an intact adrenergic nerve ending for most of its activity. Methamphetamine is approximately equal in potency to dextroamphetamine (see above) as a central stimulant and is more potent than ephedrine as a pressor agent. This drug has two principal therapeutic uses: as a pressor agent in spinal anesthesia and as a central nervous system stimulant. Its use and abuse as a stimulant are identical to that of amphetamine. In spinal anesthesia methamphetamine has certain advantages as a pressor agent. Used to prevent hypotension, it is more effective than ephedrine and seldom requires more than one dose.

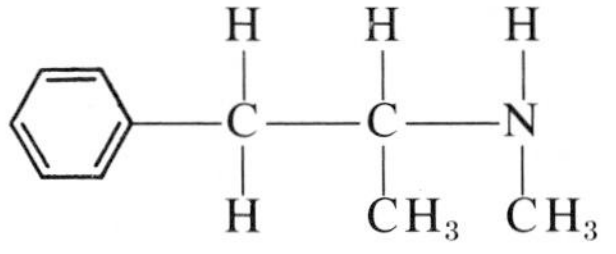

Methamphetamine

Phenylpropanolamine Hydrochloride

Phenylpropanolamine hydrochloride (Propadrine HCl) is similar in action to ephedrine but possesses somewhat greater pressor effects and causes less corticomedullary stimulation. Phenylpropanolamine is used principally as a topical and oral nasal decongestant.

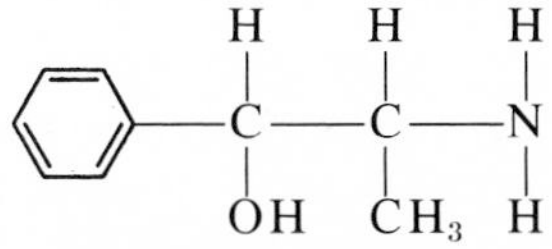

Phenylpropanolamine

Metaraminol Bitartrate

Metaraminol bitartrate (Aramine), *l*-3-hydroxyphenylisopropanolamine, is similar in action to norepinephrine. Studies on the racemic form of this amine show it to be about one-fourth as active as phenylephrine as a pressor agent. The levorotatory isomer is probably more active than the racemic mixture.

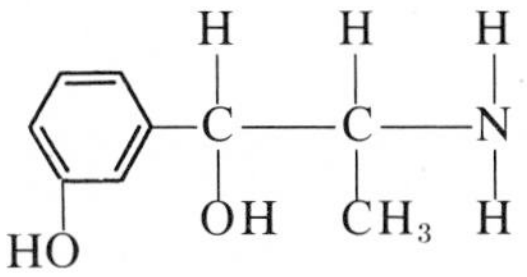

Metaraminol

In addition to producing a rise in blood pressure, metaraminol also produces an increase in myocardial contraction and cardiac output. Because of its apparent cardiac stimulant properties, metaraminol appears to resemble norepinephrine as an almost pure alpha stimulant, but is less potent. Metaraminol is principally used as a pressor agent in hypotensive states.

Methoxamine Hydrochloride

Methoxamine (Vasoxyl), racemic 2,5-dimethoxyphenylisopropanolamine, is very similar in its actions to phenylephrine. It has been used as a pressor agent and decongestant. Methoxamine is not a cardiac stimulant but produces vagal slowing. No significant stimulation of the central nervous system is caused by this drug.

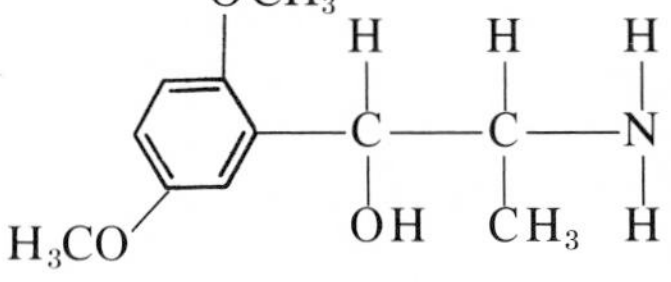

Methoxamine

Miscellaneous

Miscellaneous mixed-acting adrenergic agents include tuaminoheptane, hydroxyamphetamine, propylhexedrine, naphazoline, tetrahydrozoline, oxymetazoline, and xylometazoline.

Chapter 18

Adrenergic Blocking Drugs and Adrenergic Neuronal Blocking Drugs

The importance of the autonomic nervous system in regulating cardiovascular and visceral functions is well known and has been extensively documented. Autonomic imbalance—especially sympathoadrenal hyperactivity—is associated with many disease states. Since medical opinion has favored the view that sympathoadrenal hyperactivity is involved in cardiovascular as well as other disorders, physicians have been interested in obtaining drugs which inhibit the sympathetic nervous system.

ADRENERGIC BLOCKING DRUGS

Adrenergic blockade refers to the capacity of a chemical to antagonize some of the responses elicited in effector organs by sympathomimetic amines, especially by epinephrine and norepinephrine. Antagonism may occur at two major sites: alpha receptors and beta receptors. Drugs such as

phentolamine and phenoxybenzamine are alpha-adrenergic-receptor blocking agents. Compounds which block the beta-adrenergic receptor include propranolol and practolol. The investigational drug practolol has a greater specificity for cardiac tissue beta receptors than has propranolol. It therefore has significantly less effect on sympathomimetic amine responses in noncardiac tissue, such as the smooth muscle of the bronchioles.

Phentolamine

Phenoxybenzamine

Propranolol

Practolol

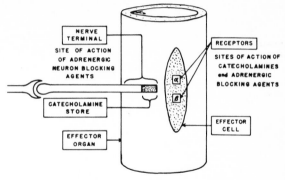

Figure 18-1 Simplified hypothetical representation of a sympathetic effector organ and an effector cell within this effector organ. Also shown is a simplified representation of a sympathetic neuron innervating the effector organ.

The diagram illustrates the sites of action of catecholamines, adrenergic blocking agents, and adrenergic neuron blocking agents as they are currently conceived.

Mechanism of Action

The sympathetic mediator norepinephrine is released from the nerve terminal during neuronal activity; it acts on the effector cells, and a response occurs. Blood-borne catecholamines elicit similar responses by impinging on the same effectors (Fig. 18-1). These effectors may be smooth muscle cells, cardiac muscle cells, or cells of exocrine glands.

Adrenergic blocking agents exert their action by combining directly with the adrenergic receptors. Agents blocking alpha responses combine with alpha receptors, and agents blocking beta responses combine with beta receptors. Such combinations reduce the availability of the alpha and beta receptors for reaction with sympathomimetic amines and therefore reduce the magnitude of the response evoked by the amines. For these reasons the blocking agents are often referred to as *alpha-receptor* and *beta-receptor* blocking agents.

Catecholamines, beta blocking agents, and the alpha blocking agents excluding phenoxybenzamine apparently are bound to the receptors by weak forces such as are obtained with hydrogen, hydrophobic, and van der Waals bondings, or by ion pair formation. Phenoxybenzamine forms a firm covalent bond with the receptor. The extent of the association of a blocking agent (or catecholamine) with adrenergic receptors seems to be determined by the law of mass action. Thus, if a concentration of blocking agent (or catecholamine) is maintained constant in the vicinity of the receptors for sufficient time, the amount of receptor-drug (or receptor-catecholamine) complex formed will reach an equilibrium value. The equilibrium value will be directly proportional to the product of the concentration of the drug (or catecholamine) and the concentration of the unoccupied receptors.

Therefore, the blocking drugs are said to produce an *equilibrium* type of blockade. Since the blocking agents act at the same receptors as the catecholamines, and the extent of both interactions is dependent on mass action, the catecholamines and the blocking drugs compete for access to the receptors. For this reason the blocking agents are termed *competitive* blocking agents. All adrenergic blocking agents discussed in this chapter, except phenoxybenzamine, are currently classified as competitive blocking agents.

However, in the initial stages of blockade, phenoxybenzamine competes with catecholamines for receptor occupancy, and here, it also can be looked upon as a competitive blocking agent. Then phenoxybenzamine, in contrast to other adrenergic blocking agents, can form a stable covalent bond with the receptor. Blockade is so persistent under these circumstances that it is sometimes loosely referred to as being "irreversible" (which is not strictly true, since recovery will be observed within a period of days or weeks). Regardless of the *non-equilibrium* nature of the blockade finally produced by phenoxybenzamine, it reacts with the same alpha receptor as do the catecholamines.

Effects on Organ Systems

Cardiovascular System Although moderate doses of alpha-adrenergic blocking agents do not usually decrease pressure in supine humans, a significant hypotension is observed when the patient stands. This postural hypotension is presumably due to blockade of sympathetic reflex compensatory mechanisms which sustain blood pressure upon standing. Large doses of alpha-adrenergic blocking agents lower blood pressure moderately in supine humans.

Alpha blocking agents antagonize the pressor response to epinephrine at a considerably lower dose than that required to antagonize the pressor responses elicited by norepinephrine or stimulation of a sympathetic trunk. Larger doses "reverse" the pressor action of epinephrine so that a depressor response is the prominent effect (Fig. 18-2). The larger doses antagonize the pressor responses to injected norepinephrine or sympathetic vasoconstrictor nerve stimulation but do not reverse them. *Epinephrine vasomotor reversal*, as it is commonly called, is best understood by remembering that epinephrine has pronounced beta-stimulant activity, notably in muscle vasculature, which is not blocked by alpha blocking agents. As would be expected, alpha blocking agents have no effect on the vasodepressor action of isoproterenol, since isoproterenol is predominantly a potent evoker of beta responses. Propranolol is quite effective in suppressing isoproterenol response (Fig. 18-2).

Heart Beta-receptor blocking agents decrease cardiac rate, contractility, and output. The concentration of propranolol required to depress the myocardium through mechanisms unrelated to beta blockade is much greater than that needed to produce significant beta-adrenergic blockade. Propranolol is an effective antagonist of catecholamine-induced cardiac arrhythmias. This action is presumably a direct consequence of beta-receptor blockade in the heart. In low doses, propranolol prevents the decrease in AV nodal refractoriness and in conduction time. Propranolol is also effective in reversing digitalis-induced arrhythmias, although not the drug of first choice. The reversal of digitalis arrhythmias is probably not due to adrenergic blockade but to a nonspecific quinidinelike action.

The physiologic responses of the heart to epinephrine and norepinephrine are not effectively blocked by alpha blocking agents and therefore have little effect on arrhythmias induced by adrenergic stimuli. Tachycardia and increased cardiac output may result as reflex responses to the decreased blood pressure induced by the alpha-adrenergic blocking agents. This is most likely the result of lack of inhibition of the cardioaccelerator effect of sympathetic nerve stimulation.

Gastrointestinal System Phentolamine increases the motility of the intact intestine. Such a stimulant action is direct and unrelated to adrenergic blockade. Phenoxybenzamine has only negligible effect on the gastrointestinal tract. Alpha blocking agents or beta blocking agents do not effectively block the response of the small intestine to epinephrine. Alpha blocking agents antagonize inhibition of the ileum if the inhibition is produced by an amine with a predominant alpha-stimulating action, for example, phenylephrine. Propranolol, on the other hand, antagonizes the inhibition evoked by a catecholamine with predominantly beta-stimulant action, for example, isoproterenol. A combination of propranolol and an alpha blocking agent is required to block epinephrine-induced inhibition. The obvious conclusion is that the intestinal smooth-muscle cells contain alpha and beta receptors, both of which subserve relaxation.

Uterus Epinephrine contracts or relaxes the uterus, depending on the hormonal influences acting on it. Catecholamine-induced contractions are suppressed by the alpha blockers, but catecholamine-induced relaxations are not.

Toxicity and Side Effects
Side effects are common with adrenergic blocking agents and are often sufficiently intense to necessi-

tate discontinuance of therapy. Phenoxybenzamine and phentolamine may elicit tachycardia, dizziness, confusion, postural hypotension, headache, gastrointestinal irritation, and disturbances of ejaculation.

Propranolol produces minor side reactions in-

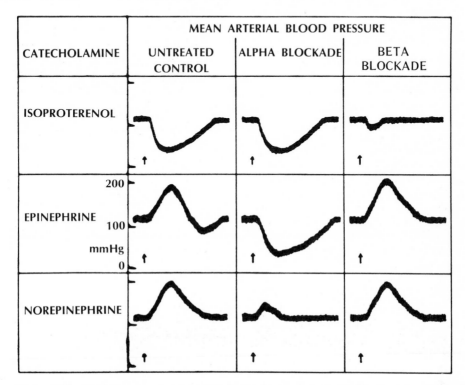

Figure 18-2 The influence of alpha and beta blocking agents on the idealized responses of the mean arterial pressure to intravenous injections of three catecholamines. The direction of the blood-pressure response is largely determined by the influence which the amines exert on total peripheral resistance. In the first column the responses in untreated animals are presented. Isoproterenol, which is predominantly an evoker of beta responses, dilates the arterioles and pressure falls. Epinephrine, which is a potent evoker of both alpha and beta responses, tends to constrict and to dilate simultaneously. The algebraic summation of these opposing effects on peripheral resistance frequently yields a biphasic effect on pressure. Pressure is first greatly increased, then falls somewhat below control level before recovering. Norepinephrine, which is predominantly an evoker of alpha responses, constricts the resistance vessels, and only a pressor response is observed.

In the presence of an effective dose of an alpha blocking agent, catecholamine-induced vasoconstriction is inhibited. Isoproterenol exerts its full depressor activity, epinephrine is purely depressor, and norepinephrine exerts only slight or no pressor effect. In the presence of an effective dose of a beta blocking agent, catecholamine-induced vasodilatation is inhibited. Isoproterenol has only slight or no depressor activity. Epinephrine is purely pressor, and the magnitude of the response is increased. Norepinephrine retains its usual pressor effect.

Arrows indicate time at which the catecholamine is injected intravenously (abscissa is time).

cluding nausea, tiredness, visual disturbances, mild diarrhea, cutaneous eruption, and insomnia, the incidence being less than 2 percent. Serious side effects resulting from the pharmacologic action of beta blockade occur relatively frequently. Severe hypotension with and without shock may occur in patients with moderately advanced cardiac disease. The hearts of these patients presumably are extremely dependent upon sympathetic support to maintain compensation. Propranolol may slow or abolish ventricular electrical activity in patients with complete AV block and idioventricular rhythm. Propranolol reduces a fall in respiratory expiration volume in asthmatic patients.

Therapeutic Uses

Peripheral Vascular Disease In its broadest sense, the term *peripheral vascular disease* applies to any disease of the blood vessels outside the heart, and to disease of the lymph vessels. The adrenergic blocking agents are used with greatest logic in peripheral vascular diseases in which vasospasm is predominant: Raynaud's syndrome, acrocyanosis, acroparesthesia, causalgia, ulceration of the extremities due to chronic peripheral vasospasm, and the sequelae of frostbite. The adrenergic blocking agents have also been used in the treatment of organic occlusive forms of peripheral vascular disease such as arteriosclerosis obliterans, thromboangiitis obliterans (Buerger's disease), and acute arterial occlusion.

Hypertension Alpha-adrenergic blocking agents have unfortunately been of little use in the treatment of hypertension. They produce mainly a postural hypotension which is often unpredictable even when the drugs are given in high doses. Tolerance to the hypotensive effects develops rapidly. Since alpha-adrenergic blocking agents do not block beta responses, the advantage gained by reduction of peripheral vascular resistance is offset by tachycardia.

Phentolamine has been found useful in the diagnosis of pheochromocytoma. Its use is based on the fact that epinephrine's action is readily blocked and reversed by these agents. Hence it is possible to select a low dose of phentolamine to selectively reduce the hypertension which is due to elevated levels of circulating epinephrine. The dose of the

blocking agent must not be too high, since blood-pressure reduction may be achieved in other forms of hypertension as the influence of the sympathetic nervous system is suppressed.

Propranolol has a mild antihypertensive effect. Initially there is a decrease in heart rate and cardiac output with a compensatory increase in total peripheral resistance. Eventually there is a progressive decrease in total peripheral resistance for no known reason. The antihypertensive effect of propranolol is apparent only with this readjustment of the circulation due to secondary peripheral arteriolar relaxation. Propranolol may also interfere with renin secretion, probably through a central mechanism. Another consequence of the central effect of propranolol is a decrease in centrally mediated sympathetic tone which may not be related to renin secretion.

Cardiac Disorders *Angina pectoris* is a paroxysmal thoracic pain associated with feelings of suffocation and impending death. The pain is considered to be due to anoxia of the myocardium and is precipitated by effort or excitement. It is usually an accompaniment to impaired coronary circulation and is frequently associated with atherosclerotic degeneration of cardiac vessels. The efficacy of the standard treatment (nitroglycerin) is presumably due to its capacity to reduce myocardial oxygen consumption. Propranolol provides symptomatic improvement in many patients with angina. The mechanism by which propranolol alleviates angina is thought to be similar to that for nitroglycerin (see Chap. 23).

In cases of *cardiac arrhythmia,* propranolol reduces or abolishes digitalis-induced ventricular premature contraction. It has also been demonstrated to slow the ventricular rate in patients with paroxysmal atrial tachycardia and partial AV block either by reducing the atrial rate or by increasing the degree of block. Propranolol also elicits a rapid and consistent decrease in the ventricular response to atrial fibrillation and flutter. Propranolol is at best partially effective, and can be completely ineffective, against ventricular arrhythmias not induced by digitalis.

Preparations and Dosage

Phenoxybenzamine hydrochloride (Dibenzyline) is

available in 10-mg capsules. The usual dosage is 20 to 60 mg daily.

Phentolamine hydrochloride (Regitine) is available in 50-mg tablets. The usual adult dosage is 50 mg 4 to 6 times daily.

Phentolamine mesylate (Regitine) is available in 5-mg ampuls. The usual dose is 5 to 10 mg.

Propranolol hydrochloride (Inderal) is available in 10- and 40-mg tablets and 1-mg ampuls. The usual oral dosage is 10 to 40 mg 3 or 4 times daily. The usual intravenous dose is 1 to 3 mg.

ADRENERGIC NEURONAL BLOCKING AGENTS

The adrenergic neuronal blocking drugs can be divided into two major categories: those drugs whose site of action is at the neuronal membrane ending, for example, guanethidine; and those drugs whose site of action is within the nerve ending, for example, guanethidine, reserpine, and methyldopa.

Guanethidine

Guanethidine

Mechanism of Action   The terminals of the sympathetic neurons contain a reservoir of catecholamines. The catecholamine store is mainly composed of bound, inactive norepinephrine. Part of the store is available for unbinding and release as a neurohumoral transmitter during postganglionic neuronal activity. The released norepinephrine impinges on the effector cells, which are adjacent to the nerve ending.

Guanethidine does not act on the effector cell, as do adrenergic blocking agents. It acts in the terminal ramifications of the sympathetic nerve fibers, where it prevents the release of the transmitter. Guanethidine exerts its nerve blockade quickly following injection. The exact mechanism by which the release of transmitter is inhibited is conjectural. It readily depletes the catecholamine stores from organs such as the heart and spleen, and from the aorta and nerve endings.

Guanethidine and norepinephrine may compete for the same storage sites in the neuron. As guanethidine increases in concentration, norepinephrine is displaced and there is a decrease in the transmitter available for release.

Effects on Organ Systems

Cardiovascular System   Guanethidine elicits sympathomimetic responses when moderate to large doses are injected intravenously. The sympathomimesis is manifested as piloerection, contraction of the spleen, and a prominent elevation of blood pressure and tachycardia. These effects last from several minutes to an hour, depending on dose, and are generally attributed to a transient discharge of norepinephrine from peripheral stores. Although elevated blood levels of catecholamines have not been demonstrated during such sympathomimetic responses, the tissues are known to be hyperresponsive to catecholamines. The pressor response can be blocked by adrenergic blocking agents and by procedures which deplete the peripheral norepinephrine stores.

Guanethidine has considerably greater hypotensive effect when patients are in the erect position than when patients are supine. Such postural hypotension is a characteristic response to agents which block the sympathetic nervous system. The hypotension is presumably due to a reduction in the capacity of vasoconstrictor fibers to bring about the usual reflex compensations upon standing. This reduces venous return and cardiac output and results in hypotension.

Guanethidine has a direct vasodilator action on blood vessels which can be observed when their indirect sympathomimetic actions have waned.

Other Systems   The predominance of the parasympathetic system following sympathetic blockade leads to gastrointestinal hyperactivity.

Weakness of the skeletal musculature is often concomitant to the use of guanethidine. It may occur in the absence of hypotension. The weakness produced may be attributed to lack of function in some of the muscle fibers within each motor unit. The drug has been observed to inhibit skeletal-muscle contraction directly. This inhibition is associated with abnormalities on the electromyographic records.

Absorption, Fate, and Excretion Guanethidine is incompletely but predictably absorbed from the gastrointestinal tract. In one study, when guanethidine was given by mouth, 36 percent was recovered from the urine in 72 h and from 20 to 25 percent recovered from the feces. Approximately 40 percent of the oral dose was unaccounted for.

Guanethidine is found in high concentrations in the cells of the kidney, liver, and lung. It cannot be easily displaced from the kidney as can other organic bases. It is possible that the protracted action of guanethidine is a result of its being firmly bound to cellular constituents.

Toxicity and Side Effects Guanethidine causes diarrhea, which often manifests itself as increased frequency of bowel movements rather than as loose stools. Muscular aching and weakness are sometimes seen with guanethidine. Excessive hypotension and syncope during muscular exercise may also occur.

Water retention is occasionally caused by guanethidine, but this is easily counteracted with thiazide diuretics. Guanethidine also produces nasal stuffiness.

Therapeutic Use Guanethidine has earned a place in the treatment of hypertension. Its important advantage is that it has a powerful antihypertensive effect similar to that of ganglionic blocking agents, but unlike the ganglionic blocking agents, it does not depress the parasympathetic nervous system. Thus, many of the unpleasant side effects associated with parasympathetic paralysis are avoided. Guanethidine reduces elevated arterial pressure in short-term therapy and is also effective in long-term management of hypertension.

Guanethidine is a very potent and long-lasting antihypertensive agent with a slow onset of activity. It primarily causes postural hypotension. The antihypertensive effect of guanethidine is usually delayed for 2 or 3 days following oral administration of an effective dose. The ensuing pressure reduction is sustained for several days. Because of its long duration of action the drug can be administered effectively in a single daily dose.

Preparation and Dosage Guanethidine sulfate (Ismelin) is available in 10- and 25-mg oral tablets.

The full effect of a given regimen of guanethidine may not be apparent for at least 1 week. The average effective maintenance dosage is 50 to 75 mg daily.

Reserpine

Reserpine is the main alkaloid found in the roots of *Rauwolfia serpentina*, and is presently isolated from the plant for medicinal purposes. It is well absorbed following oral administration; its metabolites are excreted in the urine.

Reserpine

Mechanism of Action Reserpine inhibits the binding of norepinephrine into the vesicles presumably by an action at the vesicle membrane. Since reserpine has no MAO-inhibiting action, this leads to increased intraneuronal degradation of norepinephrine by this enzyme. In addition, there is loss of amine through the nerve cell membrane. As a consequence, norepinephrine is depleted from adrenergic neurons.

Reserpine has both a central and peripheral site of action. The reduction in biogenic amine levels in subcortical areas of the brain may be responsible for its antipsychotic and sedative effects. Its depleting of norepinephrine from peripheral adrenergic nerve terminals coupled with its reducing of central sympathetic tone contribute to its antihypertensive effect.

Toxicity and Side Effects The major side effects of reserpine are sedation, psychic depressive reactions, nightmares, abdominal cramps, and diarrhea. On chronic administration reserpine may cause gastrointestinal ulceration and hemorrhage. Less severe side effects are salt and water retention, nasal congestion, extrapyramidal disturbances, and flushing of the skin.

Therapeutic Uses The only indications for the use of reserpine are in the management of certain types of hypertension, and in selected psychotic states for individuals unable to tolerate phenothiazine derivatives.

Preparations and Dosage Reserpine is available as 0.1-, 0.25-, 0.5-, and 1-mg tablets; 0.25 mg/5 ml elixir; and 2.5 and 5 mg/ml solution for injection. The usual oral adult maintenance dosage is 0.1 to 0.25 mg daily.

Related Rauwolfia Alkaloids Other drugs related structurally and pharmacologically to reserpine are deserpidine, rescinnamine, syrosingopine, and alseroxylon.

Methyldopa

Mechanism of Action The dopa-decarboxylase inhibitor methyldopa (α-methyldopa), has substantial orthostatic hypotensive activity in humans. Its hypotensive activity has been attributed to two major sites of action: (1) in the CNS and (2) at peripheral sympathetic nerve endings.

The central effect of methyldopa appears to be related to depression of sympathetic neurons within the hypothalamus and medulla. The exact mechanism is unknown although it appears to be associated with the structural similarity of methyldopa and norepinephrine. The peripheral mechanism of action of methyldopa's antihypertensive effect is the result of the formation of a false neurotransmitter. The suggestion has been that methyldopa, which is very similar in structure to dopa, might be accepted as a substrate by intraneuronal dopa-decarboxylase and that the resulting decarboxyl-

ated product would in turn be processed by dopamine-β-hydroxylase to yield α-methylnorepinephrine.

Since α-methylnorepinephrine is a weaker sympathomimetic agent than is norepinephrine, the overall effect of this substitution—should α-methylnorepinephrine be released by action potentials—would be to decrease sympathetic tone. Experiment has confirmed that these biochemical alterations of α-methyldopa do indeed occur and that α-methylnorepinephrine is released from adrenergic nerves during electrical stimulation.

Absorption, Fate, and Excretion Methyldopa can be given orally but less than 50 percent is absorbed. It is metabolized by decarboxylation and subsequent conjugation. Both the conjugated and decarboxylated derivatives are excreted in the urine.

Toxicity and Side Effects One of the major side effects of methyldopa is sedation. However, subjects become tolerant to this effect with continued usage. Vertigo, extrapyramidal reactions, and psychic depression occur much less frequently with methyldopa than with reserpine. Other adverse reactions are postural hypotension, salt and water retention with weight gain and edema, hemolytic anemia, liver damage, granulocytopenia, and thrombocytopenia.

Therapeutic Use The only clinical use for methyldopa is in the treatment of hypertension.

Preparations and Dosage Methyldopa (Aldomet) is available for oral administration in 250- and 500-mg tablets. It is also available in 5-ml ampuls (50 mg/ml) for parenteral use. The usual initial dosage is 250 mg 3 times daily.

α-Methyldopa α-Methyldopamine α-Methylnorepinephrine

Cholinomimetic Drugs, Cholinergic Blocking Drugs, and Ganglionic Stimulant and Blocking Drugs

CHOLINOMIMETIC DRUGS

Cholinomimetic agents are defined as drugs which evoke responses similar both to those produced by ACh and to those which result from activation of the parasympathetic nervous system. Excluding the stimulation produced by cholinomimetic agents of parasympathetic ganglia or the CNS, these agents produce their effects by two general mechanisms. The first mechanism involves direct activation by the cholinomimetic agents of receptor sites located on the postjunctional membranes of the nerve or effector cell. Accordingly, drugs of this class produce their effects by imitating the interactions between postjunctional elements and ACh liberated from the nerve endings. The second mechanism is an indirect process which is brought about either by the enhancement or the preservation of ACh released from the nerve terminals. Thus, the responses produced by this class of compound can be attributed primarily to the accumulation of endogenous ACh.

Pharmacologic Actions of ACh

ACh is a quaternary ammonium compound with the structural formula shown in Fig. 19-1. Because of its highly polar, positively charged ammonium group, ACh is poorly soluble in lipid-containing materials. For that reason, it is confined to the extracellular spaces of the body and does not penetrate the blood-brain barrier. Moreover, ACh is an ester and therefore readily hydrolyzed, especially by cholinesterases, into its inactive components, acetic acid and choline.

The combination of enzymatic and spontaneous hydrolysis is the reason for the relatively short-lived action of ACh.

Cardiovascular System The cardiovascular system is affected more profoundly than any other organ system by ACh administered intravenously. Doses of ACh which are too small to produce effects on the heart, skeletal muscle, glands, and other organs known to be sensitive to the drug

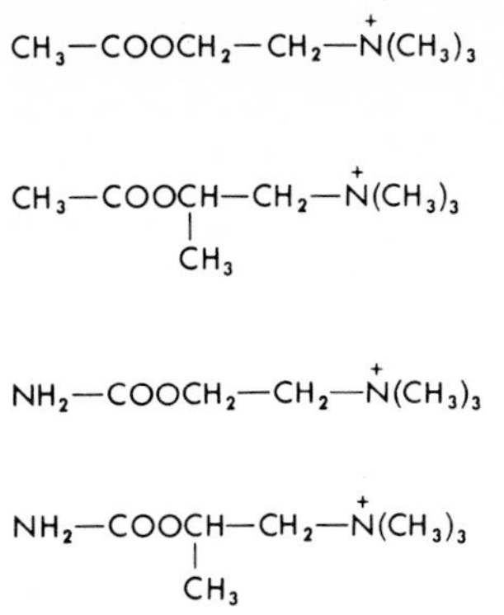

$$CH_3-COOCH_2-CH_2-\overset{+}{N}(CH_3)_3 \qquad \text{Acetylcholine}$$

$$CH_3-COOCH-CH_2-\overset{+}{N}(CH_3)_3 \qquad \text{Acetyl-}\beta\text{-methylcholine}$$
$$\underset{CH_3}{|}$$

$$NH_2-COOCH_2-CH_2-\overset{+}{N}(CH_3)_3 \qquad \text{Carbamylcholine}$$

$$NH_2-COOCH-CH_2-\overset{+}{N}(CH_3)_3 \qquad \text{Bethanechol}$$
$$\underset{CH_3}{|}$$

Figure 19-1 Structural formulas of ACh and its analogues.

produce a perceptible fall in mean arterial pressure. Not all the factors contributing to this differential sensitivity to ACh are known.

In general, ACh produces vasodilation of the major vascular beds. The presence of cholinergic innervation is not a prerequisite for this action of ACh. In fact, the vascular bed of skeletal muscle is the only area where innervation by cholinergic vasodilator fibers has been demonstrated. ACh causes vasodilation of the cerebral, coronary, cutaneous, and splanchnic vasculature, none of which is under the control of cholinergic fibers.

ACh has prominent actions on cardiac rhythm, conduction processes of the heart, and the atrial myocardium; these actions parallel almost exactly those produced by stimulation of the vagus nerve.

Both ACh and vagal stimulation cause slowing of the rate of firing of the sinoatrial node which is associated with hyperpolarization of the pacemaker membrane. On cessation of the stimulation, the membrane potential depolarizes to threshold values and the beat resumes. These effects are prevented by atropine and are exaggerated by inhibitors of the cholinesterases. Similarly depressed by ACh are other pacemaker potentials which have been observed at ectopic foci, the AV node, and in the bundle of His and Purkinje fiber complex. There is, however, a marked difference in the sensitivities of the various regions to inhibition by ACh. While the sinoatrial and AV nodes are quite sensitive to blockade by ACh, spontaneous activity in the bundle of His and Purkinje system is relatively resistant.

Atrial fibers are also inhibited by ACh and by stimulation of the vagus nerve. Unlike the pacemaker of the sinoatrial node, hyperpolarization of the membrane is not always associated with the inhibition.

In addition to the aforementioned changes in cardiac activity, the local application of ACh or vagal stimulation can also induce atrial fibrillation. The fibrillation is not due to an increase in the sinus rate or to the development of new pacemakers but appears to be due to a phenomenon called *reexcitation by reentry*. This phenomenon results from the circular movement of excitation and the reexcitation of fibers which have already passed through their refractory periods. It is favored by (1) a restriction of normal pathways due to local block, (2) a reduced refractory period, and (3) reduced conduction velocity. In addition to the various degrees of blockade described earlier, both vagal stimulation and ACh reduce the refractory period of atrial fibers by shortening the duration of the action potentials. Thus, two of the conditions which predispose the atrium to fibrillation are produced by ACh and stimulation of the vagus nerve.

Smooth-Muscle Cells In contrast with the smooth-muscle cells of the several vascular beds, those of most of the other organs respond to ACh with an increase in tone.

By a direct action, ACh causes contraction of the smooth-muscle cells of the bronchioles, uterus, ureters, bladder, stomach, small intestine, colon, and constrictor muscles of the iris. The contraction of the smooth muscle is antagonized by atropine and enhanced by the inhibitors of the cholinesterase enzymes. It has been demonstrated that the increased tone of the smooth-muscle cells is associated with depolarization of the membrane.

Neuromuscular Junction and Skeletal-Muscle System In contrast with its distinct action on the smooth-muscle cell, ACh is without significant effect on the striated muscle fiber. It has been demonstrated by means of the microscopic iontophoretic application of ACh that the chemosensitive area of the neuromuscular junction resides exclusively in the specialized subneural structure called the end plate.

Whereas extremely small amounts of ACh applied by this technique evoke an effective, super-threshold depolarization of the end plate, no electric activity is observed when ACh is applied directly to the muscle cell fiber. Accordingly, the actions of ACh at the neuromuscular junction are, in essence, the actions of ACh on the end plates.

Glands   All the glands innervated by cholinergic fibers are stimulated by ACh. These include the salivary, lacrimal, and sweat glands, in addition to the exocrine cells of the pancreas, gastrointestinal mucosa, and bronchioles.

Analogues of ACh

Acetyl-β-methylcholine (Methacholine)   As shown in Fig. 19-1, this compound differs from ACh only by the addition of a methyl group to the β-methyl position of choline. This structural change introduces two important alterations in the pharmacologic properties of the molecule. Unlike ACh, methacholine is hydrolyzed only by acetylcholinesterase, and the rate of hydrolysis of methacholine is considerably slower than that of ACh. Thus the actions of methacholine are more persistent than those of ACh. For reasons that are not clear, the introduction of the methyl group to the beta position endows the molecule with more selectivity. Methacholine acts primarily on smooth muscle, glands, and the heart and is essentially devoid of any prominent actions on autonomic ganglia and skeletal muscle. These two features, duration of response and improved selectivity, represent the primary differences between the pharmacologic actions of methacholine and ACh.

The actions of methacholine on the cardiovascular system are the same qualitatively as those described above for ACh. Its clinical use in selected cases of atrial tachycardia not responding to other forms of therapy has largely been replaced by other modalities.

Carbamylcholine (Carbaminoylcholine, Carbachol)   This compound is the most powerful of all the choline esters. In contrast with ACh and methacholine, the acid component of this ester is carbamic rather than acetic acid (Fig. 19-1). The carbamic acid–ester link is not readily susceptible to hydrolysis by the cholinesterases. Although enzymic destruction of carbachol has been dem-

onstrated, the rate of hydrolysis is too slow to be of any practical significance. Indeed, carbachol possesses anticholinesterase properties.

Carbachol has all the pharmacologic properties of ACh. In addition to producing vasodilation, cardiac slowing, increased tone and contraction of smooth muscles, and stimulation of salivary, lacrimal, and sweat glands, carbachol also stimulates autonomic ganglia and skeletal muscle. The former actions of carbachol are more resistant to blockade by atropine than are the similar actions of ACh. Because of these characteristics—lack of selectivity, potency, and resistance to atropine—carbachol has a limited place in therapy. At present, the principal use of carbachol is in ophthalmology as a miotic agent. For this purpose, carbachol is applied topically to the conjunctiva.

Bethanechol (Urecholine)   Bethanechol, the structure of which is shown in Fig. 19-1, is a choline ester with structural features common to both methacholine and carbachol. Because of these features, bethanechol has the pharmacologic properties of methacholine combined with the chemical characteristics of carbachol. Thus, bethanechol, like carbachol, is not hydrolyzed by the cholinesterase enzymes and, like methacholine, does not stimulate autonomic ganglia or skeletal muscle. Accordingly, the same contraindications that apply for methacholine apply to bethanechol.

Bethanechol appears to have a more selective action on the gastrointestinal tract and urinary bladder than do the other choline esters. Its therapeutic uses are based primarily on these actions. Bethanechol has been used in the treatment of gastric retention following vagotomy, postoperative urinary retention, postoperative abdominal distention, and other gastrointestinal disorders in which the simulation of parasympathetic stimulation may be useful.

Muscarine and Mushroom Poisoning   Muscarine, an alkaloid present in the mushroom *Amanita muscaria* (fly agaric), which has wide geographic distribution (Europe, Asia, North and South America, South Africa), is of interest because of its toxic properties and because historically it was one of the first cholinomimetic drugs to be systematically studied. Hence the term *muscarinic* has been used to describe the actions of drugs which mimic the effects of the parasympathetic nervous system. Its chemical structure is now known.

HO——
CH$_3$——O——CH$_2$—N$^+$(CH$_3$)$_3$

Muscarine

Muscarine is a very active parasympathomimetic drug, and is in a great many respects more potent than ACh. This is the result, in part, of its great stability, which renders it resistant to cholinesterase. On the other hand, it does not inhibit either acetylcholinesterase or pseudocholinesterase. Its actions are similar to those of ACh on peripheral autonomic effectors, and these actions are antagonized by atropine. Unlike ACh, it has slight atropine-sensitive effects on autonomic ganglia in very high doses, and its action on skeletal muscle is insignificant.

Mushroom poisoning is still a common occurrence. Two main types are recognized. The first type is characterized by the appearance of symptoms within a few minutes to at most a few hours. The victim shows profound stimulation of the parasympathetic nervous system. These symptoms may be treated effectively with atropine. This type of poisoning is probably the result of the actions of muscarine. It is the less common of the types of mushroom poisoning and generally is not fatal.

The second type of mushroom poisoning is due to ingestion of another species, *Amanita phalloides*. In this case the symptoms are delayed for several hours or even a day and are marked by focus on the gastrointestinal tract. Severe gastroenteritis occurs. This stage may be severe enough to lead to shock, prostration, and death. If the victim survives the initial stages, these symptoms may be followed by acute hepatic necrosis and renal parenchymal damage, eventually causing delayed death. Therapy with atropine is useless.

Pilocarpine Pilocarpine is an alkaloid obtained from the leaf of the tropical American shrub *Pilocarpus jaborandi*. Its actions are essentially the same as those of muscarine and methacholine, and, as with these compounds, its actions are antagonized by atropine. It differs from most cholino-

mimetic compounds by the absence of a quaternary nitrogen in its chemical structure.

C$_2$H$_5$——CH$_2$——N—CH$_3$
O O   N

Pilocarpine

The primary current therapeutic use of pilocarpine is in ophthalmology as a miotic. In this connection, pilocarpine is used to produce miosis in selected patients with glaucoma and to counteract the mydriasis produced by atropine. Because of its prominent actions on the salivary glands, in those situations in which salivary stimulation is desired, it is the preferred drug.

Administration of pilocarpine, like stimulation of the parasympathetic innervation of the eye, causes constriction of the pupil by activation of the sphincter muscles of the iris. The absence of a quaternary ammonium ion in its chemical structure permits a more rapid penetration of the molecule than is achieved by the previously mentioned cholinomimetic drugs.

Pilocarpine has been used in the management of nonobstructive urinary retention.

Anticholinesterase Agents

As a class, the anticholinesterase agents are probably the most important members of the cholinomimetic family of drugs. In addition to their important role in therapy, the anticholinesterase agents are used widely in the control of insects and are potential instruments of chemical warfare. It is important to note that their use in medicine, the management of their toxic manifestations, and their use as insecticides are all based on an understanding of the changes which occur in the organism following the inactivation of the cholinesterases. Before discussing the general pharmacologic properties of the anticholinesterase agents, some of the chemical characteristics of the inhibitors should be considered.

The hydrolytic cleavage by acetylcholinesterase is believed to occur by the process depicted schematically in Fig. 19-2. It is probable that the attachment of the ACh to the enzyme serves to fix and orient the molecule for enzymic attack on the ester linkage. Unlike the ionic binding between the

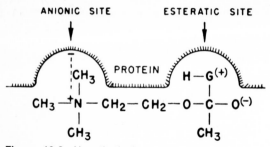

Figure 19-2 Hypothetical presentation of the complex formed by the interaction of ACh with acetylcholinesterase. At the anionic site, an electrostatic bond is formed between the enzyme and the positive charge of the nitrogen atom. At the esteratic site, a covalent bond is formed between the carbonyl group of ACh and the basic group $G^{(+)}$ of the esteratic site of the enzyme.

nitrogen atom and the enzyme, the carbonyl atom of the acetate portion of ACh forms a covalent bond with the enzyme. This results in the acetylation of the enzyme, the rupture of the ester linkage, and the elimination of choline. The acetylated enzyme then reacts with water to form regenerated enzyme and acetic acid.

The anticholinesterase agents can be divided into two groups: the reversible and irreversible inhibitors. This definition is based on the type of chemical interaction occurring between the inhibitor and the enzyme. As the name implies, the reversible anticholinesterase agents form a transient complex with the surface of the enzyme, in much the same way as does ACh. Accordingly, the inhibitors of this class compete with ACh for the active sites on the enzyme. The chemical structure of two of the classic reversible inhibitors (physostigmine and neostigmine) suggests a similarity to the structure of ACh. Like the carbonyl group of ACh, the carbonyl group of physostigmine and neostigmine forms an attachment to the *esteratic* site of the enzyme (Fig. 19-2). However, the inhibitors differ from ACh in that they are not degraded by the enzyme. In addition to binding at the esteratic site, neostigmine also has an electrostatic bond between its quaternary nitrogen and the *anionic* site of the enzyme, thus forming a two-point attachment with the enzyme. While both physostigmine and neostigmine have a very high affinity for acetylcholinesterase, the inhibition of the enzyme is reversible. Consistent with the reversibility of the enzyme-

inhibitor complex is the reversibility of the pharmacologic actions produced by the anticholinesterase agents of this class.

Pyridine-2-aldoxime methochloride (PAM) has been used to reverse the inhibition of the cholinesterases by neostigmine, physostigmine, and other reversible cholinesterase inhibitors. The reasoning for this use of PAM arises from the fact that neostigmine forms a covalent bond with the esteratic site of the cholinesterase molecule that can be disrupted by PAM.

This action of PAM is equally prominent for the irreversible organophosphorus anticholinesterase agents. Whereas the neostigminelike compounds cause a carbamylation of the enzyme, the organophosphorus compounds cause a phosphorylation of the enzyme. In effect, PAM competes with the enzyme for the carbamate and phosphorus groups of the inhibitors in such a way that the esteratic site on the enzyme is restored. When this occurs, the enzyme is able to function, and the effects of accumulated ACh begin to dissipate.

Reversible Anticholinesterase Agents

Physostigmine (Eserine) Physostigmine is an alkaloid extracted from the calabar bean, the dried ripe seed of a wood vine that grows in tropical West Africa, *Physostigma venenosum*. It is also synthesized chemically. Physostigmine has been used

Physostigmine

in ophthalmology as a miotic agent since the middle of the nineteenth century. Like most tertiary amines, physostigmine is readily absorbed from the gastrointestinal tract and also from other mucous membranes. Similarly, physostigmine readily penetrates the blood-brain barrier. Consequently, the distribution of physostigmine within the organism is widespread. All those systems which normally produce and respond to ACh are affected by physostigmine. At each of these sites, following the administration of adequate amounts of physostigmine, the resultant accumulation of the transmitter gives rise to marked cholinergic stimulation. Since these responses are essentially the same as those enumerated above for ACh and the same as those listed in Table 19-1, they will not be described here except in those instances that relate to past or present uses of physostigmine.

In ophthalmology, the physostigmine-induced miosis has been used also to antagonize the prolonged mydriasis produced by atropine. In addition, use has been made of the opposing actions on the eye of these two agents to rupture adhesions between the iris and the lens. By giving atropine and physostigmine alternately, the pupillary size can be made to shift between the extremes of dilation and constriction. The mechanical forces produced by this procedure are often adequate to break the adhesions.

One of the most striking aspects of the pharmacologic actions of physostigmine is its effect on transmission at the neuromuscular junction. When administered systemically, physostigmine produces fasciculations and, with large doses, paralysis of striated muscle. As stated earlier, these responses are due to the inhibition of acetylcholinesterase and the resulting accumulation of ACh in the neuromuscular junction. It is by this mechanism that physostigmine antagonizes the blockade of neuromuscular transmission produced by curare. Since curare blocks transmission by competing with ACh for receptor sites on the end plate, the accumula-

Table 19-1   Signs and Symptoms Produced in Humans by Anticholinesterase Agents

Site of action	Signs and symptoms	Site of action	Signs and symptoms
Following local exposure		Sweat glands	Increased sweating
Pupils	Miosis, marked, usually maximal (pinpoint), sometimes unequal	Salivary glands	Increased salivation
		Lacrimal glands	Increased lacrimation
Ciliary body	Frontal headache, eye pain on focusing, slight dimness of vision, occasional nausea and vomiting	Heart	Slight bradycardia
		Pupils	Slight miosis, occasionally unequal, later more marked miosis
Conjunctiva	Hyperemia	Ciliary body	Blurring of vision
Nasal mucous membranes	Rhinorrhea, hyperemia	Bladder	Frequency, involuntary micturition
Bronchial tree	Tightness in chest, sometimes with prolonged wheezing expiration suggestive of bronchoconstriction or increased secretion, cough	Striated muscle	Easy fatigue, mild weakness, muscular twitching, fasciculations, cramps, generalized weakness, including muscles of respiration, with dyspnea and cyanosis
Sweat glands	Sweating at site of exposure to liquid	Sympathetic ganglia	Pallor, occasional elevation of blood pressure
Striated muscle	Fasciculation at site of exposure to liquid	Central nervous system	Giddiness; tension; anxiety; jitteriness; restlessness; emotional lability; excessive dreaming; insomnia; nightmares; headache; tremor; apathy; withdrawal and depression; bursts of slow waves of elevated voltage in EEG, especially on overventilation; drowsiness; difficulty in concentrating, slowness of recall; confusion; slurred speech; ataxia; generalized weakness; coma, with absence of reflexes; Cheyne-Stokes respiration; convulsions; depression of respiratory and circulatory centers with dyspnea, cyanosis, and fall in blood pressure
Following systemic absorption			
Bronchial tree	Tightness in chest, with prolonged wheezing expiration suggestive of bronchoconstriction or increased secretion, dyspnea, slight pain in chest, increased bronchial secretion, cough		
Gastrointestinal system	Anorexia, nausea, vomiting, abdominal cramps, epigastric and substernal tightness (cardiospasm?) with "heartburn" and eructation, diarrhea, tenesmus, involuntary defecation		

tion of ACh which occurs following the inhibition of acetylcholinesterase shifts the competition in favor of the transmitter and mediates the anticurare action of physostigmine.

Neostigmine (*Prostigmin*) Neostigmine is a synthetic anticholinesterase which was developed as an outcome of the studies of the cholinesterase-inhibiting properties of physostigmine.

$$(CH_3)_2NCOO\!-\!\!\underset{}{\bigcirc}\!-\!\overset{+}{N}(CH_3)_3$$

Neostigmine

It differs from physostigmine, however, in that it contains a quaternary nitrogen. As a consequence, neostigmine differs from physostigmine in its pattern of distribution in the organism. Neostigmine is poorly and irregularly absorbed from the gastrointestinal tract. In addition, it penetrates poorly other lipoidal barriers and membranes. Thus, it is difficult to regulate plasma levels of neostigmine when the drug is given orally. On the other hand, the poor penetration by the drug of the blood-brain barrier tends to minimize any occurrence of toxicity due to the inhibition of cholinesterases of the brain.

The presence of a quaternary nitrogen in the molecule introduces another important difference between physostigmine and neostigmine. The latter compound, in addition to inhibiting the cholinesterases, also has direct actions on effector organs. Apart from these important differences, the general actions of neostigmine are like those of physostigmine and comparable to hyperactivity of cholinergic nerves.

Like other anticholinesterase agents, neostigmine possesses a powerful anticurare action. Conceptually, an anticurare effect can be brought about by: (1) increase in the amount of ACh liberated from the nerve endings, (2) preservation of the liberated transmitter by inhibiting acetylcholinesterase, and (3) direct action of the drug on the end plate. Each of these mechanisms is a distinct possibility for explaining the anticurare action of neostigmine. There is little doubt that neostigmine is an anticholinesterase agent and that this action contributes to its ability to overcome the blockade of

neuromuscular transmission produced by curare. Another contributing factor, however, is the direct excitatory action of neostigmine on the end plate. Skeletal muscles that are treated with doses of organophosphorus anticholinesterase agents adequate to inhibit completely and irreversibly the acetylcholinesterase of the end plate contract following an intraarterial injection of neostigmine. This response cannot be attributed to an anticholinesterase action. Similarly, a number of studies have shown that neostigmine and its structural analogues stimulate motor nerve endings in a manner similar to that previously described for physostigmine. It is probable that each of the three mechanisms listed above is operating in the anticurare action of neostigmine. Use is made in anesthesiology of this action of neostigmine to overcome the paralysis of skeletal muscles produced by curare and curarelike drugs.

The neuromuscular actions of neostigmine, more than those of physostigmine, have been extremely beneficial in the management of myasthenia gravis. For many years neostigmine was the drug of choice for this disorder. Although it is still used at present for this purpose, it has been displaced to some extent by newer anticholinesterases, which are better tolerated because of less intense side effects.

There are some difficulties attending the use of neostigmine for the treatment of myasthenia. First, the dosage of neostigmine is difficult to regulate. Given by mouth, it is poorly and irregularly absorbed from the gastrointestinal tract. With an overdose, the accumulation of ACh at the end plate may be excessive and paralysis of transmission may occur. This situation is termed *cholinergic crisis*. In the absence of prior knowledge of drug administrations, it then becomes necessary to distinguish between the muscle weakness of the undertreated patient, that is, *myasthenic crisis*, and the paralysis caused by an overdose of the anticholinesterase agent. This may prove difficult if the patient is receiving atropine to prevent the muscarinic side effects of neostigmine. The differential diagnosis is aided by the use of an ultra-short-acting anticholinesterase agent, edrophonium, which is described below.

A second difficulty with neostigmine is the maintenance of a stable level of strength. Since neostigmine is a reversible cholinesterase inhibitor, its actions are relatively short-lived. Accordingly, muscle strength waxes and wanes as the drug effect takes place and then diminishes. This necessitates repeated administration of the drug and incurs the risk of cumulation. For some patients it may also be necessary to interrupt their sleep for drug administration. The third problem is the ever-present one of side effects. For the anticholinesterase agents, these include excessive salivation, perspiration, abdominal distress, nausea, and vomiting. Although the side effects can be controlled by atropine, they are the indicators of cumulation and overdose of the anticholinesterase agent, and their blockade may mask an impending cholinergic crisis.

In addition to its place in the management of myasthenia, neostigmine has proven extremely valuable in the diagnosis of this disease. Improvement of muscle strength usually occurs 10 min after an intramuscular injection of neostigmine. Increased strength persists for 3 to 4 h. Nonmyasthenic patients show either no improvement of strength or increased weakness.

Neostigmine is used also as a miotic agent. In this regard it is somewhat less effective than physostigmine. This difference is related most probably to the poor penetration by neostigmine into the eye following topical application.

Other uses of neostigmine are in the treatment of postoperative atony of the intestine and urinary bladder, in suppression of paroxysmal atrial tachycardia, and as a pregnancy test. In the first two instances, the rationale is the same as that described for drugs such as methacholine and bethanechol.

Edrophonium Chloride (Tensilon)   Except for the ethyl group on the nitrogen atom, edrophonium is neostigmine lacking the ester group.

Edrophonium

The pharmacologic properties of this compound resemble qualitatively those of neostigmine. There is, however, a wider margin than exists for neostigmine between the dose of edrophonium required to produce changes in neuromuscular transmission and the dose required to stimulate the heart,

smooth-muscle cells, and glands. Accordingly, it is possible to stimulate the neuromuscular junction with doses of edrophonium that have no effect on other cholinergic structures. Two additional features distinguish the actions of edrophonium from those of neostigmine: (1) Its onset of action is more rapid than that of neostigmine and (2) its period of action is considerably shorter. These characteristics are more consistent with a directly acting agent than with one that exerts its effect by inhibiting an enzyme.

The brief duration of action of edrophonium compared with the longer-acting anticholinesterase agents is, for some purposes, a distinct advantage. It minimizes the problem of managing overdosage and reduces the possibility of cumulation of the drug. This drug, like neostigmine, is capable of paralyzing transmission at the neuromuscular junction.

Edrophonium plays a prominent role in establishing the diagnosis of myasthenia gravis and in making a differential diagnosis between myasthenic weakness and cholinergic crisis. In these situations, use is made of the transient actions of the drug. For the diagnosis of myasthenia, edrophonium is injected intravenously in divided doses. The brief duration of its effect requires that measurements of muscle strength be made quickly. The improvement in strength, if it occurs, will last for less than 5 min. The test can be repeated several times on the same day. For the differentiation between myasthenic and cholinergic crises, edrophonium is given intravenously. If the crisis is due to inadequate anticholinesterase therapy, edrophonium will result in an improvement of muscle strength. Conversely, edrophonium will further decrease muscle strength if the weakness is due to an overdose or cumulation of the anticholinesterase agent. In the case of cholinergic crisis, the short-lived actions of edrophonium will not materially prolong the crisis, and other measures, such as maintenance of airways and artificial ventilation, can be instituted.

A second important therapeutic use of edrophonium is based on its ability to antagonize curare and other curariform drugs. It is unlikely that the anticurare action is due to the inhibition of acetylcholinesterase, since doses of edrophonium which effectively antagonize the blockade of neuromuscular transmission have no effect on the sensitivity of end plate to injected ACh. An increase in the response to ACh similar to that produced by physostigmine would be expected if the inhibition of acetylcholinesterase was involved. Edrophonium has a direct excitatory action on the end plate.

Pyridostigmine Bromide (Mestinon)   Qualitatively the pharmacologic properties of pyridostigmine bromide are the same as those of neostigmine. Like neostigmine, it has anticurare, miotic, and anticholinesterase actions. However, in most pharmacologic tests pyridostigmine has about one-half the potency and about one-hundredth the anticholinesterase activity of neostigmine. Consistent with the lower potency of pyridostigmine, it is less toxic than neostigmine.

$(CH_3)_2NCOO-$

$\underset{\underset{CH_3}{|}}{\overset{+}{N}}$

Pyridostigmine

The principal therapeutic use of pyridostigmine is in the treatment of myasthenia gravis. The improvement of muscular strength following the administration of pyridostigmine is more sustained than that produced by neostigmine. Accordingly, less frequent administration is required. This is particularly important during the night. Moreover, the sustained actions of pyridostigmine permit a more even improvement of strength. As a result of its reduced potency, there is less danger of overdosage with pyridostigmine. Another advantage with pyridostigmine is the reduced severity of side effects. There appears to be a lower incidence of gastrointestinal discomfort.

Ambenonium Chloride (Mytelase Chloride)   Ambenonium chloride is an anticholinesterase agent with pharmacologic properties similar to those of neostigmine. The pharmacologic actions of ambenonium are brought about primarily through the reversible inactivation of the cholinesterases.

The principal therapeutic use for ambenonium is in the management of myasthenia gravis. Like pyridostigmine, it is claimed to have at least two advantages over neostigmine for this purpose. First, ambenonium appears to have a slightly more sustained action; and second, a lower incidence of distressing side effects, especially gastrointestinal, has been reported for ambenonium.

Other Bisymmetric Anticholinesterase Agents   Bis-neostigmine (Demecarium, Humorsol) is an anticholinesterase agent with a duration of action markedly exceeding that of the aforementioned reversible inhibitors. The inhibition of cholinesterase produced by this compound is reversible. It has a higher affinity for acetylcholinesterase than for nonspecific cholinesterase.

In the management of glaucoma, Demecarium lowers intraocular pressure when instilled into the eye. A single instillation into the conjunctival sac of normal subjects produces miosis which is apparent within 1 h, attains a maximum within 4 h, and persists for 3 to 10 days. The miosis is accompanied by spasm of the intraocular muscles of accommodation. Even though the application of the drug is confined to the eye, absorption may be large enough to bring about systemic signs of cholinesterase inhibition.

Irreversible Anticholinesterase Agents   The second class of anticholinesterase agents is the organophosphorus group of inhibitors. Only a limited number of the organophosphorus anticholinesterase agents has found a useful place in therapy. The primary pharmacologic properties of the organophosphorus inhibitors are due to the inactivation of the cholinesterases. In contrast with the anticholinesterase property of physostigmine and neostigmine, the inhibition produced by the organophosphorus compounds is, for all practical purposes, irreversible.

The organophosphorus agents have the following general formula:

$$\underset{R_2}{\overset{R_1}{}}\!\!\diagdown\!\!\underset{}{\overset{}{P}}\!\!\diagup\!\!\overset{O(S)}{\underset{X}{}}$$

The reactivity of the inhibitor with the enzyme is determined largely by the strength of the P—X bond. Although the strength of this bond varies according to the substituents on the phosphorus atom, the inactivation of the enzyme is due to the formation of a covalent bond between the phosphorus atom of the inhibitor and the *esteratic* site of the enzyme. Stated in other terms, the enzyme is phosphorylated by the organophosphorus agents. A schematic representation of the phosphorylated enzyme is illustrated in Fig. 19-3. In contrast with

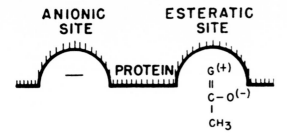

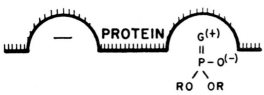

Figure 19-3 Schematic representation of acetylated acetylcholinesterase (top diagram) and phosphorylated acetylcholinesterase (bottom diagram). The symbol $G^{(+)}$ represents the basic group of the esteratic site which forms covalent bonds with the substrate and inhibitor.

the rapid regeneration by water of the acetylated enzyme produced during the hydrolysis of ACh, the phosphorylated enzyme reacts very slowly with water. It is for this reason that the enzyme-inhibitor complex is irreversible. For most of the organophosphorus compounds, de novo synthesis of the enzyme must take place for the cholinesterase activity of tissue to return. For others a limited amount of spontaneous reactivation of the enzyme occurs. Although this type of inhibition is generally regarded as irreversible, chemical agents are known which can reactivate the enzyme.

The signs and symptoms which occur following the administration of an organophosphorus anticholinesterase agent can be readily predicted and are attributable to hyperactivity of the parasympathetic nervous system, neuromuscular junction, autonomic ganglia, and cholinergic nerves of the CNS. These signs are listed in Table 19-1. Death is due primarily to depression of respiration caused by depression of the CNS, paralysis of the diaphragm and intercostal muscles, bronchospasm, and the accumulation of bronchosecretions. Each is due to the accumulation of excessive amounts of ACh. The basis of the central component of res-

piratory depression is not understood but is believed to be due also to excessive amounts of ACh.

Diisopropyl Fluorophosphate (Isoflurophate, DFP) The primary difference between DFP and agents such as physostigmine lies in the persistency of action. By the mechanism described above for the organophosphorus anticholinesterase agents, DFP produces an irreversible inactivation of the cholinesterases. Both acetylcholinesterase and "nonspecific" cholinesterase are inactivated by DFP; however, DFP has a greater affinity for the latter enzyme.

$$C_3H_7O \diagdown \atop C_3H_7O \diagup P {\diagup O \atop \diagdown F}$$

DFP

DFP is used in the treatment of certain types of glaucoma, in certain types of strabismus, and as an antidote against the harmful effects of atropine on preglaucomatous and glaucomatous eyes. The miosis occurring after a single application of a solution of DFP in peanut oil into the conjunctival sac begins within 5 to 10 min, attains a maximum (pinpoint size) in 15 to 20 min, and persists for 1 to 4 weeks. The rate of onset, intensity, and duration of action are greater for DFP than for physostigmine or neostigmine.

Tetraethylpyrophosphate ***(TEPP)*** Like DFP, TEPP is a long-acting cholinesterase inhibitor which produces a phosphorylation of the enzymes. The resulting phosphorylated enzyme exhibits all the chemical characteristics in vitro of an irreversibly inactivated enzyme. In contrast with DFP, however, limited spontaneous reversal in vivo of the enzyme-inhibitor complex occurs.

$$C_2H_5O \diagdown \atop C_2H_5O \diagup P {\overset{O}{\|}} {\diagdown \atop O} P {\overset{O}{\|}} {\diagup OC_2H_5 \atop \diagdown OC_2H_5}$$

TEPP

Echothiophate Iodide (Phospholine Iodide) Echothiophate is a phosphorylthiocholine; it is a long-acting anticholinesterase agent with pharmacologic actions on the peripheral nervous system similar to those of DFP. Spontaneous regeneration of the phosphorylated enzyme occurs more rapidly with echothiophate, as with TEPP, than with DFP.

$$(C_2H_5\text{—}O)_2 \overset{\overset{\displaystyle O}{\|}}{P}\text{—}S\text{—}CH_2\text{—}CH_2\text{—}\overset{+}{N}(CH_3)_3$$

Echothiophate

Echothiophate is used in ophthalmology for the treatment of glaucoma and other disorders of the eye amenable to therapy with anticholinesterase agents. In this regard, the water-soluble property of echothiophate affords one practical advantage over the lipid-soluble irreversible anticholinesterase agents. Lacrimation evoked by the irritation produced by solvents such as peanut oil may result in the removal of the anticholinesterase agent from the conjunctiva. Usually this does not occur with echothiophate. The use of echothiophate for these purposes is governed by the same precautions and limitations as are the other long-acting anticholinesterase agents.

Paraoxon Paraoxon actions on organ systems are the same generally as those described for other organophosphorus anticholinesterase agents. It is noteworthy also that paraoxon is the active form of the insecticide, parathion.

CHOLINERGIC BLOCKING DRUGS

Cholinergic blocking drugs act at the receptors of tissues and organs supplied by cholinergic postganglionic autonomic nerves by opposing the action of ACh liberated from these nerve endings.

Atropine and scopolamine are two of the most important cholinergic blocking drugs, and they will be discussed in more detail than some derivatives or synthetic substitutes which have specialized uses.

By blocking transmission at postganglionic parasympathetic nerve endings, atropine and scopolamine inhibit secretion of tears, sweat, and saliva, and secretions of the mucous glands of the respiratory and gastrointestinal tracts and of the pancreas. The heart rate is increased, the tone and movement of the stomach and intestines are decreased, and the bronchi are relaxed. The pupil is dilated, and the accommodation is paralyzed.

Atropine and scopolamine also act at sites other than the postganglionic parasympathetic receptors. In higher doses they have antinicotinic actions, blocking cholinergic transmission at motor nerve endings and ganglionic synapses. On the CNS, atropine first causes stimulation and then depression, whereas scopolamine has a purely depressant effect. Some of these actions may be anticholinergic and a few are not. Atropine does produce peripheral vasodilation, and this is not an anticholinergic effect.

Sources

The older drugs of the group are the various galenical preparations of belladonna, hyoscyamus, and stramonium. All these are derived from plants of the potato family, the Solanaceae. The species used as drugs include *Atropa belladonna*, one of several plants known colloquially as deadly nightshade; *Hyoscyamus niger* (black henbane); and *Datura stramonium* (jimsonweed, jamestown weed, or thorn apple). The active principles in all these plants consist mostly of *l*-hyoscyamine, with smaller and variable amounts of *l*-scopolamine (hyoscine). Atropine is *dl*-hyoscyamine. *l*-Hyoscyamine is much more active as a cholinergic blocking drug than *d*-hyoscyamine, both peripherally and on the CNS, but the racemic mixture *dl*-hyoscyamine, better known as atropine, is now preferred for most medicinal purposes because it is more stable chemically and therefore more dependable in action.

The action of scopolamine differs from that of atropine in one important respect. When given by injection, in ordinary doses, scopolamine, in addition to its cholinergic blocking effect, exerts a powerful sedative or hypnotic action.

Chemistry

Atropine is *dl*-tropyltropine and scopolamine is *l*-tropyl-*d*-scopine. They are, in fact, esters of tropic acid with the organic bases tropanol (tropine) and scopine, respectively. Scopine differs from tropine only by the oxygen bridge between C-6 and C-7.

Atropine

$$\text{Scopolamine}$$

Scopolamine

Mechanism of Action

It is assumed that parasympathetically innervated cells have specific receptors upon which ACh acts and that atropine competes with ACh for attachment to these receptors. Both atropine and ACh have a high affinity for cholinergic receptors, and both combine reversibly with the receptors. The ACh-receptor combination initiates a cholinergic response in the effector cell (high intrinsic activity), but the atropine-receptor combination initiates no such response (zero intrinsic activity).

Scopolamine acts in the same manner as atropine to block the effects of ACh, although it has not been studied in the same detail.

It is reasonable to ask why atropine does not block ACh at ganglionic synapses and motor nerve endings. A partial answer is that atropine can block at the other locations if it is administered by intra-arterial injection at sufficiently high concentration. Such concentrations are too high for medicinal use, but they show that the various receptors for ACh exhibit a quantitative rather than a qualitative difference in accessibility or susceptibility to atropine.

In general, it can be said that the muscarinic effects of ACh on smooth muscle are more easily and completely blocked by atropine than are the effects of parasympathetic nerve stimulation, but the relative susceptibility of different organs and tissues does vary.

Although the exact mode and site of action of atropine, and of the more effective scopolamine, on the CNS are not known, they probably interfere with the action of ACh at certain synapses. They do, however, have other effects. Atropine and scopolamine antagonize the actions of ACh on the CNS, and significantly reduce the brain ACh content of animals. Also, for anticholinergic drugs there is a relationship between anti-ACh potency and both antiparkinsonian activity in humans and antitremor activity in animals.

Effects on Organ Systems

Heart When atropine sulfate is administered to human subjects by mouth or by subcutaneous, intramuscular, or intravenous injection, the heart rate first shows a temporary and moderate decrease, which is followed by a more marked acceleration. This tachycardia is accompanied by an increase in cardiac output. The P-R interval is shortened by all doses of atropine. The initial bradycardia is more prolonged following small doses, and it is attributed to atropine stimulating the cardioinhibitory center in the medulla. The subsequent cardiac acceleration is due to atropine blocking the tonic vagal impulses to the heart. The acceleration of the heart rate occurs earlier, is more marked, and is more prolonged as the dose of atropine is increased.

Atropine will also prevent or reverse the decrease in the refractory period, the lengthened P-R interval, the slowing of conduction, and the decrease in cardiac output and the cardiac oxygen consumption produced by vagal stimulation or ACh. The potassium liberation from and the sodium penetration into isolated auricles produced by ACh are also reversed by atropine, and it will return the auricular fibrillation induced and maintained in animals by ACh or vagal stimulation to normal sinus rhythm.

Peripheral Circulation Normal doses of atropine, given by mouth or by intramuscular injection, have little effect on blood pressure in humans. Larger doses (2 mg or more), although causing a marked increase in heart rate, usually decrease the systolic blood pressure by a few millimeters of mercury. This fall in blood pressure is more marked in warm environments and may be caused by decreased cardiac filling due to excessive heart rate. The diastolic blood pressure shows little significant change after atropine in temperate climates, but it may show a fall in hot, dry environments.

When atropine sulfate is injected intravenously, either into conscious volunteers or anesthetized patients, the heart rate increases and the cardiac output rises, but the stroke volume, central venous pressure, and total peripheral resistance decrease. The rise in the cardiac output is dependent on the degree of increase in the heart rate and is accompanied by a rise in the arterial blood pressure; in anesthetized patients, the extent of these changes varies with the anesthetic used.

Atropine does abolish the depressor response to ACh, and it blocks the vasodilation produced by ACh in the freshly perfused rabbit ear. On its own, it has a direct vasodilatory effect on small blood vessels; this is not an anticholinergic phenomenon. Hence, a slight flushing of the skin may occur with small doses, and a pronounced reddening is a characteristic effect of toxic doses.

Central Nervous System With the usual dose of atropine sulfate, effects on the CNS are not striking, except for the slowing of the heart, mentioned above. Ordinary doses of scopolamine, given subcutaneously, have a profound soporific effect lasting 1 or 2 h. A similar dose given orally has very little soporific action, a fact which makes scopolamine given orally a possible treatment for motion sickness. Larger doses of atropine produce drowsiness, hallucinations, disorientation, and eventually coma. Similar toxic effects are produced by relatively smaller doses of scopolamine.

Medulla A normal clinical dose of atropine has neither significant stimulatory nor depressant action on respiration. Atropine is not considered effective in counteracting respiratory depression in poisoning by barbiturates or morphine. However, it is a specific antidote for the central respiratory depression occurring in poisoning with anticholinesterase agents.

Higher Centers Atropine decreases the muscle tremor and reduces the stiffness in parkinsonism (paralysis agitans). Scopolamine and many centrally active anticholinergic drugs have a similar action, and it has been suggested that their effectiveness may be due to an antagonism of ACh at central synapses. However, clinical investigations showing that large oral doses of l-dopa (l-dihydroxyphenylalanine) can relieve many of the symptoms of parkinsonism do not suggest that the disease itself is caused by a disturbance of the normal cholinergic mechanisms in the basal ganglia.

Secretions The exocrine sweat glands of the human skin are supplied by cholinergic fibers present in sympathetic nerves. Accordingly, sweating is diminished or abolished by small doses of atropine. This reduction or abolition of sweating may

be responsible for the rise in rectal temperature which sometimes follows moderate doses of atropine and is a regular consequence of toxic doses.

One of the most obvious effects of ordinary doses of atropine and scopolamine is dryness of the mouth. The copious watery flow of saliva induced by parasympathetic nerve stimulation is essentially abolished by atropine. The secretions of the nose, pharynx, and bronchi are greatly reduced by ordinary doses of atropine and scopolamine.

There are both nervous (vagal) and hormonal (gastrin and enterogastrone) mechanisms involved in the normal regulation of the secretion of gastric juice. Gastrin stimulates gastric secretion, and enterogastrone inhibits the secretion. Some believe that gastrin must be present in the blood for vagal stimulation to have a significant secretory action and that vagal stimulation also releases gastrin.

The *interdigestive secretion,* that is, the secretion when no food is in the stomach, may be caused by vagal stimulation, and atropine does inhibit this. Atropine also inhibits the chemical or hormonal phases, and the mechanism of this action is still disputed.

Atropine blocks the secretion of pancreatic juice caused by vagal stimulation or parasympathomimetic drugs, and this may be due to a blocking of the extrusion of zymogen granules. It has no effect on the secretion stimulated by secretin or pancreozymin.

Smooth-Muscle
Alimentary Tract In general the belladonna alkaloids reduce the tone, and decrease the amplitude and frequency of peristaltic contractions, of the stomach, small intestine, and to a lesser extent, the colon. The inhibitory effect of atropine on gastrointestinal motility is more pronounced and less variable than on gastric secretion. Normal motility is not appreciably altered by therapeutic doses of atropine, but hypermotility associated with peptic ulcer and certain other gastrointestinal disorders is usually reduced markedly.

Bronchi The smooth muscles of the bronchioles are slightly relaxed by atropine blocking the constrictor effects of the vagus nerves. The result is a freer airway, which is useful in anesthesia. In humans, scopolamine has a longer bronchodilator action than does atropine.

The bronchodilator action is minimal, and atropine and scopolamine are seldom used in the treatment of bronchial asthma, although they may be occasionally of value.

Biliary Tract   Atropine has little effect on secretion of bile, but it is thought to have some relaxant effect on the smooth muscle of the biliary tract, thus increasing the flow through the duct. Consequently, even though its effect is slight, it is given with morphine for the relief of biliary colic.

Urinary Bladder   Atropine decreases, but even in large doses does not abolish, the motor effects of the sacral nerves supplying the bladder. Therapeutic doses are thought to diminish the tone of the fundus of the bladder and to increase the tone of the vesical sphincter. In consequence, atropine may contribute to the retention of urine, which is often troublesome after surgical operations.

The Eye   The circular smooth muscles of the iris, which constrict the pupil, are innervated by cholinergic fibers from the third cranial (oculomotor) nerve. Fibers from the same nerve cause contraction of the ciliary muscles, thus slackening the suspensory ligament of the lens and allowing the lens to become more convex. Atropine and scopolamine block the neurohumoral mediator at both locations, causing *mydriasis* (dilation of the pupil) and *cycloplegia* (paralysis of accommodation). The ocular effects of atropine may be produced with great intensity by instilling a few drops into the conjunctival sac, or by applying an ointment. Atropine and other cycloplegics and mydriatics *should not* be used in the eyes of patients with glaucoma.

Distribution and Excretion

Since the usual doses of atropine are very small, it is hard to trace its distribution. It disappears rapidly from the blood and may be assumed to diffuse into extracellular spaces and probably into intracellular spaces.

Following the intramuscular injection of ^{14}C-labeled atropine into humans, 85 to 88 percent of the radioactivity was excreted in the urine in the first 24 h. No activity was found in the expired air, and only a trace could be extracted from the feces. About one-half of the injected dose appeared in the urine as intact atropine, more than one-third as unknown metabolites (possibly esters of tropic acid),

and less than 2 percent as free tropic acid. Neither hydroxylation of the aromatic ring nor glucuronide formation could be demonstrated.

Duration of Action and Tolerance

Duration of action depends on the dose, the mode of administration, and the action observed. Effects on the eye after local application last a long time. Some interference with accommodation may be perceptible for 3 or 4 days, and some enlargement of the pupil may persist for a week. The systemic effects of doses given orally or by injection persist only a few hours. It is usually necessary to repeat doses every 4 to 6 h for sustained action.

Patients receiving large doses of atropine for Parkinsons's syndrome for long periods require a considerable increase in dosage with time.

Toxicity

The minimum lethal dose of atropine has been stated to be 80 to 130 mg in adults and 10 to 20 mg in children, but one person is reported to have survived an oral dose of 1,000 mg. There may be some individual variation in sensitivity to the drug, but it is obvious that there is a wide margin of safety between therapeutic and lethal doses.

Excessive dosage with atropine, or one of the galenical preparations of the belladonna group, gives rise to distinctive signs, which include rapid pulse, dilated pupils, and dry, flushed skin. Patients may complain of thirst and difficulty in focusing their eyes, or may be restless, garrulous, excited, disoriented, or even delirious. If recovery ensues, there may be no recollection of the distressing episode. If the outcome is fatal, it usually follows a period of coma in which the respirations become rapid and shallow and finally cease.

The toxic effects of scopolamine are similar to those of atropine except that stupor and delirium are more prominent and excitement is less so.

Treatment

If the poisonous dose was taken orally and the patient receives attention early, the stomach should be emptied as quickly as possible and washed out thoroughly. No specific antidote is very useful, but activated charcoal or "universal antidote" should be given to adsorb or inactivate the portion of the poison remaining in the alimentary tract. Physostigmine has been shown, however, to be beneficial in the treatment of scopolamine-induced delirium. Respiratory failure is a common feature in many of the reported deaths from atropine so that, perhaps, artificial respiration should also be administered. Hyperpyrexia can be alleviated by keeping the skin wet with water until spontaneous sweating occurs.

Therapeutic Uses

Atropine is given more frequently than any other drug in preparation for surgical anesthesia. The main purpose is to minimize bronchial, nasal, and salivary secretions, which may accumulate and obstruct the respiratory passages. Scopolamine is preferred if additional sedative action is desired.

Oral administration of atropine sulfate is often useful to dry the nasal secretions for the temporary relief of common colds or hay fever. Belladonna extract is a common ingredient of the older type of "rhinitis" or "coryza" tablet.

Atropine is applied locally to the eye to produce dilation of the pupil and paralysis of accommodation for eye tests. If complete cycloplegia is important for the test, atropine is the drug of choice; otherwise the shorter-acting homatropine is preferred. Following the tests, a miotic should be instilled to constrict the pupils. Prolonged dilation of the pupil by the use of atropine is often required in the treatment of iritis, to prevent adhesion of the iris to the lens.

Oral administration with increasing doses up to the limit of tolerance is sometimes used to relieve pain in stubborn cases of peptic ulcer in which relief of symptoms is not obtained by dietary changes and antacids. Individual response varies widely, and the dose must be adjusted to the patient's needs. The accompanying effects of dryness of the mouth, blurred vision, bladder weakness, bowel impairment, and enhancement of glaucoma stimulated the search for synthetic substitutes.

Atropine is useful in treating acutely ill patients when bradycardia is associated with a low cardiac output or ventricular irritability. The syndrome of bradycardia and falling arterial blood pressure is occasionally seen in patients with acute myocardial infarction. In such cases, atropine increases the heart rate and restores the blood pressure to a normal range. Atropine is often given with morphine to relieve biliary colic.

Many older prescriptions include hyoscyamus tincture to relieve the urgency and frequency of micturition which often accompany cystitis. Atropine can also allay these symptoms, and may be useful as an adjunct in the treatment of enuresis in children, although substances such as propantheline may be more effective because they have in addition a ganglionic blocking action. Atropine may occasionally be useful for the relief of dysmenorrhea.

In parkinsonism (paralysis agitans) oral administration of atropine sulfate, with increasing doses until the limit of tolerance is reached, is often effective in relieving the muscular rigidity which impairs the speech, writing, and locomotion of patients with this disease.

Scopolamine hydrobromide in oral doses is used as a remedy for *motion sickness*. At appropriate doses taken orally it has little sedative action. It is also employed in obstetrics to promote drowsiness with amnesia, or "twilight sleep." For this purpose it is given with a sedative analgesic agent such as morphine or meperidine, or even with a barbiturate.

Atropine is recommended for the treatment of poisoning with anticholinesterase agents such as the organophosphorus insecticides and the nerve gases. In these cases atropine will block or reverse many of the toxic actions due to this abnormal concentration of ACh. If a neuromuscular blockade is present, it will not be affected by the atropine. It is important to remember that large doses of atropine may be needed for the adequate treatment of these cases of poisoning. An oxime, such as 2-PAM, should be given as an adjunct to atropine therapy.

Substitutes for Atropine

It was hoped that synthetic atropinelike drugs with greater musculotropic spasmolytic action but less anticholinergic action would be more effective than atropine for such conditions as biliary colic, renal colic, and pylorospasm, and have fewer side effects like dryness of mouth or interference with accommodation. The hopes have been fulfilled only partially.

Homatropine Hydrobromide The actions of homatropine hydrobromide resemble those of atropine, but larger doses are required to produce equivalent effects. When it is applied to the eye, a 2 percent solution is ordinarily used. Onset of mydriasis is about as rapid as with atropine, but the duration is much shorter, that is, 1 to 2 days. Cycloplegia is usually incomplete unless applications are made repeatedly. Homatropine is used in preference to atropine when a short action is desired and when complete cycloplegia is not essential for the ocular examination.

Homatropine

Homatropine Methylbromide Homatropine methylbromide is less toxic and is a less potent parasympatholytic than atropine but is a stronger depressor of ganglionic transmission. It has been recommended for internal use for the treatment of gastrointestinal spasm and hyperchlorhydria.

Eucatropine Hydrochloride Eucatropine hydrochloride is weaker and more transient in action than homatropine hydrobromide. A 5 to 10 percent solution is used for application to the eye. Satisfactory mydriasis is produced rapidly and lasts for about 24 h. Interference with accommodation is minimal. Eucatropine is satisfactory for simple ophthalmoscopic examination of the retina when cycloplegia is not required.

Methylatropine This compound results from the attachment of a methyl group to the nitrogen in the tropanol nucleus, which converts the nitrogen from the tertiary to the quaternary state and alters somewhat the pharmacologic properties. The LD_{50} is about one-third that of atropine. It is said to be more potent than atropine as a parasympatholytic and in blocking autonomic ganglia, and also to be a more rapid but shorter-acting mydriatic. The drug has been used as a mydriatic and in the treatment of congenital hypertrophic pyloric stenosis.

Methscopolamine Bromide The quaternary compound of scopolamine, methscopolamine bromide, has been investigated experimentally and therapeutically. The quaternary compound is said to lack the central sedative action of scopolamine but to be useful for treating spasm of smooth muscles in the bladder, ureters, and gastrointestinal tract. It suppresses both the volume and acidity of gastric secretion and inhibits salivary secretion and sweating.

Dibutoline Dibutoline has been used as a mydriatic and cycloplegic agent. The action is more rapid and intense but of shorter duration than that of atropine. It is ineffective by the oral route and must be given by parenteral injection. It has been used for the treatment of spastic disorders of the gastrointestinal, biliary, and genitourinary tracts.

Adiphenine Hydrochloride Adiphenine hydrochloride is a synthetic antispasmodic which acts more as a musculotropic than as an anticholinergic spasmolytic. Adiphenine is structurally similar to the local anesthetics, and it does have local anesthetic activity. It may be administered orally.

Adiphenine is proposed for the treatment of spasm in the alimentary, urinary, and biliary tracts, and for dysmenorrhea, and each dose is often combined with phenobarbital. Although it exhibits fewer adverse effects in the recommended doses than atropine, it is not so effective as atropine.

Cyclopentolate Hydrochloride This synthetic antispasmodic produces a rapid mydriasis and cycloplegia of moderate duration. It is used solely as a mydriatic.

Other Synthetic Substitutes Several of the synthetic drugs which have been introduced recently are intended particularly for the relief of pain and hyperacidity associated with peptic ulcer. The atropine substitutes discussed above have both an anticholinergic blocking effect and a direct spasmolytic action on smooth muscles; the derivatives listed below have the peripheral cholinergic blocking effects of atropine plus the ability to block the effects of ACh in automatic ganglia. The perennial hope is that these drugs will be effective in suppressing gastric secretion in doses which will not provoke undue dryness in the mouth, retention of urine, or other undesired manifestations of cholinergic blockade.

Diphemanil Methylsulfate (Prantal) This has both antimuscarinic and ganglionic-blocking activity, but is much weaker than atropine. When applied topically to the skin, it has antipruritic and anhidrotic effects.

Oxyphenonium Bromide (Antrenyl) This has weak muscarinic blocking action and in higher doses may also block ganglia. It has a sedative rather than a stimulant action on the CNS.

Methantheline Bromide (Banthine) A potent antimuscarinic, this compound has properties and side effects very similar to those of atropine.

Propantheline Bromide (Pro-Banthine) This is the isopropyl analogue of methantheline and is more active.

Pipenzolate Methylbromide (Piptal) This has muscarinic blocking activity. It produces toxic effects similar to those of atropine.

Tridihexethyl Iodide (Pathilon) This is a muscarinic blocking agent with actions similar to those of atropine, though weaker.

Miscellaneous New Preparations Other preparations for use as cholinergic blocking agents are hexocyclium methylsulfate (Tral), piperidolate hydrochloride (Dactil), isopropamide (Darbid), mepenzolate methylbromide (Cantil), oxyphencyclimine hydrochloride (Daricon), glycopyrrolate (Robinul), poldine (Nacton), mepiperphenidol (Darstine), valethamate bromide (Muvel), and dicyclomine hydrochloride (Bentyl). It has still to be shown that any of these is more useful and effective than the belladonna alkaloids, or freer of side effects if used in fully effective doses.

Treatment of Parkinsonism Another group of new cholinergic blocking agents has been introduced for the treatment of various types of parkinsonism. Such drugs are benztropine methanesulfonate (Cogentin), cycrimine hydrochloride (Pagitane), procyclidine hydrochloride (Kemadrin), and trihexyphenidyl hydrochloride (Artane). The pharmacology of these substances is discussed in Chap. 12.

GANGLIONIC STIMULANT AND BLOCKING DRUGS

Nicotine and Tobacco

Although nicotine has no therapeutic importance it has been extensively studied for several reasons. It is an important tool used to stimulate or block the autonomic ganglia. The inherent toxicity of nicotine has been applied in the control of insects. The presence of nicotine in tobacco and the recent claims that tobacco smoking is likely to cause pulmonary emphysema, pulmonary neoplasm, and heart disease have triggered an organized and systematic investigation of the medical importance of tobacco, including the pharmacologic action of nicotine.

Source and Chemistry Nicotine occurs as an alkaloid in the dried leaves of *Nicotiana tabacum* and *N. rustica* to the extent of 2 to 8 percent. The nicotine content varies from about 2 percent in the average cigarette to about 1 percent in so-called denicotinized preparations.

Nicotine

Mechanism of Action An understanding of the mode of action of nicotine depends on a knowledge of the cholinergic theory of transmission in synapses (Chap. 16). In terms of this theory, the action of nicotine is generally accepted to be a combination of nicotine with the ACh receptor of the postsynaptic membrane in the autonomic ganglion. The immediate consequence is depolarization of the membrane, with a transient stimulation of the ganglionic cells similar to the effects of ACh. If larger amounts of nicotine are used, the stimulation is followed by a prolonged blockade of transmission. Persistence of nicotine on the ACh receptor causes a depression of the effect of ACh, whether liberated by presynaptic impulses or injected.

Effects on Organ Systems
Central Nervous System The stimulation of the CNS is the result of excitation of the motor cortex.

In the spinal cord, the usual pattern is a depression of the monosynaptic patellar reflex, with no effect on the polysynaptic flexor reflex.

Autonomic Nervous System Actions of nicotine extend to all autonomic ganglia, both sympathetic and parasympathetic. These manifestations are further complicated by actions of nicotine outside the autonomic ganglia, namely, the release of epinephrine from the adrenal medulla, the stimulation of epinephrine from the adrenal medulla, and activation of visceral receptors with resulting reflex actions. The combined picture is an increase in sympathetic activity of some organs (heart, blood vessels, pupil) and in parasympathetic activity of others (salivary glands, gastrointestinal organs).

Respiratory System Nicotine initially stimulates respiration; with increasing doses the stimulation turns into depression. The minimal effective dose that stimulates respiration is dependent on intact chemoreceptors in the carotid and aortic bodies.

An intravenous injection would elicit respiratory stimulation, but this is often preceded by a brief period of apnea, which arises from stimulation of receptors in the lungs. From the toxicologic standpoint, the reflex apnea is not so important as the paralysis of respiratory muscles brought about by a direct action of nicotine on the neuromuscular junction.

Cardiovascular System Habitual smokers and nonsmokers smoking cigars, cigarettes, or pipes show an increase in pulse rate ranging from a few to over 50 beats/min. A slight rise in blood pressure may accompany this heart-rate change, but a rise in cardiac output is less constant. All these changes are in line with a generalized sympathetic stimulation. The multiple sites of action of nicotine to influence heart rate include not only the autonomic ganglia, adrenal medulla, and chemoreceptors but also the release of norepinephrine from the sympathetic nerve terminals in the heart. In humans the predominant effect of smoking is an acceleration in heart rate and increase in cardiac output.

Gastrointestinal System It has been repeatedly claimed that smoking just before a meal reduces the appetite. This action may be due to psychologic mechanisms, but it is difficult to exclude the local effects of cigarette smoke on taste buds and mucosal membranes of the upper gastrointestinal tract.

Musculoskeletal System Smoking with inhaling is followed by a large and significant rise in finger tremor. This action is another manifestation of a central nervous system action of nicotine.

Skin Smoking in human subjects causes a fall in skin temperature, an indication of vasoconstriction. This effect is not a local response but is the result of stimulation of vasomotor centers.

Urinary System The antidiuresis following cigarette smoking occurs only in the hydrated animal or human subject. The mechanism of action is temporary inhibition of vasopressin secretion from the hypophysis.

Absorption, Fate, and Metabolism Nicotine is readily absorbed from all mucosal surfaces and also via the intact skin. After absorption, this alkaloid is largely accumulated in the liver, kidney, and brain. A small portion of the absorbed nicotine is excreted unchanged in the urine. The major portion is metabolized within the body to several inactive compounds.

Toxicity

Acute Nicotine Poisoning Poisoning may occur from accidental ingestion of insecticide spray containing nicotine. The symptoms of nicotine poisoning which appear immediately include nausea or salivation, abdominal pain, vomiting and diarrhea, mental confusion, and marked weakness. The pupils become constricted and later dilated; pulse rate is at first slow and then rapid; blood pressure rises and then falls. Respiration becomes irregular when convulsions appear. Death results from respiratory paralysis.

Lobeline

Lobeline (α-lobeline; *l*-lobeline; inflatine) is the principal alkaloid of the dried leaves and tops of *Lobelia inflata*. The actions of lobeline are in many respects similar to those of nicotine, but lobeline has a potency of one-fifth to one-twentieth that of nicotine. Like nicotine, lobeline is a primary stimulant and a secondary depressant to the sympathetic ganglia, parasympathetic ganglia, adrenal medulla, medullary centers (especially the emetic centers), neuromuscular junction, and chemoreceptors in the carotid and aortic bodies. The most recent application of lobeline is as a *smoking deterrent*.

Dimethylphenylpiperazinium

Dimethylphenylpiperazinium (DMPP) was the first synthetic compound to stimulate the cholinergic areas that are responsive to nicotine, with minimal blocking action in the intact animal. This difference is not absolute; if larger quantities of DMPP are administered, blocking action on autonomic ganglia can be demonstrated. The greatest importance of DMPP lies in its use as a tool in the laboratory.

Hexamethonium and Ganglionic Blockade

The proof that hexamethonium paralyzes transmission at the ganglionic synapse has been obtained chiefly in the superior cervical ganglion of the cat. Prior to administration of the blocking drug, the preganglionic stimulation causes contraction of the nictitating membrane. This response is completely abolished by the administration of hexamethonium, yet stimulation of the postganglionic fibers is still fully effective. The blockade is therefore in the ganglionic synapse, and the postganglionic neuroeffector junction can still respond to injected epinephrine, as revealed by contraction of the nictitating membrane.

The mechanism of blockade is that of simple competition. The use of hexamethonium in humans has identified the interplay of autonomic nervous factors with nonnervous factors. Chemical blockade of the autonomic ganglia causes a fall in blood pressure which is not exclusively the result of a primary loss of vasoconstrictor tone or simple reduction of total systemic vascular resistance. Equally important is a reduction in circulatory blood volume, venous return, and cardiac output, provided the heart is not in failure. If the heart is in failure, a corresponding initial reduction in circulating blood volume from peripheral dilation is followed by an improvement in cardiac function and an increase in output.

The most surprising feature of the hemodynamic studies following hexamethonium is the improvement in allocation or distribution of cardiac output in favor of the heart and brain. Observations in humans indicate that after the autonomic nervous system is blocked, the local regulatory mechanisms (such as the metabolic control of cerebral and coronary vessels) and the local unidentified vascular (autoregulatory) factors in the kidney and splanch-

nic bed come into play. These mechanisms, which are independent of the autonomic nervous system, are active in normotensive and hypertensive individuals and account for the relative safety of the use of autonomic blocking agents in antihypertensive therapy. Without these nonautonomic mechanisms, cerebral and coronary insufficiency, manifested by fainting and cardiac arrhythmias, would be more frequently encountered.

Effects on Organ Systems

Nervous System In clinical doses, hexamethonium has no important action on the nervous system, except at the ganglion synapse.

Gastrointestinal System The administration of hexamethonium to fasting patients caused a depression in volume and acidity of the spontaneous gastric secretion. Gastric motility is inhibited, sometimes completely for many hours. The salivary secretion is also depressed. The effects on the bowel movements are variable, with either diarrhea or constipation resulting, depending on the predominance of sympathetic or parasympathetic influence.

Respiratory System The throat and larynx are sometimes noted to be drier than usual. The bronchomotor tone is relieved from a basal vagal tone, and the bronchodilation can be detected by clinical tests of pulmonary resistance.

Skin Dryness and flushing of the skin are the outcome of blockade of the sympathetic ganglion synapse.

Therapeutic Uses Until the introduction of the newer adrenergic blocking drugs, hexamethonium and other ganglionic blocking drugs were used in the long-term treatment of essential hypertension. The development of tolerance for all ganglionic blocking drugs and the erratic absorption of all of them (except mecamylamine) from the gastrointestinal tract have led to almost complete elimination of their use in prolonged management of essential hypertension.

Other Ganglionic Blocking Drugs

From the practical standpoint, the pharmacologic details outlined for hexamethonium can serve as the prototype for the other clinically useful blocking drugs.

Pentolinium Tartrate   The major difference between pentolinium and hexamethonium is that pentolinium requires a lower dose (about one-fifth) and longer duration of action (about 1½ times longer), necessitating less frequent administration. Like hexamethonium, pentolinium is more slowly and less completely absorbed orally than parenterally; thus larger oral doses are required to produce the same effect.

Mecamylamine Hydrochloride   Unlike all other ganglionic blocking drugs, mecamylamine is a secondary amine. This difference in chemical structure is significant in that mecamylamine is almost completely absorbed from the gastrointestinal tract and is exclusively given via the oral route. As with all other ganglionic blocking agents, prolonged oral administration leads to decreased effectiveness, but no cross-tolerance with quaternary ammonium compounds has been observed.

Quantitatively, mecamylamine was found to be equipotent with hexamethonium and one-fourth as active as pentolinium in inhibiting preganglionically induced contractions of the nictitating membrane of the cat. The duration of action of mecamylamine was 3 to 5 times that of the other two drugs.

Mecamylamine, with a pK_a of 11.3, has a small but appreciable fraction in the nonionized state at the pH of body fluids. Mecamylamine is therefore likely to diffuse freely across cell membranes and to be distributed within both the extracellular and intracellular compartments.

At the present time, mecamylamine is the most widely used ganglionic blocking agent administered orally. The major reason is its complete oral absorption. However, because of the development of tolerance and with the introduction of the peripheral sympathetic blocking agents such as guanethidine, the routine use of mecamylamine in severe hypertension is no longer necessary.

Trimethaphan Camsylate   The unique feature of trimethaphan is its extremely fleeting action, which makes it suitable for use as a hypotensive agent administered by continuous infusion. The rate of injection can be adjusted so that the hypotension can be controlled in its intensity or quickly terminated. Reversible hypotension has been intentionally produced during surgery to minimize bleeding. Another application has been to reduce circulating blood volume in the emergency treatment of pulmonary edema. There are technical reasons for favoring or disfavoring the use of intentional hypotension. It is important to remember that the regulation of the cardiovascular system is temporarily suspended.

Chapter 20

Skeletal Muscle Relaxants

As a group, drugs which block transmission from the motor nerve ending to skeletal muscle are known as *neuromuscular blocking agents*. Under the influence of these drugs, nerve conduction is not impaired and the muscle is capable of direct stimulation. The effect is usually transitory and recovery is complete.

Originally, neuromuscular blocking agents were extracted from curare, a paralyzing arrow poison used by South American Indians. More recently synthetic neuromuscular blocking agents have been introduced.

Other groups of skeletal muscle relaxants achieve their effects by a direct action on muscle or by an action on the central nervous system. Possessing a modulating effect only, they do not completely paralyze muscle contraction. At present, they are less important than the neuromuscular blocking agents.

PERIPHERALLY ACTING SKELETAL MUSCLE RELAXANTS

Neuromuscular Blocking Agents

Chemistry The structural formulas of representative neuromuscular blocking agents are shown in Fig. 20-1. Tubocurarine contains two quaternary nitrogen atoms approximately 1.4 nm apart, which is about twice the distance separating the two reactive groups of acetylcholine. The importance of the two quaternary nitrogen atoms was a major consideration in the synthesis of bisquaternary ammonium compounds as possible substitutes for tubocurarine. Synthetic and semisynthetic curariform drugs containing two quaternary nitrogens include dimethyl tubocurarine, pancuronium, decamethonium, and succinylcholine. Gallamine contains three quaternary nitrogens.

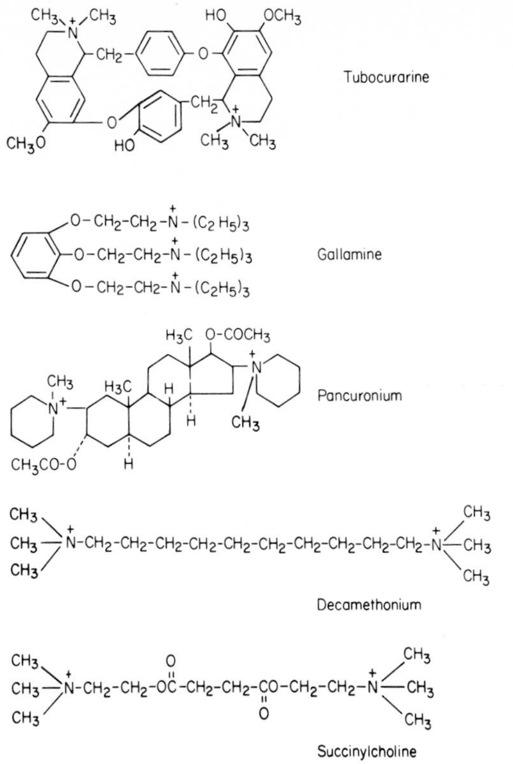

Figure 20-1 Nondepolarizing and depolarizing neuromuscular blocking agents.

Sites of Action As a consequence of a nerve impulse passing along a motor axon, the following sequence of events occurs:

1 A propagated wave of depolarization spreads over the nerve end plate.

2 Acetylcholine is released from storage vesicles in the prejunctional terminal and enters into the synaptic space.

3 Binding of acetylcholine to postjunctional receptor sites results in depolarization of the muscle end plate with associated increases in Na and K ion transport.

4 Development of a local end plate potential which eventually gives rise to a propagated muscle action potential.

5 Spread of the muscle action potential through the myofibril conduction system.

6 The muscle contracts.

7 The muscle relaxes and is refractory to another stimulus until repolarization of the muscle end plate is complete.

8 Acetylcholine is hydrolyzed by acetylcholinesterase in the synaptic cleft.

9 Repolarization of the terminal axon and muscle end plate region.

Nondepolarizing Agents

Mechanism of Action Compounds in this group, which are also referred to as antidepolarizing or competitive blocking agents, include tubocurarine, dimethyl tubocurarine, gallamine, and pancuronium. The mechanism of action is based on competition by the blocking agent with the transmitter for the postsynaptic receptors (Fig. 20-2), as in step 3 above. If sufficient receptors are occluded by the blocking agent, the number activated by the transmitter is too small to lead to the production of an end plate potential large enough to reach threshold for activation of the adjacent electrically excitable membrane. Thus transmission fails.

Potentiation of Nondepolarizing Blockade The skeletal muscle relaxant activity of nondepolarizing neuromuscular blocking agents is enhanced by certain general anesthetics such as diethyl ether, fluroxene, methoxyflurane, halothane, and cyclopropane. Consequently, when they are used together, the dose of the general anesthetic should be reduced, e.g., diethyl ether and halothane doses should be reduced 60 percent and 20 percent, respectively. The neuromuscular blockade produced is also enhanced by antibiotics such as streptomycin, neomycin, kanamycin, gentamicin, polymyxin, and colistin. Enhanced neuromuscular blockade of the tubocurarine type has occurred in antiarrhythmic therapy with quinidine and lidocaine. Fluid and electrolyte imbalances, such as acidosis, dehydration, and hypokalemia, will also enhance neuromuscular blockade. Patients with myasthenia gravis are extremely sensitive to nondepolarizing neuromuscular blocking agents.

Antagonism of Nondepolarizing Blockade An approach in the antagonism of neuromuscular blockade is to administer a cholinesterase antagonist so that acetylcholine released from the nerve ending would reach the end plate in higher concentrations and therefore compete more effectively for the receptor. (Fortunately, neuromuscular blocking agents do not interfere with cholinesterase activity.)

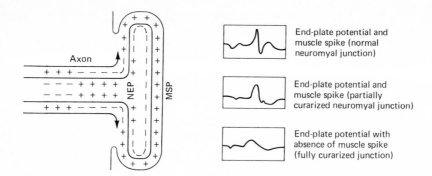

Right panel labels:
- End-plate potential and muscle spike (normal neuromyal junction)
- End-plate potential and muscle spike (partially curarized neuromyal junction)
- End-plate potential with absence of muscle spike (fully curarized junction)

Figure 20-2 *Left,* diagram of the neuromyal junction depicting the spreading wave of depolarization along the axon and end plate; (1) acetylcholine appears when the nerve end plate is depolarized; (2) the acetylcholine depolarizes the muscle end plate; (3) the wave of depolarization spreads over the muscle fiber; (4) the muscle contracts. *Right,* action potentials from normal, partially curarized, and curarized end plate regions. Tubocurarine prevents acetylcholine from depolarizing the muscle sole plate. Decamethonium, succinylcholine, and similar compounds depolarize the nerve end plate region, and the result resembles block due to failure of removal of acetylcholine.

Edrophonium and neostigmine have been tried and found to be satisfactory in the clinical situation (see Chap. 19). The choice of dose is not too critical, the antagonism is clear-cut, and the effect is well maintained (Fig. 20-3). It seems that the action of these two drugs is the result of either a presynaptic action, an action to block cholinesterase, or a combination of both. There may also be a slight contribution from a direct depolarizing action.

Depolarizing Agents

Mechanism of Action Two agents represent this group of neuromuscular blocking agents: succinylcholine and decamethonium. Decamethonium may be taken as the prototype for discussion. In contrast to the nondepolarizing agents, decamethonium is not a competitive antagonist but rather a stable agonist; that is, as far as its action is concerned, decamethonium differs from the transmitter acetylcholine only in duration of action. Both agents act at the same receptor, and with both, depolarization of the end-plate region results. Decamethonium differs only in that it produces a persistent depolarization (the normal transmitter does not, of course, because it is so quickly destroyed by the cholinesterase in the vicinity).

The persistent depolarization of the end plate leads, by local circuit action, to a persistent de-

polarization of the adjacent electrically excitable membrane of the muscle. As a result, an action potential may be produced initially; clinically, however, this appears as an initial fasciculation on administration of a depolarizing blocking agent, but the membrane around the end plate soon reaches a state of accommodation. The end plate thus finds itself surrounded by a ring of inexcitable tissue, so that signal transfer is blocked in its course to the contractile mechanism. This is *phase i* of the action of decamethonium. Although stable depolarizing blocking agents can produce a depolarization which is quite prolonged compared with that produced by the transmitter, they do not produce a depolarization of indefinite duration. Despite continued exposure to the depolarizing agent, the end plate does not stay depolarized to a constant extent and loses its responsiveness to the depolarizing agents ("desensitization"). Since the action of the transmitter is identical to that of the stable depolarizing agent, the transmitter loses its effectiveness as well. A situation is reached, therefore, where the depolarization may no longer be present but the neuromuscular block persists. This is called a *phase ii block,* a *nondepolarization block,* or *desensitization block.* The desensitization, which may result from changes in the properties of the receptor when it interacts with the depolarizing agent, has been termed a *metaphilic effect* of the agent.

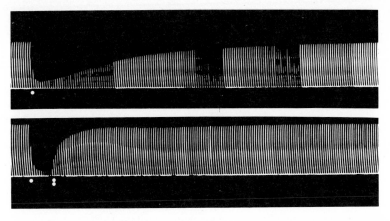

Figure 20-3 Antagonism by neostigmine of the neuromuscular block produced by tubo-curarine. Tracing of indirectly elicited twitch of cat tibialis anterior muscle. *Upper tracing, tubocuraine (200 n moles i.a.) given at ●. Lower tracing, same dose tubocurarine at ●,* followed by neostigmine at ●●.

Pharmacologic Actions

Neuromuscular Blockade   When a neuromuscular blocking agent is administered, a flaccid paralysis of the voluntary musculature develops. The muscles which produce fine movements (for example, the extraocular muscles) are said to be blocked first and the muscles of respiration, especially the diaphragm, last. However, the differences in sensitivity among muscles are so slight that interference with respiration if an appreciable block exists elsewhere must always be assumed.

When a depolarizing neuromuscular blocking agent is administered, the block is preceded by fasciculation, especially if the drug is given rapidly. Soon the fasciculation ceases, and the muscles become quiescent and superficially indistinguishable from those blocked by a competitive blocking agent.

Ganglionic Blockade   Tubocurarine is a potent ganglionic blocking agent. However, because the potency of tubocurarine is still greater at the neuromuscular junction than at the ganglia, one would not expect a side action on the ganglia during clinical use.

Histamine Liberation   Tubocurarine can liberate histamine from endogenous stores in experimental animals. There is presumptive evidence that this can occur clinically as well, but a convincing demonstration that histamine release can account quan-titatively for an episode of hypotension during anesthesia has not been recorded.

Histamine liberation can also produce bronchospasm or an increase in respiratory tract secretion, occasionally seen upon administration of tubocurarine.

Although gallamine possesses the general structural properties for activity as a histamine liberator (two nitrogenous groups separated by a bulky hydrocarbon moiety), it does not act as a potent histamine liberator, nor does succinylcholine, decamethonium, or pancuronium.

Absorption, Distribution, and Fate   Since all clinically employed neuromuscular blocking agents are charged at all levels of biologic pH, absorption from the gastrointestinal tract is negligible; therefore, these agents are usually given intravenously. Because of the charge present on the molecules, they are distributed to the extracellular space only. Finally, since the charge will prevent reabsorption across the tubular membrane in the kidney, all of the drug that crosses the glomerular membrane will be excreted.

Decamethonium contains no unstable bonds, and the only reactive groups, the charged quaternary heads, are not the type of moiety that is susceptible to conjugation, oxidation, and reduction. Decamethonium can form ionic bonds with anionic groups, but these would not be expected to lead to appreciable binding. Experimental measurements of the excretion of decamethonium confirm this picture. Gallamine is also reasonably inert. Its ether linkages are stable, and so, like decamethonium, it is removed by glomerular filtration. Such agents exert a prolonged action in patients with anuria.

A negligible fraction of tubocurarine is excreted in an altered form. There is appreciable binding to plasma proteins. The concentration continues to fall because of renal excretion. Although plasma binding will accelerate the fall in free concentration during the early phase of redistribution, the binding will, by a buffer effect, slow the second phase. The net result is a second phase with a half-life of 70 min. Because of the persistence of tubocurarine in the body and because of the margin of safety of neuromuscular transmission (which implies that a supplementary dose of tubocurarine will be given while most of the receptors are still occupied), supplementary doses of tubocurarine need not be as large as the initial dose.

Of the commonly used neuromuscular blocking agents, succinylcholine is metabolized most rapidly. It contains two ester bonds and has been found to be an excellent substrate for plasma pseudocholinesterase.

The product of the hydrolysis is succinylmonocholine, which is also broken down by the pseudocholinesterase to succinic acid and choline. Since the second stage is about 6 times slower than the first, appreciable quantities of the monocholine ester can accumulate, particularly during prolonged administration. The potency of the monocholine ester (about $\frac{1}{20}$ that of the dicholine ester) is great enough to contribute to the neuromuscular blockade.

The rapid destruction of succinylcholine not only makes the action brief but also facilitates rapid onset. A larger dose can be given so that the effective concentration at the end plate will be reached sooner, without prolonging unduly the overall duration of action. This feature has made succinylcholine popular for facilitation of early endotracheal intubation during general anesthesia.

About 1 person in 3,000 has atypical plasma cholinesterase which destroys succinylcholine less rapidly. If such a patient is given the usual dose of

succinylcholine, an overdose will result, and this will present prolonged apnea. The problem should be regarded as a form of overdosing as well as a situation in which the terminal phase of drug elimination is slowed.

Three types of individuals have been differentiated by measuring the percentage of cholinesterase inhibition produced by dibucaine ("dibucaine number"): (1) the normal homozygote with a dibucaine number of over 70, (2) the heterozygote with a value between 45 and 69, and (3) the atypical homozygote with a value below 30.

Succinylcholine also breaks down spontaneously by alkaline hydrolysis at a slow rate, but fast enough to contribute to the metabolism of the drug.

Since the neuromuscular blocking agents are charged ions, no marked transfer across the placenta would be expected. Some evidence of transfer has been reported for gallamine and tubocurarine, but it is negligible compared to the transfer of the more lipid-soluble anesthetic agents. The fate of the remaining neuromuscular blocking agents has not been determined.

Effects on Organ Systems
Cardiovascular System Cardioacceleration is seen with gallamine. This action seems to be the result of both an atropine-like action and a tyramine-like side effect of the drug, whereby norepinephrine is released from the sympathetic nerve endings supplying the pacemaker region of the heart. Succinylcholine in repeated doses has been found occasionally to lead to arrhythmias such as bradycardia, sinus arrest, or heart block. The increase in plasma potassium, which occurs when a depolarizing agent is administered, may be contributory.

Central Nervous System The charge on all these compounds makes permeation of the blood-brain barrier negligible, so that central nervous system effects are not observed in clinical practice.

Parasympathetic Nervous System Quaternary compounds can act at muscarinic receptors. Succinylcholine and decamethonium have been said to do so at concentrations that might be achieved clinically. Succinylcholine at concentrations up to at least 10^{-3} mole does not slow the rate of an isolated atrium. Succinylcholine is about 1,000 times—

and decamethonium, 100 times—less potent than acetylcholine on the guinea pig ileum.

Potassium Levels Depolarizing neuromuscular blocking agents liberate potassium from skeletal muscles. The continuous action of a depolarizing agent can lead to an elevation of the plasma potassium concentration. This should be borne in mind when patients are encountered who will need prolonged administration of a neuromuscular blocking agent and whose electrolyte concentrations are already disturbed.

Eye Depolarizing agents can cause an increase in intraocular pressure. This is usually attributed to a sustained contraction of the extraocular muscles. It occurs because the extraocular muscles are atypical in that they have many end-plate regions per muscle fiber.

Therapeutic Uses

Anesthesia The purpose of anesthesia is not only to render the patient insensible to pain but also, where possible, to facilitate surgery. Normally the motor nerves carry a constant low level of traffic to the skeletal muscles. These signals induce a contraction of only a small fraction of the muscle fibers at any time, but the activity of these fibers takes up the slack so that the muscle is ready for more intense activity at a moment's notice. This background state of slight contraction is called *muscle tone*. It can be a nuisance during anesthesia when the surgeon must struggle against it to reduce a fracture or when the tone in the flat muscles of the abdomen tends to expel the abdominal contents through an abdominal incision. Before the advent of neuromuscular blocking agents, larger doses of the anesthetic than were required simply to produce unconsciousness had to be administered in order to stop the tonic outflow at the source. General anesthetics, however, have a rather low margin of safety; the concentrations required for muscle relaxation are too close to stage IV of anesthesia. It is therefore desirable to use a second agent to abolish muscle tone so that lower concentrations of the general anesthetic can be used. The neuromuscular blocking agents have proved to be a satisfactory group of agents for this role. They abolish tone by blocking the passage of the tonic discharge from the nerve to the muscle. They have subsequently found even wider use during induction of anesthesia,

when they are given to relax the laryngeal muscles and thereby facilitate endotracheal intubation.

Electroshock Therapy When electroshock therapy is used in the treatment of psychiatric disorders, muscular contraction can be intense enough to cause fractures. Since the therapeutic effect of the convulsion does not depend on the muscular response, prior administration of a neuromuscular blocking agent can be used to abolish the muscular component. The chief hazard that may be encountered is a synergism between the drug and a postictal depression of respiration. Preparations should be made to maintain the airway and assist respiration if necessary.

Succinylcholine is the most popular agent; its short duration of action apparently outweighs its propensity to produce fasciculations and the ensuing discomfort. In practice, an intravenous injection of a somnifacient dose of a rapid-acting barbiturate is followed by an intravenous injection of succinylcholine and hyperventilation with 100 percent oxygen (to minimize the effects of hypoxia during convulsion).

Convulsive Disorders Muscle spasms, as seen in status epilepticus, tetanus, eclampsia, toxic reactions to local anesthetics, etc., may be great enough to prevent either spontaneous or controlled pulmonary ventilation. At the same time, increased muscular activity leads to increased oxygen requirements and an elevated body temperature, which add to oxygen demands. When the seizures cannot be controlled by sedatives or anticonvulsants, the use of a neuromuscular blocking agent combined with controlled respiration may be a lifesaving measure. In such an emergency, succinylcholine is the agent of choice. For prolonged therapy, a competitive blocking agent is preferred. Tubocurarine may be given by repeated intramuscular injections, but intravenous administration (continuous infusion or intermittent doses) is more reliable. In all cases, the dosage is determined by the response of the patient.

Controlled Respiration When a patient is unable to ventilate well enough to maintain a normal arterial P_{O_2} and P_{CO_2} or is becoming exhausted in his attempts to do so, it is advantageous to assist or control his respiration by means of a mechanical ventilator. Controlled respiration is often ineffective because the patient's attempts to breathe are not synchronous with the cycle of the respirator. Frequently sedation and depression of the respiratory center with narcotics will improve the situation, but occasionally it is necessary to block all respiratory effort. Intravenous competitive blocking agents are most satisfactory. Often repeated administration is not needed, since the return of arterial blood gas tensions to normal with the improved ventilation reduces the stimulus to increased respiration, and the patient no longer "fights" the respirator. Alert patients should be sedated while paralyzed.

Myasthenia Gravis Patients with myasthenia gravis are especially sensitive to the competitive neuromuscular blocking agents. Diagnosis can be facilitated in a borderline case by the use of a test dose of tubocurarine. However, tubocurarine is not used unless the more conventional tests with neostigmine or edrophonium have shown equivocal results.

Adverse Reactions The most serious adverse reaction to the neuromuscular blocking agents is apnea, which may extend into the postoperative period and may require artificial respiration over long periods. This may result following overdosage or, in the case of succinylcholine, may be due to the patient's inability to adequately metabolize the drug. The nondepolarizing blockers, such as tubocurarine and pancuronium, can be antagonized by cholinesterase inhibitors.

Neostigmine or edrophonium can be given in combination with an anticholinergic drug to minimize effects on secretions and the heart. However, the cholinesterase inhibitors will intensify the action of depolarizing neuromuscular blocking agents, e.g., succinylcholine.

"DIRECT"-ACTING SKELETAL MUSCLE RELAXANTS

Dantrolene is a substituted hydantoin reported to relieve spasticity by action on muscle. Unlike all other skeletal muscle relaxants, this agent apparently acts directly on the contractile mechanism of skeletal muscle, probably by interfering with the release of calcium from the sarcoplasm. Dantrolene is recommended for controlling the manifestations of clinical spasticity resulting from serious chronic disorders such as injury, stroke, cerebral palsy, and multiple sclerosis. It is not recommended for the treatment of skeletal muscle spasms resulting from rheumatic disorders.

Adverse Reactions The most frequent adverse effects of dantrolene are diarrhea, weakness, drowsiness, fatigue, dizziness, and general malaise. The most serious adverse reaction is potentially fatal hepatocellular disease in all females and in males over 35 years of age.

CENTRALLY ACTING SKELETAL MUSCLE RELAXANTS

Unfortunately, skeletal muscle paralysis achieved by curare-like drugs is not clinically useful in the large variety of common clinical spasticity states accompanying central nervous system lesions and local injury and inflammation. Neuromuscular block can relieve the spasm, but it also results in loss of voluntary control. The aim in conditions of muscle spasticity is to find an agent that relieves the painful muscle spasm without loss of voluntary muscle function and without impairment of cerebral function.

Many cerebral depressants cause muscular relaxation. Notable among these are the alcohols and the barbiturates, but these are ordinarily of no use, since they also produce marked sedation and other untoward effects.

The search for selective central nervous system agents capable of achieving muscular relaxation has produced a number of interesting compounds, none of which has been completely successful. Nevertheless, centrally acting skeletal muscle relaxants are widely used in the treatment of sprains, arthritis, bursitis, and similar musculoskeletal disorders. This use is based on the assumption that spasms originating through spinal cord reflexes can be depressed by these muscle relaxants. However, controlled clinical studies have not established any benefit from orally administered spinal cord depressants in these situations.

When muscle relaxation is indicated, agents such as chlordiazepoxide (Librium), diazepam (Valium), meprobamate (Equanil, Miltown), carisoprodol (Rela, Soma), chlorphenesin (Maolate), chlorzoxazone (Paraflex), or methocarbamol (Robaxin) may be used. No one agent has a significant advantage over any other of these agents.

PREPARATIONS AND DOSAGE

Tubocurarine chloride is available as 3 mg and 15 mg/ml solution for injection. The usual intravenous dose range is 0.1 to 3.0 mg/kg body weight.

Dimethyl tubocurarine iodide (Metubine) is available as a 2 mg/ml solution for injection. The usual intravenous dose range is 0.06 to 0.08 mg/kg body weight.

Gallamine triethiodide (Flaxedil) is available as 20 mg and 100 mg/ml solution for injection. The usual intravenous dose range is 0.5 to 1.0 mg/kg body weight.

Pancuronium bromide (Pavulon) is available as a 2 mg/ml solution for injection. The usual intravenous dose range is 0.02 to 0.1 mg/kg body weight.

Succinylcholine chloride (Anectine, Sucostrin) is available as 20 mg, 50 mg, and 100 mg/ml solution for injection. The usual intravenous dose range is 10 to 80 mg.

Decamethonium bromide (Syncurine) is available as a 1 mg/ml solution for injection. The usual intravenous dose is 0.04 to 0.06 mg/kg body weight.

Dantrolene sodium (Dantrium) is available as 25 mg and 100 mg capsules. The usual oral dosage range is 25 mg twice daily to 100 mg four times daily.

Part Five

The Cardiovascular-Renal System

Cardiac Glycosides

The drugs known collectively as digitalis glycosides exert a unique and valuable action on heart muscle. This action derives from active principles found in *Digitalis lanata* and *D. purpurea* as well as from various other plant and animal sources.

CHEMISTRY

The active ingredients in the digitalis plants do not contain nitrogen in their structure. It is improper, therefore, to speak of them as alkaloids; instead, these compounds are glycosides (sugar derivatives of alcohols). Their sugar components may be mono-, di-, tri-, or tetrasaccharides built from characteristic sugars which are discussed below, whereas the aglycones or genins (the nonsugar part of the glycosides) are steroids with certain typical structural features. The simplest cardiac genin is digitoxigenin

Digitoxigenin

the aglycone of one of the principal glycosides of *D. lanata* (lanatoside A) as well as of *D. purpurea* (purpurea glycoside A). The sugar component, attached to the C-3 hydroxyl of the steroid structure, is in both cases a tetrasaccharide composed of one molecule of glucose and three of *d*-digitoxose.

$$CHO$$
$$|$$
$$CH_2$$
$$|$$
$$HCOH$$
$$|$$
$$HCOH$$
$$|$$
$$HCOH$$
$$|$$
$$CH_3$$

Digitoxose

Lanatoside A carries an acetyl group attached to one of the digitoxose units. This is the sole difference between lanatoside A and purpurea glycoside A. Schematically, therefore, the structure of lanatoside A is

O—C-3 of the steroid structure
|
digitoxose—digitoxose—digitoxose—glucose
|
acetyl

The structure of two further glycosides in *D. lanata*, lanatoside B and lanatoside C, is the same, except that lanatoside B also has a hydroxyl group attached to C-16 of its genin (gitoxigenin), while in the genin of lanatoside C (digoxigenin) the extra hydroxyl is attached to C-12. *D. purpurea* also contains a glycoside B which differs from lanatoside A: the absence of an acetyl group from the sugar component of purpurea glycoside B. There is no glycoside in *D. purpurea* corresponding to lanatoside C, i.e., with a hydroxyl group at C-12. Figure 21-1 illustrates the relationships among the glycosides derived from *D. lanata* and *D. purpurea*.

Both species of *Digitalis* contain hydrolyzing enzymes which easily split off the acetyl group and the glucose. What is ordinarily extracted from both species of *Digitalis* are the partially hydrolyzed glycosides, digitoxin and gitoxin. Digoxin is obtained only from *D. lanata*.

All digitalis genins are steroids which have an unsaturated lactone ring attached to C-17 in beta orientation; a hydroxyl groups at C-14; and, most interesting, a *cis* junction of rings C and D—features unique to digitalis compounds. The main function of the sugars appears to be to solubilize the genins.

MECHANISM OF ACTION: INOTROPIC EFFECT

Digitalis is thought to affect the flux of calcium in the terminal cisternae or sacs of the sarcoplasmic reticulum in the myocardial cell (Fig. 21-2). The action potential at the membrane and at its related invaginations, the transverse or T tubules, acts to release free calcium from the terminal sacs into the cytoplasm. Calcium attaches to the troponin on the actin filaments and this action removes the barrier to actin-myosin interaction. (Normally, troponin and tropomyosin inhibit actin-myosin interaction during diastole.) These events in turn initiate contraction, activating myosin ATPase (E1 in Fig. 21-2) to provide energy from ATP (adenosine triphosphate). Following repolarization, reaccumulation of calcium by the sarcoplasmic reticulum sufficiently lowers free cytoplasmic calcium to permit relaxation.

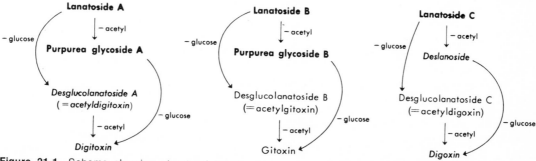

Figure 21-1 Schema showing structural relationships among some cardiac glycosides derived from *Digitalis lanata* and *D. purpurea*, and their hydrolysis products. (Native glycosides are shown in heavy print, those medicinally used in italics.)

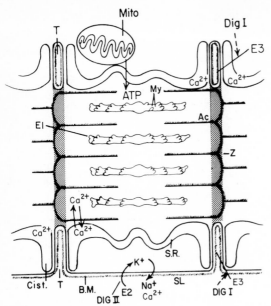

Figure 21-2 Schematic representation of proposed sites of action of digitalis in a cardiac muscle cell. SL, sarcolemma; B.M., basement membrane; S.R., sarcoplasmic reticulum or longitudinal tubular system; T, transverse tubular system (T tubules); My, myosin filaments; Ac, actin filaments; Z, Z line; Cist., terminal cisternae of S.R.; Mito, mitochondrion; EI, myosin ATPase; E2, sarcolemmal ATPase (Na "pump"); E3, T-tubular ATPase; DIG I, proposed site of action of digitalis for inotropic effect; DIG II, site for toxic arrhythmic effect.

There is some evidence to suggest that cardiac glycosides, as well as numerous other positive or negative inotropic agents, act by altering the amount of calcium stored in the sarcoplasmic reticulum. While some drugs, such as epinephrine, appear to affect calcium stores by stimulating the adenylate cyclase–cyclic-AMP system (cyclic AMP increases tubular stores of calcium), it has been suggested that digitalis works through a separate mechanism to inhibit Na^+-K^+-sensitive ATPase (E3) in the transverse tubular system. Normally, following repolarization, Na^+-K^+-sensitive ATPase restores Na^+ ions to the outside and K^+ ions to the inside of the cell. A secondary sodium-calcium exchange mechanism also functions to remove intracellular sodium. When digitalis inhibits Na^+-K^+ ATPase in the T-tubular system, the sodium-calcium exchange predominates, and the influx of

calcium ions into the cardiac cell increases. Therefore, more calcium is available to the myofibrils and a positive inotropic effect is manifested during systole.

The electrical toxic effects of the digitalis glycosides on cardiac tissue may be due to their action on sarcolemmal membrane ATPases (E2) rather than on T-tubular membrane ATPase (E3). Sarcolemmal membrane effects of digitalis are commonly interpreted as being due to a remarkably potent inhibition of Na^+- and K^+-activated ATPase (E2), which normally provides energy for the extrusion process by which sodium is removed from the cell, and is followed by a reciprocal inflow of potassium. This inhibitory effect results in a loss of intracellular potassium ions and may produce dysrhythmias. Quite possibly, the positive effect of digitalis on contractility may in time be found to be due to a combination of actions on both the sarcotubular sacs and the surface membrane.

Although many details of these various actions are incompletely established and may require further study and revision, it appears certain that digitalis has two distinct effects on the heart: (1) an effect on contractility mediated through intracellular changes in calcium stores and (2) an effect on the electrical behavior of cellular membranes mediated through changes in transport of sodium, potassium, and calcium evolving indirectly from the known inhibitory effects of digitalis on cell membrane ATPase.

Interactions between digitalis and ionic calcium and potassium at a membrane level have important clinical and toxicologic implications. There is a synergistic action between Ca^{2+} and digitalis. Sudden increases in serum Ca^{2+} may result in arrhythmias in the digitalized patient. On the other hand, digitalis and K^+ are antagonistic. Hypokalemic patients have a decreased tolerance to digitalis. In patients with digitalis toxicity, raising the serum levels of K^+ tends to alleviate the toxic effects.

ELECTROPHYSIOLOGIC EFFECTS

An explanation for the electrophysiologic effects of the commonly recognized actions of digitalis is an impressive development of recent times. On excitation of ventricular cells, a transmembrane action potential can be recorded (Fig. 21-3). This consists

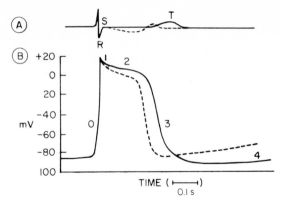

Figure 21-3 Representation of (A) electrocardiogram and (B) ventricular intracellular action potential before (solid line) and after (broken line) digitalis administration.

of rapid depolarization (phase 0) caused by increased passage of sodium into the cell and reversal of the membrane potential, so that the inside is positive in relation to the outside by 20 to 30 mV. Repolarization, involving the passage of current in the opposite direction, most of which is probably carried by potassium ions, follows at a slower rate. There is first a rapid fall (phase 1), then during repolarization the ventricular muscle fibers show a plateau (phase 2), followed by a rapid decrease (phase 3). Phase 4 is called the resting value or diastolic period of the transmembrane potential (Fig. 21-3).

The intrinsic deflection of the R wave of an ECG coincides in time with phase 0, the S-T segment with phase 2, and the T wave with phase 3. In contrast to this ventricular record, the transmembrane potential recorded from a pacemaker fiber (i.e., SA node, AV node, or His-Purkinje fibers) does not remain constant after repolarization but exhibits slow diastolic depolarization during phase 4. If this slow depolarization carries the membrane potential to the threshold potential, firing occurs. Many fibers develop this phase, but the one that first attains the threshold potential usually acts as the dominant pacemaker, and the others, with slower depolarization during phase 4, are latent pacemakers. Digitalis affects this slow diastolic depolarization of Purkinje fibers by increasing the rate of diastolic depolarization; i.e., it increases the slope of phase 4 and therefore ultimately enhances auto-

maticity with resultant ventricular ectopic beats and ventricular tachycardia.

In the atrioventricular (AV) node the cardiac glycosides slow phase 0 (depolarization), thereby diminishing conduction velocity and possibly leading to various degrees of heart block. On the surface ECG this effect is manifested as a lengthening of the P-R interval. A direct effect of digitalis on repolarization of cardiac tissue is an alteration of phases 1, 2, and 3, resulting in a shortening of the duration of the intracellular action potential and a subsequent decrease in refractoriness. In the ECG this is seen as a reduction of the Q-T interval. Furthermore, the quickening of phases 1 and 2 of repolarization are reflected as an S-T-segment depression on the ECG, sometimes referred to as the "boot heel" depression.

EFFECT ON ORGAN SYSTEMS

Cardiac Effects

At therapeutic dose levels, digitalis acts primarily by increasing the force of myocardial contraction. In the failing heart, this results in an increase in cardiac output and, usually, a decrease in heart size. In the AV node and bundle of His, the refractory period is lengthened and conduction is slowed by heightened vagal activity and possibly by reduced adrenergic activity, as well as by direct effects. This increased refractoriness is particularly beneficial in atrial fibrillation, since the number and irregularity of ventricular contractions are reduced.

Digitalis directly increases contractility of the myocardium in both the failing heart and the normal heart. In the failing, dilated heart, digitalis has been shown to double the stroke volume or cardiac output. The heightened contractility causes more complete ejection with less residual systolic volume. In this manner, the glycosides correct the depressed contractility which is responsible for ventricular failure.

The cardiac output in normal subjects who are given digitalis generally remains unchanged, although occasionally it decreases. Besides exerting a positive inotropic action on the normal (nonfailing) heart, the cardiac glycosides also produce a direct contraction of peripheral arterial and venous smooth muscle. This increased peripheral resistance along with increased contractility generally results in unchanged cardiac output. However, in congestive heart failure, there is increased peripheral resistance due to increased activity of the sympathetic nervous system, a compensatory mechanism. When digitalis is administered, enhancement of contractility, a decrease in reflex sympathetic tone, and a significant change in cardiac output are observed. The improved cardiac output results from a positive inotropic effect and a predominant indirect vasodilatation through removal of the sympathetic compensatory reflex, as opposed to the direct action of the glycosides which causes vasoconstriction. Along with the positive inotropic effect and increased cardiac output, digitalis consistently reduces the diastolic size of the heart.

The improved cardiac efficiency which occurs with digitalis suggests a relationship to some direct effect on energy production. However, extensive studies have demonstrated no direct action of this sort. Even the feature of increased energy utilization has been questioned, since oxygen consumption, which is considered an ultimate measure of this variable, reportedly does not change in proportion to cardiac work. This implies an increase in efficiency which could be attributed to some obscurely understood chemical phenomenon but is more acceptable if interpreted on the basis of the important mechanical advantage which comes from the decrease in heart size during diastole, typically caused by digitalis action.

Vagal Effects

Vagal effects occur at early stages or with minimal therapeutic dose levels and increase with higher dose levels. Pacemaker activity is slowed at the SA and AV nodes, conduction rate is decreased, and refractory intervals of the conduction tissue are increased. Vagal effects decrease contractility in the atria but have no pronounced effects on the ventricles, and apparently, the direct positive inotropic effects of digitalis overshadow these negative inotropic effects. The heightened vagal activity has been attributed to action on afferent nerves in the nodose ganglion and the carotid sinus, as well as to effects at peripheral sites and central vagal nuclei.

Early effects on conduction and refractoriness at the AV node and the bundle of His are now gen-

erally thought to be mediated almost entirely through the vagal action, except for a component of action which is antiadrenergic and which can be relatively more important under conditions of heightened sympathetic nervous system activity, as in heart failure.

Digitalis-induced vagal influences on automaticity are complicated by the marked difference in responsiveness of pacemaker or automatic cells on the one hand, and muscle fibers of the atria and ventricles on the other hand, which do not generate spontaneous action potentials. The pacemaker cells of the SA node (and possibly other specialized atrial cells) respond to vagal stimulation by a decrease in the ascending slope of the diastolic phase (phase 4) and an increase in transmembrane negativity. These effects, acting to maintain the subthreshold state, result in a pronounced reduction in heart rate, and with more intense vagal stimulation, there may be arrest of automatic activity of these cells. Under these conditions, pacemaker activity of the bundle of His and the Purkinje system may assume dominance, since automaticity in these conduction systems is not as responsive to vagal activity. This type of "vagal escape" is enhanced by adrenergic influences and by decreased levels of intracellular potassium. Release from the control of higher pacemakers and increased automaticity correspond to the later stages of digitalis arrhythmias such as induced nodal rhythms, ventricular ectopic beats, and ventricular tachycardia.

The activity at the SA node has been demonstrated by injecting cardiac glycosides into its localized blood supply; the results are predominantly bradycardia but with some occurrence of tachycardia, the latter attributed to some local release of catecholamines. Effects appear to be peripheral to strict vagal control and may be related to intracellular potassium levels.

Peripheral Vascular Effects

Rapid intravenous injection of cardiac glycosides in animals and normal human subjects leads to increased arterial pressure and increased peripheral resistance, usually of moderate degree. When more slowly administered, as by oral ingestion, digitalis does not have important effects on arterial pressure, although venous constriction may be observed. In patients with heart failure the existing sympathetic influences are more pronounced, and the relief of failure may act to reduce the sympathetic effects. However, there is undoubtedly considerable variability in the reactions of different vascular beds. Recurrent observations suggest that patients may at times be subject to congestion in the portal circulation due to constriction of the hepatic sphincters or hepatic vein.

Kidney Function and Water Balance

The present view is that digitalis is without important action on urine flow, except for improving the hemodynamics of heart failure. Improved pumping action of the heart is the most important feature of this change, but there are evidences that possible specific effects in the kidneys may contribute to the diuretic effect. Certainly the effect of digitalis in promoting excretion of NaCl and water is a prime benefit, and in instances which coincide with the forward-failure concept, the removal of salt and water may precede other features of improvement, such as lowering systemic venous pressure. The rather extreme view is that diuretics provide the best management of congestive heart failure and edema and that digitalis is an auxiliary measure to be used only in certain cases, especially the arrhythmias. Accepting the more moderate view, diuretics are of value in the management of the edema of heart failure and can be used as temporary substitutes for cardiac glycosides, for instance, when glycoside effects have reached toxic stages.

Diuretics administered to a digitalized but still edematous patient often bring on copious diuresis but coincidentally bring on the typical arrhythmias of digitalis overdose. An acceptable explanation for this phenomenon is that the diuresis lowers intracellular potassium levels, which in turn increases sensitivity to digitalis.

FATE AND DISTRIBUTION

Digitoxin and digoxin are both orally and parenterally effective. The kidney is the chief route of elimination for digoxin, and seriously depressed kidney function can result with accumulation of the drug. This is considered a major factor contributing to its toxicity. Digoxin is not biotransformed and is excreted to the extent of about 80 percent in the urine; its serum half-life is about 34 h. The time course of

elimination is slower in elderly patients with decreased kidney function. Hyperthyroidism is associated with a faster rate of elimination of digoxin, and hypothyroidism with a slower rate of elimination as contrasted with the euthyroid state. Peritoneal dialysis and hemodialysis are ineffective for removing digoxin and may precipitate toxicity if serum potassium levels are lowered by the procedure. Less digitoxin is recovered in the urine, with a greater conversion to metabolites and longer serum half-life. Digitoxin is metabolized in the liver and excreted largely in the bile. The measurements of blood levels of digoxin and digitoxin are in reasonable agreement with clinical estimates of digitalis inotropism as determined by ejection time indices. Tissue concentrations of digoxin are greatest in the kidney, the heart and liver having the next highest concentrations.

PREPARATIONS

Powdered digitalis is the dried leaf of *D. purpurea,* standardized by the pigeon assay method to correspond to the activity of an official reference powder, 0.1 g of which is equal to 1 N.F. Digitalis Unit or about 1 percent of the glycosides digitoxin, gitoxin, and gitalin. It is available as 0.1 g tablets or capsules.

Digoxin (Lanoxin) is a crystalline glycoside isolated from the leaves of *D. lanata,* available as tablets of 0.125, 0.25, and 0.5 mg; ampuls of 0.5 mg in 2 ml 10 percent alcohol.

Digoxin elixir contains 0.05 mg/ml.

Digitoxin is a crystalline glycoside from *D. purpurea* or *D. lanata* and is available in tablets of 0.1 and 0.2 mg, and ampuls of 0.05 and 0.2 mg/ml.

Deslanoside (Cedilanid D, desacetyl lanatoside C) is available in ampuls of 0.4 mg in 2 ml, and 0.8 mg in 4 ml.

The most significant difference which could exist among the various digitalis preparations would be a difference between the ratio of doses producing therapeutic effects and those producing toxic effects. In cases of progressively deteriorating cardiac function, particularly in the aged, doses of digitalis preparations must be progressively increased into the toxic range. Any superior therapeutic index of any one of these preparations would mark it the drug of choice under these conditions.

The bulk of evidence, however, demonstrates that the cardiac glycosides do not exhibit any significant difference in this vital ratio of safety. The trial-and-error method must be used and dosage should be individualized and largely empirical. Extensive clinical experience has produced some average dosages that can be used as rough guidelines (Table 21-1).

DIGITALIS ASSAY

Pharmaceutical preparations of digitoxin, digoxin, and deslanoside are assayed for their purity and content by chromatographic and spectrophotometric procedures, using specified standard preparations. The potency of powdered digitalis, as previously specified under Preparations, is determined by bioassay.

Following oral administration of digoxin or digitoxin, it is possible to determine serum concentrations of these drugs in the nanogram per milliliter (ng/ml) range by radioimmunoassay. This is essentially a competition between serum nonradioactive drug and a constant amount of tritiated drug for a constant number of drug-antibody binding sites. A liquid scintillation counter is used to measure the radioactivity of the tritiated drug-antibody complex. There is a reciprocal relationship: the lower the radioactivity of the complex, the higher the serum level of digoxin or digitoxin. The precise concentration of the glycoside in the serum is then determined from a standard curve. This radioimmunoassay is available for routine clinical use in many medical centers.

THERAPEUTIC USES

Congestive Heart Failure

The underlying cause of congestive heart failure is the failure of the heart as a pump (decrease in myo-

cardial contractility). Digitalis should first be used in an attempt to improve the function of the failing heart prior to the use of diuretics and aldosterone antagonists, salt restriction, and other measures. It is more effective in patients with low-output failure, as in hypertensive cardiovascular disease and arteriosclerotic heart disease. Though not so effective in high-output failure of the type seen in cor pulmonale and thyrotoxicosis, it should be used here together with other measures. The response to digitalis is less in conditions associated with mechanical obstruction or insufficiency, such as in valvular lesions or constrictive pericarditis, although a sufficient improvement warrants its use. In heart failure associated with acute rheumatic fever or myocarditis, digitalis should be used concomitantly with other drugs. Thus, clinical improvement may be expected in congestive failure regardless of cause, level of cardiac output, or type of cardiac rhythm.

Left-sided heart failure may develop quite precipitately as acute pulmonary edema with widely distributed rales and frothy sputum. In these cases, digitalis glycosides are given intravenously, usually in addition to morphine, oxygen, diuretics, and possibly tourniquets or venesection.

Arrhythmias

Atrial Fibrillation and Atrial Flutter In atrial fibrillation, digitalis reduces the ventricular rate by increasing the refractory period of the conduction tissue. The rapid, irregular atrial impulses showered on the AV node are extinguished in greater numbers as the refractory interval is increased by digitalis. The refractory interval of the atrial mass, on the other hand, may be shortened; this favors perpetuation of atrial fibrillation and increased atrial rate. Similarly, atrial flutter may be altered to reach

Table 21-1   Commonly Used Digitalis Preparations

Preparation	Gastrointestinal absorption	Digitalizing-dose range		Daily maintenance dosage, oral
		Oral	I.V.	
Digitalis	20%	1.2–2.0 g	—	0.1–0.2 g
Digitoxin	100%	1.0–1.6 mg	1.0–1.6 mg	0.05–0.3 mg
Digoxin	80%	0.75–1.5 mg	0.5–1.5 mg	0.125–0.5 mg
Deslanoside	Inadequate	—	1.0–1.6 mg	—

the state of atrial fibrillation. The vagal effect of digitalis is responsible for the early shortened refractory period of the atrium. General improvement in myocardial function, measured as increased contractile force, may have the later effect of converting the arrhythmias into normal sinus rhythm.

Paroxysmal Atrial Tachycardia Paroxysmal atrial tachycardia frequently responds to therapy with the glycosides. They are ordinarily used only after failure of other measures such as carotid sinus pressure, eyeball pressure, physical stimulation of the pharynx, emetics, and cholinergic drugs.

Ventricular Tachycardia Paroxysmal ventricular tachycardia presents a difficult problem because, if left untreated, patients usually develop heart failure. At the same time, one hesitates to use a drug whose severe toxic effects closely resemble the condition being treated. In some cases, however, the resemblance is only superficial and digitalis, though dangerous, may be critically helpful. Extrasystoles during heart failure may be due to anoxia and commonly disappear with digitalization and return of compensation.

Complete Atrioventricular Block In the presence of heart failure with complete AV block, digitalis can be utilized for its contractility effect. However, in patients with congestive heart failure and complete AV block, it is preferable to give digitalis after insertion of a cardiac pacemaker.

Myocardial Infarction with Failure

Digitalis is one of the inotropic agents considered in myocardial infarction associated with heart failure, and here it has an advantage over adrenergic agents in that its effects are better sustained and are associated with less of an imposed load due to pressor effects. In angina pectoris, the value of digitalis is equivocal, but any benefit has been attributed to a reduction of oxygen demand because of a decrease in heart size.

CONTRAINDICATION

Digitalis may be harmful in subaortic hypertrophic stenosis in which hypertrophied ventricular myocardium obstructs the left ventricular outflow tract. Increasing the force of contraction of the outflow tract intensifies the resistance to ventricular ejection.

TOXICITY

The prime danger with digitalis is the dose-related progressively severe arrhythmias terminating in ventricular fibrillation. The common predisposing influence is a decrease in intracellular potassium which may develop following the use of potassium-excreting diuretics, prolonged administration of corticosteroids, or any condition causing vomiting or diarrhea. Other predisposing situations occur in the elderly with decreased kidney function and correspondingly decreased renal excretion of the drug; in premature infants deficient in the usual excretory and metabolic processes; in conditions such as hypothyroidism, with decreased metabolic destruction; in any condition of decreased kidney function; and during variabilities in absorption from the alimentary tract. In refractory cases of heart failure it is expected that doses will be administered at dangerous levels.

Digitalis toxicity is common and is increasing in incidence. Some estimates indicate that 10 percent of hospitalized patients receive digitalis and that 20 percent of these develop toxicity. Patients on daily oral maintenance digoxin usually exhibit no evidence of toxicity if digoxin blood concentrations are between 1 to 2 ng/ml. Digoxin therapy is usually discontinued when blood digoxin levels are above 2 ng/ml, until the level falls below this concentration. Cardiac effects may include the various stages of AV block, premature systoles and tachycardia (especially when ventricular in origin), paroxysmal atrial tachycardia with AV block, AV dissociation with nonparoxysmal nodal tachycardia, and ventricular fibrillation. A representative summary of the incidence of signs and symptoms of digitalis poisoning is given in Tables 21-2 and 21-3.

Anorexia is usually the earliest sign of developing systemic toxicity. The subsequent nausea and vomiting is evidently a summated effect of local irritation in the gastrointestinal tract and of stimulation of the chemoreceptor trigger zone activating the emetic center. Other extracardiac effects of significance are mental disturbances and color vision changes.

Table 21-2   Symptoms and Signs in 44 Cases of Digitalis Poisoning

Symptom or sign	No. of cases
Anorexia	21
Nausea	18
Vomiting	16
Diarrhea	5
Weakness and fatigue	4
Yellow vision	6
Scotoma	3
No symptoms but ECG irregularities	17
Paroxysmal tachycardia with AV block	20
S-T and T-wave depression	15
Premature contractions, irregular	6
Bigeminy	12
Trigeminy	1
Extreme bradycardia	2
AV block	7
SA block	1
Nodal rhythm	2
Atrial fibrillation, developing during observation	10
Atrial flutter, developing during observation	1
Death, presumably due to ventricular fibrillation	2

Table 21-3   Disturbances in Cardiac Rhythm in 88 Patients

Disturbance	No. of cases
Multifocal or paired premature ventricular contractions	30
AV dissociation with and without interference	25
First-degree heart block	17
Bigeminy	15
Paroxysmal atrial tachycardia with block	9
Second-degree heart block	8
Nodal tachycardia	8
Complete AV heart block	5
Ventricular tachycardia	4
Ventricular fibrillation (terminal)	2
Ventricular fibrillation (paroxysmal)	1

TREATMENT OF DIGITALIS TOXICITY

The use of potassium salts for treating digitalis-induced arrhythmias is based on considerable clinical experience. Potassium chloride may be administered orally or by intravenous infusion. Obviously, the antidotal regimen is pointless without discontinuing all forms of digitalis or diuretics, such as thiazides or furosemide, which remove potassium.

There is broad agreement that increased extracellular potassium decreases automaticity and suppresses the ectopic beats induced by digitalis by forcing potassium into the cell. Conversely, lowered potassium levels are associated with the appearance of arrhythmias in the presence of even small doses of cardiac glycosides, and this may occur with potassium-excreting diuretics or hemodialysis. Depressed conduction due to digitalis is further depressed by increasing potassium levels or, again, by rapidly rising potassium levels. Abnormally low potassium levels also may act to depress conduction. Since many diuretic drugs produce hypomagnesemia as well as hypokalemia, and both may predispose to digitalis arrhythmias, in certain cases magnesium may also be given.

Antiarrhythmic drugs, such as diphenylhydantoin, lidocaine, and propranolol are used to correct digitalis intoxication. Ventricular premature contractions, ventricular tachycardia, and paroxysmal atrioventricular junctional tachycardia may be abolished with diphenylhydantoin.

Direct current shock may be indicated and used in certain arrhythmias such as ventricular tachycardia and fibrillation secondary to the cardiac glycosides.

Recent developments in treating digitalis toxicities involve the use of cholestyramine, digoxin-specific antibodies, and potassium canreonate.

Chapter 22

Antiarrhythmic Drugs

Treatment of cardiac arrhythmias by use of chemical agents which modify the electrical activity of the heart is based on several considerations. These are (1) an understanding of the disturbance in electrical activity which is present, that is, an accurate diagnosis; (2) a justifiable assumption that it is possible either to restore sinus rhythm or to induce a more desirable pattern of electrical activity; (3) a justifiable assumption that the intended change in electrical activity will improve either the function of the cardiovascular system or the prognosis; and (4) a reasonable probability that the therapeutic intervention to be employed will produce a desirable change without excessive risk or undesirable effects.

REVIEW OF CARDIAC ELECTROPHYSIOLOGY

There is a potential difference across the cardiac cell membrane. When the cell is quiescent, this transmembrane potential varies from 80 to 90 mV, inside negative, and is called the *transmembrane resting potential*. On excitation the transmembrane potential changes, and the inside of the membrane transiently becomes positive with respect to the outside. On recovery from excitation, the resting potential is restored. The changes in potential following excitation are called the *transmembrane action potential*. An action potential typical of a cardiac Purkinje fiber is shown in Fig. 22-1; the phase of depolarization and reversal of transmembrane potential is designated phase 0, the three phases of repolarization are labeled 1, 2, and 3, and the resting potential is designated phase 4. Not all cardiac action potentials show such clear separation between phases 1, 2, and 3; not all cells show a constant membrane potential during phase 4. Also, there are quantitative differences between the transmembrane potentials recorded from different types of cardiac cells. The following description applies to the cardiac Purkinje fiber and atrial and

225

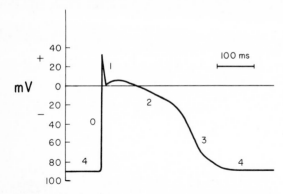

Figure 22-1 Diagrammatic representation of a trans-membrane action potential recorded from a mammalian Purkinje fiber, showing the phases of depolarization (0) and repolarization (1,2, and 3) and the resting transmembrane potential (phase 4).

ventricular muscles. A limited number of studies indicate that sinoatrial (SA) and atrioventricular (AV) nodal fibers may have somewhat different ionic mechanisms.

MECHANISMS OF ANTIARRHYTHMIC ACTION

We use the term *mechanism* to mean only the observed changes in electrical activity produced by an antiarrhythmic drug. These changes almost certainly are related to their antiarrhythmic action. One major group of antiarrhythmic compounds may be described as quinidine-like; this group includes quinidine, procainamide, propranolol, and several less important agents. These drugs have generally similar effects on the electrical properties of cardiac fibers. In addition, all these drugs possess local anesthetic activity, all directly depress mechanical activity of the heart, and all modify to some extent the effects of autonomic nerves on the heart. Effects on electrical properties will be presented in some detail for procainamide as the drug typical of this group. A second group of antiarrhythmic drugs, although somewhat more heterogeneous, includes diphenylhydantoin, lidocaine, and, under certain conditions, the catecholamines. Although these drugs share some action with the quinidine-like group, each differs in terms of several important effects on electrical properties of cardiac fibers.

Excitability

Excitability usually is measured in terms of the strength of an electrical pulse required to excite cardiac tissue at selected intervals during the cardiac cycle. Procainamide, like quinidine and propranolol, decreases the electrical excitability of atrial and ventricular muscle. This change in stimulus requirement can be noted both in diastole and during the relative refractory period. In contrast, diphenylhydantoin and lidocaine have little effect on the electrical excitability of atrial and ventricular muscle.

Automaticity

The term *automaticity* is used to describe the behavior of cardiac fibers which spontaneously generate action potentials. This mechanism can be described in terms of threshold potential and the voltage-time course of membrane potential recorded from automatic fibers. Procainamide and the other drugs with quinidine-like actions decrease the slope of phase 4 of normally automatic cells. The magnitude of this change is related to concentration. The quinidine-like drugs also influence normally automatic cells by an indirect action. The indirect effects on automaticity result from interference with the action of the efferent autonomic nerves.

The action of procainamide and the related drugs on ectopic pacemakers is more prominent than on the sinus node. However, the extent to which any automatic cell is slowed by one of these agents may depend on the complex balance between direct and indirect actions.

Refractoriness

Refractoriness is defined and measured in many ways; for the most part, we shall restrict our considerations of refractoriness to the duration of the *effective refractory period* (ERP) which is the minimum interval of time between two propagated responses.

Quinidine and procainamide modify the duration of the ERP by the following two direct actions. These agents, particularly in large doses, increase action potential duration (APD) by slowing repolarization. In addition to increasing the duration of the action potential, they shift the relationship between membrane potential and responsiveness so that repolarization must proceed further before a propagated response can be elicited. The overall effect is not just to increase the duration of the ERP but rather to increase it out of proportion to the change in APD. In contrast, propranolol decreases the APD. However, propranolol alters the relationship between membrane potential and responsiveness in the same manner as procainamide, and thus it also prolongs the ERP relative to the APD. The effects of procainamide, quinidine, and propranolol on the refractoriness and APD of atrial fibers may be modified by the indirect effects of these drugs and the resulting change in vagal action. The vagolytic effect of procainamide and quinidine would increase the duration of atrial action potentials.

Diphenylhydantoin and lidocaine, unlike procainamide, decrease the duration of the action potentials recorded from cells in the His-Purkinje system and ventricle. In addition, there is a decrease in the duration of the ERP. However, effective refractoriness is not decreased in proportion to the shortening of the action potential. It is also quite interesting that diphenylhydantoin has little or no effect on repolarization or refractoriness of atrial muscle fibers.

In summary (Table 22-1), it is evident that propranolol differs from quinidine and procainamide only in terms of its effects on APD. On the other hand, diphenylhydantoin and lidocaine resemble the quinidine-like drugs only in terms of (1) effects on automaticity, and (2) the magnitude of the change in effective refractoriness relative to the change in APD.

Conduction

Table 22-1 also contrasts the effects of these agents on conduction. In usual concentrations, procainamide, quinidine, and propranolol decrease conduction velocity in fibers of the atrium, ventricle, and His-Purkinje system. Diphenylhydantoin and lidocaine, in contrast, do not decrease conduction velocity and may at times actually increase speed of propagation. A similar contrast is demonstrated by the actions of the two groups of drugs on AV conduction time: procainamide, quinidine, and propranolol in therapeutic doses may slow AV propagation, while usual doses of diphenylhydantoin and lidocaine cause no change or speed AV conduction. These effects are more prominent if AV conduction is depressed prior to drug administration. In the

Table 22-1   Characteristic Electrophysiologic and Antiarrhythmic Actions*

	Group I		Group II
	Procainamide and quinidine	Propranolol	DPH and lidocaine
Electrophysiologic properties			
Purkinje fibers:			
Automaticity	↓	↓	↓
Responsiveness	↓	↓	→ or ↑
Conduction velocity	↓	↓	→ or ↑
ERP	↑	↓	↓
APD	↑	↓	↓
ΔERP relative to APD	↑	↑	↑
Excitability	↓	↓	→
Atrioventricular conduction time	→ or ↑	→ or ↑	→ or ↓
Experimental arrhythmias			
Digitalis-induced	+	++	+++
Coronary ligation	++	+	++?

*Abbreviations: DPH, diphenylhydantoin; ERP, effective refractory period; APD, action potential duration; +, moderately effective; ++, effective; +++, highly effective; ↑, increased; ↓, decreased; →, no change. Arrows indicate the direction and not the magnitude of change.

presence of AV block caused by digitalis, diphenyl-hydantoin and lidocaine usually improve AV conduction, unlike procainamide, quinidine, and propranolol. The ability of diphenylhydantoin to increase conduction velocity in Purkinje fibers is enhanced also by the presence of abnormally slow propagation.

CARDIAC ARRHYTHMIAS

Atrial Fibrillation

Atrial fibrillation is a rhythm characterized by irregular, disorganized depolarization of the atria at rates of 350 to 600 beats/min. These rapid depolarizations do not produce effective atrial contractions. The rapid atrial rate exceeds the ability of even the normal AV conducting system to transmit impulses; therefore, the ventricular rate is much slower, 130 to 170 beats/min in untreated cases, and is characteristically irregular. This rhythm diminishes the "cardiac reserve," produces palpitations, and is associated with an increased incidence of thromboembolization of the pulmonary or systemic arterial systems. The decrease in cardiac reserve commonly leads to the onset or aggravation of congestive heart failure, angina pectoris, or symptoms of cerebrovascular insufficiency.

Atrial Flutter

Atrial flutter is characterized by regular beating of the atria at rates between 250 and 300 beats/min; most commonly the atrial rate is precisely 300 beats/min. In adults who have not been treated, every other atrial depolarization is usually conducted to the ventricles, producing a ventricular rate of 150 beats/min. Unlike atrial fibrillation, atrial flutter produces effective contraction of the atria and thrombosis in the atria, with subsequent embolization much less common.

Paroxysmal Atrial Tachycardia

Paroxysmal atrial tachycardia (PAT) is characterized by atrial rates of 150 to 250 beats/min and most often 180 to 200 beats/min. This rhythm often occurs in the absence of demonstrable heart disease. In the absence of heart disease and drug therapy, it is common to see each atrial depolariza-

tion conduct to ventricles so that the atrial and ventricular rates are identical. Paroxysms often spontaneously terminate but also may be tenaciously persistent and cause severe anxiety and palpitations or induce heart failure even in otherwise normal hearts.

Ventricular Premature Depolarization

Ventricular premature depolarizations (VPDs) or extrasystoles originate in the ventricles, and the QRS complexes are thus wide and bizarre in configuration, prematurely interrupting the dominant rhythm. Ventricular premature depolarizations are very common both in individuals with normal hearts and in those with heart disease. Many of these cases require no treatment. If premature depolarizations are frequent or cause troublesome symptoms or signs, treatment should be considered. The decision to treat VPDs also may be based on the condition associated with the arrhythmia. For instance, digitalis in excessive doses may lead to frequent ventricular premature beats. If digitalis is continued, ventricular tachycardia or ventricular fibrillation often occurs and may prove fatal. Another example is the occurrence of VPDs during acute myocardial infarction where VPDs may presage ventricular tachycardia or fibrillation.

Ventricular Tachycardia

Ventricular tachycardia is a rapid rhythm (150 to 200 beats/min) originating in the ventricles. This site of origin produces QRS complexes in the ECG which are slurred and widened. The configuration of the QRS complexes during ventricular tachycardia is the same as VPDs originating in either right or left ventricle. The cycle length between beats is slightly irregular, and the QRS complexes are independent of the P waves. The etiologic factors and therapeutic goals are similar to those discussed under Ventricular Premature Depolarizations. However, ventricular tachycardia is much more likely to produce circulatory impairment than even frequent ventricular premature beats, and congestive cardiac failure or severe hypotension may ensue. When such catastrophic events are precipitated by ventricular tachycardia, it should be terminated immediately.

GENERAL PHARMACOLOGY

Quinidine

Quinidine is a stereoisomer of quinine; it exerts all the pharmacologic actions of quinine, including antimalarial, antipyretic, and oxytocic effects. The actions of quinidine on cardiac muscle are relatively more intense than those of quinine. Conversely, quinidine is said to be less effective against malaria than is quinine.

Chemistry Quinidine is one of the four most important alkaloids isolated from cinchona bark. Its structure is shown in Fig. 22-2. Quinidine consists of a quinoline group attached by a secondary alcohol to a quinuclidine ring. There is a methoxy side chain on the quinoline ring and a vinyl group on the quinuclidine ring. Quinidine differs from quinine only in the configuration of the secondary alcohol grouping.

Effects on Organ Systems

Cardiovascular System The major effects of quinidine on the electrical activity of the heart have been described above and are summarized in Tables 22-1 and 22-2. In general, quinidine can be described as a cardiac depressant; it decreases automaticity, excitability, and conduction velocity, prolongs refractoriness, and depresses contractility. The depressant effect on contractility has been demonstrated both in vitro and in vivo and probably is of real importance when myocardial disease is present. Large oral doses of quinidine reduce arterial pressure in man. Considerably smaller intravenous doses have the same effect. Rapid intra-

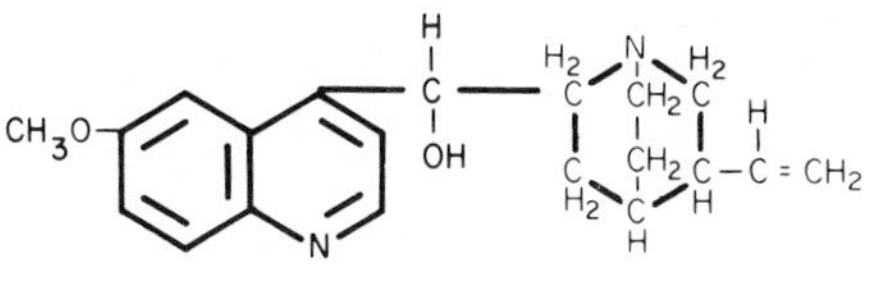

QUINIDINE

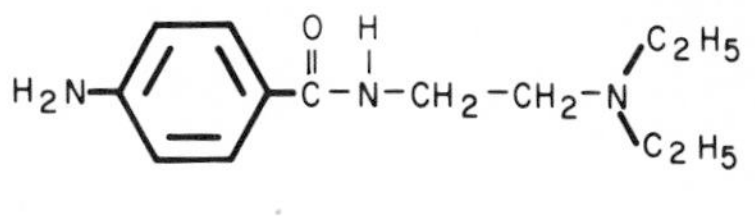

PROCAINAMIDE

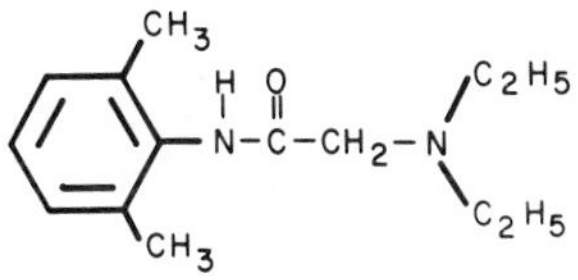

LIDOCAINE

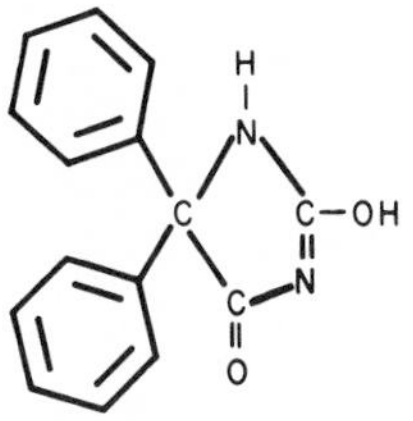

DIPHENYLHYDANTOIN

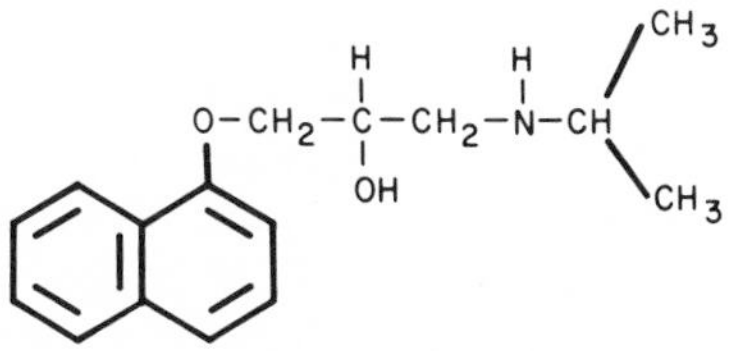

PROPRANOLOL

Figure 22-2 Structural formulas of quinidine, procainamide, lidocaine, diphenylhydantoin, and propranolol.

Table 22-2   Electrocardiographic and Hemodynamic Effects in Man*

	P-R	QRS	QT$_c$	AVRP	VR in A FIB	BP	CO	LVEDP
Quinidine	→↑	↑	↑	↑	→↑	↓	↓	↑
Procainamide	→↑	↑	↑	↑	→↑	↓	↓	↓
Propranolol	→↑	→	↓	↑	↓	→↓	↓	↑
Diphenylhydantoin	→↑	→	↓	↓	↑↓	↓	→↓	→↑
Lidocaine	→	→	→↓	→↓	↑↓	↓	→↓	→↑

*Abbreviations: P-R, QRS, QT, electrocardiographic intervals; QT$_c$, Q-T interval corrected for cycle length; AVRP, atrioventricular refractory period; VR in A FIB, ventricular rate in atrial fibrillation; BP, arterial blood pressure; CO, cardiac output; LVEDP, left ventricular end diastolic pressure; ↑, increased; ↓, decreased; →, no change. Arrows indicate the direction, but not the magnitude of change.

venous injection may cause a precipitious decrease in blood pressure and cardiac output. Although in this case the decrease in arterial pressure is due largely to peripheral vasodilatation, a decrease in cardiac output in the presence of reduced peripheral resistance shows that myocardial depression is produced by quinidine.

Many of the effects of quinidine on the electrical activity of the heart can be appreciated from the ECG. Patients in sinus rhythm may show an increase in sinus rate which presumably is caused by anticholinergic action, a reflex increase in sympathetic activity, or both. High doses, particularly in patients with atrial disease, may produce sinus arrest or sinoatrial (SA) block. Because of its effects on conduction in the His-Purkinje system and ventricle, quinidine causes a progressive prolongation of the QRS complex. Prolongation of the QRS and serious conduction disturbances are more likely when abnormality of the conduction system is present before quinidine administration. Quinidine increases the Q-T interval corrected for rate. This effect, at low doses, is due primarily to the effects of quinidine on repolarization of ventricular muscle. At higher doses, changes in the Q-T interval and in the configuration of the T wave result also from the quinidine-induced disturbances of conduction. In usual therapeutic doses quinidine has little effect on the P-R interval. This may be due to the fact that an anticholinergic action is balanced by a direct depressant effect on AV conduction. In sufficiently high concentrations quinidine can produce heart block of any degree.

Central Nervous System Quinidine first stimulates and then depresses the higher nerve centers. In man intravenous administration of quinidine may produce a sensation of warmth, profuse diaphoresis, and nausea and vomiting.

Autonomic Nervous System Quinidine appears to interfere with the effects of the parasympathetic nervous system on the heart. A vagal blocking action of quinidine would be expected to increase APD and refractoriness of atrial muscle, accelerate AV conduction (and thus shorten the P-R interval), and increase sinus rate.

Skeletal Muscle Quinidine, like the other cinchona alkaloids, increases the maximum tension developed by skeletal muscle in response to direct electrical stimulation. This action contrasts with its negative inotropic effect on cardiac muscle. Quinidine increases refractoriness of skeletal muscle. Quinidine also decreases the effectiveness of transmission across the neuromuscular junction and diminishes the response of skeletal muscle to intraarterial injections of acetylcholine.

Absorption, Fate, and Excretion Quinidine is almost entirely absorbed from the gastrointestinal tract. The extent and rate of absorption are modified by gastric acidity, amount of food in the gastrointestinal tract, and gastrointestinal motility. No significant alteration of the quinidine molecule occurs during its transport across the gastrointestinal epithelium. A single oral dose produces peak plasma concentrations between 1 and 2 h later.

Nearly 80 percent of plasma quinidine is bound to albumin. Quinidine also enters the red blood cells and is bound to hemoglobin so that, at equilibrium, similar concentrations are found in plasma and red blood cells.

Quinidine disappears from plasma with a half-life between 2 and 3 h. The drug is metabolically altered in the liver. Many of the compounds produced have not been identified, but a large proportion of the altered compounds are hydroxylated compounds. Hepatic enzymes hydroxylate either the quinoline, the quinuclidine ring, or both; in either case, the hydroxyl group attaches on the carbon atom adjacent to the nitrogen. Although the amount of unaltered quinidine and the portion of each metabolite excreted is highly variable, 95 percent of an administered dose can be recovered from the urine as the total of quinidine and its metabolic products.

Quinidine given intravenously can give effective plasma concentrations quite rapidly but is little used at present because of profound hypotension which is frequently seen after injection. Another difficulty with this method is that there is a variable lag between intravenous injection of a dose and the cardiac effect it produces.

Toxicity One of the major problems in the effective use of quinidine is its toxicity. The major undesirable side effects are listed in Table 22-3.

Cinchonism Quinidine, like the other cinchona alkaloids, cinchophen, and salicylates, can induce cinchonism. Symptoms of mild cinchonism may include tinnitus, impaired hearing, headache, mild diarrhea, or slight blurring of vision. Symptoms of severe toxicity include severe tinnitus and hearing

loss, blurred vision, diplopia, photophobia, and altered perception of color. Severe cerebral signs, such as confusion, delirium, or psychosis, may accompany the headache. Nausea, vomiting, and diarrhea may be severe and accompanied by abdominal pain. The skin is often hot and flushed.

Gastrointestinal Effects Nausea, vomiting, and diarrhea each occur alone or in varying combinations and often in the absence of symptoms involving other systems. Quinidine administration is often continued even with mild gastrointestinal symptoms; more severe reaction may force discontinuing the drug.

Blood Pressure When given intravenously, and to a lesser extent intramuscularly, quinidine may cause significant and even profound arterial hypotension. In most instances this pressure drop is primarily due to a decrease in arteriolar resistance without marked reduction in cardiac output. Severe, protracted hypotension may be treated with catecholamines or, if resistant, with angiotensin.

Cardiac Effects Quinidine in concentrations above 2.0 μg/ml causes a progressive linear increase in duration of the QRS and Q-T intervals of the ECG; the change in QRS has a higher correlation with plasma drug concentration. This relationship is useful in monitoring the cardiac effects of quinidine; the dose administered is reduced if a normal QRS duration increases by 50 percent over

Table 22-3 Characteristic Undesirable Effects*

	Cardiac			CNS	Other
	Rhythm	BP	CO		
Quinidine	V Tach V Fib Asystole	↓	↓	Cinchonism	Thrombocytopenia
Procainamide	V Tach V Fib Asystole	↓	↓		Lupus syndrome Agranulocytosis
Propranolol	Pacemaker suppression; asystole	↓	↓		Bronchospasm (asthmatics)
Diphenylhydantoin	Asystole	↓	↓	Cerebellar signs; coma	Megaloblastic anemia; lymphoma-like syndrome
Lidocaine		↓	↓	Convulsions; respiratory arrest	

* *Abbreviations:* CO, Cardiac output; V Tach, ventricular tachycardia; V Fib, ventricular fibrillation. Arrows represent the magnitude of decrease in BP and CO.

the control value. The Q-T interval is also a useful measurement to follow, and changes in this interval are easy to detect at ordinary ECG recording speeds. At plasma concentrations that may be toxic (> 8 μg/ml, true quinidine), complete SA block, high-grade AV block, or total asystole may occur. Ventricular ectopic depolarizations may become frequent and occur repetitively; ventricular tachycardia or fibrillation may ensue. Although such severe myocardial toxicity may diminish as plasma concentration declines after withholding quinidine, the ECG and hemodynamic parameters of each patient should be closely monitored. Catecholamines, molar sodium lactate, and glucagon may be useful to counteract quinidine toxicity in cases which require more active intervention.

A frequently mentioned complication of quinidine therapy for atrial fibrillation is the so-called "paradoxic" increase in ventricular rate. In many cases of atrial fibrillation, when quinidine is used alone for conversion, the atrial rate slows markedly before the change to sinus rhythm occurs. However, in a few of these cases the ventricular rate may suddenly rise as atrial rate falls because of a decrease in concealed conduction of atrial impulses in the AV junction. Even though this event is uncommon in patients treated with quinidine alone, many physicians digitalize their patients prior to using quinidine to avoid this eventuality.

Procainamide

The actions of procainamide are qualitatively similar to those of procaine. Its effects on the electrical activity of the heart, as shown in Table 22-1, are almost identical to those of quinidine. Procainamide is superior to procaine as an antiarrhythmic agent because, in contrast to procaine, (1) it is well absorbed after oral administration, (2) it has a long duration of action because it resists hydrolysis by plasma esterases, and (3) its effects on the heart are relatively strong, while its effects on the central nervous system are relatively weak.

Chemistry   Procainamide is *p*-amino-*N*-(2-diethylaminoethyl) benzamide. Its structural formula is shown in Fig. 22-2. Procainamide differs from procaine in that the ester linkage has been replaced by an amide bond.

Effects on Organ Systems

Heart   The effects of procainamide on the electrical activity of the heart have been described above and are summarized in Table 22-1. They are qualitatively the same as those of quinidine. Like quinidine, procainamide has a negative inotropic effect although, at equivalent therapeutic doses, this action may be less intense. Like quinidine, procainamide causes a decrease in systemic arterial pressure which is particularly prominent with intravenous administration. Peripheral vasodilatation and depression of cardiac contractility both contribute to the hypotensive action.

The changes in the ECG produced by procainamide are similar to those caused by quinidine. Prolongation of the QRS complex is most consistent, while prolongation of the corrected Q-T interval, changes in the morphology of the T wave, and, at high doses, prolongation of the P-R interval or production of heart block may result. As in the case of quinidine, changes in the ECG may provide some guide to the doses of procainamide to be employed. The presence of abnormalities of conduction increases the likelihood that the drug will cause further conduction delay or block.

Absorption, Fate, and Excretion   Procainamide can be given orally, intramuscularly, or intravenously. Absorption is almost complete after administration by any of these routes. Following oral doses, peak plasma concentrations are reached in 45 to 90 min. Intramuscular injections produce peak levels at 15 to 45 min, but values are more variable than after oral or intravenous doses. Procainamide is only sparingly bound to plasma proteins. However, it is bound in various body tissues in concentrations greatly in excess of the plasma concentration. Disappearance of procainamide from the plasma approximates a first-order process with a half-life of 2 to 3 h. Nearly 90 percent of procainamide and its metabolites is excreted into the urine; in man, 50 to 60 percent is excreted unchanged. When it occurs, biotransformation takes place in the liver. Unlike its homologue procaine, procainamide is highly resistant to plasma esterases.

Toxicity   The major undesirable effects of procainamide are listed in Table 22-3. Many of the undesirable effects of procainamide are related to the plasma concentration, the rate of change of plasma concentration, and the route of administration. The intravenous route of administration is more often associated with direct cardiac toxicity than is the oral route. The direct cardiac effects are expressed as progressive widening of the QRS, which may become excessive, and as ventricular ectopic beats, ventricular tachycardia or fibrillation, or as electrical asystole. High doses of procainamide may diminish myocardial contractility and cause hypotension or worsen cardiac failure.

Of special note are agranulocytosis and a syndrome resembling systemic lupus erythematosus (SLE) which may be produced by procainamide. Agranulocytosis may be severe and responsible for fatal infections. Arthralgia is the most prevalent symptom, and fever, pleuropneumonic involvement, and hepatomegaly are all common. This syndrome possesses features distinct from idiopathic SLE. There is no predilection for females. Renal and cerebral involvement are not seen. Indeed, procainamide has a greater capacity to induce a syndrome resembling SLE than any other chemical.

Lidocaine

The chemistry and effects on most organ systems of lidocaine are discussed in Chap. 7, Local Anesthetics. The major effects of lidocaine on the cardiovascular system are summarized in Tables 22-1 and 22-2.

Absorption, Fate, and Excretion When used as an antiarrhythmic drug, lidocaine is administered almost exclusively by the intravenous route as intermittent injections or by continuous infusions. The usual therapeutic range of plasma concentrations of lidocaine is 2 to 5 μg/ml of plasma, although some ventricular arrhythmias will respond favorably to concentrations of 1 to 2 μg/ml. The half-life of lidocaine in plasma ranges from 15 to 30 min. Thus, the duration of action of a single dose is short, and the steady-state plasma concentration is quickly reached on continuous, constant-rate infusion. It is therefore imperative that the infusion rate be meticulously controlled lest either ineffective or toxic concentrations result.

Intramuscular administration of lidocaine has been recommended because of its convenience in domiciliary practice or during transport of patients with arrhythmias or myocardial infarction to a hospital.

Lidocaine is bound to plasma proteins only to a limited extent. It is concentrated in many tissues, including heart muscle, relative to the plasma concentration. Rapid metabolism of the drug causes the concentration in tissues to fall rapidly after a single dose. The liver is the primary site of metabolic alteration; the hepatic microsomal enzyme system initially oxidatively de-ethylates lidocaine, then the amide bond is hydrolyzed. Only 1 to 10 percent of a dose is excreted in the urine without metabolic alteration. Plasma concentrations higher than expected can occur when usual doses are given to individuals with severe impairment of hepatic function.

Toxicity The major undesirable effects of lidocaine when it is used as an antiarrhythmic agent are listed in Table 22-3. Although circulatory collapse with fatal outcome has been seen after administration of large doses or after rapid injection, the undesirable effects of lidocaine are usually restricted to actions on the central nervous system. Central nervous system effects include drowsiness, paresthesias, decreased auditory acuity, convulsions, and respiratory arrest. Drowsiness is commonly encountered during intravenous lidocaine infusion, but is often acceptable or even desirable in patients with arrhythmias. Patients may, however, become anxious or agitated when experiencing lidocaine-induced hearing loss, paresthesias, confusion, or muscle twitching. Lidocaine-induced convulsions are related to dose and rate of administration. Respiratory arrest and death can result from the use of this drug.

Diphenylhydantoin

The chemistry and effects on most organ systems of diphenylhydantoin are discussed in Chap. 12, under Antiepileptic Drugs. The major effects of diphenylhydantoin on the cardiovascular system are summarized in Tables 22-1 and 22-2.

Absorption, Fate, and Excretion Diphenylhydantoin has been administered orally, intramuscularly, and intravenously in the treatment of cardiac arrhythmias; most frequently it has been given intravenously to abolish ventricular arrhythmias. The antiarrhythmic effect is dependent on the plasma concentration.

Intramuscular injection produces erratic changes in plasma concentration and is not recommended. Continuous intravenous infusions are not used because the extremely alkaline, irritating diluent for diphenylhydantoin causes phlebitis and pain.

Absorption of diphenylhydantoin from the gastrointestinal tract is essentially complete. Peak drug plasma concentrations may be achieved as late as 12 h after ingestion. The hepatic enzymes responsible for metabolizing diphenylhydantoin are localized in the microsomal fraction. Diphenylhydantoin is hydroxylated to 5-phenyl-5′-parahydroxyphenyl-hydantoin, conjugated with glucuronic acid, and excreted in the urine.

Other drugs given to a patient receiving diphenylhydantoin may alter its metabolism. Phenobarbital induces hepatic microsomal enzymes, and diphenylhydantoin is parahydroxylated at an increased rate during or after phenobarbital administration. Still other drugs slow its metabolism, in some cases to a marked degree. Drugs known to have this effect include bishydroxycoumarin, isonicotinic acid hydrazide, para-aminosalicylic acid, and cycloserine.

Toxicity   One of the major problems in the effective use of diphenylhydantoin as an antiarrhythmic agent is its toxicity. The major undesirable effects are listed in Table 22-3.

Undesirable effects encountered as a result of the intravenous administration of diphenylhydantoin as an antiarrhythmic agent are usually limited to the cardiovascular and central nervous systems. When it is given rapidly or in large amounts, there may be a fall in cardiac output and hypotension. This hemodynamic response is directly related to the severity of cardiac failure in the patient being treated—patients with advanced heart failure are much more likely to show marked decreases in cardiac output and arterial blood pressure. Adverse hemodynamic effects are extremely rare when diphenylhydantoin is given in repeated small doses.

Undesirable central nervous system effects are encountered more commonly. Nystagmus, vertigo, nausea, drowsiness, and obtundation all are common, and organic mental syndromes may be precipitated in the elderly. Most arrhythmias which will respond to diphenylhydantoin at all do so at plasma concentrations below those causing central nervous system effects. When given orally for prolonged control of cardiac arrhythmias, the undesirable effects seen are identical with those encountered when diphenylhydantoin is used as an anticonvulsant.

Propranolol

l-Propranolol is a β-adrenergic blocking agent which competes with β-adrenergic agonists at their receptor sites (see Chap. 18 on adrenergic blocking agents). Apart from alterations in cardiovascular function which β-adrenergic blockade itself induces, propranolol causes specific alterations in the electrical activity of myocardial cells. These membrane effects differ markedly from those exhibited by some other β-adrenergic blocking agents. It would appear that some of propranolol's antiarrhythmic effects are due to its "membrane" effects; this hypothesis is supported by the fact that *d*-propranolol, which has no significant β-adrenergic blocking action, is able to abolish certain experimental and clinical arrhythmias.

In general, propranolol is used to slow the ventricular rate in supraventricular arrhythmias and, on occasion, to abolish ventricular arrhythmias due to digitalis excess.

Absorption, Fate, and Excretion   The pharmacodynamics of propranolol in man has not been completely elucidated. Propranolol is absorbed from the gastrointestinal tract. Preliminary studies indicate that a single oral dose of 30 mg will produce maximal effects in 1 to 4 h with measurable effects lasting for 5 to 6 h. Some authors state that there is a good correlation between the propranolol concentration in the blood and its biologic activity, but admit that there is considerable variation between individual subjects. At this time, lack of a reliable method for determining plasma concentration and the low levels present in the blood after the doses usually employed in humans make it difficult to demonstrate a strong correlation between the physiologic response to propranolol and the plasma concentration. However, it has been found that plasma propranolol concentrations do correlate to some degree with the reduction in exercise tachycardia that the drug induces. Intravenous doses of 1 to 10 mg rapidly produce characteristic effects.

Toxicity Many of the undesirable effects of propranolol are related to its β-adrenergic blocking properties. When used as an antiarrhythmic drug, particularly in the setting of severe cardiovascular stress, propranolol may produce hypotension, worsening of congestive heart failure, or cardiovascular collapse. It may also lead to asystole due to severe impairment of AV conduction and depressed ventricular pacemaker activity. This agent may also induce significant bronchospasm in asthmatics and has been shown to mask the typical symptoms of insulin overdosage in diabetics, so that the first sign of hyperinsulinism may be coma. It should be noted that not only does propranolol aggravate many cases of existing heart failure, but that an occasional patient not previously known to have congestive heart failure has developed it during treatment. In some cases, propranolol-induced congestive heart failure can be controlled with digitalis; in others, the drug must be discontinued. Nausea, vomiting, insomnia, lassitude, light-headedness, mild diarrhea, and constipation all have been reported to occur during the course of clinical investigations. Propranolol can cross the placental barrier and produce low concentrations in the fetus. Table 22-3 lists the major undesirable effects of propranolol when used as an antiarrhythmic drug.

SUMMARY OF CLINICAL USE

Table 22-4 lists the effects of some pharmacologic agents against common arrhythmias.

PREPARATIONS

Quinidine *Quinidine sulfate* is available in tablets or capsules containing 100, 200, or 300 mg.

Quinidine hydrochloride is available in ampuls of 5 ml containing 0.6 g quinidine HCl for parenteral use.

Quinidine gluconate is available in ampuls of 10 ml containing 0.8 g of the salt (equivalent to 0.5 g anhydrous quinidine) for intravenous use. It is also available as *Quinaglute,* long-acting tablets containing 0.33 g.

Quinidine polygalacturonate (Cardioquin) is available in tablets containing 275 mg of the salt which has an amount of base equivalent to 200 mg quinidine sulfate. This is a long-acting preparation.

Table 22-4   Effectiveness against Specific Cardiac Arrhythmias*†

	Q	PA	P	DPH	L
Supraventricular					
Atrial premature depolarizations	4	4	2	2	1
Paroxysmal atrial tachycardia	3	3	3	2	1
Atrial flutter	2	2	2‡	1	1
Atrial fibrillation					
Conversion	4	4	2‡	1	1
Maintenance	4	4	1	1	1
AV junctional tachycardia and premature contractions	3	3	1	1	1
Ventricular					
Ventricular premature depolarizations	3	4	2	4	4
Ventricular tachycardia	2	4	2	4	4
Digitalis-induced arrhythmias					
Supraventricular	2	2	3	4	4
Ventricular	2§	2§	3§	4	4

* *Abbreviations:* Q, quinidine; PA, procainamide; P, propranolol; DPH, diphenylhydantoin; L, lidocaine.

† Scale of relative effectiveness: 1, poor; 2, fair; 3, good; 4, excellent.

‡ Propranolol is very effective in reducing the ventricular response in atrial flutter and atrial fibrillation but does not convert these arrhythmias to sinus rhythm.

§All these drugs may be effective in treating digitalis-induced ventricular arrhythmias; however, significant undesirable effects have been encountered with each of them.

Procainamide *Procainamide hydrochloride* (Pronestyl) is available in capsules that contain 0.25, 0.375, and 0.5 g; and in vials of 10 ml, containing 100 mg/ml, for intravenous use.

Diphenylhydantoin *Diphenylhydantoin sodium* (Dilantin) is available in capsules that contain 100 mg, and in sterile vials containing 100 or 250 mg.

Lidocaine *Lidocaine hydrochloride* (Xylocaine) is available in multidose vials containing 2 or 4 percent solutions. *Note:* Each concentration is provided without or with epinephrine; the solutions with epinephrine should *NOT* be used to treat cardiac arrhythmias. It is also available in vials of 5 ml, containing 100 mg for direct intravenous injection.

Propranolol *Propranolol hydrochloride* (Inderal) is available as tablets containing 10 and 40 mg and in 1 ml ampuls of 1 mg/ml.

Antianginal and Antilipemic Agents

This chapter concerns itself with two groups of drugs, those used in the therapy of angina pectoris and those used to reduce one of the factors associated with atherosclerosis—hyperlipemia. Classically, the category of antianginal agents includes compounds which are believed to owe part of their therapeutic effect to their ability to dilate the coronary vessels and thereby increase coronary blood flow. The drugs classified as antilipemic agents are used mainly to normalize altered lipid metabolism. Hopefully, these compounds may reduce the rate or reverse the progress of atherosclerosis.

ANTIANGINAL AGENTS

The Nitrates and Nitrites

Pharmacologic Classification This group includes both inorganic and organic nitrites (NO_2^- compounds) and nitrates (NO_3^- compounds). The names and formulas of two of the most commonly used compounds are shown in Fig. 23-1. As antianginal agents, the nitrites may be classified into (1) rapidly acting agents used to terminate an attack of angina, and (2) agents with prolonged action which are employed to prevent attacks of angina. Glyceryl trinitrate and amyl nitrite are rapidly acting agents with a short duration of action. Other organic nitrites used for a more prolonged action are erythrityl tetranitrate, isosorbide dinitrate, mannitol hexanitrate, and pentaerythritol tetranitrate. These agents are administered orally to prevent angina attacks. However, isosorbide dinitrate and erythrityl tetranitrate have been administered sublingually to terminate acute attacks and obtain a more prolonged effect. It is believed that all the compounds in this class have a similar mechanism of action. It was once thought that both inorganic nitrites and organic nitrates act by releasing nitrite ions (NO_2^-) in the body. Subsequent studies, however, showed that organic nitrates such as nitroglycerin, have a greater potency than can be ac-

$$CH_2-O-NO_2$$
$$CH-O-NO_2$$
$$CH_2-O-NO_2 \qquad CH_3-CH(CH_3)-CH_2-CH_2-O-NO$$

Glyceryl trinitrate   Amyl nitrite

Figure 23-1 Formulas of glyceryl trinitrate and amyl nitrite

counted for by release of nitrite ions in the body. The concentration of nitrite ions found in the blood after administration of organic nitrates is small, and there is no correlation between the nitrite concentration and pharmacologic activity. It is therefore believed now that organic nitrates have a direct effect. However, their mechanism of action appears to be qualitatively identical to that of inorganic nitrites, and therefore the entire class of compounds is generally referred to as nitrites.

Mechanism of Action Nitrites relax smooth muscles, including vascular smooth muscle, and their pharmacologic activity as coronary vasodilators is believed to be related to this property.

Nitrites produce cardiovascular effects which may account for their beneficial effect in alleviating angina. Systemic arterial pressure, pulmonary artery pressure, venous pressure, cardiac output, and cardiac size all decrease after nitrites are administered. A decrease in systemic pressure reduces the load to the heart and thus favors an improved oxygen supply:demand ratio in the coronary circulation. Similarly, a decrease in cardiac size provides for a more efficient contraction, since the necessary wall tension to produce the same intraventricular pressure is reduced when the size of the ventricle is decreased. This again would be expected to reduce the oxygen demands of the myocardium. Therefore, current evidence suggests that a decrease in oxygen requirements of cardiac tissue is probably responsible for the efficacy of these drugs.

Effects on Organ Systems Nitrites have been shown to have a more or less general vasodilator effect. Their action is generally more prominent in the postcapillary vessels, which favors pooling of blood in the systemic peripheral circulation. Venous return is thus consistently decreased and becomes more dependent on positional changes. Nitrites produce relaxation of all vascular smooth

muscle, but the magnitude of their effect varies in different vascular beds. In the skin, nitrites produce vasodilatation often associated with "flushing" of the skin of the neck and face. This effect is more prominent with amyl nitrite than with the longer-acting compounds.

In the *cerebral* vessels, nitrites produce vasodilatation and an increase in intracerebral pressure. This, coupled with the decrease in systemic pressure, results in a decrease in blood flow through the brain, which may account for the headaches that are at times associated with nitrite therapy.

Retinal vessels dilate following nitrites; this can be directly observed through the ophthalmoscope. As may be expected, intraocular tension is also increased, but with the short-acting compounds, this effect is not considered to be significant in relation to the drainage of the anterior chamber. However, caution in the use of short-acting nitrites is recommended in glaucoma.

The nitrite effect on the heart observed in man is apparently secondary to the decrease in venous pressure and venous return, or occurs as a result of the action of cardiovascular reflexes. Thus the work of the heart, and hence its oxygen consumption, are reduced. Decrease in systemic arterial pressure also decreases cardiac work and oxygen consumption.

Absorption, Fate, and Excretion Most of the nitrites used therapeutically are absorbed through the mucous membranes, and many are absorbed through the skin. Gastrointestinal absorption, however, is variable. Amyl nitrite is rapidly absorbed from the lung as well as through mucous membranes. It is partially eliminated from the lungs and partially destroyed in the body. This compound is decomposed by gastric juice and is therefore inactive orally.

Glyceryl trinitrate is absorbed from mucous membranes, from the lungs, and through the skin. It is less effective following oral than sublingual administration. It is broken down in the body and excreted in the form of various nitrites and nitrates.

Although most other organic nitrates are administered orally, absorption through the mucous membranes has been demonstrated in most cases. Some of these (for example, isosorbide dinitrate and erythrityl tetranitrate) are also available for sublingual administration. Oral preparations of organic nitrates are absorbed slowly from the gastrointestinal tract. The effect of trolnitrate phosphate (triethanolamine trinitrate diphosphate) is particularly slow in onset, and may be present for a few days after administration is stopped. The exact fate of these compounds is not entirely known, although most appear to be broken down in the body and excreted in the form of various nitrites and nitrates.

Tolerance Repeated administration of nitrites leads to the development of tolerance manifested by the need for higher doses to produce the same effect. There is cross-tolerance between various compounds of this class. The mechanism of nitrite tolerance is unknown. In general, tolerance develops quickly, within 2 to 3 weeks, but also disappears quickly, so that lack of exposure to nitrites for 1 to 2 weeks reestablishes the original sensitivity. Tolerance to nitrite-induced headache appears to develop more quickly than other nitrite effects. Headache symptoms may disappear within a few days after onset of therapy.

Selected Preparations and Doses *Amyl nitrite* is available in fragile ampuls containing 0.2 to 0.3 ml. Ampuls are crushed in a handkerchief, and the released vapor is inhaled. Usual dose is 1 ampul.

Glyceryl trinitrate (nitroglycerin) is available as sublingual tablets of various strengths. Usual dose is 0.4 to 0.8 mg; prophylactically, before any activity known to precipitate attacks, 0.3 mg or sustained-release tablets, 0.9 to 2.5 mg, once every 12 h.

Erythrityl tetranitrate (erythrol tetranitrate, Cardilate) is available in tablets, 5 mg sublingual, 10 and 15 mg oral. Usual oral dose is 10 mg three times a day.

Isosorbide dinitrate (Isordil) is available in tablets for oral (10 mg) or sublingual (5 mg) use, and sustained-release tablets (40 mg). Usual dose sublingually, 5 mg initially, can be increased as indicated; orally, 5 to 10 mg four to five times a day; one sustained-release tablet every 12 h.

Mannitol hexanitrate is available in tablets, 10 mg, taken orally; usual dose, 10 mg three times a day.

Pentaerythritol tetranitrate (Peritrate) is avail-able in tablets, 10 and 20 mg, taken orally. Usual dose is 10 to 20 mg three to four times a day; sustained-release tablets, 80 mg once every 12 h.

Toxicity Certain undesirable effects of nitrites are related to their effects on the cardiovascular system. Throbbing headaches, flushing of the face, and dizziness are common, especially at the beginning of treatment. Headache is particularly common with some of the longer-acting compounds. Usually its severity decreases with continued use, but occasionally it may be so severe as to preclude further treatment. Postural hypotension is another common reaction which is apparently due to pooling of blood in the veins of the dependent parts of the body. The hypotensive effect of nitrates is potentially dangerous in patients with renal insufficiency, since it can aggravate renal ischemia. The use of nitrates is also contraindicated in acute myocardial infarction. Similarly, administration of nitrates in patients who also receive potent antihypertensive agents requires particular caution. Marked hypotension has also been reported in patients under nitrate treatment following ingestion of alcoholic beverages.

Gastrointestinal disturbances, including nausea and vomiting, are not uncommon following orally administered nitrates. The inorganic nitrites may lead to the development of methemoglobinemia. This is due to oxidation of hemoglobin by the nitrite ion. Amyl nitrite has a similar effect, but other organic nitrates are less effective.

Acute nitrite poisoning in man is manifested by flushing of the face, marked fall in blood pressure, vomiting, cyanosis, and collapse. Death may occur from circulatory collapse or from respiratory failure.

Other Antianginal Agents

A number of agents have been introduced at various times as antianginal drugs, among which are the following selected few:

Propranolol, a β-adrenergic blocking agent, is used prophylactically to decrease the severity of pain in angina pectoris. The efficacy of propranolol may reside in its ability to reduce the oxygen requirement of the myocardium by decreasing sympathetic stimulation of the heart, thus reducing cardiac rate and contractility. Propranolol may cause nausea, vomiting, visual disturbances, mental depression, and serious hypotension. It is particularly dangerous in cases of congestive heart failure, bronchial asthma, and recent myocardial infarction.

Other drugs used as antianginal agents include dipyridamole, papaverine, and the xanthines. However, their effectiveness in this condition appear questionable.

Propranolol (Inderal) is available in 10- and 40-mg tablets. The usual adult dosage is from 10 to 80 mg every 6 h.

Therapeutic Use: Treatment of Angina Pectoris

The most common coronary artery disease in which coronary vasodilators are used is angina pectoris. The short-acting nitrites are the most potent agents known for terminating an acute attack of angina. *Nitroglycerin* is the most commonly used agent. Pain is relieved within 1 to 3 min after sublingual administration of nitroglycerin. A similar effect can be produced with inhalation of *amyl nitrite,* but side effects are usually more prominent. Sublingual preparations of long-acting nitrates (isosorbide dinitrate, erythrityl tetranitrate) are also effective in relieving the pain of angina within 3 to 5 min, and their effect may last for 1 to 2 h. Orally administered nitrates require a longer period (up to 30 min) to produce an effect which may last for 2 to 4 h. In general, oral preparations of organic nitrates are used prophylactically to reduce the frequency of attacks of angina, especially prior to activities known to precipitate angina attacks in a patient (e.g., physical exertion or emotional stress). The value of such prophylactic use of nitrates apparently varies and has not been conclusively demonstrated.

Various other drugs have been used as adjuncts to the treatment of angina. These include various sedatives (e.g., barbiturates), alcohol, and various psychopharmacologic agents (e.g., antianxiety drugs).

In general, the use of various mild sedatives and tranquilizers is considered a valuable adjuvant therapy in the treatment of angina pectoris. Similarly, therapeutic management includes the exclusion of stimulants (e.g., tobacco), the physician reassurance, and avoidance of excessive emotional or physical stress. Moderate exercise, however, is considered by some to be an important part of long-term treatment.

ANTILIPEMIC AGENTS

The evidence for any causal relationship between hyperlipemia and atherosclerosis rests upon several points. First, there is the striking correlation between the lipid composition of the early plaque and of the blood plasma. As the lesion progresses, changes in plaque lipid composition occur; e.g., older lesions accumulate large amounts of sphingomyelin. The composition of the fatty acids of the various lipid components of these plaques is under active investigation in many laboratories. In cases where a regimen of special dietary fat was maintained for several years, the fatty-acid spectrum of the arterial lipids began to resemble that of the fat. Similarly, although a number of sterols other than cholesterol have been isolated from human aortas, it is most probable that all but cholesterol, which is a normal constituent of serum, are artifacts. The lipids of the serum circulate as components of lipoproteins, and both low-density and high-density lipoproteins have been isolated from human intima. Lipoproteins containing radioactive cholesterol have been shown to penetrate the wall of the aorta in vivo. Radioactive cholesterol administered to man has been demonstrated in the circulating lipoproteins and in the aorta.

The emphasis in experimental atherosclerosis and in human epidemiology was on cholesterol, but in recent years, it has been shown that hypertriglyceridemia may be an important causative and diagnostic factor. The triglycerides are a major component of the lower-density β-lipoproteins and of chylomicrons.

In contrast, several reports suggest that there is a direct correlation between the blood lipid concentration and the advancement of atherosclerosis. However, as indicated previously, it appears that reduction of serum lipid levels is beneficial to the patient. Dietary restriction is the first measure that should be employed to decrease elevated lipid levels. Drug intervention is indicated only when diet proves unsatisfactory.

Types of Hyperlipemias

The plasma phospholipids apparently are essential for maintaining the stability of the plasma lipoprotein, which is a complex colloidal system. Plasma becomes turbid and lipemic when the plasma lipid contains less than 30 percent phospholipid. For this reason, it was once fashionable to calculate cholesterol:phospholipid (C:P) ratios for serum in all work pertaining to atherosclerosis.

However, a new way of classifying hyperlipemias has been introduced, based on an improved method for the separation of lipoprotein species by paper electrophoresis. This method provides a relatively simple, routine means of screening serum. This new procedure allows separation of hyperlipemias into five distinct classes which are presented in Table 23-1.

Antilipemic Drugs

Antilipemic drugs are employed to reduce elevated levels of triglycerides or cholesterol in patients with hyperlipemias, particularly those individuals who have had myocardial infarcts. Therefore, an increase in longevity may be expected following the use of these agents. However, a recent study sponsored by the National Heart and Lung Institute suggests that clofibrate and nicotinic acid (niacin) neither prolong the life-span of persons who have had heart attacks nor reduce the chances of recurrent episodes. This report has raised some question as to the efficacy of the antilipemic drugs in heart disease.

At the present time these initial findings should not be interpreted as a condemnation of the antilipemic drugs. Future studies will have to be undertaken before full clarification of this point is resolved. The main reason for noting the above study is to inform the reader that controversy may develop concerning the therapeutic use of antilipemic drugs.

Clofibrate   Clofibrate (Atromid-S) has the following structure:

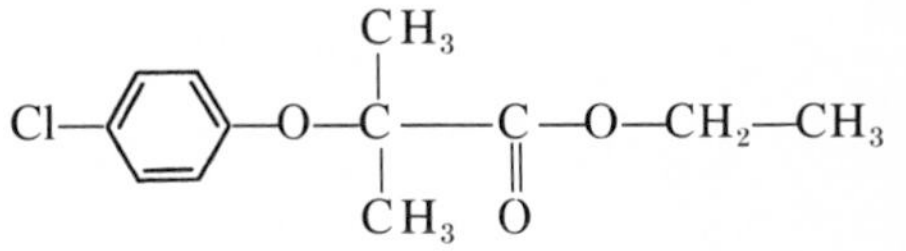

$$Cl-\underset{}{\bigcirc}-O-\underset{\underset{CH_3}{|}}{\overset{\overset{CH_3}{|}}{C}}-\underset{\underset{O}{||}}{C}-O-CH_2-CH_3$$

This agent is mainly effective in lowering triglyceride levels, primarily the triglyceride-rich lipoproteins [20 to $400S_f$ (svedberg flotation units)]. The exact mechanism of action of clofibrate is not understood at present.

Clofibrate, recently studied by a large number of clinical investigators, appears to be well tolerated and effective as an antilipemic agent. A 6-year clinical trial involving 600 patients demonstrated that only 6 percent of the group required termination of treatment due to adverse reactions. Along with dietary regulation, clofibrate is considered to be the drug of choice in type III hyperlipemia. Clofibrate also has been shown to be effective in hyperlipemias of types I, II, and IV.

Side effects associated with the use of clofibrate include nausea, vomiting, diarrhea, dermatitis, alopecia, leukopenia and muscle cramps. The drug is

Table 23-1   Classification of Hyperlipemias

Type and prevalence	Appearance of plasma	Cholesterol* elevation	Triglyceride* elevation
I Rarest	Creamy top	+	+++
II Relatively common	Clear or only slightly opalescent	+++	+
III Relatively uncommon	Moderately lactescent	++	+
IV Most common	Lactescent	+	++
V Uncommon	Creamy layer over milky infranatant	+	++

*+++, high; ++, moderate; +, low.

contraindicated during pregnancy, in nursing mothers, and in patients with impaired renal and liver function. Long-term use of the compound should be accompanied by careful monitoring of the patient. Clofibrate may also cause a transient rise in serum transaminases. Because of their competition for protein-binding sites, doses of oral anticoagulants should be reduced when clofibrate is administered concomitantly.

After termination of clofibrate therapy, cholesterol and other lipids may occasionally return to premedication levels in about 2 to 3 weeks.

Cholestyramine Resin Cholestyramine resin (Questran) is an anion exchange resin and as such is not absorbed from the gastrointestinal tract. Because of its reactive nature, cholestyramine resin binds bile acids in the intestine and enhances their rate of excretion from the body. As a result, cholesterol may be depleted, resulting in a lowering of serum cholesterol levels.

Cholestyramine appears to be a relatively safe drug. It is indicated only in type II hyperlipemia. Untoward effects associated with cholestyramine resin are nausea, vomiting, heartburn, dermatitis, and steatorrhea. The compound may reduce the absorption of the fat-soluble vitamins A, D, and K. Cholestyramine can also alter the absorption of such drugs as chlorothiazide, digitalis, thyroid, or warfarin when administered simultaneously. The usual dosage is 4 g three times a day.

Nicotinic Acid Nicotinic acid has been used successfully as an antilipemic agent by many investigators. Alteration of cholesterol biosynthesis has been suggested as a mechanism of action, but results are inconclusive. Nicotinic acid is also believed to interfere with the release of triglycerides from adipose tissue. Whatever the exact mechanism may be, the compound is effective in lowering both plasma cholesterol and triglyceride levels. It is recommended in types II, III, IV, and V of hyperlipemia.

Nicotinic acid is excreted as the glycine conjugate (nicotinuric acid). This conjugate can reduce cholesterol levels when administered in very large doses. However, the efficacy of nicotinuric acid is probably due to the fact that the compound is hydrolyzed in the body to nicotinic acid.

The major side effects associated with nicotinic acid therapy are itching and flushing. In 10 to 15 percent of patients, the flushing may persist for several weeks. Gastrointestinal upset, hyperpigmentation, abnormal liver function, decreased glucose tolerance, and elevated uric acid levels have been reported. Precaution should be exercised when nicotinic acid is used in patients with peptic ulcer, diabetes mellitus, and hypertension.

Dextrothyroxine It has been known for many years that hyperthyroidism is associated with hypocholesteremia. Although thyroid hormone enhances cholesterol biosynthesis, it has a greater effect on catabolism, and the end result is a reduction of serum cholesterol levels. Dextrothyroxine has substantially less calorigenic activity than the natural hormone L-thyroxine.

Dextrothyroxine has been recommended in hyperlipemia, types II and III. Its mechanism of action is to increase degradation of cholesterol and β-lipoproteins, resulting in a lowering of plasma cholesterol.

The side effects observed with dextrothyroxine therapy are generally related to increased metabolism. They include palpitations, loss of weight, nervousness, insomnia, excessive sweating, and diarrhea. As can be expected, this drug is contraindicated in patients with organic heart disease or cardiac arrhythmias and with advanced liver or kidney disease. In addition, dextrothyroxine may potentiate the effect of oral anticoagulants.

Other Antilipemic Agents Various agents which have been tried in the area of hyperlipemia are *estrogens, salicylates,* and *heparin.* It is generally acknowledged that premenopausal women are relatively immune to coronary disease. This observation has stimulated a search for "nonestrogenic estrogens," in the hope of finding a compound that will protect men from coronary disease without the accompanying feminizing effects of estrogens. However, to date, no such agent is available.

Salicylates, such as aspirin, in large doses (5 to 8 g/day) also lower cholesterol levels, but these dosages generally cause tinnitus, nausea, and vomiting. In light of these effects, the salicylates have been replaced by the previously discussed agents, such as clofibrate, cholestyramine and dextrothyroxine.

Heparin stimulates the release of lipoprotein lipase, an enzyme which catalyzes the hydrolysis of triglycerides, thus promoting the clearing of lipemic plasma. There is a fall in serum cholesterol and phospholipid levels because in hyperlipemics, a large fraction (up to 90 percent) of the serum cholesterol and phospholipid is associated with β-lipoproteins and chylomicrons. Moreover, there may be an increase in α-lipoproteins. Reductions in serum cholesterol levels of heparin-treated patients have been reported in some cases.

The disadvantages of heparin therapy include hemorrhage at the site of injection, lumbar pain, and various allergic reactions. The greatest disadvantage of heparin therapy is the requirement for biweekly subcutaneous injections. Sublingual heparin has been made available for clinical trial, but heparin appears to be inactive when taken in this form.

Chapter 24

Diuretics

Diuretics are drugs which increase urine flow by promoting a net loss of sodium ions and water from the body. This group of compounds (Table 24-1) can be divided into (1) agents which inhibit tubular reabsorption of sodium, thereby increasing solute excretion by the kidney, and (2) agents such as mannitol which are excreted in the glomerular filtrate to increase the osmolality within the tubular lumen.

RENAL PHYSIOLOGY

In the kidney the nephron unit can regulate reabsorption of electrolytes and water at several sites: the proximal tubule, loop of Henle, distal tubule, and collecting duct (Fig. 24-1). The glomerulus permits filtration of most of the essential constituents of the extracellular fluid and waste products. However, it prevents passage of plasma proteins, lipids, and substances bound to proteins.

Normally, the nephron unit reabsorbs 99 percent of the glomerular filtrate. In the first portion of the nephron, the proximal tubule, 60 to 70 percent of ions and water are reabsorbed. Sodium is actively transported from the lumen; chloride and water fol-

Table 24-1 Classification of Diuretic Drugs

I   Agents which increase renal solute excretion
   A   Agents which inhibit transport of Na^+
      1   Mercurials
      2   Thiazides
      3   Furosemide
      4   Ethacrynic Acid
   B   Potassium-sparing diuretics
      1   Spironolactone
      2   Triamterene
   C   Agents which depress H^+-for-Na^+ exchange
      1   Acetazolamide
   D   Osmotic nonelectrolytes
      1   Mannitol
II Agents which increase glomerular filtration rate
   A   Xanthines

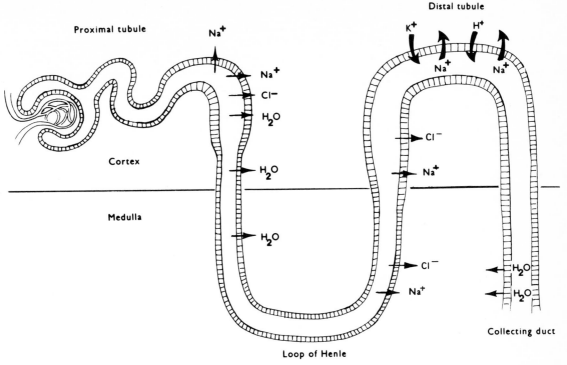

Figure 24-1 Nephron unit showing sites of electrolyte and water reabsorption.

low passively. The osmotic activity of the proximal fluid is similar to that of the interstitial fluid and plasma.

As the filtrate enters the descending limb of the loop of Henle, a concentrating mechanism operates. Water is removed and the tubular fluid becomes hypertonic as it approaches the curvature. In the ascending limb of the loop of Henle, the tubular fluid becomes diluted. This area is generally classified according to its medullary and cortical portions. In both of these segments of the ascending limb, chloride is actively transported from the lumen into the interstitium; sodium passively accompanies the chloride ion. However, water does not follow since the entire ascending limb is impermeable to it. The sodium entering the medullary interstitium maintains the hypertonicity of this tissue and is responsible for the free-water reabsorption from the collecting duct. Since sodium is removed and water remains in the lumen, the tubular fluid becomes hypotonic. For didactic purposes, the hypotonic fluid formed may be said to consist of two

hypothetical compartments: one isosmotic with plasma and the other free of solute, or so-called "free water."

In the cortical segment of the ascending limb, more sodium is transported from the lumen and further formation of free water occurs. This reabsorbed sodium from the cortical area, however, does not contribute to the hypertonicity of the interstitium. In toto, about 20 to 30 percent of filtered sodium is reabsorbed in the ascending limb of the loop of Henle.

The tubular fluid entering the distal convoluted segment is hypotonic. Filtered sodium is reabsorbed in this region and potassium is secreted. The latter mechanism is mediated by the mineralocorticoid, aldosterone. A hydrogen-sodium exchange mechanism operates here as well as in the proximal portion of the nephron unit. The tubule's permeability to water, particularly in the collecting duct, is controlled by antidiuretic hormone (ADH). The concentrations of ADH are highest in dehydration or water deprivation. As mentioned earlier, free water is reabsorbed in this area because of the hypertonicity of the medullary interstitium.

The hypertonicity of the medullary interstitium plays an important part in the hypothesis of the countercurrent multiplier mechanism. According to this theory, sodium is transported from the ascending limb of Henle's loop into the descending limb (Fig. 24-2). This establishes a small concentration gradient between the fluid contents of the ascending and descending limbs at successive levels along the course of the loop. Sodium concentration increases progressively down the descending limb because of countercurrent flow, and each unit of filtrate be-

comes more concentrated until it reaches the loop itself. This process establishes the medullary hypertonicity which provides the osmotic gradient necessary to abstract water from the lumen of the collecting duct in the final concentration of urine.

The high concentration of solute in the medulla is maintained by the vasa recta acting as a countercurrent exchanger. This process, which depends on the slow rate of medullary blood flow, maintains the $^{300}/_{1,200}$ mOsm/kg concentration differential between the cortex and the tip of the medulla. Only the water and sodium necessary to maintain the normal electrolyte concentrations of the body pass

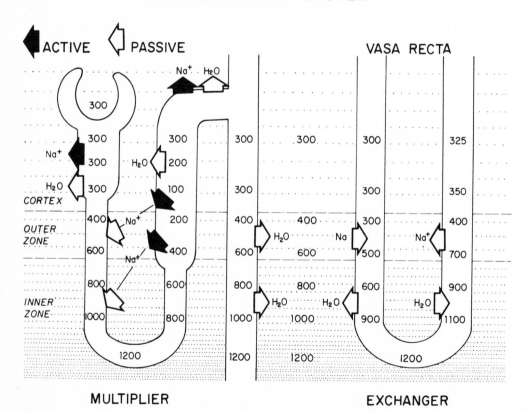

Figure 24-2 Diagram representing the countercurrent mechanism operating in the nephron and adjoining vasa recta. Extrusion of sodium by the ascending loop with subsequent diffusion into the descending limb produces a countercurrent multiplier system. Conversely, the descending and ascending loops of the vasa recta constitute the countercurrent exchange mechanism required to maintain the longitudinal concentration gradients established by the multiplier.

into the systemic circulation. The countercurrent exchange system thus prevents excessive loss of sodium from the medulla and papillae.

MERCURIAL DIURETICS

Table 24-2 lists the comparative effects of the various diuretic agents, which will be discussed individually.

The mercurial diuretics have been largely supplanted in therapy by ethacrynic acid and furosemide. However, limited use is still made of one of them and therefore their pharmacology is briefly included here.

Mechanism of Action The organomercurial diuretic, mercaptomerin, probably exerts its effect on sodium, chloride, potassium, and water by inhibiting the active reabsorption of chloride in the medullary and cortical portions of the ascending limb of the loop of Henle. The biochemical basis of this reduced sodium chloride reabsorption may be the ability of the bivalent mercury atom in this drug to bind with sulfhydryl groups present in enzymes responsible for chloride transport. This inhibition results in a decreased transport of sodium and chloride ions.

Absorption, Distribution, and Fate Mercaptomerin is usually administered by the intramuscular route. By combining the mercurial with thioglycolate, absorption from the site of injection is improved over the parent compound, thus reducing local irritation. Intravenous administration causes a higher incidence of acute systemic toxicity.

After absorption into the bloodstream, the mercurial diuretics are distributed throughout the body. The excretion rate is normally rapid, about 50 percent being eliminated in 4 to 6 h and 60 to 95 percent within 24 h. The major excretory product is a cysteine complex of the intact organomercurial molecule. Mercurial diuretics enter the intestinal tract with bile, but fecal excretion seldom exceeds 5 percent of a parenteral dose.

Therapeutic Uses Mercurial diuretics have been used principally in the treatment of edema due to congestive heart failure, the nephrotic syndrome, and in the management of Laennec's cirrhosis with ascites. Other states marked by accumulation of extracellular fluid may not materially benefit from diuretics.

Mercurial Refractoriness During treatment of congestive heart failure, the patient may not respond to mercurial diuretics and may remain edematous. Examination of plasma electrolyte patterns of such patients often reveals that chloride concentrations are low and bicarbonate and total CO_2 of the blood are high. If plasma-sodium concentrations are normal, such patients are said to be in a state of hypochloremic alkalosis. The self-limiting action of the mercurial diuretics may be overcome by acidifying salts, such as ammonium chloride.

Toxicity Organomercurial diuretics are potentially toxic and capable of producing the same cellular reactions as mercuric chloride. Organs most commonly affected in organomercurial poisoning

Table 24-2 A Comparison of Various Diuretic Groups: Urinary Excretion Patterns, Acid-Base Alterations, and Refractoriness

Drug	Urinary excretion*			Acid-base balance	Refractory
	Na+	Cl−	HCO3−		
Mercurial diuretics	+++	+++	0	Hypochloremic alkalosis	Yes
Acetazolamide	+	±`	+	Metabolic acidosis	Yes
Thiazides	++	++	±`	Hypochloremic alkalosis	No
Furosemide; ethacrynic acid	+++	+++	0	Hypochloremic alkalosis	No
Spironolactone; triamterene	+	+	0; +	None generally	No

* Substantial loss, +++; adequate loss, ++; fair loss, +; equivocal, ±; no effect, 0.

are the kidney, skin, liver, and the mucous membranes of the mouth and colon. Cardiac arrhythmias may be precipitated by I.V. injection.

Preparations and Dosage   Mercaptomerin (Thiomerin) is available in vials containing 125 mg/ml. The usual dosage is 25 to 250 mg daily.

THIAZIDE (BENZOTHIADIAZINE) DIURETICS

The thiazides are sulfonamide derivatives which were synthesized in the hope of developing a more potent carbonic anhydrase inhibitor than acetazolamide and therefore a more effective diuretic response. The first marketed drug was chlorothiazide which is capable of mobilizing edematous fluid without causing metabolic acidosis. This compound (1) promotes the renal excretion of sodium and chloride; (2) remains effective even in the presence of acidosis or alkalosis; (3) inhibits carbonic anhydrase in vitro; and (4) lowers arterial blood pressure in hypertensive patients. The structure of chlorothiazide as well as those of other thiazide diuretics are presented in Table 24-3.

Hydrochlorothiazide causes less inhibition of carbonic anhydrase, but produces 5 to 10 times more sodium diuresis than chlorothiazide. The hydrogenated ring of hydrochlorothiazide permits many possible substitutions, and the structure-activity relationships have been extensively studied in this series of compounds.

Mechanism of Action   The thiazides promote urinary excretion of water, sodium, chloride, potassium, and sometimes bicarbonate. Increased urinary loss of bicarbonate is due to inhibition of carbonic anhydrase and is primarily associated with the derivative chlorothiazide. The thiazide diuretics cause sodium excretion even in the presence of systemic alkalosis or acidosis, which is not true of mercurial diuretics.

The site of action of the thiazides is most likely the distal segment of the neprhon unit. They inhibit the reabsorption of sodium, chloride and water. The exact mechanism of action responsible for the inhibitory effect on sodium transport is not fully known. Since these diuretics do not greatly alter the hypertonicity of the interstitium, they do not decrease free-water reabsorption (see Fig. 24-1 and Renal Physiology, above). With an increased load of sodium reaching the distal convoluted tubule, the potassium-sodium exchange is enhanced, resulting in an increase in urinary potassium.

Absorption, Fate, and Metabolism   Chlorothiazide and its congeners are absorbed rapidly from the gastrointestinal tract. The thiazides appear in the bloodstream and remain in pharmacologic concentrations for several hours. They are excreted

Table 24-3   Structure and Therapeutic Dose of Various Thiazide Diuretics

Generic name	X	Y	R	Δ 3,4	Oral dose, mg/day
Chlorothiazide	Cl	H	H	Yes	500–1000
Hydroflumethiazide	CF_3	H	H	No	50–150
Hydrochlorothiazide	Cl	H	H	No	50–150
Trichlormethiazide	Cl	H	$-CHCl_2$	No	4–12
Bendroflumethiazide	CF_3	H	$-CH_2-\bigcirc$	No	5–15
Polythiazide	Cl	CH_3	$CH_2SCH_2CF_3$	No	2–4

primarily by the kidney and to a lesser extent by the liver. After intravenous injection, diuresis begins promptly but lasts only about 2 h. These drugs are therefore more suitable for oral rather than intravenous administration. Benzothiadiazines are excreted in the glomerular filtrate and by tubular secretion.

Therapeutic Uses In patients with edema, diuretic responses to the thiazides are observed within 2 to 3 h after oral administration. The duration of natriuretic action of a single dose of hydrochlorothiazide ranges between 24 and 36 h.

The thiazide diuretics are used most successfully in the day-to-day management of chronic congestive heart failure. However, the use of chlorothiazide and its congeners does not reduce the importance of other factors in the management of congestive heart failure such as bed rest and controlled salt and fluid intake. Digitalis therapy is usually continued in patients with cardiac failure who are receiving thiazide drugs. However, the dose of glycoside should be reduced to avoid digitalis intoxication in such cases, and supplemental potassium may also be necessary.

Chlorothiazide may cause a diuretic response in patients with nephrosis and other types of renal disease. In general, the efficiency of chlorothiazide is directly related to the remaining functional properties of the kidney. The therapeutic efficacy of thiazide diuretics is less than that of furosemide and ethacrynic acid. Surprisingly, the thiazides are also effective for palliative treatment of the polyuria of nephrogenic and neurohypophyseal diabetes insipidus. The mechanism by which diuretic agents exert this antidiuretic action is not completely known, but it is postulated that they indirectly decrease urinary volume by depleting body sodium, and thus may enhance the action of antidiuretic hormone (ADH).

Other conditions which may respond to thiazide therapy include edema and toxemia of pregnancy, premenstrual fluid retention, and the positive salt balance associated with glucocorticoid administration. These drugs are also effective in treating hypertension (see Chap. 25).

Toxicity Most toxic effects which develop during benzothiadiazine therapy are due to electrolyte abnormalities (hyponatremia and hypokalemia) or to a fall in arterial blood pressure. Lassitude, weakness, and vertigo occur with large doses of thiazides. Anorexia, heartburn, nausea, vomiting, cramps, diarrhea, and constipation have all been observed, but usually disappear when the dose is lowered and plasma-electrolyte abnormalities are corrected.

The most common toxic reaction to benzothiadiazine diuretics is a maculopapular skin rash. This occurs in about 1 percent of patients treated with chlorothiazide. Blood dyscrasias from chlorothiazide are rare.

Benzothiadiazine diuretics tend to precipitate digitalis intoxication in patients receiving any of the cardiac glycosides. The development of digitalis toxicity under these conditions is attributable to the enhanced excretion of potassium, which creates hypokalemia. Restoration of normal serum potassium levels usually eliminates the toxicity.

A gradual increase in blood uric acid level is commonly recorded during thiazide therapy. Acute attacks of thiazide-induced gout, however, are less common. This effect, which is caused by the thiazides as a class, is apparently due to an inhibition of renal tubular secretion of uric acid, but the possibility of increased tubular reabsorption of urate in the distal portion of the nephron has not been excluded. These drugs do not increase the rate of production of uric acid. They do cause a rise in blood glucose levels.

Preparations and Dosage *Chlorothiazide* (Diuril) is available in 250- and 500-mg tablets and in a suspension containing 250 mg/5 ml. Chlorothiazide is administered orally, the usual dose range varying between 0.5 and 2.0 g once or twice daily. Withdrawing the drug 1 or 2 days a week is recommended to avoid the occurrence of hypokalemia and hyponatremia. A lyophilized powder of chlorothiazide sodium is prepared in vials of 500 mg for intravenous injection or slow intravenous infusion.

Hydrochlorothiazide (Esidrix, HydroDiuril, Oretic) is supplied in 25- and 50-mg tablets. The usual dosage range is between 25 and 200 mg/day. Treatment should be interrupted 1 or 2 days a week to prevent the occurrence of plasma electrolyte abnormalities.

Metolazone

Metolazone (Zaroxolyn) is a relatively new diuretic agent. Chemically it resembles the thiazides in that metolazone is a sulfonamide derivative. The mechanism of action for this drug is probably similar to that of the thiazides.

Following oral administration, the onset of diuresis occurs in about 1 h and lasts from 12 to 24 h. The ability of metolazone to remove edematous fluids is equivalent to that of the thiazide diuretics but less than that of furosemide.

Metolazone is useful in the management of edema associated with liver, kidney, or heart disease and in the treatment of mild hypertension.

Side effects encountered with metolazone are similar to those of the thiazides and include hypokalemia, hyperglycemia, and hyperuricemia. Since the drug has recently been introduced and the number of patients treated with it relatively small, it is difficult to ascertain the full extent and severity of its adverse effects at present.

FUROSEMIDE AND ETHACRYNIC ACID

Furosemide and ethacrynic acid are the most potent diuretics available for the removal of edematous fluid. These agents are virtually identical in their pharmacologic actions.

Furosemide

Furosemide is a monosulfamoylanthranilic acid derivative which has greater diuretic efficacy than chlorothiazide when used at maximal therapeutic doses. Furosemide differs from most thiazide diuretics in producing a greater increase in renal chloride excretion. Despite a short duration of action, furosemide, administered once or twice daily, is capable of maintaining congestive heart failure patients in a satisfactory state of electrolyte and water balance over long periods of time.

Furosemide

Renal chloride and potassium excretion following the administration of furosemide is greater than that of sodium, and urinary pH falls. The diuretic response to furosemide is accompanied by an increase in urinary titratable acid and ammonium excretion.

Mechanism of Action Furosemide causes its potent diuretic response by inhibiting the active reabsorption of chloride in the medullary portion of the ascending limb of the loop of Henle and possibly by acting at the cortical portion. Because the chloride ion transport is decreased in the presence of furosemide, the sodium, which normally accompanies the reabsorption of chloride, is also diminished. This effect results in reduced hypertonicity of the medullary interstitium. Also, free-water absorption is reduced in the collecting duct. Along with the increased urinary sodium and chloride excretion, there is an increase in the excretion of potassium. Furosemide can produce alkalosis but refractoriness does not develop.

Ethacrynic Acid

The structure of ethacrynic acid is somewhat different from furosemide, particularly in the lack of a sulfamyl group. Administered orally or intrave-

Ethacrynic acid

nously, ethacrynic acid produces a prompt increase in renal sodium and chloride excretion and urine volume. Chloride excretion is greater than sodium excretion, and in the early phases of therapy the concentration of chloride in the urine approximates that of sodium plus potassium. Urinary titratable acidity increases after ethacrynic acid and ammonium concentration and pH fall. Loss of potassium, hydrogen, and chloride ions may lead to hypokalemic or hypochloremic alkalosis. Larger doses increase uric acid excretion, whereas lower doses cause uric acid retention.

Mechanism of Action The manner in which ethacrynic acid causes diuresis is probably similar to that of furosemide. It inhibits active reabsorption of chloride in the medullary and cortical portions of the ascending limb of the loop of Henle. Since sodium follows the chloride ion in this region, its reabsorption is also decreased.

Absorption, Fate, and Excretion Ethacrynic acid is rapidly absorbed from the gastrointestinal tract and produces a diuretic response within 2 h when given orally. After intravenous injection, plasma activity decreases rapidly for 20 min and then levels off at a rate corresponding to a half-life of 30 to 70 min. About 30 percent of an intravenous dose is excreted in the urine and 40 percent in the bile. Ethacrynic acid is secreted by the acid transport system of the proximal tubular cell. It is excreted in a conjugated form with cysteine in both urine and bile.

Therapeutic Uses of Furosemide and Ethacrynic Acid

In the treatment of fluid retention, furosemide and ethacrynic acid are recommended because of their high therapeutic efficacy. Maximum therapeutic doses produce a greater diuretic response than do the thiazide diuretics. Furosemide and ethacrynic acid are useful in treating edema associated with congestive heart failure, Laennec's cirrhosis, nephrotic syndrome, and chronic renal failure. These drugs are frequently employed in patients who do not respond to thiazides or organomercurials. Furthermore, both of these diuretics are used as adjuncts in the treatment of hypertensive crises, particularly when the hypertension is associated with acute pulmonary edema or renal failure.

Toxicities of Furosemide and Ethacrynic Acid

Adverse reactions to furosemide and ethacrynic acid usually are related to excessive fluid and electrolyte loss. Hypokalemia, prehepatic coma, hypotension, hyperuricemia, blood dyscrasias, and shock have been reported. Side effects include thirst, urinary frequency, nocturia, transient muscle cramps, and mental confusion. Other adverse reactions are transient hearing loss and gastrointestinal disturbances such as anorexia, nausea, vomiting, abdominal pains, and diarrhea.

Preparations and Dosage

Furosemide (Lasix) is supplied in 20- and 40-mg tablets. The usual dose of furosemide is 40 to 80 mg orally as a single daily dose. The total daily dose may be increased to 200 mg, administered as a single dose or in two divided doses. Furosemide is available in 2- and 10-ml ampuls, each ml containing 10 mg. The intramuscular or intravenous dose is 20 to 40 mg.

Ethacrynic acid (Edecrin) is supplied in 25- and 50-mg tablets. The usual oral dosage is 50 to 100 mg once or twice daily. Occasionally a daily dosage of up to 200 mg may be required. Sodium ethacrynate is available in vials containing 50 mg/ml to be injected intravenously. The usual dose is 50 to 100 mg.

POTASSIUM-SPARING DIURETICS

Spironolactone

Spironolactone is an aldosterone antagonist which interferes with the action of the hormone at the target organ and is most effective when circulating aldosterone levels are high. The primary action of spironolactone is on the distal segments of the nephron where sodium is exchanged for potassium and hydrogen ions.

Spironolactone

Mechanism of Action Spironolactone is believed to exert its diuretic effect by interfering with the aldosterone-mediated sodium-potassium exchange, thereby increasing sodium loss at the distal tubular site. Spironolactone presumably acts by competitive inhibition, displacing aldosterone from the receptor sites responsible for sodium reabsorption.

Therapeutic Use Spironolactone increases renal sodium excretion when prescribed alone or in combination with chlorothiazide. It is used primarily to treat those cases of Laennec's cirrhosis with ascites which are refractory to other therapy.

Spironolactone diminishes the kaliuresis induced by benzothiadiazine diuretics. It is therefore a useful adjunct in the management of patients with intractable edema in whom hypokalemia is a frequent complication. Most patients with chronic congestive heart failure, however, are satisfactorily maintained with the proper use of thiazides, furosemide, or ethacrynic acid.

Toxicity Spironolactone is contraindicated in the presence of hyperkalemia, since it may cause further elevation of plasma potassium concentrations. Potassium supplements should not be continued during spironolactone therapy.

Lethargy, drowsiness, ataxia, headache, and mental confusion have been observed during spironolactone therapy, and a few patients have developed a transient maculopapular or erythematous rash while receiving the drug. These eruptions usually disappear within 48 h after discontinuing the drug. Diarrhea and other gastrointestinal disturbances may occur during spironolactone therapy. Androgenic side effects of the drug include hirsutism, irregular menses, deepening of the voice.

Triamterene

Triamterene is a pyrazine derivative which inhibits sodium reabsorption and promotes potassium reabsorption in the distal tubule. Such a potassium-sparing diuretic causes a moderate increase in sodium and bicarbonate excretions in the urine and decreased urinary potassium and ammonia. It has little effect on urine volume, but when combined with thiazides or ethacrynic acid it enhances the diuretic response without increasing the output of potassium in the urine.

Triamterene

Its principal effect appears to be on the distal tubule where it inhibits sodium reabsorption and potassium secretion. Although the drug behaves like an aldosterone antagonist, it increases sodium excretion in adrenalectomized animals and in patients in whom aldosterone secretion is inhibited by the administration of sodium and chloride.

Therapeutic Use and Toxicity Triamterene causes a moderate increase in sodium and bicarbonate excretion and a decrease in urinary potassium and ammonia. It is a weak diuretic when used alone, but when combined with the thiazides, the combination is more effective than either drug alone. When used with hydrochlorothiazide in treating hypertension, triamterene produces a positive potassium balance and a rise in plasma potassium concentrations.

Triamterene either alone or with benzothiadiazide diuretics may cause hyperkalemia, electrocardiographic changes, and death. Triamterene has also been reported to decrease glomerular filtration rate and increase blood urea concentrations.

Preparations and Dosage

Spironolactone (Aldactone) is supplied in 25-mg tablets. An initial schedule of 25 mg two to four times daily is recommended.

Triamterene (Dyrenium) is available in 100-mg capsules. The recommended initial dosage is 100 mg twice daily.

ACETAZOLAMIDE

A variety of aromatic sulfonamides with a free sulfamyl group ($-SO_2-NH_2$) are specific inhibitors of carbonic anhydrase. An example of such a compound is acetazolamide which increases renal sodium and bicarbonate excretion and was the first carbonic anhydrase inhibitor to have clinical value as a diuretic. The drug produces an alkaline urine with increased concentrations of sodium, potassium, and bicarbonate ions, thus demonstrating the reciprocal relationship between hydrogen and potassium-ion excretion and sodium reabsorption in the renal tubules.

Mechanism of Action The diuretic action of acetazolamide is due to inhibition of carbonic anhydrase in the renal tubule. Following administration of acetazolamide, reabsorption of sodium ions in exchange for hydrogen ions is depressed throughout the nephron; sodium bicarbonate excretion increases and chloride output falls. Bicarbonate excretion is increased because the carbonic anhydrase inhibitory effect of the drug also suppresses the reabsorption of CO_2 from the glomerular filtrate. Chloride ions are retained by the kidney to offset the loss of bicarbonate and maintain ionic balance. Because of decreased availability of hydrogen ions in the distal tubule, potassium is excreted in exchange for sodium, and urinary potassium output increases.

The renal electrolyte excretion pattern of patients receiving a carbonic anhydrase inhibitor is characterized by increased amounts of sodium, potassium, and bicarbonate, with only moderate increases in water output. The urine becomes alkaline and the plasma bicarbonate concentration decreases. If therapy is continued, the patient develops a metabolic acidosis. Plasma chloride levels increase. Urinary ammonia concentrations drop when hydrogen ions present in the tubule are insufficient to convert ammonia to NH_4^+.

Absorption and Excretion Acetazolamide is absorbed rapidly from the gastrointestinal tract: peak plasma levels are reached within 2 h after oral administration. Acetazolamide is excreted unchanged in the urine, about 80 percent of a single oral dose appearing in the urine within 8 to 12 h.

Therapeutic Uses Acetazolamide is a weak diuretic with limited use since the introduction of the thiazides. However, there are four indications for carbonic anhydrase inhibitors: (1) in edema, to promote a diuretic response; (2) in glaucoma; (3) in petit mal epilepsy; and (4) in premenstrual tention.

Toxicity Acetazolamide produces reversible side effects which include flushing, headache, drowsiness, dizziness, fatigue, irritability, and excitability. Instances of polydipsia and polyuria, paresthesias, ataxia, hyperpnea, anorexia, vomiting, and gastrointestinal distress have been reported during therapy with carbonic anhydrase inhibitors. Such manifestations disappear when dosage is reduced.

Like antibacterial sulfonamides, acetazolamide may cause fever and blood dyscrasias such as leukopenia, agranulocytosis, thrombocytopenia, and aplastic anemia. Allergic skin reactions, including exfoliative dermatitis, may develop during acetazolamide administration. Genitourinary complications of acetazolamide therapy include crystalluria, calculus formation (chiefly calcium phosphate and citrate) with renal colic, and secondary renal lesions.

Preparations and Dosage *Acetazolamide* (Diamox) is available in 125- and 250-mg tablets, and 500-mg sustained-release capsules. The usual oral dosage is 250 mg two to four times daily. Sodium acetazolamide is supplied in 500-mg vials. The usual intravenous or intramuscular dosage range is 0.5 to 1.0 g daily.

OSMOTIC NONELECTROLYTES

Today the most clinically used member of this category is mannitol. In the presence of normal cardiorenal function, mannitol causes a solute or osmotic diuresis. This agent is not metabolized or reabsorbed by the tubular cells; it is excreted by the glomeruli and, being osmotically active, retains water in the tubular fluid to increase urine volume.

Therapeutic Uses Mannitol is primarily used as an adjunct in the prevention or treatment of oliguria and anuria. It may also be employed to reduce intraocular pressure pre- and postoperatively in ophthalmic procedures.

Toxicity Mannitol does not penetrate the cells, and its only method of excretion is via the glomerular filtrate. Intravenous infusions of mannitol, therefore, increase blood volume. Expansion of blood volume in patients with congestive heart failure may cause further decompensation. When given to patients with renal failure, mannitol produces vascular overfilling with hyperosmolality and hyponatremia. Clinically, there is a picture of tissue dehydration accompanied by signs of congestive heart failure. Hyperosmolality has been reported after mannitol infusions in patient with cirrhosis and ascites. Peritoneal dialysis may correct the overhydration produced by mannitol infusions, but deaths due to vascular overfilling, hyperosmolality, and hyponatremia have also been reported.

Preparation and Dosage *Mannitol* is a polyhydric alcohol which must be infused intravenously to produce a diuretic response. The usual dosage is 25 to 100 g/day, prepared in a 10 percent aqueous solution.

XANTHINE DIURETICS

The naturally occurring xanthines have mild diuretic properties. Of the various xanthines available for diuretic therapy, theophylline is preferred, since caffeine and theobromine cause restlessness and insomnia. Aminophylline (theophylline ethylenediamine) may promote diuresis when other therapeutic measures fail. It is also capable of increasing the natriuretic response to other diuretics.

Mechanism of Action Theophylline and aminophylline increase cardiac output. Their diuretic action has been attributed to an increase in renal plasma flow and a higher glomerular filtration rate. There also is evidence that aminophylline inhibits sodium reabsorption from the glomerular filtrate in the renal tubules.

Therapeutic Uses Aminophylline may be used either alone or in combination with other classes of diuretic drugs to achieve a negative water and sodium balance in patients with congestive heart failure. The intravenous administration of aminophylline 90 to 120 min after injecting an organomercurial increases renal plasma flow, glomerular filtration rate, and the filtered load of electrolytes. In the presence of the organomercurial, aminophylline augments the diuretic response. Blood theophylline levels of 0.5 mg/100 ml are required to increase urine flow.

Toxicity Toxic effects of aminophylline include signs of central nervous system stimulation such as dizziness, restlessness, headache, increased reflex excitability, and clonic and tonic convulsions.

Patients with aminophylline toxicity develop severe, persistent vomiting with dehydration, fever, and hematemesis. Cardiovascular side effects consist of palpitation, flushing, hypotension, and circulatory collapse. Aminophylline should be infused slowly when given parenterally because fatal cardiovascular reactions may occur suddenly after intravenous injection.

Preparation and Dosage *Aminophylline* is supplied in ampuls containing 0.25 and 0.5 g for intravenous injection. The usual dosage is 500 mg one to three times daily. Aminophylline is a mixture of theophylline (75 to 82 percent) and ethylenediamine (12.3 to 13.8 percent). The drug must be slowly infused intravenously, since sudden deaths have occurred during acute intravenous injections.

Chapter 25

Antihypertensive Drugs

CLASSIFICATION OF HYPERTENSION

It should be noted that hypertension with sustained diastolic pressures above 115 mmHg is considered severe, since such pressures herald morbid events that will occur in 40 percent of hypertensive patients within 20 months. Patients with diastolic pressures below 105 mmHg appear to be in the mildest category. Patients with diastolic pressures above 130 mmHg or with evidence of necrotizing vasculitis on funduscopic examination constitute medical emergencies. Classification of hypertension on the basis of severity is presented in Table 25-1.

PRINCIPLES OF DRUG THERAPY

A main principle of antihypertensive therapy is that patients may require multiple drugs attacking the three major sites of increased peripheral vascular resistance: the central vasomotor sympathetic cen-

ter; the peripheral sympathetic nervous system; and the arteriolar smooth muscle directly. Three classes of drugs are used—depending on the severity of hypertension (Table 25-1)—which are introduced in a specific sequence. All patients are started on an oral antihypertensive diuretic as the first line of therapy. Although the mechanism by which diuretics lower blood pressure is not clear, they are the most useful antihypertensive drugs. Generally well tolerated, these drugs enhance all other antihypertensive therapy. The second group of drugs is the adrenergic blocking agents, given either after a diuretic has been started or concurrently with it. Finally, after adrenergic blockade has been established, peripheral vasodilators may be added. Peripheral vasodilators are started only after adrenergic blockers because the former drugs cause two troublesome side effects—increased cardiac output and tachycardia—which occur when blood pressure falls in response to peripheral vasodilatation in the presence of an intact sympathetic nervous system.

255

Table 25-1   Classification of Diastolic Hypertension by Degree of Severity

Degree	Diastolic pressure (mmHg)	Outlook
Severe	130 or above; grade III or IV retinopathy	Medical emergency
Moderately severe	115–129	40 percent of the patients can be expected to have morbid events within 20 months
Moderate	105–114	One-half of the patients may have morbid events within 5 years
Mild	90–104	Excessive cardiovascular disease over long term

ORAL ANTIHYPERTENSIVE DIURETICS

The various diuretics and usual doses employed in patients with hypertension are listed in Table 25-2. As a rule, patients are started on a diuretic from the thiazide or thiazide-like group. The three main side effects associated with this group are hyperuricemia and attacks of gouty arthritis; worsening of diabetes mellitus; and electrolyte abnormalities characterized by hypokalemia, metabolic alkalosis, and hypochloremia.

Spironolactone is a competitive inhibitor of aldosterone but does not have side effects such as potassium wasting, hyperuricemia, or deterioration of glucose tolerance. Spironolactone is utilized as a first-line diuretic for patients with gout or diabetes mellitus or for those who have shown hypokalemic responses to the thiazide group of diuretics.

Furosemide and ethacrynic acid, although more potent diuretics, have not demonstrated a more potent antihypertensive action than the standard thiazide-like group. Furosemide and ethacrynic acid are used for those patients who show evidence of hypervolemia and decreased glomerular filtration rates, manifested in elevated serum creatinine or BUN concentration. Occasionally a patient with renal insufficiency, on a thiazide diuretic, will exhibit deterioration of renal function and a rising BUN; this has not been noted with furosemide or ethacrynic acid.

Table 25-2   Oral Antihypertensive Diuretics

Classification and generic name	Trade name	Daily dosage (mg)
Thiazides		
Chlorothiazide	Diuril	500–1000
Hydrochlorothiazide	HydroDiuril	50–100
	Esidrix	
	Oretic	
Benzthiazide	ExNa	50–100
Hydroflumethiazide	Saluron	50–100
Bendroflumethiazide	Naturetin	5–10
Methyclothiazide	Enduron	5–10
Trichlormethiazide	Naqua	2–4
	Metahydrin	2–4
Polythiazide	Renese	2–4
Cyclothiazide	Anhydron	1–2
Phthalimidine		
Chlorthalidone	Hygroton	50–100
Quinazolines		
Quinethazone	Hydromox	50–100
Metolazone	Zaroxolyn	2.5–5
Aldosterone antagonist		
Spironolactone	Aldactone	75–400
Organic acids		
Furosemide	Lasix	80–160
Ethacrynic acid	Edecrin	50–100

ADRENERGIC BLOCKING DRUGS

Reserpine is a commonly used adrenergic blocking agent in antihypertensive therapy. Its principal advantages are that it is effective in patients in either the supine or the erect position and that side effects are generally mild. Its antihypertensive effect is also mild. The most common side effect of reserpine is psychic depression, occasionally progressing to severe disturbances including nightmares and severe depressive reactions. It also causes some nasal stuffiness and some increased gastric acid secretion.

Another commonly used adrenergic blocking

agent is methydopa. It has a substantial orthostatic effect. The main side effects include sleepiness and tiredness, which usually last only through the first 2 weeks of use. In addition, it has been associated with Coombs-positive red cells and, rarely, Coombs-positive hemolytic anemia.

The adrenergic blocking agent guanethidine is a long-acting drug. Its antihypertensive action is almost exclusively orthostatic, with very little effect on blood pressure when the patient is supine. Its most distressing side effect is orthostatic hypotension; severe orthostatic symptoms require reduction in drug dosage. Impotence in men is a substantial problem with guanethidine. Occasional mild diarrhea occurs, but this is rarely a contraindication to administration. Dual adrenergic blockade is sometimes used, with guanethidine added to high-dose methyldopa therapy.

Propranolol and clonidine are two other adrenergic blockers which are available as antihypertensive drugs. The beta-adrenergic blocking agent propranolol has certain advantages: (1) no central nervous system depression and (2) few complaints of sleepiness. Therefore, it has proved useful in patients who must maintain a high degree of mental alertness in their work. Given alone, propranolol is only modestly antihypertensive and is almost always used in conjunction with a diuretic and a vasodilator such as hydralazine. It causes substantial bradycardia and a decrease in cardiac output. Propranolol is contraindicated in patients with bronchial asthma or heart block, or in those pa-

tients in whom the risk of congestive heart failure is great. Several reports have shown it to be more effective in patients with elevated plasma renin levels.

Clonidine sulfate is a potent adrenergic blocking agent, acting predominantly on the central sympathetic vasomotor centers. It is effective in microgram (μg) doses, and its main side effects are sleepiness, dryness of mouth, and orthostatic hypotension.

Although the MAOI pargyline has substantial potency and the advantage of no soporific side effects, it has proved difficult to use in clinical practice because of two major problems: (1) a considerable orthostatic effect and (2) an extremely long duration of action. This leads to cumulative drug effect and, occasionally, severe orthostatic effects, even though the dosage is not increased. Because it is a potent MAOI, patients must be warned against ingestion of cheese, wines, and beers which may contain tyramine and cause severe paradoxic hypertensive responses. Available adrenergic blocking drugs, their doses, and mechanisms of action are listed in Table 25-3.

PERIPHERAL VASODILATORS

Hydralazine (Table 25-4) is a short-acting drug with direct smooth-muscle vasodilatating effects. The side effects of hydralazine are tachycardia, increased cardiac output, palpitations, and headache. All of these can be prevented if the patient under-

Table 25-3 Adrenergic Blocking Drugs

Generic name	Trade name	Dosage range (mg/day)	Mechanism
Reserpine	Serpasil	0.25–0.50	Depletes peripheral catecholamines; suppresses CNS sympathetic activity
	Sandril	0.25–0.50	
	Reserpoid	0.25–0.50	
Whole root	Raudixin	100–300	
Alseroxylon fraction	Rauwiloid	2–4	
Methyldopa	Aldomet	250–2000	False transmitter accumulates at sympathetic nerve endings; suppresses CNS activity; inhibits catecholamine synthesis
Guanethidine	Ismelin	10–200	Depletes peripheral catecholamines
Propranolol	Inderal	160–320	Uncertain
Clonidine	Catapres	0.1–2.0	Suppresses CNS sympathetic activity
Pargyline	Eutonyl	10–200	Uncertain; MAOI

Table 25-4 Peripheral Vasodilators

Drug	Daily dose range (mg)	Side effects
Hydralazine	40–300	Tachycardia; increased cardiac output; palpitations; headache
Prazosin	5–20	Headache; palpitations
Guancydine	500–1500	Headache; palpitations
Minoxidil	5–70	Hirsutism; arrhythmias

Table 25-5 Hypertensive Emergencies and Preferred Treatment

Situation	Drugs of choice
Dissecting aneurysm of the aorta	Trimethaphan Reserpine Methyldopa Propranolol
Pheochromocytoma	Phentolamine Phenoxybenzamine
Hypertension with hypovolemia	Volume expander
Hypertensive encephalopathy	Diazoxide Trimethaphan Sodium nitroprusside
Accelerated hypertension with acute left ventricular failure	Diazoxide Trimethaphan Furosemide
Accelerated hypertension with intracranial hemorrhage	Diazoxide Trimethaphan Sodium nitroprusside
Severe hypertension with acute and chronic renal disease	Diazoxide Methyldopa Hydralazine Furosemide
Severe hypertension in pregnancy	Diazoxide Hydralazine Methyldopa Reserpine

goes prior or simultaneous adrenergic blockade. Long-term administration may produce an arthritis-like syndrome leading to a clinical picture simulating acute systemic lupus erythematosus. A single dose of hydralazine may precipitate angina pectoris or a myocardial infarction.

Peripheral vasodilators under investigation include prazosin, guancydine and minoxidil. Prazosin is a vasodilator with intrinsic adrenergic blocking activity; therefore, the concomitant use of a primary adrenergic blocking drug is not required. Guancydine appears to be an effective peripheral vasodilator, more potent than hydralazine. It has been used in patients with severe and refractory hypertension, those undergoing renal dialysis, and those in transplantation programs. Its chief side effect is hirsutism. Some cardiac arrhythmias have also been reported.

HYPERTENSIVE EMERGENCIES

The patient with hypertensive emergencies requires constant monitoring of blood pressure in an intensive-care setting or its equivalent. The availability of diazoxide and nitroprusside has considerably enhanced our ability to deal with hypertensive emergencies. Diazoxide is a nondiuretic thiazide which reduces blood pressure by selective precapillary vasodilatation. Its use may lead to reflex adrenergic discharge, resulting in tachycardia and increased cardiac output. Hyperglycemia is a frequent adverse reaction encountered with diazoxide. The antihypertensive effects of nitroprusside are due to peripheral vasodilatation as a result of direct action on the smooth muscle of blood vessels. This action is independent of autonomic innervation and is probably due to the nitroso (NO) group. Tables 25-5 and 25-6 are lists of hypertensive emergencies and preferred treatments.

Table 25-6 Drugs for Hypertensive Emergencies

Drug	Dose and method of administration	Onset
Trimethaphan	1000 mg/ml in intravenous infusion; titrate	Instantaneous
Sodium nitroprusside	50–100 mg/l intravenous infusion; titrate	Instantaneous
Diazoxide	300–600 mg as rapid intravenous push	Instantaneous
Hydralazine	10–60 mg intramuscularly	30 min
	20–40 mg/20 ml intermittently intravenously	10 min
	50–100 mg/l intravenous infusion	10 min
Methyldopa	250–500 mg/100 ml intravenous infusion	3 h
Reserpine	2.5–10 mg intramuscularly	3 h
Phentolamine*	5–30 mg intravenously	Instantaneous

* Specific for pheochromocytoma.

Part Six

The Hematopoietic System

Chapter 26

Antianemia Agents

DRUGS EFFECTIVE IN PERNICIOUS ANEMIA AND OTHER MEGALOBLASTIC ANEMIAS

Pernicious anemia and other megaloblastic anemias are macrocytic anemias associated with the presence of abnormal erythrocyte precursors, megaloblasts, in the bone marrow. The most common causes of megaloblastic anemias are deficiencies of vitamin B_{12} and folic acid. In these cases repletion of the lacking vitamin corrects the anemia and restores bone marrow morphology to normal. Occasionally megaloblastic anemia has other causes, for example, antimetabolite therapy, such as 6-mercaptopurine and 5-fluorouracil, hereditary orotic aciduria or refractory anemia. In these cases vitamin therapy is ineffective.

Current evidence suggests that the megaloblast is a cell in a state of "unbalanced growth" due to impaired synthesis of one or more deoxyribonucleotides, the precursors of DNA. Hence, the RNA:DNA ratio rises, since the replication of DNA and cell division are blocked, while the synthesis of cytoplasmic components proceeds normally. The roles of vitamin B_{12} and folic acid in deoxyribonucleotide synthesis will be discussed later.

Vitamin B_{12}

Foods in the human diet that contain vitamin B_{12} are essentially those of animal origin—liver, seafood, meat, eggs, and milk. Though the chemical structure of vitamin B_{12} relates it to a group known as *corrinoid* compounds, the term *cobalamin* (introduced before the structure was known) is frequently used to refer to the vitamin B_{12} molecule minus the cyano group (see Fig. 26-1). Vitamin B_{12} itself then becomes cyanocobalamin. Cobalamin, in either the cyano or hydroxy form, is readily converted to deoxyadenosylcobalamin in tissues by a "coenzyme synthetase" system. In this reaction, the deoxyadenosyl moiety of ATP is transferred intact to the vitamin to form the coenzyme.

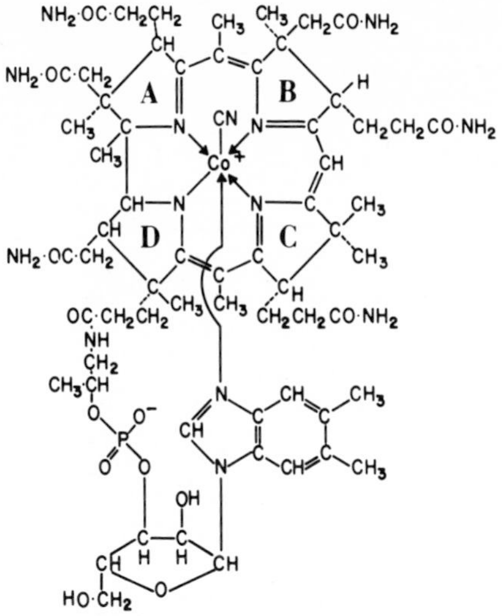

Figure 26-1 Chemical structure of vitamin B_{12}.

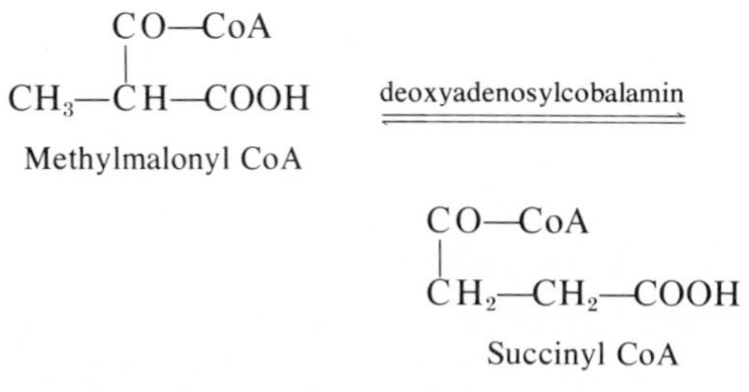

Propionic acid metabolism, resulting from fatty acid oxidation, in animal tissue involves the biotin-dependent carboxylation of propionyl CoA to methylmalonyl CoA. After a racemization step, methylmalonyl CoA mutase catalyzes the reversible conversion of methylmalonyl CoA to succinyl CoA, which can then enter the tricarboxylic acid cycle after conversion to succinate. Nondividing nerve cells are not engaged in DNA synthesis, but they do synthesize myelin and other lipids. Vitamin B_{12}-deficient humans excrete abnormal quantities of methylmalonate and acetate. Preliminary data suggest that the presence and severity of neurologic symptoms correlate with the degree of acetic aciduria, but not of methylmalonic aciduria. These results, as well as evidence from recent isotopic studies of propionate metabolism in human vitamin B_{12} deficiency, are compatible with the view that distorted lipid metabolism may be responsible for neurologic damage.

Metabolic Functions It appears that the three most significant biochemical systems impaired in human vitamin B_{12} deficiency are (1) deoxyribosyl and thus DNA synthesis; (2) methylmalonyl CoA and thus propionate catabolism; and (3) methionine methyl synthesis and thus N^5-methyltetrafolate demethylation. Impairment of the first accounts for megaloblastic erythropoiesis and related phenomena. The ribonucleoside triphosphate reductase reaction, in which ribonucleotides are converted to deoxyribonucleotides is dependent upon a vitamin B_{12} cofactor, deoxyadenosylcobalamin.

It is conceivable that impairment of methylmalonyl CoA conversion accounts for the neurologic damage of human vitamin B_{12} deficiency. The cobamide-dependent isomerization of methylmalonyl CoA is a step in the catabolism of propionic acid.

$$\begin{array}{c} CO\!-\!CoA \\ | \\ CH_3\!-\!CH\!-\!COOH \end{array} \quad \xrightarrow{\text{deoxyadenosylcobalamin}}$$

Methylmalonyl CoA

$$\begin{array}{c} CO\!-\!CoA \\ | \\ CH_2\!-\!CH_2\!-\!COOH \end{array}$$

Succinyl CoA

Absorption, Fate, and Excretion Gastric intrinsic factor binds dietary vitamin B_{12} and small oral doses of the pure vitamin cyanocobalamin. Intrinsic factor carries the bound vitamin down to the ileum, attaches to specific sites on the microvilli, and releases vitamin B_{12} into the mucosal cells. With small doses of vitamin B_{12}, there is a delay of several hours before the vitamin appears in the blood. Larger oral doses are absorbed by simple diffusion, both in normal and pernicious anemia subjects. In these instances, the vitamin appears almost immediately in the blood.

Intrinsic factor has been highly purified from human gastric juice and hog stomach. In both species it is a glycoprotein of molecular weight 114,000 to 119,000. The dimeric molecule binds two molecules of vitamin B_{12}. Normal plasma contains at least two vitamin B_{12}-binding proteins, termed transcobalamins I and II. The former, an α_1-globulin, binds most of the circulating endogenous vitamin B_{12}. The latter, a β-globulin, binds most of the vitamin B_{12} ingested or injected. Small injected doses are almost completely retained, whereas injections of more than 50 μg lead to increased urinary loss.

The average daily diet in Western countries contains 5 to 30 μg of vitamin B_{12}. The vitamin is widely distributed throughout body tissues. The average total body content is about 4 mg, of which approximately 1 mg is in the liver. Kidney and adrenals also have high vitamin B_{12} levels. The forms in which the vitamin exists in tissues are incompletely studied, but in the liver the majority exists as deoxyadenosylcobalamin.

There is an active enterohepatic circulation of vitamin B_{12}. The total amount of vitamin B_{12} in feces exceeds the sum of that excreted in the urine plus the unabsorbed vitamin because there is some new synthesis by colon bacteria. Vitamin from this source is apparently not available to the human host. As yet, there is little information concerning the degradation of vitamin B_{12} in human tissues.

Clinical Aspects of Vitamin B_{12} Deficiency   Vitamin B_{12} deficiency is usually due to intestinal malabsorption of various causes. The most common is pernicious anemia in which a gastric mucosal defect decreases intrinsic factor synthesis. Other and less common causes of malabsorption include (1) total (and occasionally subtotal) gastrectomy; (2) the overgrowth of intestinal bacteria which occurs in the "blind loop" syndrome, strictures, anastomoses, diverticula, and other conditions producing intestinal stasis; (3) parasitic infestation with the vitamin B_{12}-devouring fish tapeworm *Diphyllobothrium latum*, a common condition in Scandinavian countries; and (4) organic disease of the bowel wall.

Vitamin B_{12} deficiency due to increased requirements is seen mainly in pregnancy.

The large body stores of vitamin B_{12} must be depleted before a deficiency state develops. Since the daily requirement is only 1 μg, an interval of several years elapses before deficiency symptoms develop after total gastrectomy or abrupt cessation of adequate treatment in pernicious anemia.

The major clinical manifestations of vitamin B_{12} deficiency are (1) megaloblastic anemia and its many sequelae; (2) gastrointestinal symptoms including glossitis and the dyspepsia of gastric mucosal atrophy; and (3) diverse neurologic abnormalities with degenerative changes of the dorsal and lateral columns of the spinal cord and peripheral nerves and associated disturbances of vibratory sense, proprioception, and pyramidal tract function. Optic atrophy and mental aberrations, ranging from mood changes to frank psychosis, may occur, and toxic amblyopia may be associated with vita-

min B_{12} deficiency. Neurologic symptoms may dominate the clinical picture, occurring sometimes in the absence of anemia.

Preparations and Dosages   Vitamin B_{12} is usually administered intramuscularly or subcutaneously as Cyanocobalamin (vitamin B_{12}) Injection, preparations of which are ordinarily marketed in solutions containing 100 or 1,000 μg/ml. The vitamin is also available in other concentrations and in crystalline form.

Hydroxocobalamin, an analogue of cyanocobalamin, is equal to cyanocobalamin in hematopoietic activity. Its duration of action may be somewhat longer than that of cyanocobalamin, but it apparently has no intrinsic advantage over cyanocobalamin.

The response of the patient with vitamin B_{12} deficiency to initial therapy is usually dramatic. Within 48 hours, there is a change in mood and a sense of well-being, followed shortly by increased appetite and strength. Characteristically, the reticulocyte concentration first rises appreciably on the third or fourth day of therapy, increases sharply to "peak" value on the fifth to eighth day and then more gradually diminishes as the erythrocyte count and hemoglobin rise to normal levels. The magnitude of the reticulocyte response is proportional to the severity of the anemia. The milder peripheral neurologic defects may also improve, whereas most manifestations of spinal cord injury, although arrested, are reversed slightly or not at all. Mental changes, including psychotic manifestations, may or may not improve rapidly.

The oral route should be reserved for treating nutritional vitamin B_{12} deficiency. This route should not be used for treating pernicious anemia, because oral preparations of cyanocobalamin are unreliable for obtaining an adequate or sustained therapeutic response.

Toxicity   No toxic effects have been found even with doses far in excess of the therapeutic range of usefulness. There are no known contraindications for the use of vitamin B_{12}.

Therapeutic Use   The only valid indication for vitamin B_{12} therapy is vitamin B_{12} deficiency. The most important part of any therapeutic regimen is to make the patient with pernicious anemia understand that injections of vitamin B_{12} are necessary at regular intervals or irreversible neurologic damage will develop.

Folic Acid

Chemistry and Nomenclature Folic acid, the common name for pteroylglutamic acid, is a parent compound for a large group of growth factors and coenzymes collectively referred to as "folates." The folic acid molecule contains three structural units: (1) a pteridine derivative; (2) *p*-aminobenzoic acid; and (3) glutamic acid. (See diagram below.) Pteroylglutamic or folic acid (F) is involved in enzyme reactions only after conversion to its coenzyme form, 5,6,7,8-tetrahydrofolic acid (FH_4). Reduction of F to FH_4 is believed to occur in two steps: F is reduced to 7,8-dihydrofolic acid (FH_2), and this is reduced further to FH_4, both reactions being catalyzed by a single NADPH-linked enzyme, dihydrofolate reductase.

Because reduced derivatives of folic acid are extremely sensitive to oxidation in air, they are unstable and difficult to preserve. A notable exception is the stable compound N^5-formyl FH_4, which was isolated from liver and yeast soon after the discovery of folic acid. It was first recognized as a growth factor for *Leuconostoc citrovorum* (since renamed *Pediococcus cerevisiae*) and thus it was named *citrovorum factor*. Leucovorin and folinic acid are other common names for this compound.

Sources The many compounds of the folate group are widely distributed in nature. Green leaves which are especially rich in the vitamin are presumed to be sites of active synthesis. Though the vitamin is also synthesized by many bacteria, the principal sources in the average diet are leafy vegetables, liver, and fruits. Excessive cooking, particularly with large amounts of water, can remove or destroy a large fraction of the folate in foods.

Absorption, Fate, and Excretion When 0.2 to 2.0 mg folic acid is administered orally to a normal person, more than 65 percent is usually absorbed. About 5 percent of the 0.2-mg dose and 15 percent of the 2.0-mg dose is excreted in the urine. After a 1-mg oral dose, serum levels can be detected within minutes and reach a peak in about 1 h.

Although various folates are synthesized by intestinal bacteria, little of the material is absorbed since most of the synthesis occurs in the colon, which is distal to the major absorption site, the proximal small intestine.

Folates have been found in all analyzed body tissues. The principal form of the vitamin in serum, red blood cells, and liver has been thought to be N^5-methyl FH_4, but recent work indicates that one-third or more of the serum folate is N^5-methyl FH_2.

The urine is the route of disposition of folates and their cleavage products. Filtered folic acid is actively reabsorbed by the renal tubule, although at low concentrations it is not transferred back into the circulation, but remains in the tubule cells. With doses of folic acid greater than 15 μg/kg, considerable amounts are excreted unchanged. Doses of folic acid lower than 15 μg/kg or folates from dietary sources are excreted in the urine in reduced forms, particularly as N^{10}-formyl FH_4. The urine also contains *p*-aminobenzoylglutamate arising from cleavage of the vitamin. The fate of the pteridine portion of the molecule is not known.

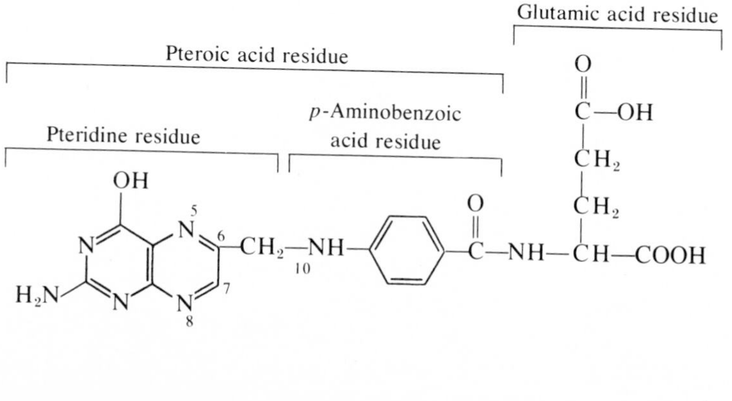

Metabolic Functions In metabolism, FH_4 is a catalytic self-regenerating acceptor-donor of one-carbon units in reactions involving one-carbon transfers from a carbon-containing donor compound, X—C, to an acceptor, Y:

$$X—C + FH_4 \longrightarrow X + C—FH_4$$
$$C—FH_4 + Y \longrightarrow Y—C + FH_4$$

Sum: $X—C + Y \longrightarrow Y—C + X$

The varieties of $C—FH_4$ differ only in the identity of the one-carbon unit and the site of its attachment of FH_4. One-carbon units can attach to either N^5, N^{10}, or to both nitrogens. Formyl, hydroxymethyl, methyl, and formimino containing nitrogen groups are found among the one-carbon units carried by FH_4. Specific enzymes are known which interconvert many of these compounds. In human folate deficiency, the reaction whose impairment produces the major clinical manifestations is thymidylate synthesis. The methylation of deoxyuridylate to thymidylate, catalyzed by the thymidylate synthetase, is an essential preliminary step in the synthesis of DNA, which requires thymine instead of uracil present in RNA. The coenzyme of this reaction N^5, N^{10}-methylene FH_4 transfers a one-carbon group and also acts as a hydrogen donor in reducing the transferred group to a methyl group. This reaction generates FH_2 which dihydrofolate reductase must reduce to FH_4 before it can again be utilized as a folate coenzyme. Limitation of thymidylate synthesis in folic acid deficiency results in defective DNA synthesis manifested by megaloblast formation.

Clinical Aspects of Folic Acid Deficiency The minimum daily requirement for folic acid in the normal adult is approximately 50 μg. Although the average diet contains several times this amount in the form of various folate compounds, body reserves of folic acid are relatively smaller than are those of vitamin B_{12}. Switching the folic acid intake from normal to a low daily intake of 5 μg per day results in the development of megaloblastic anemia in about 4 months. The principal causes for folate deficiency are inadequate dietary intake, defective intestinal absorption, abnormally increased requirements, and impaired utilization in the tissues. In contrast to the vitamin B_{12} deficiency syndromes,

malnutrition is an important cause of folic acid deficiency. Various forms of malabsorption, tropical and nontropical sprue, are also common causes of folic acid deficiency. Tropical sprue may be due to a deficiency of dietary folate, the malabsorption resulting from secondary gastrointestinal changes. Treatment with folic acid alone usually reverses all abnormalities, including the defective absorption of the vitamin itself. In nontropical sprue, as in most other forms of malabsorption, folic acid treatment corrects only the deficiency without affecting the absorptive defect. Low serum folate levels in patients receiving diphenylhydantoin and other anticonvulsants have been attributed to a reversible drug-induced malabsorption of folate.

Increased requirements for folic acid occur in certain hemolytic anemias, leukemia, and other malignant diseases and in pregnancy, which increases requirements threefold to sixfold. Finally, a major mechanism of folic acid "deficiency" is the inhibition of folic acid reduction caused by various pharmacologic agents. For example, the 4-aminofolic acid analogues, such as methotrexate, are powerful inhibitors of dihydrofolate reductase.

It is essential to distinguish between folic acid and vitamin B_{12} deficiencies so that the pathogenetic mechanism may be understood and appropriate therapy given. The hematologic manifestations of the two deficiencies are indistinguishable. The gastrointestinal features may also be similar to those of pernicious anemia. Neurologic abnormalities are thought to occur only in vitamin B_{12} deficiency, although scattered recent reports have suggested that neurologic changes may occur in pure folic acid deficiency. It should be remembered that neuropathies can result from deficiencies of other vitamins that may accompany a deficiency of folic acid.

Preparations and Dosages Although the oral replacement dose of folic acid is 0.25 to 1.0 mg daily, 100 μg daily produces an adequate hematologic response in patients with uncomplicated folate deficiency. Daily doses greater than 1 mg do not appear to enhance the hematologic effect. The sodium salt of folic acid (folate sodium) may be given by intramuscular, intravenous, or deep subcutaneous injection. Although parenteral administration of folic acid has no advantage over oral administration, it may be preferred when the folate deficiency is caused by malabsorption rather than by ingestion of inadequate amounts. Doses of 500 to 1,000 μg daily are considered adequate for parenteral therapy.

Calcium leucovorin injection is the therapeutic preparation of N^5-formyl FH_4. Its main clinical indication is severe intoxication by folic acid antagonists (such as methotrexate) which act by blocking the reduction of FH_2 to FH_4. In the absence of such inhibition, no purpose is accomplished in ordinary folate deficiency by giving this compound in place of folic acid. Suggestions that impaired reduction of folate in liver disease may respond to leucovorin await confirmation. Leucovorin is available as a sterile solution containing 3 mg/ml calcium salt. The usual dose is 3 to 6 mg/day administered intramuscularly.

Toxicity Signs of toxicity from folic acid have not been observed even with doses several times higher than the usual therapeutic levels. A few instances of apparent allergy have been reported, but this is exceedingly rare. Moreover, studies have not been undertaken to rule out the possibility that the active allergen is an impurity.

Therapeutic Use As in the case of vitamin B_{12}, the sole indication for folic acid therapy is folic acid deficiency or, as in pregnancy, anticipated folic acid deficiency. All therapeutic effects are attributable to reversal of the deficiency state.

DRUGS EFFECTIVE IN IRON-DEFICIENCY ANEMIAS: MICROCYTIC ANEMIAS

Of the elements found in the body, iron is one of the most multifunctional and essential. Iron is generally associated with hemoglobin, myoglobin, storage compounds (ferritin and hemosiderin), transport iron bound to transferrin, and parenchymal iron.

The major component of body iron is in hemoglobin, a protein of mol. wt. 64,458, which contains approximately 0.35 percent iron by weight. Divalent iron is bound in stable covalent linkage within the porphyrin ring of heme, with additional coordination positions attached to the globin peptide chains. Molecular oxygen is bound reversibly by the iron of hemoglobin for transport throughout the body. Oxidation of the iron to the ferric state (as in methemoglobin) causes hemoglobin to lose its capacity to carry oxygen.

Myoglobin, with a mol. wt. of 16,500, is the protein-bound heme of skeletal and cardiac muscle. The concentration of this protein varies greatly in different muscles and is only about 1 percent of the concentration of hemoglobin in blood. The affinity of myoglobin is much greater than that of hemoglobin for oxygen, especially at low oxygen tensions, and it readily accepts and stores oxygen released from hemoglobin.

Transferrin, which is a β_1-globulin of mol. wt. 90,000, has the specific property of binding iron, in which each transferrin molecule combines with two atoms of ferric iron. The combination is reversible. It serves to transport iron from the gastrointestinal tract to the bone marrow and tissue storage organs.

Iron is stored in the body as ferritin and hemosiderin. Ferritin is composed of a protein, apoferritin, within whose matrix iron in amounts up to about 23 percent by weight is bound in the form of hydroxide and phosphate complexes. The distinctive brown crystals after treatment with $CdSO_4$ (cadmium sulfate) and the electron microscopic structure of ferritin have made it easy to identify in tissues. Its major function is as a storage compound, although with its iron in the reduced form it has vasodepressive and antidiuretic properties. Hemosiderin is distinguishable from ferritin by its lack of solubility in water and its increased iron concentration—up to 35 percent iron by weight.

In cells, iron is an integral part of the heme enzymes (catalases, peroxidases, the cytochromes, and cytochrome oxidase) and of the ferroflavoproteins (succinic dehydrogenase, xanthine oxidase, and NADH cytochrome reductase). It also serves as a necessary cofactor for some enzymes. Iron is present in small amounts in a variety of other cell components, including red hair pigment, the muscle proteins myosin and actomyosin, a protein of human milk, and an unknown compound of brain.

Iron Absorption, Transport, and Storage

In human subjects the absorption of inorganic iron salts can occur from any level of the gastrointestinal tract. Ferrous iron is better absorbed than is the ferric form. Virtually all iron that is absorbed by the intestine enters the body via the bloodstream rather than by lymphatics. Uptake into the mucosal cell is unidirectional, with no excretion of iron into the gut except by cell desquamation. Absorption of iron normally balances excretion, with maintenance of fairly constant body levels. Iron absorption appears to be an active transport process dependent on oxidative metabolism sharply localized to the proximal duodenum. A number of studies report data consistent with a two-stage process of intestinal iron absorption. The initial rapid stage is virtually complete within an hour and is mediated by nonprotein, small molecular weight iron compounds. The second slower stage involves iron bound to protein, identified in part as ferritin. However, in contrast to the original "mucosal block" theory, ferritin serves as a storage compound rather than a carrier substance; iron not mobilized within the 2- to 3-day life-span of the mucosal cell is lost to the body by desquamation of the cell from the villous tip.

Iron absorption from different foods varies greatly, but averages between 5 and 10 percent in normal subjects and about 20 percent in iron-deficient subjects when it is given in amounts normally present in the diet (1 to 17 mg). Since the American diet contains about 6 mg iron/1000 calories, which amounts to 10 to 18 mg iron per day, normal subjects may absorb 0.5 to 1.8 mg and iron-deficient subjects absorb 2 to 4 mg of iron from their daily food.

Most food iron is bound in organic complexes. Heme iron, a major component in the American diet, is probably absorbed as the porphyrin complex, without conversion to the free ionized form. Other food iron complexes require processing to simple ferrous compounds for optimal absorption to occur. Acid gastric secretions aid in the ionization of food iron, which is subsequently reduced by ascorbic acid, sulfhydryl groups, or cysteine. The presence of hydrochloric acid in gastric secretions is not essential to iron absorption, though an acid medium helps maintain iron in a soluble form. On the other hand, ascorbic acid enhances nonhemoglobin food iron absorption.

Iron in plasma under normal circumstances circulates entirely bound to transferrin. Ordinarily, the iron-binding capacity of this protein is about one-third saturated.

Decrease in plasma iron level with increase in total iron-binding capacity is characteristic of iron deficiency and late pregnancy; high levels of plasma iron, almost totally saturating the transferrin, are seen in hemosiderosis and hemochromatosis; reduction of both plasma iron and iron-binding capacity are characteristic of infectious and inflammatory diseases. Oral contraceptives produce a rise in both iron-binding capacity and plasma iron.

Normal iron stores in the adult male range from 0.5 to 1.5 g. Normal women have smaller stores, in the range of 0.1 to 0.5 g, which are present in the bone marrow, liver, spleen, and in other areas with reticuloendothelial components. Storage iron is present in the form of ferritin and hemosiderin. Ferritin predominates, except in conditions where excessive amounts of storage iron are present. Both forms are available for mobilization and utilization for heme synthesis in response to blood loss. Iron stores are virtually absent in patients with iron-deficiency anemia.

Iron Excretion

The capacity of the body to excrete iron is usually limited. Most excretion is by desquamation of iron-containing cells from the bowel, skin, and genitourinary tract, although some iron is contained in fluids such as bile, urine, and sweat. The total daily iron loss for an adult male or nonmenstruating female is about 0.5 to 1.0 mg; an additional daily increment of 0.5 to 0.6 mg is added for normal menstrual loss.

Iron loss as hemosiderin granules in the urinary sediment is found in many patients with massive iron overload and in some patients with brisk intravascular hemolysis. During pregnancy iron is lost from the mother to the fetus and the placental tissues; there is further loss at delivery; and normal iron excretion (minus menstrual losses) continues.

Iron Requirements

Requirements for iron vary during different periods of life and are associated with the demands of growth, menstruation, or pregnancy. The effects of these variations superimposed on the baseline excretion are listed in Table 26-1. In the United States, with a dietary intake of 10 to 18 mg food iron, from which 5 to 10 percent is absorbed, men and postmenopausal women normally can maintain an adequate iron balance. Women during their reproductive years and adolescent girls, who must

Table 26-1 Estimated Dietary Iron Requirements

	Absorbed iron requirement, mg/day	Daily food iron requirement,* mg/day
Normal men and non-menstruating women	0.5–1	5–10
Menstruating women	0.7–2	7–20
Pregnant women	2–4.8	20–48†
Adolescents	1–2	10–20
Children	0.4–1	4–10
Infants	0.5–1.5	1.5 mg/kg‡

* Assuming 10% absorption.

† This amount of iron cannot be derived from diet and should be met by iron supplementation in the latter half of pregnancy.

‡ To a maximum of 15 mg.

cope with both growth and menstruation, are constantly in precarious iron balance and readily become iron-deficient. Similarly, infants from six to twenty-four months of age during this period of rapid increase in body size often outrun their dietary iron intake.

The kinetics of the daily turnover of iron bound to plasma transferrin for a normal subject is schematically summarized in Fig. 26-2.

Iron-Deficiency States

Initially, iron deficiency depletes tissue iron stores and in this stage is not associated with clear-cut functional derangements. Further body-iron depletion has been associated with a variety of symp-

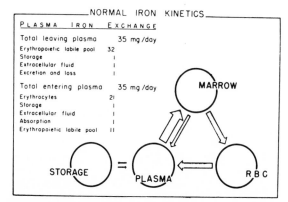

Figure 26-2 Summary of iron kinetics of a normal adult subject.

toms, usually of an ill-defined, subjective nature, such as easy fatigability, lack of appetite, headache, dizziness, and palpitations, even before a significant anemia appears or before there is definite abnormality of the plasma iron. With more severe and prolonged iron depletion, a hypochromic microcytic anemia ensues, associated with a low plasma iron level and elevated plasma iron-binding capacity. Epithelial changes such as cheilosis, hypopharyngeal webs associated with dysphagia, and gastritis with hypochlorhydria (Plummer-Vinson syndrome) may be seen with severe iron deficiency.

Iron-deficiency anemia in its fully developed form is characterized hematologically by the presence of small erythrocytes (microcytosis) poorly filled with hemoglobin (hypochromia) and many cells of bizarre shapes (poikilocytosis) and variable size (anisocytosis). Iron-deficiency anemia is the major type of hypochromic microcytic anemia.

Clinically, iron-deficiency anemia is a symptom rather than a disease. In adult males and postmenopausal females it usually signifies the presence of significant blood loss, the cause for which must be diligently sought, most often by careful examination of the gastrointestinal tract. For women of child-bearing age, excessive menstrual flow and multiple pregnancies are the most common causes. Infants and children with rapid growth demands on limited dietary iron intake may suffer from insufficient iron, though bleeding may add to their iron depletion in a significant percentage of cases. Malabsorption of iron due to diseases or surgical alterations of the gastrointestinal tract may be an additional cause of iron-deficiency anemia. Rare in this country is the dietary insufficiency of iron as the sole cause of iron-deficiency anemia in adults.

In the treatment of iron-deficiency anemia there are two basic points to consider: (1) correction of the hemoglobin and tissue iron deficiency and (2) recognition and, if possible, correction of the underlying cause. Of the two aims the second is often overlooked and is usually of greater importance. The first may be accomplished with remarkable ease and efficiency if one applies the principles of iron metabolism just reviewed.

Since ferrous salts are better absorbed than are ferric iron compounds, the former is most often used in the treatment of iron-deficiency anemia. Most iron compounds given orally to adults are compounded as tablets, with sugar coatings to retard the oxidation of iron to the ferric state. Liquid preparations of iron, such as elixirs or concentrated solutions to be given in drop form, are used primarily to treat infants and small children.

Acute Iron Toxicity

The ingestion of large doses of soluble iron compounds, especially by small children, often results in acute iron intoxication, leading to severe symptoms and death in a high proportion of cases. Lethal doses of ferrous sulfate have varied from 3 to 18 g, although survival has been reported after doses as high as 15 g.

The clinical effects of ingesting toxic doses of iron have been divided into four phases chronologically. The first phase begins with abdominal pain, nausea, and vomiting about 30 to 60 min after the iron tablets are taken. Partially dissolved iron tablets may be vomited together with brown or bloody stomach contents. Irritability, pallor, and drowsiness appear, along with frequent black or bloody diarrhea. Signs of acidosis and cardiovascular collapse may become prominent; coma and death ensue within 4 to 6 h in about 20 percent of children taking large doses of iron. The second phase is a period of improvement, with subsidence of the initial signs and symptoms spontaneously or in response to treatment. This period, lasting 8 to 16 h, may herald the onset of progressive improvement. Often, however, this lull in symptoms is shattered by a third phase of progressive cardiovascular collapse, convulsions, coma, and high mortality about 24 h after iron ingestion. Finally, a fourth phase of gastrointestinal obstruction from scarring of the stomach or small intestine may occur weeks or months after the initial episode of iron intoxication.

In combating iron toxicity in children, the most important measure is prevention. However, a rational plan of treatment for acute iron intoxication can be outlined: (1) Rid the stomach of its contents by inducing emesis and by lavage with a large-bore tube to remove undissolved iron tablets. With the tube still in place, instill a 1 percent solution of sodium bicarbonate or preferably an iron-binding chelate, such as deferoxamine (5 to 10 g), to bind residual iron in a poorly absorbable form. Follow the gastric lavage with an enema to remove iron from the lower bowel. (2) Institute measures to combat peripheral vascular collapse, including early replacement of body fluids and electrolytes using isotonic saline solution, Ringer's lactate solution, plasma, dextran, or whole blood. Bind iron circulating in the plasma in excess of transferrin-binding capacity to hasten its excretion. (3) Additional measures of frequent value include treating metabolic acidosis with appropriate solutions of sodium bicarbonate and using oxygen and vasopressor substances to help combat shock. The use of barbiturates, paraldehyde, or diphenylhydantoin may be required to control convulsions.

Chronic Iron Overload

Excessive amounts of iron may accumulate in the body under a variety of conditions, as shown in the following list of major types of iron-storage diseases.

1 Idiopathic hemochromatosis
2 Transfusion iron overload
3 Dietary iron overload
  a Bantu siderosis
  b Kaschin-Beck disease
4 Medicinal iron overload
  a Oral
  b Parenteral
5 Hemolytic iron overload
  a Refractory anemias
  b Thalassemia

Much confusion results from the nomenclature of clinical disorders of iron overload which reflects the incomplete understanding of the pathogenesis of excessive body iron storage and associated tissue damage. For the sake of discussion, *hemosiderosis* is defined as an increase in storage iron without associated tissue damage; the term *hemochromatosis* is used to denote increased storage iron with associated tissue damage.

Idiopathic Hemochromatosis

Idiopathic hemochromatosis is a rare disease manifested by excessive deposits of iron in parenchymal cells of many organs, especially the liver, pancreas, thyroid, adrenals, and stomach, with the clinical triad of pigmented cirrhosis, diabetes, and skin pigmentation. The disease occurs primarily in men fifty to seventy years of age and is only one-tenth as prevalent in women. Most studies suggest that hemochromatosis occurs as an inborn error of metabolism due to an autosomal dominant gene with incomplete penetrance or expressivity, resulting in increased iron absorption throughout life. Diagnosis is usually established by the demonstration of cirrhosis and excessive iron deposits on biopsy of liver; increased iron in skin, gastric mucosa, or urine sediment are confirmatory findings. Elevated plasma iron level with completely saturated iron-binding capacity is generally observed.

Transfusion Hemosiderosis

Because of the limited capacity of the body to excrete iron, multiple blood transfusions given for a variety of types of anemia (e.g., aplastic anemia and thalassemia) result in the deposition of storage iron, primarily in cells of the reticuloendothelial system. Eventually, after a patient has received 100 or more pints of blood, amounts of iron approaching those in patients with idiopathic hemochromatosis accumulate. However, chemical analysis of hepatic iron content in some cases shows much more iron than can be accounted for by transfusions alone, suggesting the additional factor of increased intestinal iron absorption that may modify the distribution and effects of excess iron stores. Many investigators have tried ways to remove these excess iron deposits or prevent their accumulation in the hope that fibrosis, cirrhosis, and diabetes might be prevented. Phlebotomy, as used in idiopathic hemochromatosis, is not feasible in these anemic patients receiving blood transfusions. Alternate means of iron removal involve the use of iron-chelating substances. Chelating agents such as DTPA (diethylenetriaminepentaacetate), EDDHA (ethylenediamine di-o-hydroxyphenylacetic acid), or deferoxamine have been administered therapeutically to patients with transfusion hemosiderosis.

Iron Compounds for Oral Administration

Ferrous Sulfate   Over the years ferrous sulfate has been the standard to which new iron preparations have been compared. Two forms of ferrous sulfate are generally used therapeutically: (1) The hydrated salt ($FeSO_4 \cdot 7H_2O$) contains 20 percent iron by weight and is dispensed in 0.3-g tablets; and (2) the exsiccated form (80 percent anhydrous $FeSO_4$) contains 30 percent elemental iron and is compounded in 0.2-g tablets. Dosage of either form is three or four tablets daily.

Careful studies indicate that gastrointestinal intolerance occurs only in 5 to 10 percent of patients given the usual therapeutic dose.

Liquid forms of ferrous sulfate are available, primarily for pediatric use. Ferrous sulfate syrup contains 40 mg ferrous sulfate (8 mg iron)/ml. The usual pediatric dose for treatment of iron-deficiency anemia is 5 ml twice or three times daily.

Ferrous Gluconate   Ferrous gluconate was introduced in an effort to reduce the side effects of ferrous sulfate. It contains 12 percent elemental iron. Ferrous gluconate is marketed as 0.3-g tablets or capsules, each providing 36 mg iron. The adult dose to provide the requisite amount of iron is five or six tablets daily. An elixir of ferrous gluconate containing 36 mg iron/5 ml is also available. Hemoglobin regeneration is comparable to that after ferrous sulfate therapy. The smaller iron content per tablet and the frequently used lower total dosage of iron may account for the clinical impression of a better-tolerated medication.

Ferrous Fumarate   Ferrous fumarate is a reddish-brown iron salt of fumaric acid containing 33 percent elemental iron. It is relatively resistant to oxidation, even in uncoated tablets, and is relatively insoluble in aqueous solutions except at low pH. The major use of ferrous fumarate is in iron-multivitamin-mineral mixtures, although 200-mg tablets and 300-mg sustained-release capsules are commercially available. Recommended adult dosage is three or four tablets per day. The incidence of gastrointestinal side effects have been reported to be about the same as with ferrous sulfate and ferrous gluconate.

Ferric Choline Citrate   Known also as ferrocholinate, this material is a chelate of ferric hydroxide and choline dihydrogen citrate, containing 12 percent elemental iron by weight. It is marketed in 0.33-g tablets (40 mg iron) and in pediatric drops containing 25 mg/ml. Average adult dosage is five tablets daily. The frequency of gastrointestinal side effects in patients is approximately the same as that after taking comparable doses of ferrous sulfate. Absorption of a similar chelate, ferric choline isocitrate, was found to be about half that of ferrous sulfate.

Iron Compounds for Parenteral Use

The great majority of patients with iron-deficiency anemia can best be treated with orally administered iron. However, the use of a parenteral preparation of iron may be desirable for certain patients: (1) those unable to tolerate or unwilling to take iron orally, e.g., those with ulcerative colitis, regional enteritis, colostomies, or extensive bowel resections, as well as those who for various reasons cannot be relied on to take medications prescribed for them; (2) those unable to absorb iron given orally, e.g., patients with idiopathic or postresection malabsorption syndromes; and (3) those with severe iron deficiency for whom it is impossible to provide iron quickly enough by the oral route.

Iron Dextran   Iron dextran is a complex of ferric hydroxide and low molecular weight dextran (5,000 to 20,000 average mol. wt.). It contains 50 mg elemental iron/ml. The pH of the solution is 6.0, and when injected intramuscularly it produces little local reaction in most patients. Intradermal injection produces prolonged skin staining. Recent experience with direct intravenous injection of 10 ml iron dextran, or infusion of the total iron requirement in isotonic saline solution at a rate of 20 to 60 drops/min, has been effective, with only a 1 to 2 percent incidence of minor reactions.

Dextriferron   Dextriferron is a complex of ferric hydroxide and partially hydrolyzed dextrin, of about 230,000 mol. wt., containing 20 mg elemental iron/ml of solution. It is administered only by the intravenous route, with a starting dose of 1.5 ml (30 mg iron) increased by daily increments of 1.5 ml until a maximum dose of 5 ml (100 mg iron) has been reached.

Iron-Sorbitol-Citric Acid Complex   Iron-sorbitol-citric acid complex is a preparation of about 5,000 mol. wt., containing 50 mg iron/ml. Many investigators have shown that this drug administered by the intramuscular route produces a therapeutic response comparable to that of iron dextran. Toxic side effects occur with about the same frequency as with iron dextran; skin staining is not a problem, although some patients show evidence of renal irritation.

Chapter 27

Anticoagulant and Coagulant Drugs

The clotting of blood is an important defense mechanism which normally is constantly available for protection against excessive hemorrhage.

However, should a clot develop in an intact vessel, the problem of thrombosis arises, and unless an effective clot-resolving mechanism or collateral circulation is available, the thrombus (clot) may lead to infarction, with subsequent necrosis of the tissue supplied with blood by the thrombosed vessel. Emboli which break off from the blood clot may lodge in vital areas of the body. Death may occur from either the original thrombosis or the subsequent embolization.

In the opposite situation, blood clotting may not occur normally and a patient may bleed excessively from minor injuries.

Adequate treatment of hemorrhagic and thrombotic disorders involves drug therapy. The rational use of drugs which influence the clotting mechanism of the blood is based on an understanding of the existing fundamental concepts of the mechanism of coagulation and resolution of the blood clot. The following discussion presents the most acceptable fundamental concepts of blood clotting as related to the action of drugs.

FORMATION OF BLOOD CLOTS

The formation of a clot is the result of a complicated series of biochemical reactions and interactions, many of which are not clearly defined. In fact, the order in which the various factors react to produce the final blood clot is not well defined, and it is probable that several of the factors exist in the blood in inactive precursor form. Table 27-1 consists of a list of the various factors by number and common name, for reference purposes.

Figure 27-1 schematically depicts the sequence of reactions which leads to the formation of the clot. This mechanism may be divided into three distinct stages: (1) the formation of an active prothrombin-converting substance (thromboplastin),

Table 27-1 Blood-clotting Factors

Factor numbers	Common name
I	Fibrinogen
II	Prothrombin
III	Thromboplastin
IV	Ionic calcium
V	Hereditary labile factor
	Activator (AC) globulin
	Proaccelerin
VI	(No factor described)
VII	Proconvertin
	Serum prothrombin conversion accelerator (SPCA)
VIII	Antihemophilic factor
IX	Plasma thromboplastin component (PTC)
	Christmas factor
X	Stuart-Prower factor
XI	Plasma thromboplastin antecedent
XII	Hageman factor
XIII	Fibrin-stabilizing factor

(2) the conversion of prothrombin to thrombin by thromboplastin, and (3) the conversion of fibrinogen to fibrin by thrombin.

The circulating blood contains all the factors necessary for the formation of the blood clot, but it is now apparent that active prothrombin-converting material can be derived from two sources: (1) the *intrinsic source*, because it involves only components of blood, with the exception that a surface other than the natural endothelium of the blood vessel must be present (a surface such as glass enables the reaction to take place between factors V, VIII, IX, X, calcium ions, and blood platelets, leading to the formation of an active prothrombin-converting substance); and (2) the *extrinsic source*, involving an intracellular substance which is present in all tissues, which is liberated after cell injury, and which then reacts with the clotting factors V, VII, X, and calcium in plasma to form a potent active prothrombin-converting material. The active prothrombin-converting materials derived from these two sources are probably not identical, but they serve the same purpose in that they are both capable of converting prothrombin to thrombin; in this text they will be referred to as *active thromboplastin*.

When active thromboplastin becomes available

in plasma, the second stage of coagulation takes place and prothrombin is converted to thrombin.

In the absence of calcium ions this reaction is slow; therefore, ionic calcium is considered necessary for optimum activity. When a small amount of thrombin is once formed, the activity of factor V is increased and the rate of formation of thrombin increases.

When thrombin becomes available in the blood, the third stage in the formation of the clot can occur. This reaction is the conversion of fibrinogen to fibrin. The action of thrombin as a catalyst promotes the conversion of fibrinogen to a fibrin monomer and subsequent polymerization of the monomer occurs, resulting in the formation of the insoluble filaments of fibrin. Fibrin is the matrix of the blood clot, giving it its gel-like nature.

RESOLUTION OF BLOOD CLOTS

The mechanism of resolution of the clot involves the existence in the plasma of an additional globulin protein known as *profibrinolysin* (or plasminogen). Profibrinolysin is the inactive precursor of a lytic enzyme known as *fibrinolysin* (or plasmin). Fibrinolysin is capable of causing the lysis, or resolution, of fibrin. The conversion of profibrinolysin to fibrinolysin occurs spontaneously in the presence of cell fragments or may be brought about more rapidly by the enzyme streptokinase. Fibrinolysin then enzymatically converts the insoluble fibrin of a clot to smaller, soluble protein fragments so that the final result is a resolution of the clot (Fig. 27-1).

ANTICOAGULANT DRUGS

Heparin

Heparin has the property of prolonging the clotting time of blood either in vivo or in vitro. Heparin is a naturally occurring mucoitin polysulfuric acid consisting of equal parts of hexuronic acid and acetylated glycosamine, with sulfuric acid ester groups. A principal characteristic of its molecule is its strong negative charge. The site of formation of heparin in the animal is not established, but it is stored in the mast cells as granules which exhibit metachromatic activity.

The commercial source of heparin is the lungs of

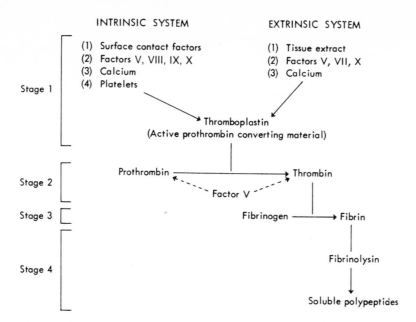

INTRINSIC SYSTEM   EXTRINSIC SYSTEM

Stage 1

(1) Surface contact factors
(2) Factors V, VIII, IX, X
(3) Calcium
(4) Platelets

(1) Tissue extract
(2) Factors V, VII, X
(3) Calcium

Thromboplastin
(Active prothrombin converting material)

Stage 2

Prothrombin   Thrombin

Factor V

Stage 3

Fibrinogen ⟶ Fibrin

Stage 4

Fibrinolysin

Soluble polypeptides

Figure 27-1 Schematic representation of the blood coagulation mechanism and clot resolution.

domestic animals used for food by man. The heparin extracts obtained from different animals and different tissues vary in potency, so that the final preparations must be biologically standardized.

The commercial preparations which are available in the United States are labeled with their activity in units as well as with the approximate weight of the heparin contained therein. References in the literature frequently refer to doses of heparin in terms of milligrams of the sodium salt. One unit of heparin represents the activity in approximately 0.01 mg, so that 100 mg of heparin is approximately equal to 10,000 units. Since there is biologic variation, the dose of heparin should be ordered by units.

Mechanism of Action Heparin serves to prevent the formation of fibrin in the coagulation of blood by (1) retarding the conversion of prothrombin to thrombin; (2) an antithrombin action; and (3) decreasing the agglutination of platelets. The first effect of heparin on the clotting mechanism, and probably the most significant clinically, is its ability to interfere with the conversion of prothrombin to thrombin by thromboplastin. This has been called the *antiprothrombin action* or the *antithromboplas-*

tin action of heparin. The term *antithromboplastin action* is preferred.

It is interesting that the antithromboplastin activity of heparin is not manifested unless plasma is present. The identity of the plasma cofactor necessary for this action of heparin to take place has not been definitely established.

The second action of heparin is its effect in antagonizing the ability of thrombin to bring about the conversion of fibrinogen to fibrin. This function has been called the *antithrombin action* of heparin.

Maximum antithrombin action of heparin is not obtainable unless plasma is present in the reaction mixture. Therefore, a plasma cofactor is necessary for this action of heparin to be manifested.

The present concept of the antithrombin action of heparin is that heparin acts by developing an antithrombin in the blood, either by combining with a plasma cofactor or by converting an inactive precursor to an active antithrombin.

Finally, heparin also has the property of being able to reduce the degree of adhesiveness of platelets. This is of particular interest in connection with the rationale for the use of heparin, since the number of platelets, as well as their adhesiveness, increases in the immediate postoperative and puerperal periods.

An action of heparin which may be of importance when this drug is used in the therapy of thrombotic disorders is the facilitation of clot resolution by preventing extension of an existing intravascular clot. However, it should be pointed out that there is no evidence indicating that heparin has a direct lytic action on the well-formed fibrin of a clot.

Hyperlipemia and Heparin   After a high-fat meal the plasma becomes cloudy with fat particles and is therefore in a state of hyperlipemia. Five minutes following the injection of heparin in such a hyperlipemic subject the cloudiness (Tyndall effect) of hyperlipemic plasma will be absent. This action is called the *antichylomicronemic action* of heparin and is observed after doses of heparin which are so small that there is no concomitant anticoagulant effect.

This effect of heparin has been shown to be due to an ability of heparin to bring about a shift in the distribution of low-density lipoproteins of blood.

Since heparin lowers the low-density lipoproteins and accelerates removal of fat from the bloodstream, efforts have been made to alter the development of atherosclerosis in experimental animals and in human beings by administration of heparin. However, the clinical usefulness of heparin's antihyperlipemic action in atherosclerosis has yet to be demonstrated.

Route of Administration and Duration of Action Aqueous solutions of sodium heparin are usually administered intravenously or subcutaneously. Heparin is not effective via the oral or rectal route, and a report indicating a definite sublingual absorption of heparin has not been confirmed.

A single dose of 100 units (approximately 1 mg) per kg given intravenously will cause the clotting time to be four or five times longer than normal. The onset of action is almost immediate, maximum effect being manifest within 5 to 10 min, and the clotting time will then gradually return to normal over the subsequent 2 to 4 h.

The action of heparin may be prolonged by the use of repository preparations containing heparin in a gelatin-dextrose menstruum. This preparation may cause tissue reaction and pain at the site of in-

jection, with definite tenderness lasting from 2 to 4 days.

Excretion   Following intravenous administration, from 20 to 25 percent of a single dose of heparin can be recovered as active material from the urine. This low amount recovered as a result of urinary excretion fails to account for the rapid loss of heparin from the circulation. However, the mast cells may act as a storage depot for exogenously administered heparin. Because of the highly reactive nature of the heparin molecule, it is probable that heparin combines with plasma proteins and thereby is not available for passive excretion by the kidney.

Toxicity   Toxicity of heparin is due to overdosage. The toxicity manifests itself as bleeding from mucous membranes and from open wounds. Because of the short duration of action of aqueous heparin, treatment of such hemorrhagic phenomena involves decreasing the dose or frequency of injections. All the actions of heparin on the clotting mechanism can be directly reversed by the administration of protamine (salmine) sulfate. This compound reacts directly with heparin, forming an inactive complex as indicated by in vitro tests. Protamine is a strongly basic protein, and it should be given slowly, although this drug only rarely produces headache or an anaphylactoid reaction. Long-term use of heparin has been reported to cause osteoporosis.

Coumarin Derivatives

The coumarin compounds are orally effective anticoagulants. Among the most important are ethyl biscoumacetate (Tromexan), sodium warfarin (Coumadin), acenocoumarol (Sintrom), and phenprocoumon (Liquamar). Dicumarol, the first coumarin derivative, is compared for similarity of structure to vitamin K and phenindione (Fig. 27-2).

Mechanism of Action   Unlike heparin, the therapeutic action of the coumarin compounds depends on their ability to prolong the prothrombin time by suppressing the formation of prothrombin and factors VII, IX, and X by the liver. The effect of these compounds occurs only in vivo. Synthesis of prothrombin and factors VII, IX, and X occurs in the

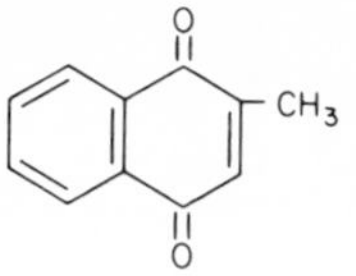

Vitamin K
(Menadione)

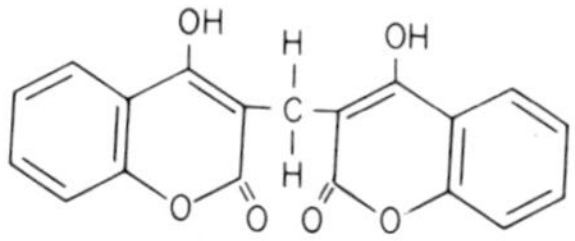

Bishydroxycoumarin
(Dicumarol)

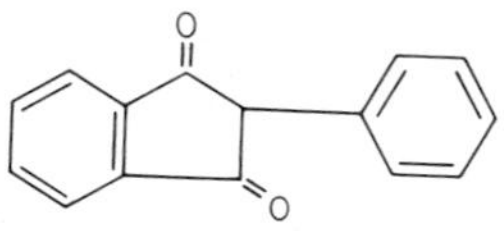

Phenindione
(Hedulin, Danilone)

Figure 27-2 Structural relationships between vitamin K and the hypoprothrombin-inducing drugs.

liver and requires the presence of vitamin K. The similarity in the structure of vitamin K and the coumarin compounds, particularly bishydroxycoumarin (dicumarol), has suggested that these compounds act as antimetabolites to block the utilization of vitamin K by the liver. The drugs, which act by interfering with the synthesis in the liver of the proteins which require the presence of vitamin K, are commonly referred to as "hypoprothrombin"-inducing agents, or as having prothrombinemic action.

Route of Administration and Excretion The coumarin drugs are well absorbed following oral administration. Sodium warfarin is the only drug of this group which may be administered parenterally. The various coumarin derivatives differ chiefly in the time required to produce hypoprothrombinemia, and the time required before the blood coagulation factors determined by the prothrombin-time test will return to normal when the drug is discontinued. Although with a sufficiently high dose, synthesis of the vitamin K-dependent factors

by the liver is probably decreased almost immediately following absorption of the drug, a period of time is required before blood levels of the factors fall as a result of normal utilization. Therefore, following administration of the drugs, there is a latent period before the prothrombin time becomes prolonged.

To obtain as rapid an onset of activity as possible, the initial doses of these drugs are higher than subsequent maintenance ones. The time required for blood prothrombin time to return to normal when therapy is discontinued varies more than the time required to produce an effect and, depending on the drug, may be from 1 to 8 days.

The rate of metabolism of the coumarin drugs varies from person to person, but in a given individual it is quite constant even at different times. These drugs are biotransformed by the microsomal enzyme system in the liver, which explains their interaction with other drugs capable of inducing or inhibiting these enzymes.

These drugs do not appear in any significant amounts per se in the urine, but unidentified metabolic products of the drug are excreted in the urine.

Toxicity The principal toxicity of these compounds is the direct effect of overdosage, resulting in marked hypoprothrombinemia. The toxicity manifests itself as ecchymoses and purpura. The hemorrhages may be major in character and may result in death of the patient. The hypoprothrombinemia produced by all the coumarin drugs can be combated by fresh whole-blood transfusions which supply the needed vitamin K-dependent blood coagulation factors to the patient. Large doses of vitamin K_1 oxide will similarly combat such hypoprothrombinemias by supplying the vitamin needed to enable the liver to synthesize the clotting factors, thereby decreasing the effect of the coumarin compounds. Following the intravenous administration of vitamin K_1 oxide, there is a latent period of several hours before its effect on prothrombin time is obtained; the action of vitamin K_1 begins within half an hour. Therefore, when hemorrhage occurs, the coumarin drug should be discontinued and fresh whole-blood transfusions and vitamin K_1 should be administered.

Vitamin K_1 is an oily liquid which is available as an emulsion for intravenous use, and a dose of 100 to 150 mg will return the prothrombin time to safe levels in approximately 6 h. A prothrombin-time determination should be performed within 6 h after the injection of vitamin K_1 to determine if additional doses are needed.

The role of vitamin K_1 in antagonizing the action of the coumarins and their similarity in structure have lent support to the theory that the coumarins compete with the utilization of vitamin K by the liver in the production of prothrombin and with factors VII, IX, and X.

Drug Interaction Perhaps no other group of drugs is more subject to drug interaction than the oral anticoagulants. This is because the hypoprothrombinopenic effect is directly related to the plasma level, and this level is determined not only by the dose but also by the rate of biotransformation of the drug. Thus all the other drugs which induce increased activity of the liver microsomal enzyme system cause an increased inactivation of the oral anticoagulants. This decreases their effect for a given dose, so that the clinician observing this effect tends to increase the dose. If at this point the inducing drug is stopped, the anticoagulant will have a much greater effect, and serious toxicity from hemorrhagic accidents may result. Among the many drugs which can induce the microsomal enzyme system are phenobarbital, chloral hydrate, glutethimide, meprobamate, griseofulvin, and haloperidol.

Agents such as phenylbutazone, diphenylhydantoin, and salicylates tend to displace the coumarins from their plasma protein-binding sites and thus have the effect of increasing the blood level for a given dose. Also of importance is the fact that antibiotics such as chloramphenicol and the sulfa drug sulfisoxazole interfere with the intestinal bacteria which synthesize vitamin K.

In their own right the coumarins are known to increase the blood level of diphenylhydantoin and to increase the hypoglycemic effect of tolbutamide.

Indandione Derivatives

Certain indandione derivatives produce an anticoagulant effect similar to that produced by the coumarin series of compounds. The indandione ring structure is comparable to that of the coumarins (see Fig. 27-2). These compounds act by decreasing the formation of the vitamin K-dependent coagulation proteins by the liver. They are well absorbed following oral administration.

The recommended initial dose followed by maintenance doses will usually maintain the blood-prothrombin levels between 10 and 30 percent of normal. The onset of maximum therapeutic effect is usually within 24 h after the initial dose. After single doses the prothrombin concentration of the blood returns to normal in 48 to 96 h.

Toxicity Toxicity to the indandiones is similar to that produced by the coumarin agents. Overdose of the drug leads to excessive lowering of the level of factors VII, IX, X, and prothrombin in the blood, and may result in hemorrhagic complications. Large doses have also been reported to produce polyuria, polydipsia, and tachycardia. Hematuria is usually the earliest manifestation of incipient hemorrhagic complications. At the first indication of the presence of hematuria the drug should be discontinued until the prothrombin content of the blood rises to safe levels. In the presence of excessive hemorrhagic complications the drug should be discontinued and vitamin K_1 plus fresh whole-blood transfusions should be administered. Granulocytopenia and a jaundice-producing liver dyscrasia have been reported as additional toxic effects resulting from indandione medication. These latter toxic effects probably represent a hypersensitivity reaction rather than a consistent toxicity of the drugs.

Therapeutic Uses of Anticoagulant Drugs

The anticoagulant drugs have the following clinical indications:

1 In the treatment of thromboembolic diseases to prevent clot extension and subsequent embolism. Treatment should also be accorded thrombophlebitis which may develop spontaneously, following surgery, trauma, or disease processes, such as coronary occlusion and congestive heart failure.

2 Prophylactically, to prevent thromboembolic complications following surgery, in certain cases of trauma such as fractures, in patients with acute coronary thrombosis, and in certain patients with congestive heart failure. Whether or not prophylactic treatment is instituted depends on many factors such as age of the patient, the degree of bed rest,

the history of previous thromboembolic disease, and the absence of specific contraindications.

3 Prophylactically, to prevent arterial embolization in certain patients with atrial fibrillation and mural heart thrombi and to prevent thrombus formation following vascular surgery.

4 To prevent clotting during transfusion.

PROTEOLYTIC ENZYMES

Some proteolytic enzymes are known to have a clot-accelerating effect. Examples are trypsin and certain proteolytic enzyme-containing snake venoms, among which the Russell viper venom (Stypven) is the most potent. Minute quantities of these agents promote clot formation by accelerating the activation of prothrombin to thrombin. They can activate the conversion of prothrombin to thrombin even in the absence of thromboplastin, although the presence of thromboplastin considerably improves their effectiveness. However, a paradoxical effect on clotting occurs when the concentration of snake venom is high, because under this condition the rate of clot formation is inhibited. This effect is currently believed to be due to the formation of an anticoagulant with antithrombin activity.

Fibrinolysin

Active fibrinolysin from human blood is available as *actase* and *thrombolysin*. The preparation is made by allowing streptokinase to activate the profibrinolysin fraction obtained from human blood plasma. It is standardized on the basis of units of fibrinolytic activity determined in vitro. It has been used by intravenous injection in an attempt to promote resolution of blood clots, but the effectiveness of the lytic action in human beings remains to be established. Its use is accompanied by several undesirable effects: (1) a degradation of fibrinogen, as shown by a decreased plasma level of fibrinogen in human beings who have received fibrinolysin; (2) a febrile response, which is possibly the result of impurities in the preparation, such as streptokinase; (3) the antigenic effect of the preparation, which after repeated administration may produce severe allergic reactions.

Streptokinase and Streptodornase

Streptokinase and streptodornase, together with certain other enzymes such as hyaluronidase and ribonuclease, are produced and excreted into the culture medium by group C hemolytic streptococci.

Streptodornase is probably not a single enzyme but consists of a mixture of enzymes produced by the streptococci. Its principal value in the clinic is to catalyze the breakdown of deoxyribonucleoprotein, which constitutes 30 to 70 percent of the sediment in thick purulent exudates. Preparations of streptokinase and streptodornase consist of the lyophilized, partially purified, bacteria-free filtrate of culture media.

Only freshly prepared solutions should be used. The available preparation is Varidase, which is a sterile vacuum-dried powder having the equivalent of 100,000 units of streptokinase and 25,000 units of streptodornase. Four to six hours of contact is required for the enzymes to be effective.

Streptokinase given intramuscularly or by the buccal route is capable of producing a generalized systemic anti-inflammatory effect, the mechanism of which has not been clarified.

The mixture of streptokinase and streptodornase is used to aid in the resolution of exudates containing both fibrin and purulent material.

The presently available preparation must not be administered intravenously, since it may result in a pyrogenic reaction. The enzymes are antigenic, and proper precautions should be taken in this regard. The antigenic and febrile responses are the most common reactions, and the patient may experience a rise in temperature of 1 to 5°F within 12 h after the administration of Varidase. This preparation has been used successfully in hemothorax, in thoracic empyema, in bladder clots and wound sloughs, and in general hematomas.

A mixture of fibrinolysin and deoxyribonuclease prepared from bovine source material is also available as Elase. This mixture of enzymes is effective in lysing fibrin and in liquefying pus. In ointment form it is used to liquefy debris in vaginitis and cervicitis, as well as for the purposes described for the streptokinase-streptodornase preparation.

AGENTS USED TO PROMOTE THE COAGULATION OF BLOOD
Thrombin

Thrombin is obtained from bovine plasma. It can be used only by topical application. Clinically it is used principally when blood continues to ooze from abraded or otherwise open vessels, and it is impractical to use ligation or pressure techniques or when they are unsuccessful. Thrombin has been used orally to control upper gastrointestinal bleeding, as from a peptic ulcer.

Fibrin

Fibrin is the protein formed from fibrinogen in the presence of thrombin. It is the netlike mesh which gives the blood clot its characteristic gel-like structure. It is commercially obtained from human blood and is available in the dehydrated form as sheets from which segments of any desired size may be cut for use on bleeding surfaces. It is occasionally packaged together with a solution of thrombin. The purpose of the fibrin is to act as a mechanical barrier to hold the thrombin in position over the bleeding area. The sheet of fibrin acts as a preformed network to enmesh the oozing blood from surface areas. The presence of thrombin facilitates the clotting of the enmeshed blood. This leads to a cementing together of the fibrin with the bleeding surface.

Gelfoam

Gelfoam is a specially prepared form of gelatin which has been processed to give it a porous nature. Like fibrin, it is generally used in conjunction with thrombin and serves to stay the oozing of blood from surface wounds. Gelfoam in powdered form has also been used in the treatment of bleeding peptic ulcer.

Oxycel

Oxycel is surgical gauze which has been treated with nitrogen dioxide. It retains about half the original tensile strength of surgical gauze if it remains dry, but when it is wet with tissue juice it rapidly loses its tensile strength and becomes rather sticky and gummy. Its hemostatic action is due to its sticky mechanical blockage, which simulates an artificial clot over the surface of a wound that tends to ooze blood.

Antihemophilic Globulin

The present concept of the causation of hemophilia indicates that it is a sex-linked hereditary disease characterized by a lack of normal amounts of factor VIII (antihemophilic globulin). The bleeding time in hemophilic patients may be normal, because when the skin is pierced to conduct a bleeding-time test, tissue juice supplies the lacking thromboplastin and factor VIII is not needed for extrinsic formation of thromboplastin.

It is interesting that 1 mg of the antihemophilic globulin will cause hemophilic blood to clot more rapidly, but even 200 times this amount of the globulin will not cause the blood of a hemophiliac to clot in the normal time. Because of this, fresh whole-blood transfusions, even if small, will be effective in shortening the clotting time in hemophilic patients, but unless massive transfusions are given, the clotting time will not be completely returned to normal.

Antihemophilic globulin is available. It is prepared from pooled, normal, human blood plasma by the low-temperature-alcohol fractionation method of Cohn or by a similar procedure. This globulin is sometimes referred to as fraction 1. It is not completely free of other globulins and is therefore standardized on the basis of its ability to shorten the clotting time of hemophilic blood.

Aminocaproic Acid

Aminocaproic acid (Amicar) is administered orally or intravenously. This drug is effective in decreasing hemorrhage associated with certain surgical procedures. Its mechanism of action primarily involves competitive inhibition of plasminogen activators.

Part Seven

Allergy Drugs

Chapter 28

Histamine and Antihistamines

HISTAMINE

Demonstration of the natural occurrence of a pharmacologically potent substance has always prompted an intensive investigation of the role that agent might play in the physiologic and pathologic processes of the organism. However, though histamine was first synthesized and its natural occurrence described more than 50 years ago, the role(s) of this biogenic amine in such processes remains to be resolved.

Distribution, Localization, and Binding

There is scarcely a tissue or organ which does not contain histamine. The gastrointestinal tract and skin are particularly rich in histamine, and moderate amounts are present in the liver in man. Histamine has also been demonstrated in nervous tissue.

Most tissue histamine is found in the granules of the mast cell (labrocyte). Heparin is associated with histamine in the mast cell and has been considered

a binding site for histamine. Generally, histamine becomes pharmacologically active only when the cells are lysed.

Formation

There has long been controversy concerning the origin of body stores of histamine. One theory proposes the enzymic decarboxylation of histidine by several tissues. This enzyme-catalyzed decarboxylation proceeds as follows:

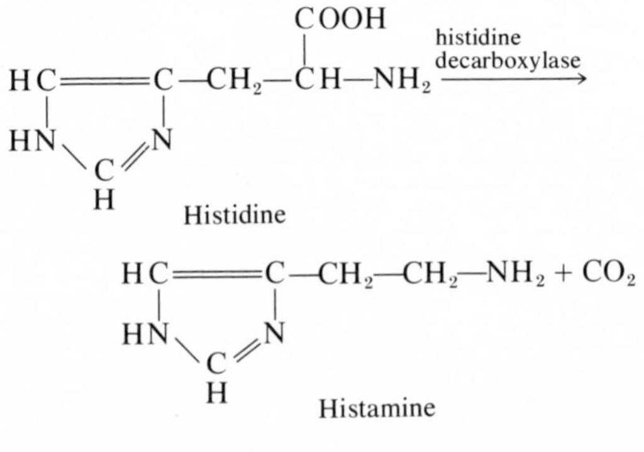

Histidine

Histamine

The enzyme histidine decarboxylase is present in many tissues. However, there are conflicting data supporting the tissue histidine decarboxylase theory. An alternative theory proposes that histamine is formed in the gastrointestinal tract by bacterial action and then is absorbed. Urinary histamine excretion is decreased following sterilization of the gastrointestinal tract, while ingestion of histidine increases urinary histamine excretion; these observations tend to support the absorption theory of the origin of tissue histamine.

Metabolism and Fate

The principal pathway of histamine inactivation involves methylation of the ring to form 1-methylhistamine (reaction 1, Fig. 28-1). A major fraction of this inactive metabolite is converted to the primary urinary metabolite 1-methylimidazole-4-acetic acid by the enzyme monoamine oxidase (MAO) (reaction 2, Fig. 28-1). A secondary route of histamine degradation involves oxidative deamination of the side chain by diamine oxidase (histaminase) to

yield imidazole-4-acetic acid (reaction 3, Fig. 28-1). Much of the metabolite is conjugated with ribose (reaction 4, Fig. 28-1) and excreted as 1-ribosylimidazole-4-acetic acid. Small amounts of free histamine and varying proportions of the intermediate and ultimate metabolites are excreted in the urine. The third and probably least important route of metabolism is the acetylation of histamine (reaction 5, Fig. 28-1). Histamine present in ingested food or derived from dietary histidine by the decarboxylating activity of intestinal bacteria is largely catabolized by this route.

Release

A variety of agents has been shown to cause histamine release from bound storage sites. These include tissue irritants, surface-active substances (e.g., Tween 20), polymers (e.g., dextran), drugs (e.g., morphine and d-tubocurarine), and certain enzymes, such as chymotrypsin, trypsin, and phosphatidase A.

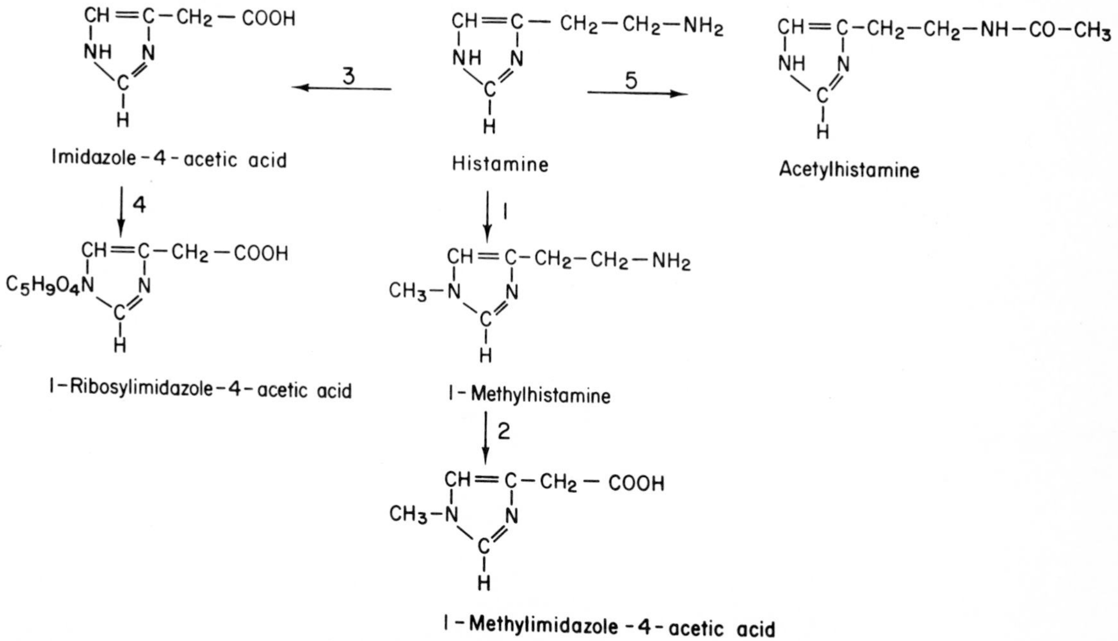

Figure 28-1 Reaction 1: A major pathway of inactivation catalyzed by the enzyme imidazole-N-methyltransferase. Reaction 2: Oxidation by monoamine oxidase. Reaction 3: Diamine oxidase (histaminase) catalyzes this reaction. Reaction 4: Enzyme which catalyzes this reaction not definitively characterized. Reaction 5: A pathway of questionable significance.

There are various theories concerning the circumstances under which histamine is liberated. One hypothesis requires the participation of an intracellular, heat-labile, calcium-requiring enzyme system which is transiently activated by the antigen-antibody reaction or the presence of 48/80, a mixture of p-methoxy-N-methylphenethylamine moieties.

The release of histamine is blocked by various esterase inhibitors, inhibitors of enzymes involved in energy production, and other types of interfering agents. Cromolyn sodium, an agent presently employed as an adjunct in the management of severe perennial bronchial asthma, apparently acts at the cellular level, since there is a definite inhibition of the release of histamine from mast cells, possibly by stabilizing the mast cell membrane or its granules.

Itching, anaphylactoid crisis (characterized by extensive urticaria, edema of the mucous membranes, fall in blood pressure, and peripheral circulatory failure), bronchospasm, and increased gastric acid secretion are manifestations of the release of histamine. These systems are suggestive of those observed in anaphylactic shock due to antigen challenge in a previously sensitized subject. Thus, the release of histamine by organic agents is similar to but not necessarily identical with anaphylaxis in many respects.

Actions

The actions of histamine considered to be of importance are those on the cardiovascular system, smooth muscle, and exocrine glands.

Cardiovascular System   The cardiovascular effects of histamine appear to be related to four general actions: (1) relaxation or constriction of arterioles and alteration in venous tone, (2) potent capillary dilatation, (3) cardiac muscle effects, and (4) release by reflex or other means of adrenergic mediators from the adrenal medulla and other tissues.

Blood Pressure   The intravenous or intraarterial administration or infusion of high concentrations of histamine elicits a fall in the systemic blood pressure. The fall in systemic pressure may be observed in arteries of various caliber almost immediately after administration of the drug; it is a result of the potent dilatation of capillaries and the relaxation of arteriolar tone.

The histamine-induced systemic hypotension is transitory. Recovery is rapid since the amine is rapidly detoxified and compensatory reflexes come into play (e.g., cardioacceleration, vasoconstriction, and increased cardiac output), part of which is due to release of adrenergic mediators from the adrenal medulla by histamine itself.

Histamine shock has been attributed primarily to excessive dilatation of capillaries which permits plasma to leave the capillaries, thus decreasing the circulating blood volume. The reflex discharge of epinephrine maintains good chronotropy and inotropy, but cardiac output remains low because of a stasis of blood in the capillaries, poor venous return, and decreased blood volume. Histamine hypotension can be prevented, to various degrees, by epinephrine and antihistamines.

Capillaries   Histamine can induce permeability alterations which lead to loss of plasma protein and fluid through the capillary wall to the extracellular space. Local injection of histamine into the skin of man (10 to 20 μg intracutaneously) increases capillary permeability and is manifested as the "triple response," described as follows: (1) a prompt reddening at the site of injection, due to local vasodilatation; (2) followed by a wheal or disk of localized edema, induced by the increased capillary permeability, which obscures the red spot; and (3) succeeded by the bright crimson flare or halo surrounding the wheal, which may be as large as 5 cm and may last approximately 10 min. Since degeneration or section of the peripheral sensory nerves prevents flare formation, it is probable that flare is a local phenomenon mediated by an axon reflex involving peripheral sensory nerves.

Smooth Muscle   In general, histamine stimulates smooth muscle. The uterus and bronchus are the most susceptible; the intestinal and arteriolar muscles are intermediate; and the urinary bladder, gallbladder, and iris are least susceptible to histamine effects. Histamine causes a marked bronchial constriction when administered to asthmatic subjects.

Histamine consistently stimulates ureteral smooth muscle, a tissue which does not respond to cholinergic or adrenergic challenge. Moreover, antihistamines abolish ureteral contractions, whether spontaneous or induced.

Exocrine Glands

Gastric Glands   Histamine stimulates the glands of the gastrointestinal tract (gastric, salivary, pancreatic). It also increases bronchial and lacrimal secretions. However, the gastric glands are most affected, and, indeed, this is thought to be one of the physiologic actions of histamine. Histamine administration to man causes proportionate increases in pepsin and gastric acid secretion. The rate of gastric secretion is directly influenced by changing the rate of blood flow; this probably accounts for the depressant effect of epinephrine and sympathetic nervous system stimulation. Histamine-induced gastric secretion is poorly antagonized by atropine and by most antihistaminic drugs, but acid secretion induced by other means is attenuated by the administration of inhibitors of histidine decarboxylase. It has been suggested that no chemostimulator is interposed between histamine and the parietal cell, implying thereby that many substances (for example, gastrin) which increase gastric secretion do so by releasing histamine. Histamine has been found in the mucosa and in the gastric juice. The ability of histamine to cause gastric acid secretion has been utilized to diagnose achlorhydria.

Tissue Growth

Tissues which are undergoing rapid growth (for example, embryonic, reparative after wounds, malignant) synthesize increasing amounts of histamine to enhance growth. This histamine, called "nascent" histamine, is not replaced by exogenous histamine. High histamine-forming capacity has been demonstrated in wound and granulation tissue in man, and wound healing can be facilitated or attenuated by manipulating histamine formation.

Receptors

Histamine apparently exerts its action via two types of receptors, H_1- and H_2-receptors. Contraction of the smooth muscle of the gastrointestinal tract and bronchi have been classified as being mediated through H_1-receptor activation. These smooth muscle responses to histamine are effectively antagonized by classical antihistamines such as pyrilamine. Stimulation of gastric secretion, inhibition of uterine contraction and an increase in heart rate have been shown to involve H_2-receptors. These are pyrilamine-insensitive actions of histamine. The identification of H_2-receptors has been made possible by the development of burimamide and metiamide, specific H_2-histamine receptor antagonists. Burimamide is the prototype of this new class of antihistamines and metiamide is now being tested clinically to diminish gastric acid secretion.

The cardiovascular responses to histamine have been shown to involve activation of both H_1- and H_2-receptors. It has been suggested that both H_1- and H_2-receptors can exist on a single blood vessel. Further investigation is necessary to establish if individual smooth muscle cells of certain blood vessels may possess both types (motor and inhibitory) of histamine receptors, just as they may possess both types of adrenergic receptors.

Because the H_2-receptor antagonists are not currently commercially available, the second section of this chapter is devoted exclusively to the classical antihistamines.

Toxicity

The symptoms of histamine toxicity can be easily predicted on the basis of its pharmacologic activities. The primary finding is a precipitous fall in blood pressure accompanied by generalized vasodilatation with skin temperature rise, headache, and visual disturbances. In addition, smooth-muscle stimulation leads to bronchial constriction, dyspnea, and diarrhea. Further effects noted are vomiting and a metallic taste. In severe cases, shock may supervene, and appropriate measures must be taken to treat this serious complication. In general, nonshock cases can best be treated with epinephrine. Antihistamines do not provide adequate therapy in cases of severe histamine toxicity.

Therapeutic Uses

The ubiquitous distribution of histamine throughout the various body tissues suggests that it serves some function and that small quantities of this amine may have some therapeutic effect. This may be especially true if there is a deficiency of histamine in the tissue. Though a deficiency has generally not been noted, many investigators have attempted to ascertain whether this amine might have any therapeutic efficacy. These efforts have met with little success.

Clinical use of histamine has thus been confined

to two areas: (1) *The gastric function test*. The gastric secretory response to an effective dose of histamine phosphate injected subcutaneously is approximately related to the functional parietal cell mass. If the total amount of gastric acid produced is lower than the expected normal values following histamine administration, it is indicative of true achlorhydria associated with the loss of parietal cell function. (2) *Histamine desensitization*. Repeated doses of histamine may reduce the sensitivity (desensitize) in an individual with an allergic disorder in which histamine may be an important factor. This procedure has rarely been successful.

Preparations and Dose

Histamine Phosphate Injection   Histamine phosphate injection contains histamine phosphate equivalent to 1 mg of histamine base in 1 ml. This requires the use of 3.07 mg of salt, since it is a diphosphate. The usual dose is 0.01 mg/kg of the histamine base, subcutaneously.

Betazole Hydrochloride   Betazole hydrochloride (Histalog) is a synthetic analogue of histamine, 3-(2-aminoethyl) pyrazole dihydrochloride. This drug effectively stimulates the secretion of gastric hydrochloric acid, with fewer side effects than are observed with histamine. Betazole produces less of a fall in blood pressure and has less tendency to increase heart rate. In certain patients, qualitatively similar histamine side effects are produced, such as flushing, sweating, and headache. Also, as with histamine, urticaria, faintness, and syncope are occasionally encountered. The drug is to be used with great caution in patients with bronchial asthma.

$$HC{=}\!\!=\!\!\!=\!\!\!=\!\!\!=\!\!C{-}CH_2{-}CH_2{-}NH_2 \text{ HCl}$$

Betazole hydrochloride

Betazole is available in ampuls containing 50 mg in 1 ml. The dose is 0.5 mg/kg intramuscularly or, preferably, subcutaneously to produce an equivalent response of 0.01 mg/kg histamine base. Because of the wide margin of safety, 50 mg is often used in normal-sized adults.

ANTIHISTAMINES

Antihistamines do not influence the formation or release of histamine, but selectively and competitively antagonize most of the actions of histamine at H_1-receptors. Antihistamines may also possess other less significant properties, for example, anticholinergic, antispasmodic, adrenergic blocking, and local anesthetic actions. Newer antihistaminic agents with "multiple blocking" actions (e.g., cyproheptadine, trimeprazine, and methdilazine) have been highlighted for their significant antiserotonin action in experimental animals, a characteristic known to be present in the older drug promethazine.

The predominant antihistaminic action probably explains the clinical utility of this class of compounds in general. Their other blocking actions, however, have become useful laboratory tools in a constant search for drugs that may have wider and more effective therapeutic utility.

Chemistry

Three naturally occurring amines, acetylcholine, epinephrine, and histamine possess an ethylamine

$$-\!\overset{|}{\underset{|}{C}}\!-\!\overset{|}{\underset{|}{C}}\!-\!N\!\!\big\langle \text{ group. Correspondingly, the ethyl-}$$

amine grouping may be quite regularly found not only in most antihistamines but also in many anticholinergic, ganglionic blocking, and adrenergic blocking agents. The same is evident in certain local anesthetics and antispasmodics. It is not too surprising, therefore, that many antihistamines exert various combinations and degrees of such actions coupled with the dominant antihistamine activity. Conversely, it is not uncommon for other classes of compounds, structurally related to antihistamines, to exhibit some lesser degree of the latter action.

The greater potency of the *d*-isomer of chlorpheniramine compared with that of the *l*-isomer or racemic mixture emphasizes the significance of optical isomerism in those antihistamines possessing an asymmetric carbon atom.

Most of the more active antihistamines may be represented by the general formula:

$$\begin{matrix} R_1 \\ \\ R_2 \end{matrix}\!\!\!\big\rangle X\!-\!\overset{|}{\underset{|}{C}}\!-\!\overset{|}{\underset{|}{C}}\!-\!N\!\!\big\langle\!\!\!\begin{matrix} R_3 \\ \\ R_4 \end{matrix}$$

where R_1 and R_2 (the nucleus) are carbocyclic or heterocyclic aromatic systems, one of which may or may not be separated from X by a methylene group, and X is oxygen, nitrogen, or carbon connecting the side chain to the nucleus. The ethylene group of the side chain may also be a 2-carbon fragment of a nitrogen-heterocyclic system (e.g., in cyclizine). Optimum activity is found when R_3 and R_4 are methyl groups. Activity may usually be increased by introducing para substituents into one of the rings of the nucleus (e.g., in chlorpheniramine).

The compounds depicted and described in Table 28-1 have been arranged as follows:

1 Ethylenediamines: when X is nitrogen.
2 Aminoalkyl ethers: when X is oxygen.
3 Alkylamines: when X is carbon.
4 Piperazines: when X is carbon in conjunction with a piperazine ring.
5 Phenothiazines: when X is nitrogen as part of the phenothiazine nucleus.

6 Miscellaneous: structures representing a departure from the above classification.

Pharmacologic Actions

Antihistamine Action   It is essential to the understanding of the classification and mode of action of these drugs that they be recognized as *specific* antagonists of the pharmacologic effects of histamine. The antihistaminic drugs block most of the actions of injected or endogenously released histamine without inducing diametrically opposite pharmacologic activities of their own. On the other hand, *nonspecific* action, sometimes referred to as "physiologic antagonism," would be characteristic of histamine antagonism by epinephrine since the latter amine produces prominent effects such as bronchodilation, vasoconstriction, and inhibition of intestinal motility, all of which tend to offset the opposite actions of histamine at these tissue sites.

Table 28-1   Common Antihistamines

Official or generic name	Trade name	Structure	Single oral dose for adults and remarks
1 Ethylenediamines			
Methapyrilene HCl	Histadyl Thenylene Semikon	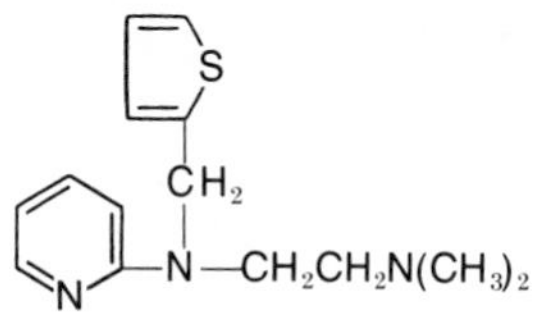	50–100 mg Sedation slight
Pyrilamine maleate	Neo-Antergan Paramal Stangen Thylogen	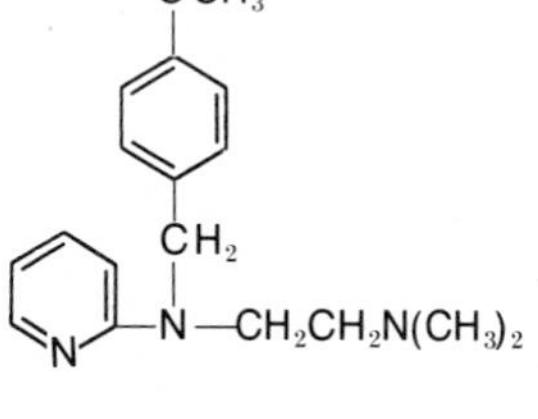	25–50 mg Sedation slight
Tripelennamine HCl	Pyribenzamine	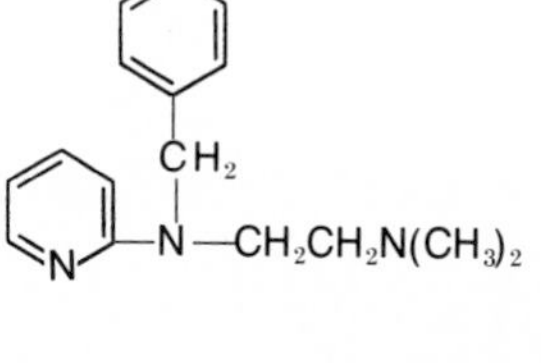	25–50 mg Sedation moderate

Table 28-1 Common Antihistamines (*Continued*)

Official or generic name	Trade name	Structure	Single oral dose for adults and remarks
		2 Aminoalkyl Ethers	
Dimenhydrinate	Dramamine (Chlorotheophyllinate of Benadryl)		50 mg Sedation marked Primarily used for motion sickness
Diphenhydramine HCl	Benadryl		25–50 mg Sedation marked
		3 Alkylamines	
Chlorpheniramine maleate	Chlor-Trimeton		4–8 mg Sedation slight
Dexchlorpheniramine maleate	Polaramine (*d*-isomer)		2–6 mg Sedation slight
		4 Piperazines	
Cyclizine HCl	Marezine		50 mg Sedation slight Primarily used for motion sickness
Meclizine HCl	Bonine		12.5–50 mg Sedation slight Primarily used for motion sickness

Table 28-1   Common Antihistamines (*Continued*)

Official or generic name	Trade name	Structure	Single oral dose for adults and remarks
5 Phenothiazines			
Trimeprazine tartrate	Temaril	(structure) $CH_2CHCH_2N(CH_3)_2$ CH_3	2.5 mg Sedation moderate Emphasis on pruritus
Promethazine HCl	Phenergan	(structure) $CH_2CHN(CH_3)_2$ CH_3	12.5–25 mg Sedation marked Preanesthetic adjunct Treatment of motion sickness, nausea, and vomiting
6 Miscellaneous			
Cyproheptadine HCl	Periactin	(structure) CH_3	4 mg Sedation moderate Emphasis on pruritus

Indeed, such responses result from the activation of receptors which differ from those for which histamine has a strong affinity. However, the antihistamines may be considered to have particular affinity for the specific receptors activated by the agonist histamine. In this case, they antagonize the action of histamine on certain tissue systems by means of a reversible union with a common receptor site but without eliciting an intrinsic action of their own at that site. This relationship of antagonist and agonist at similar receptor sites is also referred to as *competitive inhibition.*

There is no evidence that the action of antihistamines is in any way due to chemical or physical inactivation of histamine or to interference with its synthesis. Since the available antihistamines only antagonize the H_1-receptor actions of histamine, they should not be expected to prevent histamine-induced gastric secretion. Recent studies show that the parietal cells of the stomach have H_2-receptors only, which are appropriately antagonized by burimamide and metiamide.

The failure of antihistamines to relieve the bronchial spasm of asthma is probably because this disease is not mediated by histamine alone. Peptides such as kinins, slow-reacting substance–anaphylaxis (SRS–A), and acetylcholine are also involved. The success of cromolyn sodium in certain types of asthma is due not only to its prevention of the release of histamine but also of SRS–A from the mast cells.

Other Actions   Most of the known antihistamines exert some degree of *local anesthetic* action.

Numerous clinical studies have utilized diphen-hydramine or tripelennamine in the form of oint-ments or solutions for topical application.

Many antihistamines possess varying degrees of *anticholinergic* action, and more recent compounds also have considerable *antiserotonin* effects. None of these ancillary actions appears to be in any way related to antihistamine activity or potency.

The effects of antihistamines on the CNS (cen-tral nervous system) are complex and dose-related. Sedation and drowsiness are the most commonly encountered central manifestations following thera-peutic doses of antihistaminic drugs. There is no apparent correlation between peripheral antihista-minic effectiveness and central nervous system suppressant activity. Ordinary doses of antihista-mines may occasionally produce restlessness, ner-vousness, and insomnia. Toxic doses of antihista-mines produce an initial central nervous system depression followed by marked excitation associ-ated with sensory and motor disturbances and, in many instances, convulsions. Young children are especially sensitive to the central stimulant action of these drugs. After the excitatory phase, depres-sion or paralysis of vital centers may occur with administration of extremely large doses of anti-histaminic drugs.

Absorption, Fate, and Metabolism

The antihistamines as a class are generally well absorbed following oral or parenteral administra-tion. Although some decrease in effectiveness has been noted with prolonged usage, the development of any significant degree of tolerance has not been a problem with these drugs. Some tolerance, how-ever, to the sedative effects of certain antihista-mines has been observed. Metabolism and excre-tion is rapid without evident cumulative effects, and doses of most of these drugs must be repeated in about 4 h. Exception to this apparent rapid con-version to inactive metabolites is provided by mec-lizine, since the effects of a single dose may per-sist for 8 to 24 h. Only generalizations can be made about the fate of antihistamines in the body, since the sensitivity of chemical methods of analysis has not been great, and thus investigations appear to have been limited to a few compounds.

Toxicity

In man, the predominant central action is sedation, except in some children and certain adults in whom agitation, nervousness, delirium, tremors, and even convulsions may occur. The more commonly ob-served sedative action is noted in 20 to 50 percent of patients and varies from diminished alertness and impaired ability to concentrate to muscular weakness and marked drowsiness, even in a thera-peutic dose range. In some instances the physi-cians may make therapeutic use of this action to afford the allergic patient some relief when con-siderable loss of sleep has been a problem. A num-ber of more or less well-known antihistamines have recently become available as over-the-counter, "non-habit-forming" sedatives or "tranquilizers." The dangers inherent in this form of self-medica-tion as far as probable neglect of the need for proper diagnosis are evident.

Lesser side actions of antihistamines may mani-fest as loss of appetite, nausea, vomiting, epigastric distress, constipation, or diarrhea. Other untoward effects include possible dryness of the mouth, fre-quent urination, palpitation, hypertension or hypo-tension, headache, faintness, tightness of the chest, and visual disturbances. In spite of their antiallergic properties, these drugs may themselves cause urti-caria and dermatitis following topical or oral use. More serious but quite rare, hypersensitivity reac-tions are leukopenia and agranulocytosis.

The antihistamines generally possess high thera-peutic indices (toxic dose/therapeutic dose), and it is relatively rare to note serious toxicity from their use. Most of the lesser untoward actions may be alleviated by reducing the dose, change to another compound, administering the dose only at meal-time, etc. Perhaps the most serious potential hazard of the injudicious use of these drugs is accident-proneness (while driving vehicles or operating ma-chinery, for instance) as a result of drowsiness.

Administration of two of the antihistamines cyclizine and meclizine during pregnancy or to women who may become pregnant is contraindi-cated in view of the teratogenic effect of the drugs in laboratory animals.

Therapeutic Uses

Allergic diseases represent a complex series of dis-orders with acute and chronic manifestations which may vary from mild urticaria or rhinitis to severe and possibly fatal anaphylactic shock. It has been estimated that approximately 10 percent of the population suffers from some form of allergic disease, which places allergy third in prevalence among the chronic diseases in this country. Specific therapy directed toward removal of the offending allergen from the patient's environment (or vice versa) and treatment by desensitization is not always practical or successful. Difficulties in adequate diagnosis have been, in part, responsible for this situation. In a number of allergic disorders, the causative allergen(s) cannot be demonstrated, and associated chronic infection often complicates possible approaches to therapy. Therefore, in conjunction with direct treatment, symptomatic management with a variety of drugs has been common practice.

Because of differing criteria involved in estimating drug effectiveness and the basic variability inherent in using the patient's subjective interpretation of response, it is difficult to assess many of the clinical reports on the therapeutic efficacy of these drugs. However, acceptance of efficacy has developed over years of experience with most of the established antihistamines.

Dermatoses The antihistamines are probably most effective in the treatment of acute and chronic urticaria, the itching and wheal reactions usually being rapidly relieved in 70 to 80 percent of patients. Angioneurotic edema also responds favorably. Effectiveness may vary with the nature of the provoking antigen, as well as idiosyncratic or hypersensitive reactions to drugs. Good responses to oral or topical antihistamines may also be achieved following insect bites or stings. The antihistamines are effective in only about 50 percent of patients with atopic dermatitis or eczema and seem principally to alleviate the characteristic pruritus. Some antihistamines, such as trimeprazine and cyproheptadine, have been reported to be effective especially against pruritus. The sedative effect of some of these and other agents may reduce the urge to scratch by decreasing the associated anxiety and tension. Similarly, the itching and urticaria as a consequence of serum sickness may be considerably relieved by antihistamines, although the joint involvement and fever may require other therapy.

Allergic Rhinitis Seasonal rhinitis ("hay fever" or pollinosis) is partially or completely relieved in about 80 percent of patients suffering from pruritus of the nose, eyes, ears, and throat as well as from rhinorrhea, sneezing, and nasal mucous membrane congestion. Antihistamine therapy is especially effective when used in conjunction with successful desensitization and in combination with decongestants such as phenylephrine or pseudoephedrine. The antihistamines also are useful in the prevention of systemic allergic responses resulting from desensitization procedures.

In vasomotor or perennial rhinitis, at least partial relief is afforded some 50 percent of the patients. The chronic nature of this form of rhinitis requires the particular use of more direct therapy as well as other palliative measures for better efficacy in relieving congested sinuses and headache.

Bronchial Asthma The development of specific and potent antagonists of histamine held great promise for more effective treatment of bronchial asthma. Unfortunately, none of the newer antihistamines has changed the relatively unsatisfactory results of these drugs in asthmatic patients. A small percentage of those afflicted (especially children) are helped when an allergic component is the predominant feature of this complex disease.

Common Cold Unfortunately, a somewhat negative attitude developed toward the antihistamines when the short-lived saga of their "curative" effect on the common cold was discredited by controlled placebo studies. When the excitement over exaggerated claims and conflicting statements subsided, it was evident that the antihistamines were generally considered as simple palliative agents instead of "miraculous cures." Of the latter, in pharmacotherapy, there are few; of the former, there are many utilized in accepted standard therapeutics. Although it is now well established that the common cold has a viral etiology, an allergic component probably exists, and of course, many purely allergic conditions are easily confused with the common cold. Low doses of selected antihistamines combined with other traditional agents will continue to provide some degree of symptomatic relief to many common cold victims while producing relatively mild, if any, side effects.

Motion Sickness and Emesis The antimotion and antiemetic sickness actions of certain antihistaminic drugs seem to be more related to central anticholinergic activity than to peripheral antihistamine activity. Moreover, the central nervous system depressant action of antihistamines in man may be a basic factor in their effects on the vertigo, giddiness, dizziness, tinnitus, nausea, vomiting, and prostration which may be present in airsickness, seasickness, or swingsickness. These and other forms of labyrinthine disturbances have generally been ameliorated by treatment with anticholinergic agents such as atropine or related belladonna alkaloids. The barbiturates have also been used with some success. Particular antihistamines (usually piperazines or phenothiazines) such as meclizine, cyclizine, promethazine, and dimenhydrinate have been found especially helpful in alleviating most symptoms of disturbed equilibrium while producing minimal side effects. Various degrees of effectiveness as antiemetic agents have been reported for many of the phenothiazine tranquilizers. Most of these drugs possess only slight antihistaminic and anticholinergic actions.

Miscellaneous Several other uses of antihistamines relate to the prevention and treatment of allergic reactions to blood transfusion or reactions to intravenously administered x-ray contrast media. The drugs are less effective when such reactions are particularly severe, especially if they are anaphylactoid in nature.

Drugs such as diphenhydramine, which possesses both antihistaminic and anticholinergic activity, have had some utility as adjuncts in the therapy of Parkinson's disease.

Preparations and Doses

Table 28-1 lists twelve common antihistamines. Many physicians familiar with the advantages and disadvantages of each prefer to have a working pool of antihistamine drugs for selection and variation as indicated by individual patient need in terms of efficacy and side effects. Few other classes of drugs possess such depth in type and number for choice by the physician and acceptance by the patient.

Part Eight

Endocrines

Chapter 29

Thyroid and Parathyroid Drugs

THYROID HORMONES AND ANTITHYROID DRUGS

The thyroid gland exerts a profound metabolic control over the body through two iodine-containing amino acid hormones, triiodothyronine (T_3) and thyroxine (T_4). These hormones regulate general body metabolism by controlling the rate of the cellular oxidative processes. The activity of the thyroid gland is directly regulated by a pituitary thyroid-stimulating hormone (TSH), thyrotropin.

Anatomically, the thyroid is a bilateral organ in the neck. It consists of vesicles lined by cubical epithelium surrounding a follicular cavity containing a colloidal iodinated protein, thyroglobulin. In addition to T_4 and T_3, the thyroid gland secretes a third hormone, calcitonin.

Normal Thyroid Function

The absorption of iodide, as well as biosynthesis, secretion, and degradation of active thyroid hormones, occur by means of complex metabolic pathways. The major steps are described below and summarized in Table 29-1.

Dietary Intake Dietary inorganic iodide (I^-) is absorbed as such. Molecular inorganic iodine (I_2) is reduced in the gut to iodide and is then absorbed. Nonthyroidal organic iodine compounds are absorbed and then biotransformed by reductive dehalogenation in the liver, yielding inorganic iodide to the iodide pool.

Human dietary intake varies considerably according to the local iodine content of the soil and water, and the variations among culturally determined eating habits. The euthyroid individual may ingest 150 to 200 μg of iodine daily and eliminate the same amount in the urine and feces. About 80 to 90 percent of the iodine is excreted in the urine, while 10 to 20 percent is eliminated in the feces. The metabolic products of the thyroid hormones are excreted in the feces.

Table 29-1 Steps In Iodide Oxidation, Organification, and Secretion

Step	Stimulated by	Inhibited by
1 Uptake of circulated iodide ion by thyroid	Thiocyanate, nitrite, and perchlorate ions	
2 Enzymatic oxidation of iodide ion to active iodine	TSH	Thiocarbamides
3 Reaction of active iodine with tyrosine groups on thyroglobulin to form monoiodotyrosine and diiodotyrosine groups		
4 Combination of monoiodotyrosine and diiodotyrosine groups on thyroglobulin to form T_4 and T_3		
5 Storage of the iodinated thyroglobulin in the colloid of the thyroid gland		
6 Proteolysis of iodinated thyroglobulin and secretion of T_4 and T_3	TSH	Iodide ion (high concentrations)
7 Circulating T_4 and T_3 on alpha globulin and prealbumin inhibits secretion of TSH by anterior pituitary		

Iodide Uptake by Thyroid Usually about half of the daily intake of iodine (approximately 150 to 200 μg) is "trapped" by the thyroid gland, while most of the remainder is excreted by the kidney. In the normal thyroid, this active transport system is capable of sustaining an intracellular iodide concentration 25 to 40 times higher than that of the extracellular fluid; TSH stimulates this uptake. The iodide "trapping mechanism" of the thyroid requires energy which is supplied by actively respiring thyroid cells, and has been linked to potassium transport. Since there is little free iodine in the thyroid gland (less than 0.2 percent of the total thyroidal iodine), this trapping process can be regraded as the rate-limiting step in thyroid hormone formation.

Iodide Oxidation and Organification The sequential reactions involved in iodide oxidation and organification are: (1) oxidation of iodide ion to a form that serves as an iodinating reagent; (2) iodination of tyrosyl groups in preformed thyroprotein to form iodotyrosines; and (3) coupling of two peptide-bound iodotyrosines to form peptide-bound iodothyronine.

The oxidation of iodide probably is catalyzed by an iodide-peroxidase in the microsomal fraction since the reaction requires molecular oxygen and a source of hydrogen peroxide. The product of this peroxidation has not been identified because of its extreme reactivity, which results in instantaneous iodination of the tyrosyl groups. Hypoiodite (IO^-) or iodinium ion (I^+) have been postulated as the intermediate. Tyrosine groups of thyroglobulin readily react with the highly active iodine, forming monoiodotyrosine (MIT) and diiodotyrosine (DIT) (see Fig. 29-1). Two DIT molecules or one DIT and one MIT molecule aerobically condense to form T_4 and T_3 (Fig. 29-1), respectively, in the approximate ratio of 3:1. Two MIT molecules do not condense because the nature of the biosynthetic reaction is such that DIT must remain in peptide linkage during the coupling reaction; consequently DIT must be at least one of the two reaction partners. T_3 and T_4 are stored in the colloid of the follicular cavity as a moiety of the thyroglobulin molecule.

Thyroglobulin is a large protein (mol. wt. 670,-000) containing approximately 5,000 amino acid residues of which 110 to 120 are tyrosyl residues. As the thyroglobulin molecule is folded, only about 10 percent of the tyrosines are iodinated and of these, only a few are coupled to form thyronine. Thus there are only about 3 thyronines per molecule of thyroglobulin. The iodine in thyroglobulin is distributed approximately as follows: 30 percent in T_4, 10 percent in T_3, 20 percent in MIT, and 40 percent in DIT.

Secretion of T_3 and T_4 The thyroglobulin molecule is too large to leave the thyroid and hence secretion follows proteolysis, removing the T_4 and T_3 from the thyroglobulin molecules. T_4 and T_3

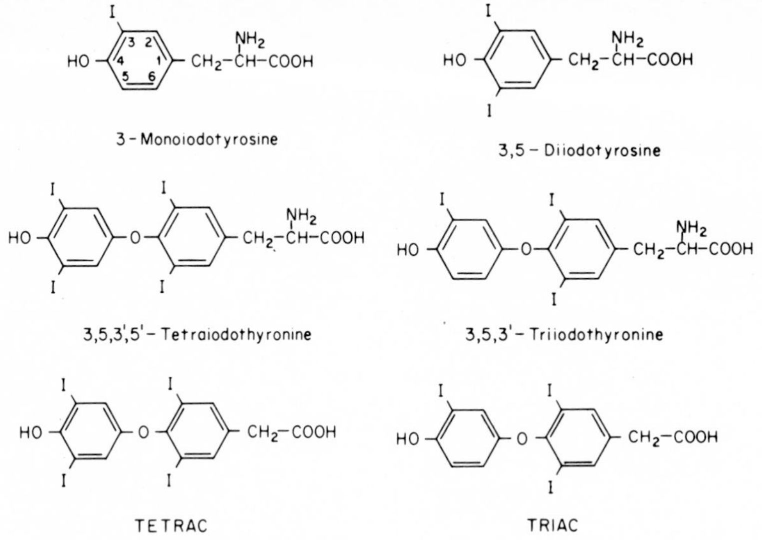

Figure 29-1 Thyroid iodoamino acids and metabolites.

then enter the bloodstream. This step is blocked by large doses of iodide and enhanced by TSH. Normally, 75 μg of T_4 and 25 μg of T_3 are released daily.

Plasma Binding and Transport of Thyroid Hormones T_4 and T_3 are transported in the bloodstream bound firmly but reversibly to plasma proteins. Most of the thyroid hormones are bound to an α_2-globulin called thyroxine-binding globulin (TBG) or to a prealbumin called thyroxine-binding prealbumin (TBPA), while only approximately 1 percent of T_4 and T_3 circulates unbound. One indication of the blood levels of bound hormone is the serum protein-bound iodine (PBI). The binding protects the thyroid hormones from loss in the urine and also serves as a reservoir which regulates the peripheral supply of hormone in the free active form. Tissue utilization of thyroid hormones results in a reduction in the peripheral level of T_3 and T_4, shifting the balance to favor dissociation of the protein-bound complex. By this mechanism it is possible for the free hormone to be delivered to the peripheral tissues at rates proportional to the metabolic requirement of each tissue.

Metabolism and Excretion Thyroxine has a half-life of 16 to 17 days in a euthyroid person. The rate

of removal of circulating hormone is reduced in hypothyroidism, but the rate of secretion is reduced even more. In hyperthyroidism the rate of removal is greater than normal, but the rate of secretion is greater than that. The three major sites of metabolic alteration of the iodothyronine molecules are the phenolic hydroxyl group, the carbamino grouping of the side chain, and the carbon-iodine linkages.

Of the physiologically important reactions, all can be carried out by the liver, both in vivo and in vitro. Kidney and muscle are other sites of one or more of the degradative processes. In the liver, T_4 is conjugated mainly as the glucuronide while T_3 is conjugated mainly as the sulfate. After excretion via the bile duct, the conjugates are hydrolyzed in the intestine, possibly by bacterial enzymes, and most of the T_4 and T_3 reenter the blood via the hepatic portal vessel. Approximately 10 to 20 percent is excreted in the feces.

Two other important products of liver and kidney metabolism, tetraiodothyroacetic acid (TETRAC) and triiodothyroacetic acid (TRIAC) are measured in diagnostic tests. These metabolites are products of oxidative deamination, transamination, and decarboxylation of the alanine side chain of T_4 and T_3. They are subject to conjugation and deiodination just as are the parent compounds.

Hormonal Actions of T_3 and T_4 At very low concentrations, the thyroid hormones initiate normal growth and development. The mechanism of this growth-promoting quality is throught to be initiation of the incorporation of amino acids into specific proteins. At higher concentrations, the thyroid hormones have been shown to induce many oxidative enzymes and to uncouple oxidative phosphorylation. This results in increased heat production and oxygen consumption. Although liver, muscle, kidney, and heart, among others, are involved, some, such as the brain, lymph nodes, spleen, and testes, are apparently not stimulated in this manner by the thyroid hormones.

Many aspects of carbohydrate and lipid metabolism are affected by thyroid hormones, either alone or in combination with other hormones. These include:

1 Increased intestinal absorption of glucose and galactose
2 Potentiation of the glycogenolytic-hyperglycemic and lipolytic actions of epinephrine
3 Potentiation of insulin-induced glycogen synthesis and glucose utilization
4 Reduced serum cholesterol level
5 Increased uptake of glucose by adipose tissue
6 Increased mobilization of free fatty acids from adipose tissue (in part through potentiation of epinephrine)
7 Maturation of the CNS

Thyroid hormones decrease the level of serum cholesterol by stimulating cholesterol degradation in excess of biosynthesis. These hormones also increase coenzyme and vitamin requirements probably indirectly through increased metabolic demand.

Disorders of Thyroid Function

Thyroid hormone disease states may be the result either of overproduction of thyroid hormone, *hyperthyroidism,* or underproduction of thyroid hormone, *hypothyroidism.* In either case, the physical manifestations can be a goiter or swelling of the thyroid glands. In hypothyroidism, due to insufficient iodine intake, the negative-feedback mechanism of the thyroid hormones on the pituitary does not function and an increase in TSH secretion results, causing the gland to hypertrophy. In

hyperthyroidism, goiter may or may not be present. A goiter indicates that either the negative-feedback system that shuts off TSH does not function or that another hormone that stimulates the thyroid is being secreted, namely long-acting thyroid stimulating hormone (LATS) which is not controllable by the feedback mechanisms of the thyroid. LATS and TSH have identical stimulatory effects on thyroidal growth and iodine metabolism.

Hypothyroidism A variety of causes may produce hypothyroidism. Thyrotic cretinism may be due to failure of the gland to develop, to synthesis failure, or to defects in the releasing mechanism. At birth, cretins may be recognized by a puffy expressionless face and reduced general body metabolism. If not treated immediately, irreversible brain changes may occur. Treatment is by replacement therapy with the various thyroid hormones in the pure or impure forms. Failure of thyrotropin secretion by the pituitary may also occur, and replacement therapy with thyroid hormones is again indicated. Myxedema or severe thyroid deficiency in the adult can be recognized by thick, dry skin, dullness, and generally lower body metabolism. Here, depending on the cause (i.e., lack of dietary iodine, thyroiditis, or autoimmune disease), treatment varies.

Drugs Used in Hypothyroidism Several thyromimetic preparations are available for the lifelong management of the irreversibly hypothyroid patient, or for interim treatment of reversible endemic goiter.

Preparations and Dosage

Thyroid (Desiccated Thyroid) The U.S.P. specifications require 0.2 percent organic iodine content, although some preparations with the specified iodine content may prove to be inactive. Both T_4 and T_3 are present and account for its activity. The usual replacement dose is 15 to 600 mg/day.

Thyroglobulin (Proloid) Partially purified, this drug is standardized chemically by its iodine content, and biologically by the stimulation of metabolic rate in test animals. The dosage is the same as for thyroid, although some preparations of thyroglobulin may be less active on a weight basis than thyroid.

Levothyroxine Sodium (L-T_4) This is a pure synthetic substance. The usual replacement dose is 25 to 400 μg/day.

Liothyronine Sodium (L-T_3) This is a pure synthetic substance which has the most rapid action of all the thyromimetic preparations. The usual replacement dose is 50 to 75 μg/day given in divided doses.

Liotrix This preparation is a mixture of L-T_4 and L-T_3 at a 4:1 ratio. It mimics the natural secretion of the thyroid gland and provides an onset and duration of action similar to the natural hormone. The usual replacement dose is 150 to 200 μg/day.

Although the euthyroid state may be maintained with any of the above preparations, the serum PBI varies with the therapeutic agent. The low PBI observed with T_3 therapy results from the low plasma binding and rapid metabolic turnover of this agent. However, the use of T_3 is indicated when rapid results are required, as in the treatment of myxedema coma or in correcting the severe myalgia of iatrogenic hypothyroidism which occasionally occurs in overtreatment of thyrotoxicosis.

The L-enantiomorphs of the main thyroid hormones, T_4 and T_3, have the greatest goiter-preventing and basal metabolic rate (BMR)-raising potency. On the one hand, the D-form has 5 times more cholesterol-lowering capacity than does the L-form. L-Triiodothyronine has approximately 8 times the BMR-raising and goiter-preventing capacity of L-thyroxine.

Toxicity Untoward effects of thyroid hormone therapy may result from relative overdosage. These take the form of symptoms of hyperthyroidism variably accompanied by psychotic behavior, angina pectoris, cardiac decompensation, myalgia, severe diarrhea, or adrenal insufficiency.

Other Uses for Thyroid Hormone Thyroid hormones have been used somewhat uncritically in the treatment of female infertility, menorrhagia, habitual abortion, and obesity. In the euthyroid woman, the ingestion of a replacement dose of desiccated thyroid (120 to 180 mg/day) inhibits endogenous thyroid hormone production without altering the plasma-free T_3 level. Thus the exogenous material merely substitutes for the endogenous and does not alter the euthyroid state. However, in the habitual

aborter with decreased thyroid reserve, treatment with thyroid hormone in early pregnancy may prevent spontaneous abortion.

In order to obtain weight loss in the euthyroid obese patient, it is necessary to administer large amounts of thyroid hormone, sufficient to produce hypermetabolism and iatrogenic thyrotoxicosis. However, such a practice is to be condemned.

Hyperthyroidism Excessive production of the thyroid hormones may be due to an excess of TSH, lack of inhibition of TSH release, or the presence of LATS. Clinical symptoms include loss of weight and generally increased metabolism with increased appetite, heat production, perspiration, tachycardia, muscle weakness, and anxiety.

Drugs Used in Hyperthyroidism Each step in the synthesis, release, and blood transport of thyroid hormone is subject to pharmacologic interference, generally leading to a reduction in the activity of the thyroid gland. Antithyroid drugs are used to decrease the production of thyroid hormones in hyperthyroidism. In less intense cases, iodine or a thiocarbamide agent (see below) may control the excessive thyroid hormone production. Drugs which cause a reduction of thyroid hormone synthesis or secretion may be classified and used as follows.

Iodide Iodide may be supplied in the form of strong iodine solution (Lugol's solution) or potassium iodide solution. Although small amounts of iodide are required for hormone synthesis, larger amounts block synthesis. The action of iodide is primarily to inhibit the release of thyroid hormone, and secondarily to block the organic binding of iodine. When used for long periods of time, however, the inhibition of thyroid hormone release is overcome and the thyroid hormone stored in the gland pours out, causing an acute hyperthyroid condition known as thyroid storm. This may occur after a few weeks or months of use. Iodide use in hyperthyroidism is now usually limited to preparation for surgery. Iodide before surgery renders the gland less vascular by shrinking it, and hence facilitates surgical removal.

Radioactive Iodine (^{131}I) ^{131}I has been employed at low doses for diagnosis of thyroid function, although it has been found useful in some cases of hyperthyroidism for partial or full destruction of the gland at higher doses. [131]I has a half-life of 8 days, and emits both beta and gamma rays. The beta rays have ionizing properties and thus destroy cells, but their poor penetration (1 to 2 mm) renders them undetectable by instruments outside the body; gamma rays penetrate much further, and can be used for diagnostic purposes.

Certain types of thyroid cancer may respond to radioiodine therapy because they take up iodine; however, the anaplastic type does not take up iodine and therefore does not respond. However, radioiodine therapy does not dispense with the ultimate need for surgical removal of the primary growth.

Ionic Inhibitors Competitive inhibition of the iodide-trapping mechanism of the thyroid occurs with a group of monovalent hydrated anions, including thiocyanate (SCN^-), nitrite (NO_2^-), and perchlorate (ClO_4^-). Excessive amounts of iodide can reverse these inhibitions. Potassium perchlorate, at daily doses of 0.6 to 1.0 g, may be used where toxic reactions from the thiocarbamide-type drugs have occurred.

Thiocarbamide (Thiouracil)-type Drugs These drugs (Fig. 29-2) inhibit the organification of iodide in the thyroid gland by interfering with the oxidation of iodide to active iodine and by inhibiting the coupling of iodotyrosines. Since all these compounds are strong reducing agents, it is thought that they act by reducing active iodine back to iodide.

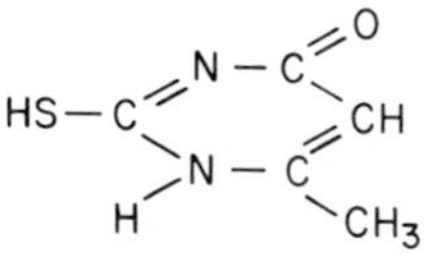

Methylthiouracil

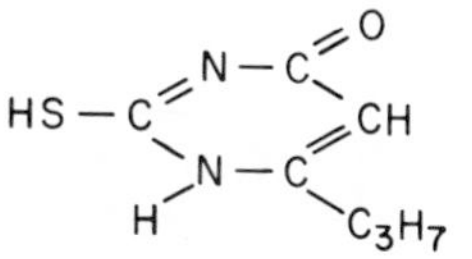

Propylthiouracil

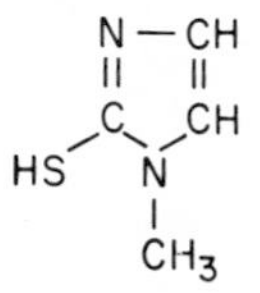

Methimazole

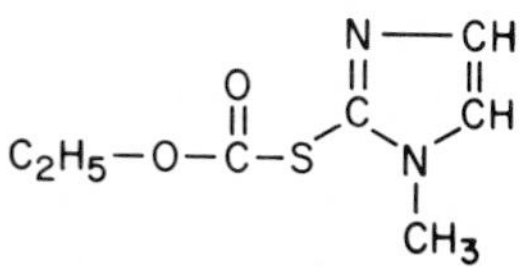

Carbimazole

Figure 29-2 Structures of thiocarbamide agents.

Thiocarbamides may be employed as the sole therapeutic agent in the treatment of hyperthyroidism. Prolonged administration (for 1 to 2 years) is often accompanied by gradual remission of the disease, with no return of the hyperthyroidism even after withdrawal of the drug. Administration of a full blocking dose of antithyroid drug along with 60 to 120 mg desiccated thyroid to the hyperthyroid pregnant woman prevents the development of goiter in the newborn infant. However, since thiocarbamides may enter the milk, mothers who are ingesting these drugs should refrain from breastfeeding their infants.

After a prolonged course of antithyroid drug therapy, a trial without the drug may be attempted when there is evidence of reduced thyroid size and vascularity (loss of bruit), and the patient appears to be in good health. The long-term remission rate has been reported to be 40 to 70 percent.

If the patient is extremely toxic, the antithyroid drug should be given to induce partial remission prior to the administration of a therapeutic dose of radioiodine. This will obviate thyroid storm. Furthermore, if a patient has received radioiodine therapy and remains hyperthyroid, the thiocarbamide derivatives may be given during the 3-month waiting period prior to the administration of a second therapeutic dose of radioiodine.

Untoward reactions to thiocarbamides consist of fever, skin rash, edema, urticaria, myalgia, jaundice, gastrointestinal upset, lymphadenopathy, arthralgia, agranulocytosis, and possible death. Although many of the reactions may be exceedingly severe, they usually disappear within a week or two of cessation of medication. Sore throat and high fever during the early months of treatment may indicate the development of agranulocytosis.

Preparations and Dosage Propylthiouracil is available in 50-mg tablets. The usual dosage range is 100 to 900 mg/day.

Methimazole (Tapazole) is available in 5- and 10-mg tablets. The usual dosage range is 5 to 60 mg/day.

Methylthiouracil is not available in a pharmaceutical dosage form. The usual dosage is 50 mg, 4 times daily.

Carbimazole is not available in a pharmaceutical dosage form. The usual dosage is 10 mg, 3 times daily.

PARATHYROID HORMONE, CALCITONIN, VITAMIN D, AND CALCIUM

Calcium metabolism in the body is controlled by parathyroid hormone, vitamin D, and calcitonin (Fig. 29-3).

An adult human contains approximately 1200 g of calcium; about 10 g is found in the extracellular fluid and soft tissues, while the remainder (approximately 99 percent) is deposited in bone. The normal concentration of total plasma calcium, which is divided about equally between free ionic calcium and calcium loosely bound to plasma proteins (Table 29-2), is 8.8 to 10.3 mg/100 ml plasma. This range of concentrations of calcium in plasma also is apparently ideal for normal growth and development of the skeleton and dentition and for the maintenance of healthy bone.

One of the principal functions of calcium is at the cellular membrane—a decrease causing less stability, an increase causing greater stability. For in-

stance, nerve fiber membranes in the presence of low calcium become partially depolarized and therefore transmit repetitive and uncontrolled impulses. Spasm or tetany of skeletal muscles may result. Very high concentrations of calcium ions depress neurons in the CNS presumably because membranes will not depolarize. Serum calcium homeostatis is intimately related to calcium metabolism in bone and also, to some extent, to calcium absorption and excretion.

Parathyroid Hormone

Source and Chemistry Parathyroid hormone (PTH) is secreted by four parathyroid glands, each about 30 to 35 mg in weight. They are situated near the thyroid. Histologically, the normal human parathyroid gland consists of closely packed sheets of chief cells which measure 6 to 8 μ in diameter, usually with a rather eosinophilic cytoplasm. There are also present a large number of oxyphil cells

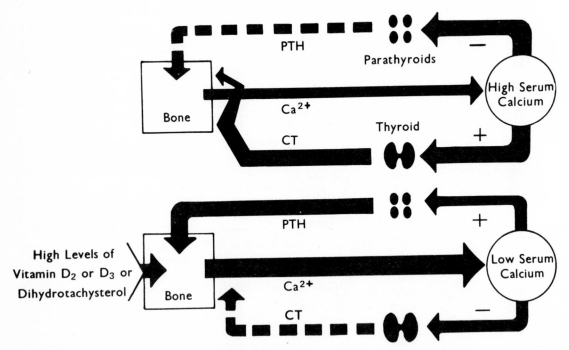

Figure 29-3 PTH and calcitonin act in opposite directions to provide the key elements in a reciprocal control system that regulates serum calcium. Calcitonin with phosphate (above) acts to inhibit bone resorption, while PTH with vitamin D or dihydrotachysterol (below) acts to stimulate it.

Table 29-2 Distribution of Calcium in Human Plasma

Form	% of total
Ionized	48
Protein-bound	46
Complexed	3
Unidentified	3

(large cells with eosinophilic cytoplasm). Both types of cells contain secretory granules.

PTH is a polypeptide chain of 84 amino acids. Human porcine, and bovine hormones are of the same size but exhibit some differences in amino acid composition. Its release is regulated by the blood calcium level; a drop in serum calcium stimulates PTH secretion.

Effects of PTH The major physiologic function of PTH is to raise the concentration of calcium ion in the plasma to the optimum level for efficient neuromuscular activity. On removal of the source of parathyroid hormone, the plasma calcium may fall within a few days to 7 mg/100 ml; if therapy is not instituted promptly, tetany (tonic spasms of the muscles) may ensue which could lead to death, usually from respiratory paralysis. If, on the other hand, there is an excess of circulating PTH, either as in spontaneous hyperparathyroidism or following administration of PTH, the plasma calcium rises above the normal level (see Fig. 29-3).

The sites of action of PTH are bone, kidney, and intestine. It increases the resorption of bone and thus the calcium and phosphate in the serum. PTH has a phosphaturic effect on the kidney, since it inhibits the reabsorption of inorganic phosphate from the renal tubule, and has also been reported to increase calcium reabsorption. PTH, in conjunction with vitamin D, increases the absorption of calcium in the intestine. Vitamin D, however, is the principal factor for intestinal calcium absorption.

Bone The most important source of calcium for the increase in plasma calcium effected by PTH is bone. The calcium of the teeth is not available for resorption by the hormone. Effects on calcium absorption from the intestine and on reabsorption of calcium by the renal tubule, although not insignificant, are relatively secondary in importance.

Most of the calcium and phosphate in bone exists in a highly crystalline form similar but not identical to hydroxyapatite, which has the composition $Ca_{10}(PO_4)_6(OH)_2$. The process of bone calcification involves the crystallization of the calcium phosphate complex in the bone matrix, which consists largely of collagen arranged in a highly organized manner.

Based on current evidence, it seems likely that both mechanisms of bone resorption, osteocytic and osteoclastic, are physiologically important. Osteocytic osteolysis may be the principal mechanism for rapid mobilization of calcium from bone, particularly in response to the initial action of parathyroid hormone. The role of the osteoclast may be more important in the normal remodeling of bone and in long-term effects of continued stimulation of bone resorption due to PTH and other metabolic agents. The effect of PTH on the blood-calcium level thus is dependent on the dynamic state of calcium, both in blood and bone. Calcium is constantly leaving the blood to participate in the formation of new bone and constantly entering the blood from bone as the result of resorption. In the adult the two processes are normally in balance. When circulating PTH increases, the rate of bone resorption increases. Therefore, without a corresponding increase in bone formation, the blood-calcium level increases. When circulating PTH decreases, as after parathyroidectomy, bone resorption decreases and, since there is no corresponding decrease in bone formation, the blood-calcium level decreases.

Kidney The phosphaturic effect of PTH has been shown to result from a direct inhibitory action on the reabsorption of inorganic phosphate by the renal proximal convoluted tubule. Purified PTH, unlike the crude extract, has no effect on the renal clearance of calcium.

Intestine Vitamin D is the principal factor responsible for promoting the absorption of calcium from the intestine. However, there are a few investigations utilizing both in vivo and in vitro systems which indicate that PTH may also stimulate calcium absorption. The long lag in onset of action and persistence of the action as PTH disappears from blood suggests that the effect is indirect.

Preparation and Administration The only commercially available parathyroid hormone preparation for medical use is Parathyroid Injection. It is given subcutaneously or intramuscularly. An elevation of the serum calcium is usually evident within 4 h if at all, reaching a maximum in 8 to 16 h and returning to the control level in 20 to 24 h. If continued effect is desired, the dose may be repeated at intervals of 12 h. Parathyroid Injection may also be administered intravenously for more rapid onset of effect, but the duration of the effect is much shorter after subcutaneous or intramuscular injection.

There is a very limited market for PTH because of the length of time required to reach the peak effect, the short duration of action, and the possible antigenicity of the animal preparations. In addition, calcium injections can substitute more effectively where a rapid increase in serum calcium is necessary; for long-term treatment the vitamin D derivatives are more effective, since they can be given orally and antigenicity is not a factor.

Calcitonin

When hypercalcemic blood is perfused through the thyroid gland, a hypocalcemic hormone, called calcitonin or thyrocalcitonin, is secreted. The cell of origin in the thyroid gland appears to be the light or C cell. Calcitonin has been isolated from the thyroid gland of humans and many other mammals, as well as from the ultimobranchial gland of birds and fish. It is also prepared synthetically. In all cases it is a polypeptide consisting of a 32 amino acid chain. The first 25 amino acids from the N terminus appear to be necessary for full activity. The amino acids appear to differ in different species.

Mechanism of Action Calcitonin is hypocalcemic and hypophosphatemic. However, the normal output of thyrocalcitonin by the thyroid gland is not sufficient to produce hypocalcemia. Removal of the thyroid gland does not result in elevation of the blood-calcium level under usual circumstances. Replacement therapy of calcitonin in the absence of the thyroid gland would consist of enough hormone to prevent hypercalcemia in the face of a calcium challenge, but not so much as to produce hypocalcemia.

The major site of action of calcitonin is bone, where it inhibits resorption, and thus calcium is retained in bone. The ionized calcium of the plasma, approximately 50 percent of the total plasma calcium, is in rapid equilibrium with the surface mineral phase of bone. However, a portion of the calcium leaving the blood is not exchanged; it enters into the process of bone accretion, which occurs constantly due to bone remodeling even after the growth period is over. Normally the calcium lost from the blood for bone accretion is balanced by an equal amount returned to the blood from bone due to resorption.

Absorption, Metabolism, and Fate Calcitonin is inactive orally, probably because of its polypeptide nature which makes it nonabsorbable and susceptible to the action of proteolytic enzymes. It is active when administered intravenously, intraperitoneally, or subcutaneously. Porcine calcitonin is rapidly inactivated by one or more heat labile factors in serum, which may contribute to the rapid disappearance rate. The eventual fate of calcitonin is uncertain. It has not yet been identified in urine.

Regulation of Secretion The rate of secretion of calcitonin is regulated by the calcium concentration of the blood flowing through the thyroid gland, rising as the level of calcium increases, and falling as it decreases. The thyrocalcitonin-secreting cells probably respond to ionic calcium rather than to total calcium in the blood.

Toxicity Nausea and vomiting have been noted in about 10 percent of patients treated with calcitonin. Local inflammatory reactions at the subcutaneous or intramuscular site of injection have been observed. Because calcitonin and gelatin (diluent) are protein in nature, the possibility of a systemic allergic reaction is always present.

Preparation, Dosage, and Administration Calcitonin (Calcimar) is available as a lyophilized powder, 400 MRC (Medical Research Council) units per vial, with 20 mg of hydrolyzed gelatin. The recommended starting dosage in advanced Paget's disease is 100 MRC units daily administered subcutaneously or intramuscularly.

Vitamin D

Vitamin D (calciferol) is formed from plant and animal precursors. Ultraviolet radiation of skin converts 7-dehydrocholesterol (formed in animals) to cholecalciferol (vitamin D_3) and also converts ergosterol (formed in plants) to ergocalciferol (vitamin D_2). The major storage form of vitamin D in humans is cholecalciferol.

Pharmacology of the Vitamin D Preparations Various vitamin D preparations such as D_2 (ergocalciferol), D_3 (cholecalciferol), and dihydrotachysterol have been used with success in hypocalcemic states. The effects of these vitamin D preparations are compared with PTH in Table 29-3.

Vitamin D_2 or D_3 in pharmacologic doses of 50,000 to 250,000 units/day or dihydrotachysterol at 1 mg/day have been used to replace PTH. Serum calcium is increased to normal levels by increased gastrointestinal calcium absorption rather than by the resorption of bone with these preparations (see Fig. 29-3). In the case of vitamin D excess, a hypercalcemia is produced with metastatic calcification to soft tissues.

Hypoparathyroidism

Hypoparathyroidism is a metabolic abnormality characterized by hypocalcemia and consequent neuromuscular symptoms. The disease results from a deficiency of PTH production or, more rarely, end-organ resistance to the action of the hormone.

The most common cause of hypoparathyroidism is removal of the parathyroid glands or trauma to the glands or their vascular supply during thyroid surgery. In *idiopathic hypoparathyroidism*, the parathyroid glands are usually absent or atrophied.

Many of the symptoms of hypoparathyroidism reflect altered neuromuscular irritability due to decreased concentration of ionized calcium in the plasma; they can be abolished by restoring the blood calcium toward normal.

In hypoparathyroidism, tetany and convulsions, which are caused by hypocalcemia, represent the most serious complications. Increased mineral density of the bones, or osteosclerosis, is the most common skeletal abnormality. Late complications of untreated hypoparathyroidism include cataracts, calcification of basal ganglia, papilledema, and dystrophic changes in skin and nails.

Emergency treatment of hypocalcemic tetany requires the use of an intravenous calcium preparation. The beneficial effect of parenteral calcium in hypoparathyroidism is short-lived because of rapid deposition of the calcium in the skeleton and excretion. Therefore, oral therapy with the slower but longer-acting vitamin D_2 (ergocalciferol), vitamin D_3 (cholecalciferol), or dihydrotachysterol should be instituted.

Dihydrotachysterol, a synthetic compound similar chemically to vitamin D and an alternative to the vitamin in the therapy of hypoparathyroidism, has the advantage of a more rapid onset and a shorter duration of action.

Further improvements in the clinical pharmacology of vitamin D are likely to result from the identification of 25-hydroxycholecalciferol and 1,25-dihydroxycholecalciferol metabolites of vitamin D_3, which, unlike D_3, act directly on gut and bone. These compounds may represent an improvement in therapy in regard to shorter duration and broader spectrum of actions.

Vitamin D is active as an antirachitic substance

Table 29-3   Effect of Vitamin D Preparations Compared with PTH on Calcium and Phosphate Homeostasis

Preparation	Calcium absorption	Phosphate excretion	Bone resorption	Onset of action
Vitamin D (D_2 or D_3) (physiological dose 500–1,000 units/day)	3+*	...	+	2+
Vitamin D_2 or D_3 (pharmacological dose 50,000–250,000 units/day)	4+	2+	3+	2+
Dihydrotachysterol (1 mg/day)	3+	3+	3+	+
PTH	+	4+	4+	4+

* 4+ = high; 3+ = moderate; 2+ = low; + = slight.

in very small amounts, mainly because it promotes the absorption of calcium from the intestine. When much larger amounts are used, as in the treatment of hypoparathyroidism, the property of increasing the absorption of calcium is not lost, and is of some significance, but this effect by itself would not be sufficient. The major effect of vitamin D in large doses, the effect that adequately substitutes for the missing PTH, is stimulation of bone resorption. It is partly for this reason that dihydrotachysterol, which is only one-fiftieth as potent as vitamin D in stimulating calcium absorption, but 3 times as active as vitamin D in promoting resorption, can be recommended in hypoparathyroidism.

Hyperparathyroidism

This is a generalized disorder of calcium, phosphate, and bone metabolism resulting from an increased and autonomous secretion of PTH caused, in almost 90 percent of cases, by benign tumors called adenomas. The elevated concentration of circulating hormone usually results in hypercalcemia and hypophosphatemia. In *secondary hyperparathyroidism,* like the primary form of the disease, there is excessive secretion of parathyroid hormone; however, unlike primary hyperparathyroidism, it can be inhibited by elevation of the blood calcium. Secondary hyperparathyroidism, a feature of osteomalacia, pseudohypoparathyroidism, and chronic renal disease, is characterized by mild hypocalcemia (due to resistance to the action of the hormone or other causes) and an elevated concentration of circulating PTH as determined by radioimmunoassay.

The largest number of patients with primary hyperparathyroidism seeking medical attention do so because of the occurrence of renal calculi. (However, only a slight percentage of patients with renal calculi have hyperparathyroidism.) The most reliable diagnostic observation is hypercalcemia (above 10.5 mg/100 ml).

Once the presumptive diagnosis of primary hyperparathyroidism has been carefully made, surgical excision, usually of an adenoma, is the treatment of choice. Postoperative hypocalcemia may occur and should be treated with calcium and/or vitamin D.

Phosphate, intravenous or oral, has become widely employed as an effective treatment for hypercalcemic states, including hyperparathyroidism. When phosphate is given intravenously, the blood-calcium-lowering effect is seen within 24 h. Severe complications have occurred as a result of intravenous phosphate, including metastatic calcification, severe hypotension, and renal failure. These complications may also occur with oral phosphate therapy, but they do not appear to be as common or as severe. The reduction in the hypercalcemia does not occur until after several days.

Calcitonin might be expected to be unusually effective in combating hypercalcemia caused by excessive parathyroid hormone. Inhibition of bone resorption would be preferred over other methods of control of hypercalcemia, yet experience with calcitonin has not been highly successful.

Other Hypercalcemic States

A variety of nonparathyroid tumors have been associated with hypercalcemia. Hypercalcemia is the most common "endocrine" abnormality associated with neoplasia. However, in many patients, the hypercalcemia is associated with metastatic invasion of bone by tumor; presumably the hypercalcemia results from the osteolytic lesions in bone. In a smaller number of patients with malignancy and hypercalcemia there is no evidence of bone metastatis.

Osteoporosis

Osteoporosis, the most frequently occurring metabolic bone disease, is characterized by a generalized decrease in bone mass. Through an unexplained failure of the normal mechanisms that govern skeletal homeostasis, a progressive decrease occurs in skeletal mass with a marked thinning of cortical bone and a reduction in the number and size of trabeculae in cancellous bones. The structure of the residual bone appears to be normal, when assessed histologically and chemically. Symptomatic osteoporosis, with sufficient demineralization to cause pain, deformities, and pathological fractures, seems to represent an exaggeration of the normal aging process. The most frequently occurring form of osteoporosis is the idiopathic form usually seen in the aged population. Idiopathic osteoporosis is often termed *postmenopausal osteoporosis* in the female and *senile osteoporosis* in the male.

Attempts at therapy of patients with osteoporosis have rarely been successful and are frustrating to physician and patient alike. In high doses, fluoride stimulates the formation of bone of greatly increased density. Unfortunately, the resultant bone may be mechanically deficient and susceptible to fractures.

Calcitonin is theoretically attractive for the treatment of osteoporosis because of its demonstrated ability to inhibit bone resorption and possibly also to stimulate bone accretion. Dietary phosphate supplements for sustained increase in bone formation with concomitant use of calcitonin are also a possibility. Such approaches are currently being evaluated. However, it must be recognized that not only must a net increase in bone mineral deposition be achieved, but the new bone formed must be remodeled to be of suitable mechanical strength.

Preparations and Dosage

Dihydrotachysterol (Hytakerol) This drug is available in 0.125-mg capsules, 0.2-mg tablets, and 0.25 mg/ml solution. The usual adult dosage range is 0.75 to 2.5 mg/day.

Ergocalciferol Ergocalciferol (vitamin D_2, Deltalin, Drisdol, Geltabs) is available in 0.625-mg (25,000 units) and 1.25-mg (50,000 units) capsules and 0.250 mg (10,000 units)/ml solution. The usual adult dosage range is 1.25 to 25 mg daily.

Chapter 30

Insulins and Oral Antidiabetic Agents

Diabetes mellitus is a metabolic disease associated with high blood-glucose levels and alterations in lipid and protein metabolism. Ketoacidosis is its most severe biochemical disturbance. The vascular complications of diabetes mellitus consist of progressively advancing microangiopathies involving the extremities, eyes, kidneys, and heart. The clinical manifestations of this vascular degeneration include gangrene of the foot, blindness, uremia, and coronary artery disease.

CLASSIFICATION OF HUMAN DIABETES

Diabetes mellitus can be classified as: (1) prediabetes or potential diabetes, (2) latent or stress diabetes, (3) chemical or asymptomatic diabetes, and (4) clinical or overt diabetes.

Prediabetes is a prediction term, applied to the period preceding glucose intolerance. There are no known symptoms, but the probability of falling into this category can be predicted from a genetic relationship to known diabetics. A latent or stress diabetic shows a high blood glucose only during periods of stress, including infection, pregnancy, myocardial infarctions, etc. In chemical or asymptomatic diabetes, there is usually a normal fasting blood-glucose level but an elevated postprandial blood-glucose level. With clinical or overt diabetes the blood-glucose levels are elevated at all times.

Diabetes is also classified according to whether the syndrome has a juvenile or adult onset. Juvenile-onset diabetes is usually a rapidly progressing disease due to partial or complete absence of insulin production by the pancreatic beta cells. Adult-onset diabetes in many cases is a slowly progressing disease usually due to subnormal production of insulin by the beta cells. In this case inadequate insulin production is usually associated with secretory dysfunction or receptor abnormalities.

The obvious clinical symptoms of diabetes are usually those due to hyperglycemia (nocturia, polyuria, polydipsia, polyphagia, and pruritus); in the adult-onset disease, there is also usually a history or evidence of recent weight gain. Although human diabetes was originally defined, because of ease of measurement, as a hyperglycemia with subsequent glucosuria, it was subsequently recognized that the metabolic alterations of fats and proteins were not only interrelated with those of carbohydrates, but were of profound importance. These metabolic alterations include overproduction of glucose by the liver from glycogen and other sources, under-utilization of glucose peripherally, depression of oxidation of glucose in muscle and fat, and the almost complete disappearance of lipogenesis in fat. Glucose disposal is decreased in regard to both Embden-Meyerhof and pentose-phosphate pathways. Protein in peripheral tissues is broken down excessively, and the amino acids are taken into the liver and converted into glucose. Similarly, there is a decrease of protein synthesis from amino acids in muscle, with eventual inhibition of growth. Fat synthesis is blocked at one or more sites early in the normal sequence of reactions. Conversion of glucose to glycerol is inhibited in fat tissue, with defective esterification of fat and a rise in serum-free fatty acids. The inability of liver and muscles to cope with the defect in lipid metabolism results in excess fat catabolism and the production of both ketonemia and ketonuria. The hyperglycemia and ketonemia eventually result in profound water and electrolyte disturbances and cause alterations of acid-base content of blood as well as losses of total fixed bases which clinicially constitute diabetic acidosis. With acidosis, the proper functioning of the brain tissue is impossible, and coma and death may result.

INSULIN

Insulin is a protein composed of 51 amino acids arranged in two chains (A and B) linked by two disulfide bridges (Table 30-1). The amino acid composition of these chains may differ in different species (Table 30-2) and may explain the various antigenicity and serum binding of different sources. A precursor of insulin in the beta cell, proinsulin, contains the A and B chains of insulin connected by a large peptide. This connecting peptide in humans is approximately 33 amino acids long and links the threonine of the B chain to the glycine of the A chain.

Secretion and Metabolism

The pancreas secretes and releases insulin constantly at a rate which varies with the blood-glucose level. Insulin concentration in blood varies from approximately 20 microunits/ml during fasting to 5 times that amount after eating or glucose infusion. The normal range for whole-blood glucose during the fasting state ranges between 70 to 110 mg/100 ml. After secretion into the portal venous blood, some insulin is probably bound by liver and the remainder is associated with an alpha and a beta (and slightly with a gamma) globulin carrier in the serum. Insulin is not stored in the body, and its destruction depends on an insulinase–anti-insulinase system which is present mainly in liver, kidney, and muscle. This system has great reserve and does not appear to be altered in diabetes.

Mechanism and Locus of Action

The mechanism of action of insulin is to facilitate the penetration of monosaccharides and amino acids through the cell membrane of insulin-sensitive tissues which would otherwise have a low permeability to these substances. Glucose is the sugar primarily affected by insulin action. Insulin is not required for glucose transport into the liver, brain, and erythrocytes (insulin-insensitive tissues) as opposed to skeletal and heart muscle, fat, and leukocytes (insulin-sensitive tissues). The plasma membrane of insulin-sensitive cells contains specific receptors for this hormone. A signal from this receptor site sets off a number of biochemical events. Glucose is carried across the cell membrane and phosphorylated by hexokinase to glucose 6-phosphate. Insulin has also been shown to increase the synthesis of enzymes unique to glycolysis and to decrease the enzymes unique to the pathway of gluconeogenesis. Thus an insulin-induced signal will stimulate glycolysis and produce a relative decrease in gluconeogenesis, while lack of a signal will produce the opposite. As for the nature of the signal, it is theorized that an intracellular mediator substance is generated; evidence points to cyclic 3',5'-AMP as this substance. Some of the consequences of this signal generation via the insulin receptor are rapid, and include the effects on the transport of many substances into the cell such as inorganic ions, amino acids, and sugars. Other

Table 30-1   Structural Formula of Mammalian Insulin

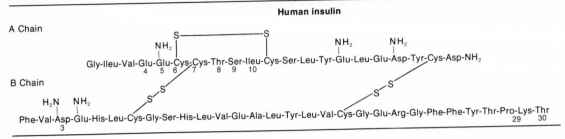

Human insulin

A Chain

$$\text{Gly-Ileu-Val-Glu-Glu-Cys-Cys-Thr-Ser-Ileu-Cys-Ser-Leu-Tyr-Glu-Leu-Glu-Asp-Tyr-Cys-Asp-NH}_2$$

B Chain

$$\text{Phe-Val-Asp-Glu-His-Leu-Cys-Gly-Ser-His-Leu-Val-Glu-Ala-Leu-Tyr-Leu-Val-Cys-Gly-Glu-Arg-Gly-Phe-Phe-Tyr-Thr-Pro-Lys-Thr}$$

consequences of the signal are relatively slow and include the synthesis of the enzymes for glycolysis as well as the enzymes for protein and fat synthesis, thus leading to acceleration of growth.

Preparations Used in Diabetes

Because of its protein nature, insulin is destroyed if administered orally; therefore it is administered parenterally, usually by the subcutaneous route. In order to delay absorption and prolong its action, insulin is combined with certain proteins and/or suspended in specific buffers as shown in Table 30-3.

All preparations of insulin are supplied in 10-ml vials and marketed in concentrations of 40, 80, and 100 units/ml. Eventually, however, only 100 units/ml will be made available in order to (1) decrease the risk of error involved in measuring different unitages, (2) standardize the syringes used, (3) reduce injection volumes, and (4) make the dosage and dilutions more metric. Insulin injection is also supplied at 500 units/ml for emergency use.

Insulin Injection (Crystalline Zinc Insulin, Regular Insulin)   The first insulin developed for clinical use was the amorphous form of insulin. Rapidly acting insulin (regular, crystalline zinc insulin) is

Table 30-2   Amino Acid Sequences of Insulin from Various Mammalian Sources

Source	A Chain			B Chain
	8	**9**	**10**	**30**
Human	Thr	Ser	Ileu	Thr
Pig	Thr	Ser	Ileu	Ala
Beef	Ala	Ser	Val	Ala
Sheep	Ala	Gly	Val	Ala

purified, crystallized, and stabilized by being produced at a neutral pH. Regular insulin is usually administered subcutaneously 1 to 2 h before each meal so that availability will coincide with need (see Fig. 30-1). It is also used in the management of diabetic coma. The duration of action is from 6 to 8 h; this short duration of action constituted the rationale for the 6-h management program whereby the diabetic consumed a meal and administered insulin every 6 h.

Protamine Insulins

Protamine Zinc Insulin Suspension   Mixing insulin, protamine, and zinc with a phosphate buffer yields protamine zinc insulin suspension buffered to pH 7.2. When the protamine cation is added to the insulin anion the two together flocculate out as a fine suspension containing 1.25 mg of protamine

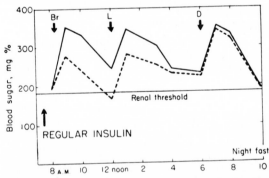

Figure 30-1   The duration of action of regular insulin. One moderate-size dose of regular insulin was given in the morning to a patient with moderately severe untreated diabetes who was eating three meals a day—breakfast (Br), lunch (L), and dinner (D). The solid line indicates the blood-sugar curve before insulin and the broken line the curve after the single dose of regular insulin. Note the limited effectiveness of one dose of this type of insulin.

Table 30-3   Insulin Preparations

Types of insulin	Action		Buffer	Added protein	
	Onset	Duration, h		Type	mg/100 units
Insulin injection* (regular, crystalline zinc)	Rapid	6–8	None	None	...
Isophane insulin suspension (NPH)	Intermediate	24–28	Phosphate	Protamine	0.5
Protamine zinc insulin suspension	Slow	36+	Phosphate	Protamine	1.25
Prompt insulin zinc suspension (semilente)	Rapid	10–14	Acetate	None	...
Insulin zinc suspension (lente)	Intermediate	22–26	Acetate	None	...
Extended insulin zinc suspension (ultralente)	Slow	36+	Acetate	None	...

* A clear solution, all others are turbid.

and 0.2 mg of zinc per 100 units of insulin. The addition of the zinc stabilizes the preparation and prevents clumping. Its onset of action is slow (2 h), and its duration of action is long (more than 24 h). The clinical application of protamine zinc insulin (PZI) is shown in Fig. 30-2.

Isophane Insulin Suspension (NPH Insulin)   This preparation is an example of a type of insulin with intermediate action. It is a suspension of a crystalline form of protamine zinc insulin which is almost neutral (pH 7.2) and contains 0.50 mg protamine per 100 units insulin. This is just enough protamine to bind the regular insulin. Its action is similar to a mixture having one part protamine zinc insulin and two parts regular insulin. The action of NPH (neutral protamine hagedorn) insulin starts in about 2 h, reaches a peak of activity in 8 to 10 h, and wanes by 24 h.

Insulin Zinc Suspensions (Lente Insulins)   In order to slow down the action of insulin without combining it with a basic protein which may be antigenic, a method was discovered whereby the size of the insulin particles could be varied by substituting an acetate buffer at pH 7.2 instead of the usual phosphate buffers. At present there are three available forms:

1 Prompt insulin zinc suspension or semilente insulin (Table 30-3) is a crystalline form with small crystals which dissolves rapidly, producing a prompt, short action.

2 Extended insulin zinc suspension or ultralente insulin is composed of large crystals and hence is long-acting.

3 Insulin zinc suspension or lente insulin is an intermediate-acting preparation which is a mixture of 30 percent prompt insulin zinc suspension and 70 percent extended insulin zinc suspension.

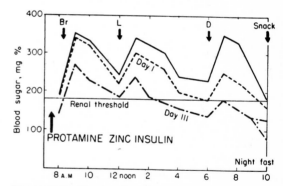

Figure 30-2   The duration of action of protamine zinc insulin. A moderate-size dose of protamine zinc insulin was given to a patient with moderately severe untreated diabetes who was eating three meals a day as in Figure 30-1. The solid line indicates the blood-sugar curve before treatment and the broken lines the curve on the first and third days of treatment. The progressive effect of this type of insulin upon the blood-sugar curve during a given day may be noted, with a maximum effect at night. A small amount of food (snack) is interposed at bedtime to avoid hypoglycemia. The progressive improvement in the blood-sugar curve from the first day to a maximum effect on the third day is a characteristic response of this type of insulin.

Variations can be custom-mixed from the prompt and extended insulin zinc suspensions to suit the needs of particular patients.

Dosage

The dose of insulin to be used is ultimately determined by clinical trial in a given patient on a given diet as the amount which accomplishes the therapeutic objective set by the physician. Such objectives vary from a minimum of eliminating diabetic symptoms to a maximum of attaining normoglycemia. The normal pancreas produces from 30 to 50 units of insulin per day, so most diabetics with insulin deficiency require somewhat less than this dosage of insulin.

Factors that may alter insulin requirements include: (1) the metabolic needs of the body, for example, thyrotoxicosis, fever, myxedema, etc.; (2) stress conditions, for example, surgery, injury, myocardial infarction, anesthesia, infection, etc.; (3) allergic response to insulin; (4) muscular exercise; (5) psychic stress; and (6) drugs administered, for example, thiazides, salicylates, etc.

Toxicity Due to Overdosage

Prevention of hypoglycemia is an important aim in insulin therapy. Regularity in eating and avoidance of wide variations in diet are important. Warning symptoms of milder degrees of hypoglycemia must be watched for, and the insulin dose reduced or food interposed at such times. Hypoglycemia can be anticipated according to the peak action of the insulin. A severe prolonged hypoglycemic reaction can, if untreated, lead to permanent cerebral damage or death.

The prime clinical manifestations of insulin overdosage are due to the effects of hypoglycemia on the nervous system. Once the blood sugar drops below 50 to 60 mg/100 ml, symptoms of hunger, faintness, sweating, tremors, muscular weakness, nausea, psychic disturbances, and finally loss of consciousness may occur (insulin shock).

Fortunately, the mammalian body has corrective factors available to counteract hypoglycemia by providing glucose from the liver by gluconeogenesis from noncarbohydrate sources and by glycogenolysis. These factors include adrenal corticosteroids, epinephrine, and pituitary growth hormone. All these hormones also decrease peripheral utilization of glucose. Glucagon secreted by pancreatic alpha cells also has glycogenolytic action. These hormonal factors are elicited promptly by hypoglycemia.

Differential Diagnosis and Treatment of Hypoglycemia

Diabetic acidosis due to ketone body production from lack of effectiveness of insulin may be confused with severe insulin hypoglycemia, especially that due to the long-acting varieties of insulin. Table 30-4 shows the differential points of diagnosis. Intravenous glucose therapy should not be delayed for the results of laboratory findings.

When a patient suffering from insulin-induced hypoglycemia is conscious, the patient should be given sugar-containing foods such as orange juice, sweet drinks, or lump sugar. It may take ½ or ¾ h for an effect. For more severe degrees of hypoglycemia with unconsciousness, glucose intravenously is the treatment of choice. Glucagon may also be used therapeutically for hypoglycemia.

Glucagon

Another pancreatic hormone, glucagon, is a protein composed of a single chain of amino acids. It is secreted by the alpha cells of the pancreas in response to hypoglycemia, is detectable in blood by radioimmunoassay at a level of about 500 pg/ml in the fasting state, and is destroyed by the liver. The main function of glucagon is to help maintain blood-sugar level by hepatic glycogenolysis. It acts by reactivating hepatic phosphorylases and is effective within 15 min after intravenous infusion at a dosage level of 2 μg/min, or 1 to 2 mg administered by the deep subcutaneous route.

Adjuncts to the Treatment of Diabetes

In practice, full agreement on the ultimate objectives of therapy in human diabetes is still lacking. Most physicians aim for aglycosuria, and a substantial proportion for normoglycemia, if possible, in the belief that this may help prevent complications of diabetes. Dietary restriction is still the cornerstone of therapy. A diabetic diet should aim for restoration and maintenance of ideal weight; daily constancy in the proportions of carbohydrate, protein, and fats; and convenience for the patient.

Table 30-4 Differential Diagnosis of Severe Insulin Reactions and Diabetic Acidotic Coma

	Insulin reaction	Acidotic coma
History		
Regulation	Frequently unstable with previous reactions	Usually poor, with metabolic symptoms
Immediate precipitating factors		
Food	Acutely insufficient	Ample or excessive
Complications		Infection, especially with vomiting or diarrhea
Insulin	Excess	Too little, acutely or chronically
Other	Extra exercise	
Symptoms		
Metabolic	None	Usually present
Vomiting	Absent	Common
Abdominal pain	Absent	Frequent
Vision	Double	Dim
Signs		
Respiration	Normal	Deep "Kussmaul"
Tremors	Frequently present	Absent
Convulsions	Occasionally	Rare
Dehydration	Absent	Dry skin and tongue, soft eyeballs
Blood pressure	Normal or elevated	Subnormal or in shock
Laboratory findings		
Urine		
Glycosuria	May be + but negative in second specimen	4+*
Ketonuria	At most ± in first specimen	4+*
Blood		
Sugar	Low (below 70 mg/100 ml)	Elevated (usually above 200 mg/100 ml)
Ketones	Normal	Elevated
Response to therapy	Immediate, minutes after 5 to 20 g glucose intravenously or orally	No immediate response; requires insulin, water, and electrolytes

* In rare instances, in the presence of shock with oliguria, both glucose and acetone may disappear from urine.

Special noncarbohydrate sweetening agents are used: sorbitol in the manufacture of food and saccharin added by the patient as desired.

Saccharin is the anhydride of *o*-sulfamidobenzoic acid. It has no food value, and is almost entirely excreted in the urine and stool within the first 24 h after ingestion. It has a sweetening power 400 times that of sugar. Above concentrations of one ten-thousandth the sweetness is partly replaced by a bitter taste; some persons detect this and find it objectionable even at commonly used concentrations. The bitter taste is increased by heating.

Sodium or calcium cyclohexylsulfamate (Sucaryl), a cyclamate, is a sweetening agent with about 30 times the sweetening power of sugar and was previously used in many foods and soft drinks. Cyclamates have been withdrawn from the market because they potentially cause bladder cancer.

ORAL ANTIDIABETIC DRUGS

Drugs which may be useful in individuals who have some endogenous insulin secretion are the sulfonylureas, since the main action of these orally effective drugs is to force the pancreatic beta cells to release insulin. Phenformin is another orally effective drug which appears to be effective in patients whose carbohydrate metabolism in muscle and fat tissue needs to be increased. When these drugs are employed, concomitant dietary regulation is of utmost importance in order to decrease obesity, loss of body protein, or acidosis.

The effectiveness and safety of oral antidiabetic agents has recently been questioned. A group of 800 diabetics on tolbutamide and/or diet therapy compared with insulin and diet therapy were studied at 12 university medical centers for up to 8 years. A significantly greater number of cardiovascular deaths were recorded in the tolbutamide-treated groups than in any other group, including placebo-treated controls. Increased mortality also occurred in the phenformin-treated groups. This study has been criticized as defective in design by some competent diabetologists, while others claim that diet and weight control are much more effective in controlling diabetes than are the sulfonylureas.

Sulfonylurea Drugs

The four sulfonylurea antidiabetic agents in current use in the United States are tolbutamide, chlorpropamide, acetohexamide, and tolazamide. These sulfonylureas (Table 30-5) have the same mechanism of action but differ in their metabolic fate, potency (Table 30-6), and toxicity.

Mechanism of Action The major action of all sulfonylurea drugs is to promote increased insulin output by pancreatic beta cells. In *acute* experiments, it has been shown repeatedly that the sulfonylureas markedly increase the plasma insulin level. This insulin rise results from direct stimulation of pancreatic beta cells to release insulin. This stimulating effect is dependent on the functional state of beta cell reserve. After acute stimulation with a sulfonylurea drug, there is a rise in blood insulin and the normal pancreas can respond again in 4 h, but that of the adult diabetic may be refractory for as long as 24 h. Since the action of the drugs requires a minimum amount of functioning beta cell tissue (at least 30 percent of normal), this effect does not occur in pancreatectomized individuals or in patients with an absolute deficiency of insulin (that is, juvenile diabetics).

Table 30-5 The Sulfonylureas

Generic name	Trade name	Structural formula and chemical name
Tolbutamide	Orinase	CH_3—⟨ ⟩—SO_2—NH—CO—NH—C_4H_9 *N*-(*p*-Tolylsulfonyl)-*N'*-butylcarbamide
Chlorpropamide	Diabinese	Cl—⟨ ⟩—SO_2—NH—CO—NH—C_3H_7 *N*-propyl-*N'*-*p*-chlorophenylsulfonyl-carbamide
Acetohexamide	Dymelor	$CH_3C\overset{O}{\overset{\|}{C}}$—⟨ ⟩—$SO_2$—NH—$\overset{O}{\overset{\|}{C}}$—NH—⟨ ⟩ *N*-(*p*-Acetylphenylsulfonyl)-*N'*-cyclohexylurea
Tolazamide	Tolinase	CH_3—⟨ ⟩—SO_2—NH—$\overset{O}{\overset{\|}{C}}$—NH—N⟨ ⟩ *N*-(Hexahydro-1-azepinyl)-*N'*-*p*-tolylsulfonylurea

Table 30-6 Dosage and Pharmacologic Properties of the Oral Sulfonylureas

	Tolbutamide	Acetohexamide	Tolazamide	Chlorpropamide
Common dosage, g/day	1.5	0.75	0.25	0.25
Range dosage, g/day	0.5–3.0	0.25–1.25	0.1–0.75	0.1–0.5
Blood peak, h	3–5	2–4	4–8	2–4
Chief metabolites in urine	Carboxytolbutamide	Hydroxyhexamide	1 *p*-Carboxytolazamide 2 4-Hydroxymethyl-tolazamide 3 3,4-Hydroxy on azepinyl ring	Unchanged
Biologic half-life, h	5.6	4.7–5.3	7	35
Metabolic half-life, h	4.7	6–8	10	*
% in urine in 24 h	90	80	85	30
Peak hypoglycemic activity, h	4–6	3	4–6	10
Duration of action, h	6–12	12–24	12–24	Up to 60
Onset of action, h	2–4	1–2	4–6	4

* Drug blood level reaches sustained level after 3 to 5 days of therapy.

Absorption, Fate, and Metabolism When administered orally, the sulfonylurea drugs are absorbed promptly from the small intestine and appear in the blood within 1 to 2 h. However, these drugs have differences in rates of absorption, metabolic degradation, and duration of action, as shown in Table 30-6. Tolbutamide is rapidly metabolized to an inactive product, and therefore the biologic half-life approximates the metabolic half-life. With acetohexamide and tolazamide, however, the metabolic products also have considerable hypoglycemic activity, and the metabolic half-life is considerably longer than the biologic half-life for these agents. Chlorpropamide is not metabolized and therefore has only a biologic but not a metabolic half-life.

Preparations

Chlorpropamide (Diabinese) Supplied in tablets of 100 and 250 mg for oral use. The recommended dose is 100 to 500 mg/day given as a single dose.

Tolazamide (Tolinase) Supplied in tablets of 100 and 250 mg for oral use. The recommended dose is 100 to 750 mg/day.

Acetohexamide (Dymelor) Supplied in tablets of 250 mg and 500 mg for oral use. The recommended dose is 250 to 1500 mg/day.

Tolbutamide (Orinase) Supplied in tablets of 500 mg for oral use. The recommended dose is 0.5 to 3.0 g/day in divided doses. The *powder* sodium tolbutamide is available in vials containing 1.0 gm; this is recommended for intravenous use for testing purposes.

Toxicity All the sulfonylurea drugs have some toxicity. The incidence is usually less than 10 percent, depending on the subjects selected for therapy and the dosage regimens. Cross-reaction among the drugs is infrequent, and sensitivity to one drug usually does not preclude trial with the others. Hypoglycemia is the most common untoward reaction and seems to occur more frequently with the longer-acting drugs. The greater the possibility of hypoglycemia, the milder the diabetes and the more elderly the patient. A *central nervous system syndrome* of muscular weakness, vertigo, ataxia, and mental confusion has been described following administration of very high doses of these drugs, particularly chlorpropamide. However, these effects on the CNS are reversible on withdrawal of the drug and are definitely related to dosage. Gastrointestinal symptoms in susceptible individuals consist of heartburn, upper abdominal discomfort, nausea, lower abdominal cramps, and diarrhea. Exacerbation of peptic ulcer may occur. Accordingly, a history of gastrointestinal disease requires low dosage or avoidance of sulfonylurea drug therapy. A reaction reminiscent of the reaction to disulfiram after the ingestion of alcohol may occasionally occur in patients receiving any of the sulfonylurea drugs.

Hypersensitivity reactions have been described with all the sulfonylurea drugs. The incidence is about 1 to 5 percent and may involve a variety of systems. Skin reactions consist of photosensitivity, erythema, and morbilliform or maculopapular rashes. The hematopoietic effects consist of leukopenia, thrombocytopenia, pancytopenia, agranulocytosis, hemolytic anemia, and aplastic anemia. The hepatic reaction may be a simple elevation of alkaline phosphatase (which may occur without drug therapy in diabetes), or jaundice of the cholestatic variety. These reactions usually occur within the first 6 to 8 weeks of therapy.

Contraindications The sulfonylurea drugs should not be used alone for the management of patients with an absolute or severe deficiency in endogenous insulin action. Such patients are prone to ketoacidosis and constitute a majority of juvenile-onset diabetics. The use of sulfonylureas is contraindicated in the presence of ketosis or of complications likely to increase severity of the diabetes (see above). Following surgical intervention, except for minor procedures, sulfonylureas must be supplemented by or replaced with insulin. The long half-life of chlorpropamide makes it necessary to stop the drug at least 2 days prior to a major surgical procedure. If an emergency surgical procedure precludes this, provision must be made for continuous postoperative intravenous therapy with glucose-containing solutions for a similar period. The sulfonylurea drugs should be used with great caution or not at all in the presence of peptic ulcer, extensive liver disease, or renal disease. These drugs may not be used in pregnancy, since their safety has not yet been established. Similarly, consideration should be given to the possible hazards of their use in women of the childbearing age who might become pregnant.

Therapeutic Action The acute hypoglycemic action of the sulfonylurea drugs in maturity-onset diabetes is dependent upon a minimal effective blood (and tissue) level of the drug or its active metabolites. This level is somewhat different for each of the sulfonylureas but rises roughly in proportion to the dose. Even for the responsive diabetic pancreas, there is a maximum effective dose which is characteristic for each drug and beyond which no further action occurs. The functional capacity of the beta cells to synthesize and release insulin in response to a chemical stimulus is variable in diabetic patients and must be considered in dose-response evaluations.

In maturity-onset diabetics, the pattern of hypoglycemic response induced by sulfonylurea drugs is prolonged when compared with that of insulin. Two mechanisms may determine the prolonged hypoglycemia after administration of sulfonylureas: (1) a prolonged beta cell stimulation, and (2) an inhibitory effect on hepatic gluconeogenesis. Furthermore, the hypoglycemic effect of sulfonylureas is relatively delayed in responsive diabetics when compared with normal subjects.

Phenformin

The only clinically useful oral antidiabetic agent which is not related chemically to the sulfonylureas is phenformin (DBI). It is a biguanide and has the following structure:

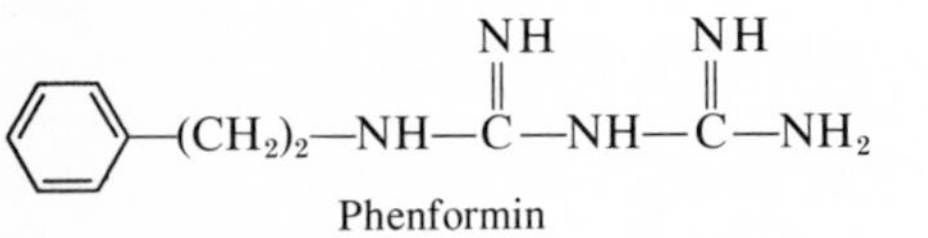

$$\text{\textcircled{\hexagon}}-(CH_2)_2-NH-\underset{\underset{NH}{\|}}{C}-NH-\underset{\underset{NH}{\|}}{C}-NH_2$$

Phenformin

Mechanism of Action Even though the mechanisms of the blood-sugar-lowering effect of phenformin in humans are not yet understood, it is quite clear that these mechanisms are entirely different from those of the sulfonylureas. Indeed, in normal humans phenformin has not been found to lower the blood sugar. In adult diabetic patients, it has further been shown to decrease the inordinate rise in blood-insulin level which occurs after administration of glucose. It does not stimulate pancreatic beta cells physiologically or histologically, nor does it have an effect after pancreatectomy. Thus, phenformin is the only oral antidiabetic drug that lowers blood sugar without stimulating the release of insulin from the pancreas.

Studies have shown that, in vitro, the main effects of phenformin are to increase the uptake and oxidation of glucose by the adipose tissue and to increase anaerobic glycolysis to lactic acid in muscle in the presence of insulin. In vivo studies also show that this drug promotes disposal of glucose and requires the presence of insulin. The therapeutic range of dosage is 50 to 200 mg/day.

Absorption, Fate, and Metabolism After oral administration, the phenformin is pooled in and absorbed from the gastric juice. Its degradation occurs by removal of the phenyl group; 30 percent of the degraded drug is recovered in the urine in 5 h and 90 percent in 24 h.

Toxicity Acute lethal doses cause paralysis of the respiratory center or death from hypoglycemia. Chronic toxicity has not been observed. In the presence of adequate insulin and in routine treatment of properly selected diabetic patients, striking abnormalities of blood lactic acid do not usually occur. Gastrointestinal symptoms such as bitter taste, dryness of mouth, anorexia, nausea, and vomiting may occur. These symptoms are a matter of individual idiosyncrasy. They are dosage-dependent, occurring mainly at dosage levels above 100 mg/day, and are reversible within several hours by even a slight reduction in dosage. Phenformin does not aggravate peptic ulcer as may the sulfonylurea drugs.

No evidence of organ tissue or functional toxicity has been observed to date in diabetic patients given phenformin in therapeutically effective daily doses for varying periods up to and beyond 4 years. There have been no adverse renal or hematologic effects with continued use of phenformin and no undesirable changes in liver function. No undesirable changes in adrenal, thyroid, cardiac, or respiratory functions have occurred during prolonged therapy, nor have dermatologic manifestations unequivocally related to the administration of phenformin been observed.

Contraindications The biguanides should be replaced with insulin (as should the sulfonylurea drugs) when surgical procedures, infection, and other complications ensue. They should not be used in severe hepatic disease, renal disease with uremia, or during cardiovascular collapse (shock). At present, the use of any oral antidiabetic drug, including phenformin, is to be avoided in pregnancy.

Therapeutic Management Significant gastrointestinal symptoms may be uniformly avoided if the starting dose is low, and if subsequent doses are not increased. All diabetics of the ketoacidotic-prone type, and those suffering onset of diabetes before twenty years of age who are being treated to decrease lability of the disease, should receive adequate amounts of insulin. Replacement of too much insulin by phenformin in such patients may result in ketonemia. Ketonuria in the presence of relatively normal blood sugars and low or absent glycosuria suggests the "starvation" phenomenon and must be differentiated from the ketoacidosis of insufficient insulin. The latter is demonstrated by marked elevations of blood sugar and glycosuria in the presence of ketonemia or ketonuria. For starvation ketosis, reduction in the dose of phenformin by 25 to 50 mg/day and/or a liberalization in carbohydrate intake quickly restores metabolic balance and eliminates the ketosis. Naturally, in ketoacidosis, insulin dosage must be increased. Therefore, the presence of ketonuria does not always indicate the need for more insulin. Blood or urine sugars should be checked prior to giving insulin to these patients.

The minimal effective dose of phenformin is probably 50 mg/day. When supplementing insulin, the reduction of the dose of insulin after each increment of phenformin need not be made for 3 to 5 days.

Chapter 31

Male Sex Hormones, Anabolic Steroids

The term *male sex hormone,* or *androgen,* implies that such a compound is the principal substance secreted by the sex glands of the male. By common usage, androgens—and particularly testosterone—are considered as compounds which have masculinizing effects. The designation of a steroid as a male sex hormone is probably poor, since both the male and female members of the species have varying amounts of both male and female sex hormones in their body. Nevertheless, the term male sex hormones has usually referred to the androgenic compounds or masculinizing substances. The so-called anabolic steroids are also included in this chapter, since all the steroids available to date with this property have definite androgenic activity when used in sufficiently high doses.

CHEMISTRY

All androgens known at present possess the cyclopentanophenanthrene nucleus. Testosterone is the

Testosterone

major naturally occurring androgen which is the 17β-hydroxy-3-one derivative of Δ^4-androstene. The principal source of endogenous testosterone in the male is the Leydig cells. This steroid, and the many related compounds used clinically, are no longer extracted from the gonads of domestic animals but are prepared synthetically from plant sterols.

EFFECTS OF ANDROGENS ON ORGAN SYSTEMS

Male Reproductive Tract

When androgens are administered in adequate doses, suppression of pituitary gonadotropic secretion occurs, resulting in inhibition of testicular function and growth. Testosterone also induces discernible cytologic effects in the prostate gland. There is cellular hypertrophy of the glandular elements followed by increased glandular secretion and enlargement of the gland.

Androgens affect the penis of hypogonadal males by an increase in size and frequency of penile erections. Penile growth is usually expected following androgen therapy up to the time that epiphyseal closure takes place. Except for the patient with Klinefelter's syndrome or frank hypogonadism, the small penis of an adult with normal testicular function usually fails to show any evidence of further increase in size after epiphyseal closure has taken place. Androgen will cause priapism in the young male, whether he is hypogonadal or eugonadal. The penis of the young adolescent is an unusually sensitive indicator of androgenic activity. The initial response of the young male to androgens would be expressed by an increased degree of penile rubor and priapism, then by an increase in penile size, scrotum redundancy and rugae, and amount of pubic hair.

Female Reproductive Tract

Androgens indirectly influence ovarian anatomy and function by inhibition of pituitary gonadotropic secretion. The inhibitory action of androgens upon gonadotropic secretion is not as effective as that attributed to estrogens. Nevertheless, once the steroid has been withdrawn, pituitary gonadotropins are released, and stimulation of ovarian function follows. A direct effect of androgens on the myometrium and vaginal mucosa has also been demonstrated. In the myometrium, there is an increase in mucification with a reduction in the degree of cornification.

Nonendocrine Organs

Striated muscle in general increases in mass with androgen, a clinical finding evident when one considers the relatively poor muscle development of castrates versus that of noncastrates. Stimulation of muscle growth with androgens is inhibited by cortisone.

The anabolic and androgenic steroids exert a pronounced effect upon bone tissue. Whereas these steroids promote and enhance protein activity of the osteoid matrix and thereby increase osteoblastic activity, androgens also promote linear growth by their action upon the epiphyses. However, the growth-stimulating effects of androgens are encumbered by the fact that these steroids may also hasten epiphyseal closure. Nevertheless, it should be emphasized that androgens are considerably less active than estrogens in closing the epiphyses. The anabolic steroids have greater growth-stimulating effects and are less active in closing the epiphyses than the so-called pure androgens.

The male sex hormones also show an influence on skin and hair. The effect of androgens upon the skin is characterized by an increased rate of secretion of the sebaceous glands, resulting in an enhanced oiliness of the skin plus an increase in amount of inspissated material blocking the ducts of the sebaceous or sweat glands. The skin also tends to become somewhat coarse and thickened. The changes seen in the skin are characteristic of those seen in the young male at puberty.

The effect of the sex steroids on hair growth on the body is dependent upon the fact that there are two spheres of influence in the human concerning hair growth and loss. The growth of hair on the scalp is enhanced by estrogens and progesterone and inhibited by the action of androgens. In contrast, growth of hair on the body is enhanced by androgens and is either not influenced by estrogens, or may even be inhibited by estrogens.

Absorption, Metabolism, and Excretion

The rate of absorption of androgens depends upon their mode of administration. Testosterone is almost completely inactivated when ingested because of passage of the steroid through the liver. Chemical modification of the androgen, such as methylation, however, results in a considerable degree of protection of the compound against metabolic destruction by the liver so that it may be administered orally with significant clinical efficacy.

The effectiveness of parenteral administration of

solutions of the steroid in oil or as aqueous suspensions depends upon the delay in absorption of the material from the site of injection. The free compounds, such as unesterified testosterone in oil solution, are readily and quickly absorbed from the intramuscular site. On the other hand, if the compound is esterified and then injected as an oil solution, there is a delayed absorption from the site of injection resulting in an increase in, or prolongation of, effect. The rate of dissipation of the drug is also retarded. The duration of the androgenic activity of such a preparation would depend upon the choice of the esterifying acid. A significant degree of retardation of absorption may be achieved by the use of aqueous suspensions of the free steroids or of certain esters. Aqueous suspension of testosterone will considerably delay the rate of absorption of the steroid from the site of injection and is well tolerated by the patient. On the other hand, aqueous suspension of testosterone propionate has usually been associated with a marked degree of pain and discomfort at the site of injection.

The relatively slow absorption of material from the site of injection results in a sustained but enhanced clinical response. This principle emphasizes an important point, which may be stated as follows: A specific dose of a drug—when administered in such a manner as to result in continuous availability of the substance over a period of several days, albeit in small amounts—will achieve a much greater effect than that noted if the same amount of drug is administered at daily intervals or twice a day over the same period of time in a short-acting menstruum.

The complexity of the problem of steroid excretion is accentuated, since not only does more than one organ produce a common metabolite, but the parent substance may also be produced by one or more of the steroid-secreting organs. In addition, after its elaboration from the ovary or adrenal, dehydroepiandrosterone may be converted in the periphery into testosterone. However, categorically one can say that the 11-hydroxy-17-ketosteroids are only of adrenal origin. Very little testosterone is secreted as such from the adrenal gland, so that most of this steroid is either of ovarian or testicular origin. Normally, since testosterone is secreted by the testes and dehydroepiandrosterone and Δ^4-androstenedione arise from both the adrenals and the gonads (testes or ovaries),

the total neutral desoxy-17-ketosteroid represents end products of gonadal and adrenal cortical steroids.

Testosterone is the most potent androgen of this group; androstenedione and dehydroepiandrosterone, which contribute heavily to 17-ketosteroid levels, are relatively poor androgenic substances. Δ^4-Androstenedione may be the key intermediate in the metabolism of testosterone. Testosterone is probably converted to androstenedione by oxidation of its 17-hydroxyl group to a ketone.

The level of 17-ketosteroid metabolites in the urine depends greatly upon the metabolic functions of organs such as the liver and kidney, and on how these organs influence the circulating endogenous androgens. Certain androgenic steroids, however, including methyltestosterone, methylandrostenediol, and the group of the 17-nortestosterone derivatives, are not excreted as 17-ketosteroids.

Preparations

A large number of preparations are available for clinical use (see Table 31-1).

Adverse Reactions and Precautions

The most frequent side effect of androgenic steroids is virilism. Signs of virilism in the prepuberal male include growth of pubic hair, increased occurrence of erections, and an increase in penile size. In females untoward effects of androgen therapy include hirsutism, clitoral enlargement, acne, deepening of voice, and menstrual irregularities. Other undesirable effects associated with these agents are premature epiphyseal closure, liver dysfunction, hypercalcemia, and retention of sodium and water which may cause edema.

The androgenic compounds are contraindicated in pregnant women, in men with prostatic carcinoma, and in patients with nephrosis.

Therapeutic Use in the Male

The primary use of androgenic steroids is in the treatment of definite testicular deficiency or absence of testosterone production in the male. Primary testicular failure may be due in part to infection, to trauma following surgical procedure, or to inadvertent ligation of the spermatic cords in the repair of an inguinal hernia. Also, mumps orchitis

Table 31-1 Preparations of Male Sex Hormones

Steroid	Preparation and form	Anabolic dose, mg/kg	Relative activity	
			Androgenic	Anabolic
Testosterone (free and esters)	Intramuscular and linguet		1	1
Methyltestosterone	5- and 10-mg tablets and linguet		1	1
Fluoxymesterone	2-, 5-, and 10-mg tablets		1	1
Methandrostenolone	5-mg tablet	0.25	1	1
Nandrolone phenpropionate	25 mg/ml in oil	0.75–1.0 mg/week	1	2.0
Nandrolone decanoate	50 mg/ml in oil	1.0–2.0 mg every 3–4 weeks	1	3.0
Oxymetholone	5- and 10-mg tablets	0.75–1.0	1	2.0
Stanozolol	2-mg tablets	0.05–0.1	1	3.0
Oxandrolone	2.5-mg tablets	0.1–0.2	1	3.0
Dromostanolone propionate	50 mg/ml in oil	3.0 mg/week	1	3.0

may destroy testicular function sufficiently to nullify seminiferous tubular activity.

There are many different variants of hypogonadism where the defect may be primary in the testes or secondary because of hypogonadotropism. The diagnosis of either primary or secondary hypogonadism is mainly of theoretical importance, since the therapeutic approach will invariably involve the administration of androgenic substances. Although the hypogonadotropic hypogonadism would theoretically benefit from the use of gonadotropic preparations, these preparations are notoriously lacking in effectiveness, difficult to obtain, and fairly expensive for the patient. The same type of treatment as is suggested above for the hypogonadal male would also be employed in patients with panhypopituitarism.

Other than in definite testicular deficiency or absence of testosterone production, adrogenic compounds are used in selected cases of advanced or metastatic breast carcinoma and for their anabolic effect.

Therapeutic Use in The Female

The only indication for large-dose, long-term androgen therapy in females is in selected cases of premenopausal metastatic or advanced breast carcinoma. Androgens also have been used in the treatment of selected noncarcinogenic gynecologic

conditions, but estrogens and progestins are now used most commonly to treat these conditions.

ANABOLIC ACTIONS OF ANDROGENS, OR ANABOLIC STEROIDS

The use of these steroids for stimulating growth has been widely promulgated in the past decade. The anabolic steroids of choice, however, may change as the years go by since better preparations are constantly being made available—preparations which display a lesser degree of androgenic effects and greater promise of anabolic activity alone. The growth-stimulating effect with steroids may be achieved after the use of either parenteral or oral preparations. The oral preparations which are said to possess greater anabolic than androgenic activity include methandrostenolone, stanozolol, fluoxymesterone, and oxymetholone.

The anabolic steroids have been recommended for patients in a negative nitrogen balance, particularly during the postoperative period. Also, the anabolic steroids have been used to enhance weight gain in children and adults who are underweight. These steroids have been employed in premature infants in an attempt to increase the rate of weight gain and thereby prevent some of the complications of prematurity. The various preparations and suggested dosages are listed in Table 31-1.

Chapter 32

Female Sex Hormones, Oral Contraceptives, Fertility Agents

Estrogens are used primarily as replacement therapy in the treatment of hypoestrogenic diseases and certain metabolic conditions, and for their ability to bring about certain anatomic changes. One of the most important uses of progestational steroids has been in the area of contraception. In order to understand more fully the pharmacology of the female sex hormones and related compounds, a brief review of the physiology of the monthly ovarian cycle is presented.

MONTHLY OVARIAN CYCLE

The pituitary gonadotropic hormones involved with ovarian stimulation and functions are follicle-stimulating hormones (FSH) and luteinizing hormones (LH). A third gonadotropin, luteotropic hormone (LTH) might be implicated in the menstrual cycle, but its precise role is open to question at present.

The first events in the ovarian cycle are initiated by FSH. Early in the cycle FSH brings about stimu-

lation of follicle growth and enlargement of the ovum itself, along with increased proliferation of granulosa and theca cells. The theca interna cells produce estrogen under the influence of LH. In addition, FSH increases the amount of fluid in the graafian follicle to form the mature follicle.

When the follicle matures sufficiently and the appropriate level of estrogen is achieved, a brief excessive release of LH occurs, resulting in ovulation. The combined action of FSH and LH is needed for rupture and liberation of the ovum from the follicle. The vacated follicle then undergoes various changes to form the corpus luteum; this is followed by the elaboration of progesterone by the granulosa cells. Again, estrogen continues to be released from the theca cells.

LH, and perhaps LTH, maintain the functioning of the corpus luteum for approximately 10 days postovulation. If fertilization does not take place, the corpus luteum will begin to reduce hormone production and eventually cease functioning altogether. The onset of menses will then follow at about the twenty-eighth day of the cycle. Figure 32-1 illustrates the levels of estrogen and progesterone during the 28-day period of a typical monthly ovarian cycle.

Simultaneously with ovulation in the ovary, the endometrium of the uterus manifests cyclic alterations (Fig. 32-1). These changes result from the influence of estrogen and progesterone on the tissues. In the first part of the cycle, as estrogen is being secreted, the endometrium enters its proliferative phase (approximately 11 days). During this phase the tissue increases in thickness, with progressive growth of glandular and vascular elements. Under the combined influence of estrogen and progesterone on the endometrium following ovulation, the secretory phase (approximately 13 days) is established. During this period there is further development of blood vessels and glandular structures, and an elaboration of the contents of the

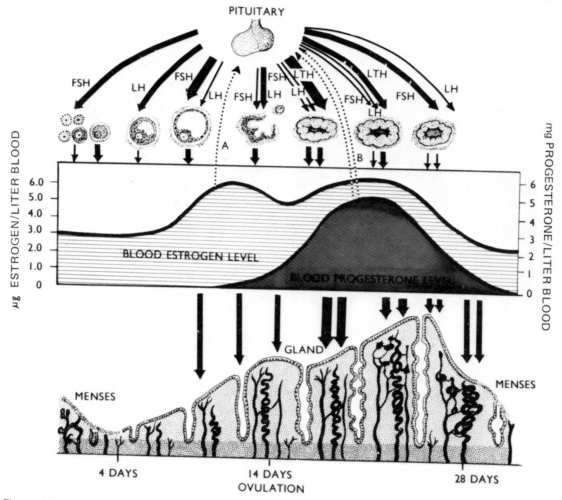

Figure 32-1 Variations in pituitary and ovarian hormone secretion, and endometrial morphology during the menstrual cycle. The widths of the arrows indicate the relative circulating levels of the hormones. (A) indicates inhibition of FSH and stimulation of LH secretion by estrogens. (B) indicates the net inhibitory influence of estrogens and progesterone on LTH secretion. These influences are probably mediated via the CNS.

glandular epithelial cells. If implantation of a fertilized ovum does not occur, the levels of progesterone and estrogen gradually decrease. The endometrium then begins to undergo desquamation, and menses ensue.

ESTROGENS

Chemistry

Estrogens may be divided into two chemical categories: those with a steroid nucleus and those without one. The so-called *naturally occurring estrogens* possess the cyclopentanophenanthrene nucleus and include 17β-estradiol, estrone, and estriol (see Fig. 32-2). Note that they all contain an aromatic A ring.

The biosynthesis of estrogens in all the organs capable of producing them is essentially the same, regardless of the site of secretion. The process of estrogen synthesis in vivo involves the conversion of cholesterol via intermediate products to 17β-estradiol. It is interesting to note that testosterone, the androgenic steroid, must be considered a necessary precursor for estrogen.

Absorption and Distribution

Estrogens may be absorbed via the skin and mucous membranes as well as from subcutaneous and intramuscular sites. The rate of absorption from parenteral areas is delayed by esterification of the estrogen. Absorption from the skin may be of such proportion that when adequate amounts of material are used, systemic effects may occur.

Oral administration of estrogens results in rapid absorption but also in prompt inactivation via the liver. In general, one may state that because of rapid absorption, excretion, and inactivation, the oral route is the least effective way of achieving a therapeutic effect. There are, however, several exceptions. One is where the presence of an ethinyl group (ethinyl estradiol) may result in a decreased rate of liver inactivation. Another unusual exception is chlorotrianisene, where the parenteral form is less active than comparable doses administered orally. It has been suggested that the liver converts the synthetic estrogen into a more active form; hence chlorotrianisene has been referred to as a proestrogen.

Metabolism and Excretion

The physiologically active and major estrogen in the body is 17β-estradiol. This steroid may be converted as follows:

$$17\beta\text{-Estradiol} \rightleftharpoons \text{estrone} \longrightarrow \text{estriol}$$
$$\Updownarrow$$
$$17\alpha\text{-estradiol}$$

Estrogens circulate in the blood in both conjugated and unconjugated forms. Steroids are generally conjugated through the hydroxyl group at C-3 with inorganic sulfate or glucuronic acid. Conjugation takes place in the liver. The conjugated and unconjugated forms are usually bound (50 to 80 percent) to certain of the plasma proteins. The conjugated steroids are more water-soluble and thus their excretion into the urine is facilitated.

Large amounts of estrogen in the free form are also excreted by the liver in the bile. This is rapidly conjugated in the intestinal tract, where some of the estrogen may be degraded by bacteria present. In addition, there is considerable reabsorption of the bile-excreted estrogen, which results in an enterohepatic circulation of the steroid. The mate-

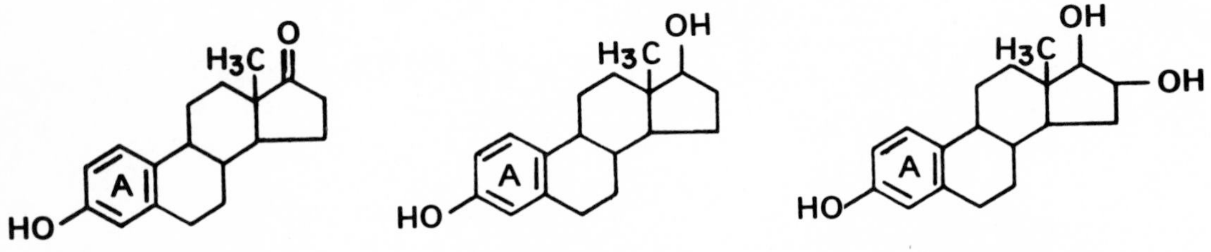

Figure 32-2 The structural formulas of the three primary estrogen compounds.

rial reabsorbed from the intestine is transported to the portal system and is further degraded in the liver cells.

Estrogen is also excreted in the feces. The fecal estrogen probably represents the sum total of the unabsorbed estrogen and that excreted in the bile.

The effect of the kidney upon circulating estrogen is not one of excretory function alone. Although estrogen metabolites are removed by the kidney in the form of glucuronates and cleared like creatinine, the kidney is also active in the conjugation of estrogen.

Effects of Estrogen on Organ Systems

The effect of estrogen on different tissues in the body helps to explain some of its apparently divergent actions.

Genital Action In addition to its influence on pituitary gonadotropin secretion, there is some evidence to show that estrogen may have a direct effect upon the ovary which is manifested by ovarian hyperemia. The secondary effects of estrogens upon the ovary are mediated via the pars distalis where estrogens appear to have a twofold effect: one to inhibit FSH secretion and the other to influence the release of LH from the adenohypophysis. In principle, it would appear that the primary effect of estrogens upon pituitary gonadotropin is probably not a direct one upon the pituitary gland itself, but that the estrogens act indirectly, through the influence of the steroid upon the hypothalamus.

The action of estrogen on the oviduct is similar to that on the uterus in that the steroid will produce an increase in muscle and mucosal growth. However, the marked increase in secretion by the mucosal cells noted at the time of ovulation is probably a manifestation of response to both estrogen and progesterone. It should also be pointed out that estrogens primarily affect the epithelial layers of the mucosal lining of the vagina and cause an increase in numbers of mitotic figures in the cells of the basal layers, followed by an increase in cell thickness. Moreover, the number of epithelial papillae along the basement membranes increases after estrogen therapy.

There have been divergent opinions on the precise role played by estrogens on the growth and development of breast tissue. However, it would appear that estrogen alone can induce almost complete mammary development.

Clinically, it should be noted that high doses of estrogens are effective in preventing postpartum lactation. The necessary factors required to depress lactation are not basically dependent on the estrogenic properties of the preparation being used but must be attributed to the ability of the hormone to suppress anterior pituitary secretion of milk-stimulating factors. Estrogens cause increased pigmentation of the areolae and accentuate Montgomery's tubercles.

Nongenital Action The nongenital action of estrogens may involve the thyroid gland, blood, hair, skin, bone, and electrolytes. The administration of estrogens increases the plasma protein-bound-iodine level without significantly changing the radioactive iodine uptake. The increase in the protein-bound iodine is due to the increase in thyroxin-binding protein. Estrogens do not affect the release of thyrotropin (TSH). The influence of estrogens on the thyroid may be inferred by the fact that the thyroid enlarges at puberty, at menstruation, and during pregnancy.

Estrogens apparently diminish blood cholesterol and phospholipids when these are elevated. By lowering blood cholesterol, estrogens may prevent the formation of atheromatous plaques of blood vessels by decreasing the level of circulating lipids which enhance the deposition of such plaques. These steroids decrease cholesterol/phospholipid and β-lipoprotein/α-lipoprotein ratios, at the same time increasing serum phospholipids and plasma triglycerides.

Estrogens also increase the amount of elastic elements in the skin, a change which may inhibit some of the process of aging one sees in the skin of the elderly female. Estrogen does not increase seborrheic activity. The hormone may actually enhance hair growth on the scalp where hair loss may have taken place because of increased androgenic activity.

The female sex hormones have a marked effect on bone tissue and electrolytes. The effect upon bone is twofold: calcium deposition and epiphyseal closure. The influence of estrogens upon calcium deposition may be indirect and is attributed to the stimulating properties of these steroids on the protein matrix of the bone which permits increased calcium deposition. Estrogens act on the epiphyses by accelerating epiphyseal closure. Although the initial response of the open epiphyses to estrogen is increased growth, rapid closure of the epiphyses would normally be expected with excessive doses of estrogens. The initial growth-stimulating response may be inhibited if large enough doses of the steroid are used to inhibit pituitary growth hormone.

Finally, estrogens can promote sodium retention, with associated fluid retention and edema. This is more likely to occur when only high doses of estrogen are used. However, the effects of estrogen upon fluid retention are less severe than are those following testosterone or glucocorticoid therapy.

Preparations and Doses

The presently available preparations, and the average doses, are listed in Table 32-1.

PROGESTERONE

There is no single comprehensive definition of a progestin. It is a substance with a cyclopentano-phenanthrene nucleus (to date there are no known synthetic progestational compounds that do not possess this chemical structure) which simulates the activity of progesterone upon the estrogen-primed endometrium. The properties of the various progestins differ in that some of the synthetic steroids will simulate the action of progesterone upon both the stroma and endometrium. In contrast, the 19-norsteroids (19-nortestosterone derivatives)

Table 32-1 Selected Estrogenic Compounds

Generic name	Route of administration	Average dosage, mg
Ethinyl estradiol	Oral	0.05–0.1/day
Mestranol	Oral	0.1–0.2/day
Conjugated estrogens (equine)	Oral	1.25–2.5/day
Diethylstilbestrol	Oral	0.3–0.6/day
Chlorotrianisene	Oral	12–24/day
Estradiol valerate	Intramuscular	10–20/every 2 weeks

have a far greater effect on the stroma than on glandular development. This dichotomy of effect might have some useful therapeutic application when progesterone itself may be of little value. The structural formulas of two progestational agents are shown in Fig. 32-3.

Source and Metabolism

Since progesterone is a vital precursor in the endogenous synthesis of all steroids, one would expect to find progesterone elaborated by all organs involved in steroidogenesis, that is, the ovaries, testes, adrenals, and placenta. Secretion of progesterone has been demonstrated from all these organs except the testes. There are three physiologically active progestins secreted by the ovary and the placenta. These include progesterone and Δ^4-pregnene-3-one-20α or 20β-ol, which have biologic activity of their own, albeit less than progesterone, but are also effective augmentors of progesterone itself.

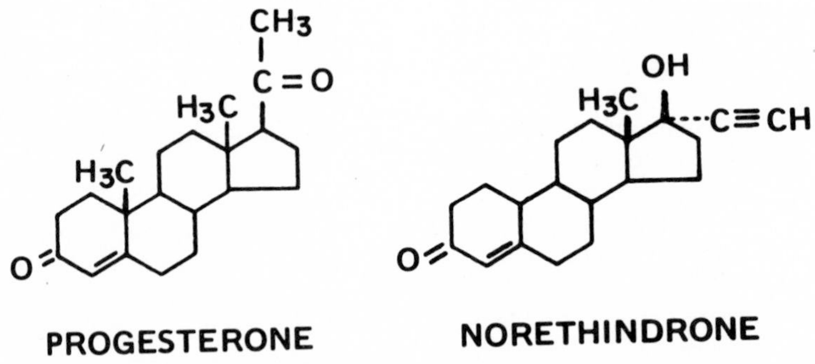

Figure 32-3 Progesterone and norethindrone.

Progesterone is synthesized from both tissue and blood cholesterol, with the tissue cholesterol derived from acetate. It is released into the bloodstream and circulated in association with plasma protein. The hormone is taken up by the fat depots in the body and stored there. It is metabolized by the liver, where it is also conjugated with glucuronic acid to form the glucuronide of pregnanediol, the form in which its excretory product appears in the urine. As with the estrogens, there is an important enterohepatic circulation of progesterone. However, unlike the estrogens, a large part is not reabsorbed and is excreted via the feces.

Effects on Organ Systems

Genital Tract The effects of progesterone upon the ovary are primarily inhibitory, occurring by suppression of pituitary gonadotropin. Progesterone appears to inhibit the release of luteinizing hormone, and thereby would appear to be an effective agent for inhibiting ovulation. It is this inhibitory effect upon ovulation that led to the use of oral progestins as contraceptive agents.

The principal site of action of progesterone is the uterus, both the mucosal and myometrial portions. Progesterone is not a growth-stimulating substance but will mature those glands which have been stimulated toward proliferation by estrogen. Progesterone can induce an adequate response only after proliferative phase activity has been accomplished by estrogen. Progesterone acts on the myometrium as a muscle relaxant to decrease the amplitude of estrogen-induced contraction. The decreased contractile activity of the myometrium under the influence of progesterone may be due to the fact that myometrial cells have a decreased intracellular concentration of potassium ions and an increased sodium ion content. This change in ionic gradient across the cell membrane may be responsible for the altered resting potential.

Progesterone appears to have an effect upon the vaginal mucosa somewhat opposite to that of estrogen. It does not produce the rapid growth of the vaginal epithelium one sees with estrogen therapy. Indeed, after estrogen treatment, progesterone will increase the rate of desquamation of the vaginal cells, so that instead of the cells remaining attached until full cornification occurs (complete maturity),

they are cast off long before the stage of cornification. Progesterone also has three other specific effects upon the vaginal mucosa: (1) It increases the degree of mucification; (2) it causes cellular folding of the desquamated cells, a characteristic finding in the ovulatory phase; and (3) it increases the number of polymorphonuclear neutrophils.

Preparations and Doses

Preparations, routes of administration, and usual dosages for progestational agents are given in Table 32-2.

THERAPEUTIC USES OF THE FEMALE SEX HORMONES

Hormonal Deficiency States

Estrogens have been used for extended periods in the management of the climacteric syndrome in the female. This syndrome, which is associated with various complaints and symptoms, is presumably due to a decrease in estrogen level and is not attributed to the increase in FSH which many of these patients show. Control of such symptoms is accomplished very easily by the use of oral estrogenic substances. The only complication to the use of estrogen in this syndrome is that uterine bleeding may occur. However, this can be controlled by using progesteronal therapy primarily to produce bleeding at desired intervals according to plan. This type of therapy may be continued for years and

Table 32-2 Selected Progestational Agents

Generic name	Route of administration	Usual dosage
Progesterone	Intramuscular	5–50 mg/day
Hydroxyprogesterone caproate	Intramuscular	375 mg/month
Medroxyprogesterone acetate	Intramuscular	50 mg–1 g/week
	Oral	2.5–10 mg/day for 5 to 20 days
Dydrogesterone	Oral	10–20 mg/day for 5 to 20 days
Norethindrone	Oral	5–40 mg/day

apparently has been instrumental in preventing some of the processes of aging and associated adverse effects that may be seen in older females.

Primary Amenorrhea or Premature Ovarian Failure

In patients with primary amenorrhea, the lack of ovarian activity may be congenital; that is, the ovaries may be completely absent. The patient with premature ovarian failure is actually precipitated into an early climacteric. Patients with primary amenorrhea require therapy not only to prevent some of the adverse effects caused by a hormonal deficiency, but also to allow adequate development of secondary sexual characteristics. Accepted therapy requires estrogen taken continuously along with intermittent treatment with the progestational steroids. Such treatment creates a eumorphically mature female who is able to participate in normal sexual relationships.

Osteoporosis

Decreased calcium deposition in bone (osteoporosis) is frequent in patients with an absence of ovarian activity. The degree of osteoporosis is markedly accentuated if patients in the climacteric are given concomitant doses of corticoids. Management of these patients requires use of estrogen for an extended period.

Inhibition of Lactation

Estrogens, or some of the newer progestational steroids, may be employed effectively to inhibit lactation during the postpartum period.

Cystic Disease of the Breasts

This usually cyclic condition can be controlled by the use of progestational steroids, particularly those having little estrogenic activity, which indirectly induce an estrogenic effect by virtue of the metabolic breakdown of the steroid into an estrogenic component. The progestogen should be administered premenstrually, beginning 7 days before the expected onset of the period.

Excessive Growth in Females

Estrogens may be used to close the epiphyses of females who are excessively tall and show poor secondary sexual development. However, high doses of estrogen must be used continuously together with concomitant but cyclic administration of a progestational steroid.

Habitual Abortion

From recent studies it would appear that when adequate controls are used, the progestational steroids are effective in maintaining pregnancy in patients with a progesterone-deficiency syndrome.

Dysmenorrhea

The management of dysmenorrhea with progestational steroids depends upon their ability to inhibit ovulation. The use of progestational agents premenstrually in patients with bona fide dysmenorrhea could accentuate the degree of dysmenorrhea rather than improve it. Ovulatory suppressive doses of such steroids twice a day from the tenth day of the cycle until the twentieth day usually ameliorate the pain of functional dysmenorrhea.

Sexual Precocity

Control of sexual precocity, particularly in the female, has in the past been very difficult because the steroids employed to inhibit ovarian activity can in their own right have an adverse effect upon accelerating closure of the epiphyses. More recently, the use of depot medroxyprogesterone parenterally was found to be an effective means of inhibiting endogenous gonadotropic hormone secretion, thereby preventing sexual precocity from continuing. Sexually precocious patients should be treated, since they will suffer adverse physiologic effects from precocious catamenia. In addition, if treatment is not instituted, premature closure of the epiphyses will take place, causing such individuals to be unusually short as adults.

Endometriosis

Endometriosis may be treated successfully by regimens employing the 19-norsteroids or depot medroxyprogesterone.

Functional Uterine Bleeding

Since the major cause of functional uterine bleeding is probably anovulation, this is most likely to occur at the time of the menarche or climacteric. Provided that all organic causes have been eliminated, patients with functional uterine bleeding are managed by the use of a progestational steroid to induce deciduation of the endometrium.

During the acute phase of menstrual bleeding, the hemorrhage may be controlled by intravenous estrogens in the form of a solution of conjugated estrogens (equine). The hemostatic effect of intravenous estrogen is quickly achieved, although the manner by which the effect is accomplished is not known.

Local Action of Estrogens

Vaginal administration of estrogens may bring about a desired therapeutic effect upon the mucosal membrane of the vagina without causing any generalized systemic changes. This is of some advantage in senile vaginitis where a systemic effect may not be desirable. The local effect of the estrogens would correct the disturbance and leave the body otherwise free of estrogenic activity.

Contraindications

There are no contraindications to the use of progestins except for steroids with strong androgenic potential (ethisterone, norethisterone) in gravid patients because of possible masculinizing effects such steroids may have on the external genitalia of the female infant.

Specific contraindications to the use of estrogens would be in patients with an active anaplastic lesion of the uterus excluding the cervix and breasts. In addition, it has been said that these steroids should not be used in the older female patient where there is a family history of breast or uterine carcinoma. Diethylstilbestrol (DES) used during pregnancy has been found to cause uterine cancer in female offspring as much as twenty years later.

ORAL CONTRACEPTIVES

One of the most important uses of progestational and estrogenic steroids has been in the area of fertility control. The estrogen-progestin oral contraceptives are designed to have the pharmacologic effect of suppressing ovulation with a minimum of side effects. The simultaneous oral administration of estrogen-progestogen combinations has been found to be almost completely effective in preventing conception. The sequential oral administration of estrogens followed by estrogen-progestogen combinations has also been highly effective. Continuous oral administration of a low-dose progestogen, however, has been found less effective than the first two dosage regimens.

The *mechanism of action* of oral contraception may possibly involve any or all of these areas: (1) interference with pituitary function through blockade of LH and FSH release; (2) alteration of fallopian tubular motility, which would discourage fertilization; (3) modification of endometrial maturation with subsequent determent of nidation; and (4) rendering cervical mucus hostile to sperm migration.

Three main types of therapy are currently in use: *combination, sequential,* and *single-entity* therapy. Examples of selected available oral contraceptives of each type are presented in Table 32-3. Combination therapy uses tablets containing both a progestogen and estrogen. These are taken orally for 20 or 21 days of each menstrual cycle, beginning on day 5 and terminating on day 24 or 25 (day 1 corresponds to the onset of menstrual bleeding). Withdrawal bleeding generally occurs 3 to 4 days after the last dose is taken. The sequential type uses two separate tablets. Estrogen (alone) is taken orally for 14 to 16 days of each cycle beginning on day 5; then a progestogen is taken with the estrogen for the next 5 to 6 days. Withdrawal bleeding generally occurs 3 to 4 days following administration of the last dose. In single-entity therapy, one tablet of a low-dose progestogen is administered daily.

Toxicities

Thromboembolic phenomena, vascular headaches, and visual disturbances have been ascribed to the use of oral contraceptives. In particular, thromboembolism has been a major source of controversy. Several statistical studies have shown an association between the use of these compounds and thromboembolic accidents; other studies by eminent authorities have failed to confirm a distinct relationship. Nevertheless, the oral contraceptives should not be used in a female with a thromboembolic history or tendency. Increased systolic and diastolic blood pressure have developed during use of oral contraceptives. Termination of therapy

Table 32-3 Selected Available Oral Contraceptives

Progestogen, mg : Estrogen, μg	Trade name
Combination formulations	
Ethynodiol diacetate 1 : Mestranol 100	Ovulen
Ethynodiol diacetate 1 : Ethinyl estradiol 50	Demulen
Norethindrone 2 : Mestranol 100	Norinyl, 2 mg
	Ortho-Novum, 2 mg
Norethindrone 1 : Mestranol 80	Norinyl, 1 + 80
	Ortho-Novum, 1/80
Norethindrone 1 : Mestranol 50	Norinyl, 1 + 50
	Ortho-Novum, 1/50
Norethindrone acetate 1 : Ethinyl estradiol 50	Norlestrin, 1 mg
Norethynodrel 2.5 : Mestranol 100	Enovid-E
Norgestrel 0.5 : Ethinyl estradiol 50	Ovral
Sequential formulations	
Dimethisterone 25 : Ethinyl estradiol 100	Oracon
Norethindrone 2 : Mestranol 80	Norquen
	Ortho-Novum SQ
Single-entity formulation	
Norethindrone 0.35	Micronor
	Nor-Q.D.
Norgestrel 0.075	Ovrette

usually resulted in a return to normal blood pressure.

Untoward side effects due to oral contraceptive compounds are as follows:

Estrogen excess
Nausea
Chloasma
Monilia vaginal infections
Mucoid leucorrhea (without odor)
Increase in pigment of areolae
Increase in size of leiomyoma
Edema

Progestogen Excess (with Androgenic Potential)
Increased appetite with weight gain
Acne
Hirsutism
Seborrhea
Cholestatic jaundice (also with estrogens)

Progestogen Excess (without Androgenic Potential)
Decreased libido
Delayed onset of menses
Fatigue
Decreased menstrual flow
Depression
Uterine cramps

Estrogen and Progestogen Deficiency
Vasomotor symptoms
Irritability
Decreased menstruation
Breakthrough bleeding and spotting

FERTILITY AGENTS

Clomiphene

In the search for antifertility compounds, several very weak estrogenic agents have been synthesized. The theory was that these weak agents would attach to estrogenic receptor sites and thus block activity. This proved to be a rather unsuccessful venture, but one of the compounds turned out to be interesting for a different reason. Clomiphene citrate, Clomid, is a relative of chlorotrianisene. It stimulates the release of pituitary gonadotropins, thus inducing follicular development and ovulation. The exact mechanism by which the gonadotropins are released is unknown but may involve direct stimulation of the hypothalamic-pituitary axis, or reduction of the inhibitory influence of endogenous estrogen. The latter action may be by competitive antagonism for sites involved in suppression of gonadotropin-releasing factors at the hypothalamic level.

$$(C_2H_5)_2NCH_2CH_2O-\!\!\!\bigcirc\!\!\!-C\!\!=\!\!\underset{|}{\overset{Cl}{C}}-\!\!\!\bigcirc\!\!\!\cdot C_6H_8O_7$$

Clomiphene citrate

Therapy consists of oral administration of tablets for 5 days starting on the fifth day of the menstrual cycle or at any time in amenorrheic women. If ovulation occurs without conception, or if ovulation does not occur, a second and possibly third course of cyclic therapy may be instituted. A minimum of 30 days should elapse between each treatment period.

Since clomiphene does not possess intrinsic gonadotropic activity, clinical effectiveness requires a hypothalamic-pituitary system capable of adequate FSH and LH secretion and an ovary capable of follicular maturation and ovulation in response to these secretions. Failure to respond to clomiphene does not, therefore, preclude the possibility of satisfactory response to exogenous gonadotropins, that is, menotropins.

Adverse Reactions The major adverse reaction to clomiphene is ovarian overstimulation resulting in ovarian enlargement, formation of ovarian cysts, ascites, acute lower abdominal pain, and ovarian hemorrhage. Relatively frequent and generally dose-related reactions include nausea, abdominal discomfort, headache, skin rash, breast soreness, reversible visual disturbances, vasomotor symptoms, and mood changes. A high incidence (10 to 15 percent) of multiple pregnancies has followed induction of ovulation by clomiphene. Transient impaired liver function and rare cases of biliary stasis have been reported. Clomiphene is potentially teratogenic, and clomiphene therapy should never be instituted until the absence of pregnancy has been ascertained.

Gonadotropins

Human menopausal gonadotropin (menotropins, HMG) is a purified preparation of gonadotropins extracted from the urine of postmenopausal women. It contains LH and FSH activity. Menotropins is used to treat anovulatory women whose ovaries are capable of responding to pituitary-gonadotropins but whose gonadotropin levels are inadequate. Menotropins administered for 9 to 12 days produces ovarian failure. Since treatment with menotropins in most instances results only in follicular growth and maturation, human chorionic gonadotropin (HCG) must be given following the administration of menotropins in order to affect ovulation. There is considerable variation in individual response to menotropins, and different dosage regimens have been used; consequently, the results of clinical experience are varied.

Chapter 33

Corticotropin and Corticosteroids

The adrenocorticotropic hormone (ACTH, corticotropin) is a pituitary hormone whose clinical effects are essentially the same as those of corticosteroids since the main action of ACTH is stimulation of production of these adrenal hormones.

CORTICOTROPIN

Sources and Chemistry

ACTH hormone is a polypeptide thought to be secreted by the microsomes of the corticotropic cells of the anterior pituitary gland. This gland also secretes an adrenal growth factor, which may modify adrenal responsiveness to ACTH.

Commercial ACTH is obtained from extracts of animal pituitary glands by chromatographic or electrophoretic technics. Although the entire ACTH polypeptide molecule has been synthesized, this method is not yet practical for commercial production.

Human ACTH contains 39 amino acids and has a molecular weight of about 4,500. Its structure is shown in Fig. 33-1. ACTH from various animal species is similar except in the sequence between amino acids 29 and 33. Synthetic corticotropinlike compounds have been prepared which are active with as few as 13 amino acids. However, for appreciable activity, a minimum of 20 amino acids is necessary.

Regulation of Secretion and Mechanism of Action of ACTH

Regulation of Secretion Secretion of ACTH is regulated by corticotropin-releasing hormone (CRH), which is formed in the area of the median eminence of the hypothalamus. It traverses the hypothalamic-portal venous system to the anterior pituitary, where it acts upon certain cells to cause increased synthesis and release of ACTH. Several mechanisms are involved in the regulation of this basic neurobiochemical process. Cortisol (hydrocortisone) in the blood acts to inhibit ACTH secre-

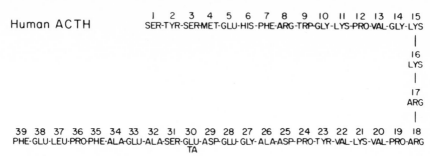

Figure 33-1 Amino acid sequence of human ACTH.

tion through a negative-feedback mechanism controlling CRH secretion. Cortisol may also have some direct pituitary and adrenal inhibitory effect.

Mechanism of Action on the Adrenal Cortex The primary action of ACTH is to increase adrenal synthesis of glucocorticoids through a pathway involving cyclic 3'5'-AMP. Apparently, the hormone acts on adenylate cyclase on the cell membrane, increasing the production of cyclic 3'5'-AMP. Associated with this is depletion of adrenal cortical lipids and ascorbic acid. Oxidative phosphorylation and protein synthesis in the adrenal cortex are increased as measured by oxygen uptake, incorporation of ^{32}P, incorporation of acetate and amino acids into protein, and formation of RNA.

Extraadrenal Effects of ACTH Perhaps the most prominent extraadrenal action of ACTH is its effect on lipid metabolism. Nonesterified fatty acids and neutral fats are mobilized from adipose depots, and increased amounts of fat appear in the liver. Ketogenesis increases, but oxidation of fat is also increased since the respiratory quotient decreases. Increased lipolysis can even be demonstrated in vitro, presumably due to activation of an adipose tissue lipase. ACTH also has a direct effect on carbohydrate metabolism which leads to reduction in blood sugar, increase in tolerance to glucose, and an increase in muscle glycogen which may be due to increased secretion of insulin.

Absorption, Fate, and Excretion

ACTH is destroyed by proteolytic enzymes; therefore, it is ineffective when given orally. The main route of administration is intramuscular, although occasionally the intravenous route is used. On intravenous injection, ACTH disappears rapidly since the plasma half-life is about 15 min. Blood and tissue proteolytic enzymes, possibly fibrinolysin, hydrolyze ACTH and thus destroy its activity. A negligible amount appears in the urine. The adrenal cortex fixes only a very small amount; much more is recoverable (10 to 20 percent) from kidney tissue. Since a target organ responds best when it is subjected to a continuous concentration of stimulating hormone, intramuscular injection is preferred. Even more efficacious are long-acting preparations of a repository type such as ACTH in a gelatin matrix.

Bioassay

Because commercial corticotropin is prepared from porcine, bovine, and cetacean pituitaries it must be bioassayed against a standard preparation of the hormone. The activity of a corticotropin preparation is expressed in U.S.P. units.

Therapeutic Use

At present, corticotropin is rarely used in therapy since its therapeutic usefulness can be accomplished with corticosteroids. Moreover, the production of antibodies may limit its therapeutic usefulness.

As a diagnostic agent, corticotropin infusion is employed to distinguish between excessive production of ACTH by the adenohypophysis and that caused by an extrapituitary neoplasm or adrenal neoplasm. Corticotropin can be used to assay adrenal cortical function. In classical Addison's disease there is no response as measured by urinary excretion of 17-ketosteroids. Corticotropin has also been used in tests of adenohypophyseal dysfunction.

Toxicity

There are rare anaphylactic reactions to corticotropin. Apart from this, corticotropin toxicity is the result of increased rate of corticosteroid secretion.

Preparations and Dose

Corticotropin Injection (Acthar) is a lyophilized powder for intravenous use. Ordinarily 20 U.S.P. units are infused over an 8-h period.

Corticotropin Repository is purified ACTH in gelatin solution for subcutaneous or intramuscular injection. An average dose is 40 units once daily.

Corticotropin, Zinc Hydroxide Suspension, is given in dosages of 40 units, once daily, by intramuscular injection.

CORTICOSTEROIDS

The corticosteroids cause a wide variety of pharmacologic activities in mammalian organisms. Two major systems are affected by these agents. The liver glycogen deposition system is stimulated (the activity is commonly referred to as *glucocorticoid* activity); and sodium ions and water are retained within the body's electrolyte and water balance system by the action of these drugs (*mineralocorticoid* activity).

The corticosteroids are classified into two groups, depending on their source. The natural corticosteroids, which are prepared from the adrenal gland, include cortisol, cortisone, corticosterone, 11-desoxycorticosterone, and aldosterone. The synthetic corticosteroids include such compounds as 9α-fluorocortisol, prednisolone, prednisone, and triamcinolone. Corticosteroids are also divided according to their glucocorticoid and mineralocorticoid activities. The order of decreasing glucocorticoid activity is 9α-fluorocortisol, triamcinolone, prednisolone, cortisol, and cortisone. The order of decreasing mineralocorticoid activity is aldosterone, 9α-fluorocortisol, and 11-desoxycorticosterone.

Chemistry and Commercial Source

The naturally occurring steroids having corticosteroid activity are pregnane derivatives (Fig. 33-2), which have ketone groups on C-3 and C-20, are unsaturated between carbons 4 and 5 of ring A (de-

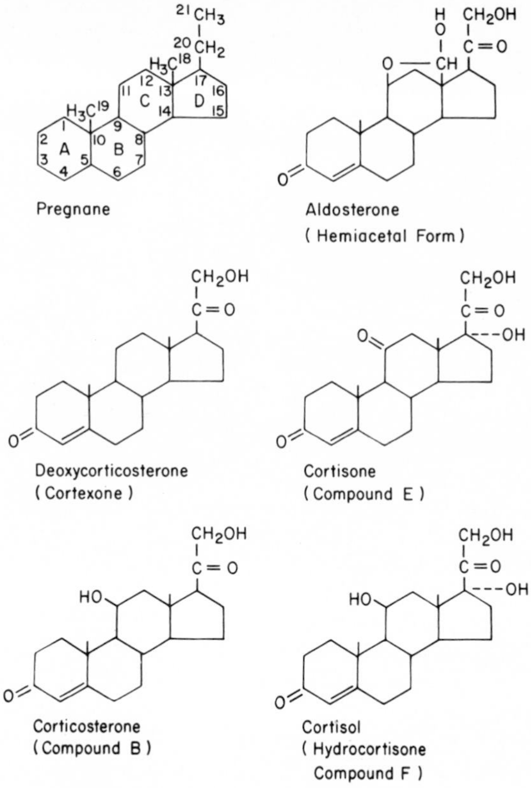

Figure 33-2 Structural formulas of pregnane and naturally occurring corticosteroids.

noted as Δ^4), and have a 17β-CO—CH$_2$OH side chain. The natural adrenal steroids vary in the presence or absence of an 11-keto, 11β-hydroxyl, 17α-hydroxyl group, and/or 18-oxygen function, and this determines their main physiologic and pharmacologic action.

Corticoids for medicinal use have been synthesized from steroid sapogenins. Although many chemical processes are involved, the discovery and use of various fungi and other microorganisms to introduce the 11β-hydroxyl group and Δ^1 unsaturation have contributed greatly to synthetic production.

Relation of Structure to Function

Figure 33-3 shows the structural formulas of the main synthetic corticosteroids. The relationship of chemical structure to function of corticosteroids is extremely complex, but a number of basic generali-

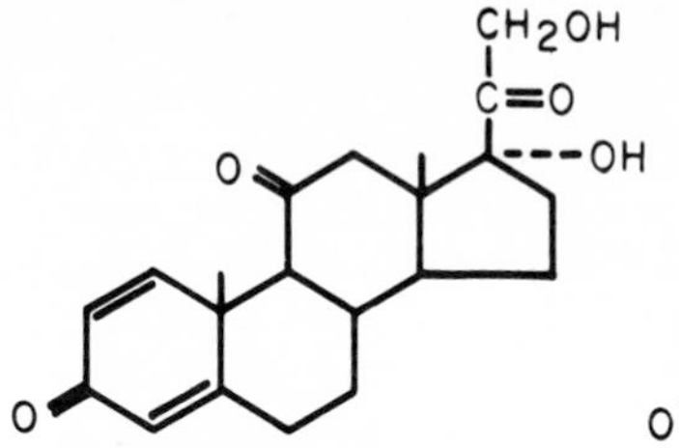

PREDNISONE
(Δ^1, CORTISONE)

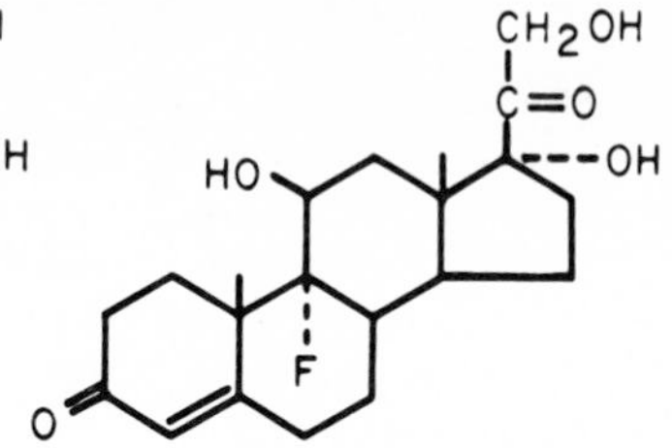

9α-FLUOROHYDROCORTISONE

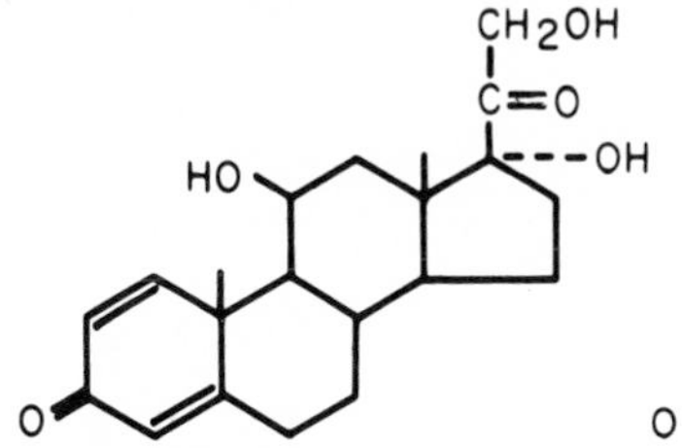

PREDNISOLONE
(Δ^1, CORTISOL)

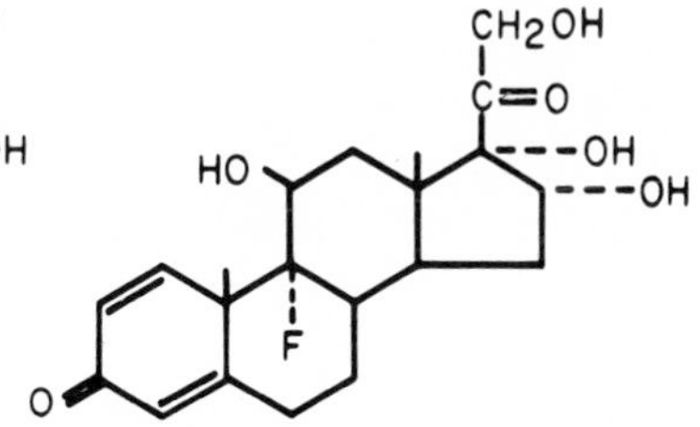

TRIAMCINOLONE
(9α-FLUORO, 16α-HYDROXY, PREDNISOLONE)

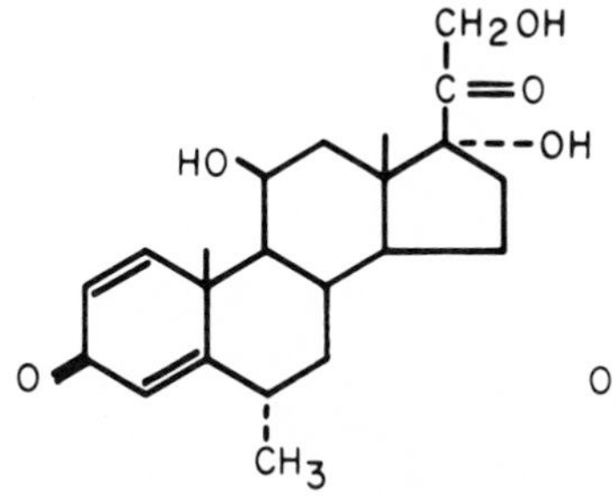

6α-METHYL PREDNISOLONE

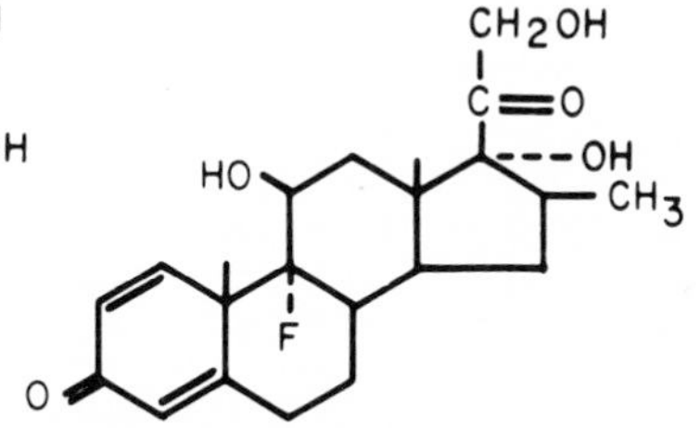

BETAMETHASONE
(9α-FLUORO, 16β-METHYL, PREDNISOLONE)

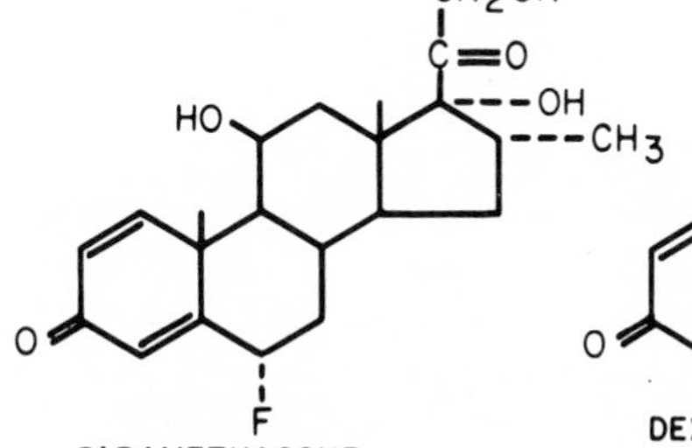

PARAMETHASONE
(6α-FLUORO, 16α-METHYL,
PREDNISOLONE)

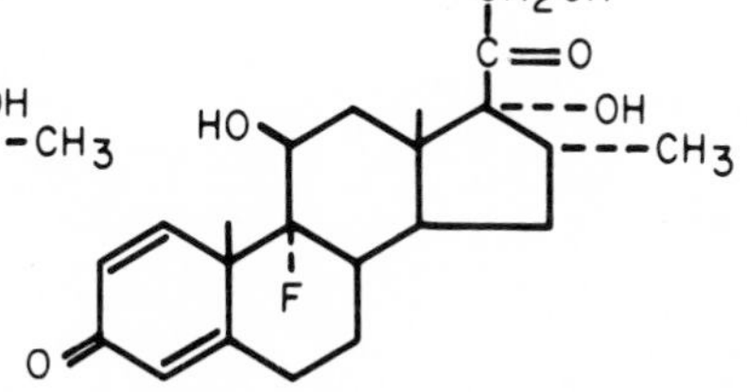

DEXAMETHASONE
(9α-FLUORO, 16α-METHYL,
PREDNISOLONE)

Figure 33-3 Structural formulas of commonly used synthetic corticosteroids.

zations can be made. Generally, structural modifications alter receptor affinity, the rate of biotransformation of the compounds, and conversion to mineralocorticoid or glucocorticoid actions.

All corticosteroids ideally must possess a 3-keto group, a 17β side chain with a 20-carbonyl group, and a 21-hydroxyl group. For glucocorticoid activity, the 11β-hydroxyl and 17α-hydroxyl groups are important. For adequate mineralocorticoid activity, the presence of oxygen at C-11 and C-18, or absence of oxygen at both C-11 and C-17, is required. In general, glucocorticoid binding occurs on the surface of the molecule, especially involving the 11β-hydroxyl and 17β-CO—CH_2OH groups which project above the plane of the ring. Since the 11β-hydroxyl group is generally essential for glucocorticoid activity, it seems likely that this group is involved in the primary steroid-receptor combination, with a secondary combination with the 17β-CO—CH_2OH side chain. Thus, bulky beta substituents would interfere with binding and decrease activity, while equatorial or alpha substituents would not.

Since 11-desoxycorticosterone has no glucocorticoid activity but is a potent mineralocorticoid and has only two potentially reactive substituents, receptor combination must involve the 3-keto and/or the 17β-CO—CH_2OH groups. Some association with the alpha-surface of the molecule of rings A, C, and D may also be involved. The fact that modifications affecting the D ring markedly affect mineralocorticoid activity suggest that the 17β-CO—CH_2OH side chain may be more important. 9α-Fluorination increases the mineralocorticoid potency of both 11-hydroxy (cortisol) and 11-desoxy (desoxycorticosterone) compounds. Furthermore, the influence of the 18-aldehyde group as in aldosterone is unknown. Conceivably it influences the reactivity of the 11-oxygen function but could also change the D ring or influence the 17β side chain.

General Physiologic and Pharmacologic Effects

The corticosteroids do not confer upon any tissue any capacities or attributes which they do not inherently possess. They do influence the rate at which the function of a particular tissue is performed. In this respect they are similar to other regulatory hormones.

Destruction of the adrenal cortex in a human results in an individual who at best can only survive under optimal conditions. Excess sodium chloride must be ingested, infection must be rigidly avoided, and any stresses such as trauma cannot be tolerated. Even under these circumstances, weight loss, protein wastage, lassitude, and inanition are inevitable consequences. In such cases, a small dose of cortisol restores the individual to normal health. Larger doses produce pharmacologic effects such as weight gain, hypertension, salt and water retention, diabetes mellitus, and abnormal fat deposits mimicking exactly the syndrome of adrenocortical hyperfunction (Cushing's syndrome).

Effects on Organ Systems

The effects of corticosteroids on organ systems are generally the indirect effects of the actions on carbohydrate, protein, fat, mineral, and water metabolism. Some may be direct actions on the target organ. The effects to be described are mainly those of the glucocorticoids cortisol, cortisone, and corticosterone, and synthetic steroids such as prednisone and triamcinolone. Desoxycorticosterone and aldosterone have effects restricted almost exclusively to mineral metabolism.

Carbohydrate and Protein Metabolism In the absence of cortisol, a brief period of starvation depletes carbohydrate reserves, since the concentration of glycogen in the liver and muscles is marginal. As a consequence, there is an extreme sensitivity to insulin. The administration of cortisol restores blood-glucose levels and the glycogen stores of the liver and muscles. The evidence is that gluconeogenesis is promoted in the liver and the periphery. Increased excretion of nitrogen suggests that protein is converted to carbohydrate.

Large doses of cortisol produce hyperglycemia, increased liver glycogen, and resistance to insulin. A catabolic effect on protein metabolism is reflected in reduced muscle mass, osteoporosis due to loss of bone matrix, thinning of skin, and a general wasting of tissues. Large amounts of amino acids are excreted in the urine.

Lipid Metabolism The actions of cortisol on fat metabolism are complex and not entirely understood. Every phase is affected: transfer, mobilization, oxidation, synthesis, and storage. Analysis of the effects of glucosteroids is difficult because they are often indirect, working through a mechanism involving other hormones. For example, the mobilization of fat from the peripheral fat depots by epinephrine is markedly impaired by the absence of glucocorticoids. Also, growth hormone from the pituitary requires the presence of glucocorticoids to promote lipolysis.

The dramatically visible effect of large doses of cortisol in humans is a peculiar alteration of fat distribution. Fat is deposited in the neck and in the supraclavicular areas on the cheeks giving rise to descriptive names such as "buffalo hump" and "moon face." Accompanying these changes is a loss of fat in the extremities.

Electrolyte and Water Metabolism Deficiency of adrenal cortical hormones leads to sodium loss, hyponatremia, hyperkalemia, reduction of extracellular fluid, and cellular hydration. Excess of cortical hormones results in the opposite picture: sodium gain, normal or slightly elevated plasma sodium, hypokalemia, and increase in the extracellular fluid compartment. The importance of the electrolyte- and water-metabolism effects of adrenal hormones is emphasized by the fact that the patient with Addison's disease may be kept alive simply by the administration of sodium chloride and water. The effects of adrenal hormones reside largely in the renal tubules; however, every cell in the body is affected.

Aldosterone is the most potent endogenous mineralocorticoid. The evidence is that the main action of aldosterone is on the distal renal tubule. Aldosterone is believed to play a major role in the normal control of electrolyte and fluid balance.

Desoxycorticosterone, another mineralocorticoid, is secreted by the adrenal cortex in relatively small amounts. It is only about one-thirtieth as potent as aldosterone, but qualitatively its effects on salt and water metabolism are similar.

Fludrocortisone is a halogenated derivative of hydrocortisone which differs from other corticoids because it has potent mineralocorticoid as well as glucocorticoid effects. It is used in the replacement therapy of salt-losing forms of congenital adrenogenital syndromes.

Some glucocorticoids, such as hydrocortisone and cortisone itself, do have sufficient salt and water metabolic effects to be used as complete replacement therapy in uncomplicated cases of Addison's disease. The newer synthetic glucocorticoids are essentially devoid of mineralocorticoid actions and are therefore considered more suitable for anti-inflammatory therapy.

Central Nervous System It is clear that changes in the concentration of circulating glucocorticoids have an effect on thought processes and central nervous system metabolism, because patients with Addison's disease (primary adrenocortical insufficiency), especially those with Cushing's syndrome (adrenocortical hyperfunction) and those receiving large doses of glucocorticoids, are apt to have abnormal mental reactions. The EEG may be abnormal in the presence of an excess or a deficiency of cortisol and, in the latter case shows slowing. Glucocorticoids, in contrast with desoxycorticosterone, increase the excitability of the brain and lower the electroshock-seizure threshold.

Cardiovascular System Following adrenalectomy, a decrease in cardiac output, stroke volume, myocardial contractility, and mean blood pressure, and an increase in pulse rate and peripheral vascular resistance occur. Myocardial atrophy can be demonstrated in about 2 weeks. Administration of corticosteroids or volume expansion tends to restore function. Studies with isolated heart-lung preparations show a reduction in cardiac work and blood pressure when blood used for perfusion is obtained from an adrenalectomized animal, and function is increased when cortisol, corticosterone, aldosterone, or 9α-fluorocortisol is added to the perfusate in low concentrations. Large doses of glucocorticoids and mineralocorticoids may have a negative inotropic effect and produce degenerative lesions in the myocardium. The participation of cortisol in blood pressure homeostasis is the result of several actions, including maintenance of normal blood volume, sodium and protein concentration, and normal peripheral vascular reactivity. Blood pressure response to norepinephrine, which is subnormal in adrenal insufficiency, is rapidly restored by the administration of cortisol.

Gastrointestinal System Glucocorticoids may stimulate excessive production of acid and pepsin and tend to reduce the gastric mucous protective barrier; therefore, the incidence of peptic and particularly gastric ulcer is greatly increased in patients treated with glucocorticoids. The stomach and duodenum appear to be quite sensitive to this effect.

Musculoskeletal System Muscle weakness may occur as a result of corticosteroid deficiency or excess, but due to different mechanisms. In adrenal insufficiency, there is rapid muscular exhaustion; work capacity of normal muscle is not increased by corticosteroids. Although the mechanism of action is unknown, corticosteroids may directly influence the metabolic processes necessary for maintenance of normal muscle contraction.

Glucocorticoid excess may cause steroid myopathy. Antianabolic and catabolic effects on protein metabolism and potassium depletion appear to be the significant factors in its development. Interestingly, thigh and gluteal muscles seem to be more affected than others.

Abnormalities in calcium and bone metabolism, including development of osteoporosis, can be demonstrated in humans or animals as a result of glucocorticoid therapy, and are also observed in Cushing's syndrome. Cortisol reduces absorption of calcium from the gastrointestinal tract, perhaps in part because of antagonism with the action of vitamin D.

Skin and Connective Tissue In Addison's disease, the skin is cool and dry and exhibits a purplish-brown pigmentation due to increased amounts of melanin or its metabolic products. Pigmentation is not the direct effect of cortisol deficiency but is due to increased ACTH and/or MSH (melanocyte stimulating hormone) secretion resulting from loss of cortisol inhibition. These changes can be reversed by administration of cortisol, but it is not uncommon that some degree of pigmentation persists.

In Cushing's syndrome, or during chronic high-dose glucocorticoid therapy, the skin may become atrophic, and purplish-red striae may develop on the abdomen and upper thighs and, in women, around the breasts. Acne and hirsutism are not infrequent in Cushing's syndrome but probably are more the result of androgenic 17-ketosteroid production than of excessive cortisol production.

Hematologic Effects The optimal blood-cortisol concentration for greatest migratory activity of neutrophils appears to be 0.4 to 1.0 μg/ml, and both migratory properties and the phagocytic index are decreased in adrenal insufficiency. At higher cortisol levels of 10 to 100 μg/ml, neutrophils increase in number and survival rate is prolonged, but there is a decrease in cellular "stickiness," diapedesis, ameboid activity, phagocytosis, digestion, and glycolysis. Since normal plasma-cortisol levels are in the range of about 0.1 to 0.2 μg/ml, it is obvious that the protective functions of the neutrophil would be enhanced by the moderate elevations in plasma-cortisol levels occurring in stress but inhibited by the extremely high levels obtained when very large doses of glucocorticoids are given.

The phagocytic activity of monocytes is reduced by low plasma-cortisol levels, increased by normal to moderately elevated levels, and inhibited by very high levels. High levels also decrease mitotic activity, diapedesis, digestive power, and participation in granuloma formation, and increase intracellular parasite survival time. Participation of lymphocytes in certain allergic phenomena, such as active delayed allergy and antibody formation, is also altered by glucocorticoids.

Metabolism of plasma cells is depressed by excessive amounts of cortisol, especially at the stage of rapid cellular development. As a result, mitotic activity and antibody formation in response to a primary antigenic stimulus are depressed. Response to a secondary antigenic stimulus is less affected.

Even small amounts of cortisol depress the number of circulating eosinophils, possibly as a result of increased sequestration in the lungs and spleen; larger doses cause a reduction of the eosinophils in the bone marrow. The effect on basophils is similar.

Excesses of glucocorticoids also tend to increase the number of circulating red blood cells and platelets and to shorten blood clotting time.

Immunologic Effects In most of the studies on immunologic processes, relatively large doses of glucocorticoids have been used, and relatively little is known about the effect of physiologic doses. Pharmacologic doses reduce antibody production by lymphocytes and plasma cells, and administration of ACTH or cortisone during active immunization reduces the amount of measurable antibodies compared with untreated controls. This is chiefly due to inhibition of antibody synthesis rather than to increased destruction of antibody.

Effects on the Endocrine System The most obvious effect of the glucocorticoids on the endocrine system is suppression of pituitary ACTH secretion, which results in adrenal cortical atrophy. There may also be an adrenal inhibitory effect not mediated through ACTH suppression. The degree of adrenal atrophy is dose-dependent but may be severe if moderate or high doses are given for more than 2 to 4 weeks. The atrophy is primarily of the reticular and fascicular zones of the adrenal cortex, but the glomerular, being only slightly under ACTH control, changes very little. Clinically, ACTH suppression is reflected by a decrease in urinary 17-ketosteroids, unless a very high dose of the glucocorticoid, which in itself can be partly metabolized to 17-ketosteroids, is used. Adrenal atrophy, so produced, may be only slowly reversed after withdrawal of steroid therapy, and clinical adrenal insufficiency may occur. Secretion of MSH is also suppressed by glucocorticoids, and pigmentation in treated addisonian patients may decrease.

Metyrapone

A number of drugs have been discovered which block steroidogenesis. Metyrapone, the most important of the series, blocks 11β- and 18,19-hydroxylases. Unfortunately, although metyrapone has a low toxicity, it does not have a permanent effect on adrenal hyperfunction.

Metyrapone

Metyrapone (Metopirone) is marketed for use as a diagnostic test of hypothalamic pituitary function. An ACTH test should be done first to ensure that adrenal function is present. Metyrapone is then administered and urinary output of steroids observed. The excretion of 17-hydroxycorticosteroids (17-OHCS) and 17-ketogenic steroids (17-KGS) is increased when pituitary function is normal. If pituitary function is decreased, there is no significant increase in 17-hydroxycorticosteroids or 17-ketogenic steroids.

Spironolactone

The 17-spirolactosteroids are a group of synthetic compounds capable of blocking the sodium-retaining effects of aldosterone, desoxycorticosterone, and cortisol. The most important of these is spironolactone (Aldactone). It appears to compete with aldosterone, desoxycorticosterone, and cortisol for binding sites in the distal renal tubule, thus reducing binding of these sodium-retaining compounds to tubular receptors. Since spironolactone inherently has only weak sodium-retaining activity, the resultant effect is sodium diuresis. The potassium-excreting effect of mineralocorticoids is also blocked. Although spironolactone is not indicated in the treatment of primary aldosteronism, it may be of value in secondary aldosteronism. The primary use of spironolactone is as a diuretic (see Chap. 24).

Spironolactone

Therapy with Glucocorticoids

Most clinicians consider using these drugs only when other agents offer no relief and the benefits outweigh the risks. Techniques of administration such as local instillation into the eye or injection into the knee joint may achieve local relief without risking systemic toxicity.

In general, the new synthetic glucocorticoids which have little or no sodium-retaining activity are preferred and may be used almost interchangeably in equivalent anti-inflammatory doses, since with two or three exceptions, there is no convincing evidence that one steroid is more effective than another at a practical clinical level. Similarly, toxicity from commonly employed doses, again with two or three exceptions, seems to be about the same when equivalent doses are used (Table 33-1).

Table 33-1 Equivalent Anti-inflammatory Doses of Glucocorticoids

Glucocorticoid	Dose, mg
Cortisone	25
Cortisol	20
Prednisone	5
Prednisolone	5
Methylprednisolone	4
Triamcinolone	4
Paramethasone	2
Dexamethasone	0.75
Betamethasone	0.6

Ordinarily, therapy is initiated with large or massive doses of glucocorticoids, and the dose is gradually reduced to the minimum amount which controls the manifestations of the disease, using adjunctive therapy or more specific drugs when these are available. The intermittent dosage regimen is worthy of consideration and should be tried more often. Short-acting steroids, such as cortisone, cortisol, prednisone, prednisolone, or methylprednisolone, should be used for this purpose. Administering steroids on three consecutive days a week has been effective in some situations, and toxicity is lessened.

Substitution Therapy Corticosteroids do not cure any disease: they are replacement therapy for either acute or chronic adrenal insufficiency. Fortunately, such diseases are rare.

In acute adrenal insufficiency water, salt, glucose, and hydrocortisone are indicated. Care must be exercised not to cause an excessive salt and water load.

In chronic adrenal insufficiency when the adrenals are totally destroyed either by disease or surgery, substitution must be carried out for the lifespan of the individual. Usually 5 to 15 mg/day of hydrocortisone is adequate. In addition, some patients require small doses of a mineralocorticoid. Others get along quite well merely by adding dietary salt.

Pharmacologic Use of Corticosteroids

Rheumatoid Arthritis When feasible, therapy should be restricted to a localized area. In acute stages, where no other therapy is effective, corticosteroids may be used for brief periods (2 to 3 weeks). Intermittent therapy has been tried with some success. Severe cases of osteoarthritis may also be treated by local instillation into the affected joint.

Rheumatic Carditis In severe cases acute rheumatic carditis may be brought under control with corticosteroids. However, this therapy is reserved for cases which do not respond to salicylates.

Bronchial Asthma In status asthmaticus corticoids may be life-saving. However, the use of these agents in chronic asthma is reserved only for the most resistant cases.

Eye Diseases Perhaps one of the most successful uses of corticosteroids has been in various inflammatory diseases of the eye. Diseases which respond are allergic blepharitis, uveitis, iritis, choroiditis, sympathetic ophthalmia, and conjunctivitis.

Miscellaneous A number of other specific diseases have responded to corticoid therapy. These are nephrosis, acute stages of nephritis, lupus erythematosus, eczematoid skin diseases, various allergic skin disorders, pemphigus cerebral edema, leukemias, and Hodgkin's disease.

Toxicity

Pharmacologic doses of corticosteroids *always* provoke toxic manifestations. It is impossible to achieve a clinical benefit without incurring some unpleasant and even dangerous side action. Continued use of large doses results in iatrogenic Cushing's syndrome. The most dangerous aspects of corticosteroid therapy are peptic ulceration, with or without hemorrhage, and increased susceptibility to infection. Psychoses are frequent and may be a most dangerous complication. Osteoporosis may be induced by chronic use in the elderly, especially in postmenopausal women. Myopathy is an uncommon but serious complication.

The incidence of serious complications is a function of time. Rarely does toxicity become dangerous with therapies lasting less than 2 weeks. On the other hand, with intermittent dosage and fastidious care, serious toxicity may be minimized and therapy continued even for years.

In intensive corticosteriod therapy even for short periods, sudden cessation results in withdrawal symptoms consisting mainly of the signs of adrenal insufficiency, but sometimes also including fever, myalgia, arthralgia, and malaise. For this reason, it is advisable to reduce corticosteroid dosage gradually rather than terminate therapy abruptly.

Preparations

Cortisone Acetate (Cortisone Acetate, Cortogen Acetate, Cortone Acetate) Ointment (ophthalmic), 1.5 percent. Suspension (injection), 25 and 50 mg/ml; suspension (ophthalmic), 0.5 and 2.5 percent. Tablets, 5, 10, and 25 mg.

Dexamethasone (Decadron, Deronil, Dexameth, Gammacorten, Hexadrol) Aerosol (topical), 10 mg/ 90 g. Elixir, 0.1 mg/ml. Tablets, 0.25, 0.5, 0.75, 1.5, and 4 mg.

Hydrocortisone (Cortef, Cortril, Hycortole, Hydrocortone) Cream (topical), 1 and 2.5 percent. Lotion (topical), 0.5, 1, and 2.5 percent. Ointment (topical), 1 and 2.5 percent. Solution (injection), 25, 50, and 100 mg/ml. Suspension (oral), 2 mg/ml. Tablets, 5, 10, and 20 mg.

Prednisone (Deltasone, Deltra, Meticorten, Paracort, Delta-Dome) Tablets, 1, 2.5, 5, 10, 20, and 25 mg.

Triamcinolone (Aristocort, Kenacort) Syrup, 0.2 and 0.4 mg/ml. Tablets, 1, 2, 4, 8, and 16 mg.

Triamcinolone Acetonide (Aristocort, Aristoderm, Kenalog, Kenalog-IM) Cream (topical), 0.1 and 0.5 percent. Foam, 0.1 percent. Lotin, 0.025 and 0.1 percent. Ointment, 0.025 and 0.1 percent. Spray, 0.007 percent. Suspension (injection), 10 and 40 mg/ml.

Triamcinolone Diacetate (Aristocort, Aristocort Forte) Suspension (injection), 25 and 40 mg/ml. Syrup, 0.4 and 0.8 mg/ml.

Fludrocortisone Acetate (Florinef Acetate) Tablets, 0.1 mg.

Part Nine

Antineoplastic Agents

Chapter 34

Cancer Chemotherapy

An intensive search is under way to discover drugs which will specifically interfere with the growth of cancer cells. In recent years this goal has been pursued with increasing vigor, in large part because of financial support provided by the United States government. Large-scale programs have been established to screen drugs of all types and origins for anticancer activity.

The drugs discussed in this chapter have been selected principally because of their therapeutic activity against some forms of cancer. Their effects, however, are not specific against neoplastic cells since in most instances they act by similar mechanism on related normal cells.

ANTIMETABOLITES

Antimetabolites are structural analogues of physiologically occurring substances (metabolites) which can produce evidence of deficiency of the metabolites in a biologic system. This does not imply that

all structural analogues are antimetabolites, since many are metabolically inert and some may even substitute for the corresponding metabolite. This definition implies that the analogue interferes with the function of the corresponding physiologic substance. Figure 34-1 gives examples of the proved or potentially useful antimetabolites discussed below compared structurally with the corresponding metabolite.

Folic Acid Antagonists

The mechanism of action of the folic acid antagonists in producing cellular injury must be considered in relation to the biologic functions of folic acid. In order to exert its biologic effect, folic acid (F) must be reduced to its active coenzyme form, 5,6,7,8-tetrahydrofolic acid (FH_4) (Fig. 34-2). This conversion occurs in two steps: The first is an NADPH-dependent reduction of folic acid to 7,8-dihydrofolic acid (FH_2), and the second is an NADH- or NADPH-dependent reduction of FH_2 to

FH_4. Folate reductases are necessary for catalyzing both of these reductions.

Several derivatives of FH_4 are involved in the transfer of one-carbon groups in a number of essential reactions in the biosynthesis of nucleic acids and amino acids. Although several folic acid antagonists have been synthesized and studied, *methotrexate*, 4-amino-N^{10}-methylpteroylglutamic acid, is the most widely used (Fig. 34-1).

Methotrexate

Mechanism of Action The principal action of methotrexate is to competitively inhibit dihydrofolate reductase, thereby preventing the formation

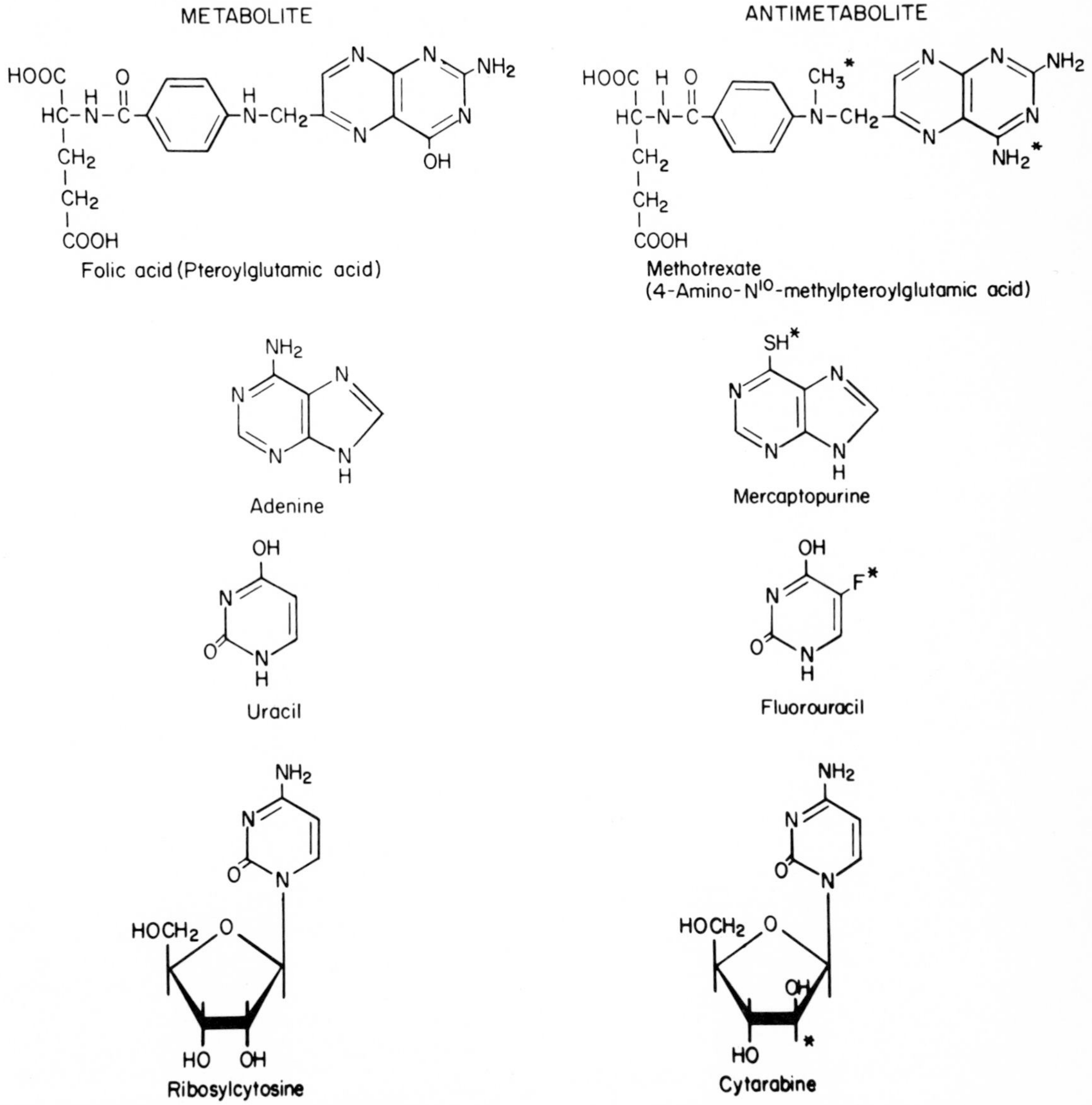

METABOLITE

ANTIMETABOLITE

Folic acid (Pteroylglutamic acid)

Methotrexate
(4-Amino-N^{10}-methylpteroylglutamic acid)

Adenine

Mercaptopurine

Uracil

Fluorouracil

Ribosylcytosine

Cytarabine

Figure 34-1 Examples of antimetabolites compared with the corresponding metabolites. (The asterisk indicates *structural change*.)

(1) Folic Acid $\xrightarrow{+2H}$ Dihydrofolic Acid (FH_2)

(2) $FH_2 \xrightarrow{+2H}$ Tetrahydrofolic Acid (FH_4)

(3) $FH_4 \xrightarrow{\text{formate}} N^{10}$-formyl FH_4

Figure 34-2 Steps in the conversion of folic acid to tetrahydrofolic acid (FH_4).

of FH_4 from FH_2. The affinity of dihydrofolate reductase for the antimetabolite is far greater than its affinity for the normal substrate (FH_2). Because of the marked affinity of the enzyme for methotrexate, even very large doses of folic acid given simultaneously fail to reverse the toxic effects of methotrexate in vivo. If folic acid is given 1 h prior to methotrexate, the toxic effects can be prevented since this allows time for the reduction of folic acid to the active derivatives. Citrovorum factor, however, if given with or shortly after methotrexate, will prevent its toxic effects, since citrovorum factor (N^5-formyl FH_4) is a derivative of the product (FH_4) of the blocked reaction. There is, however, no selective block of toxic effects, and except in special circumstances, the use of citrovorum factor prevents all the effects of methotrexate.

Physiologic Fate and Distribution   Methotrexate is absorbed rapidly from the gastrointestinal tract, and peak blood concentrations occur within 1 h after oral ingestion in humans. It is rapidly excreted in the urine, and the blood concentration in humans falls to negligible levels 3 to 7 h after administration of usual therapeutic doses.

Methotrexate penetrates the blood-brain barrier poorly, and its concentration in the cerebrospinal fluid is less than 10 percent of that in the blood. When given intrathecally, a concentration can be maintained in the cerebrospinal fluid for as long as 6 days following a single injection.

Toxicity   With conventional dosage schedules, methotrexate may produce myelosuppression, mucositis, and gastrointestinal symptoms. At high dose regimens and after prolonged use, hepatic necrosis may develop.

Treatment of Toxicity   At the first signs of toxicity, the drug must be temporarily discontinued. If an excessive dose has been given, folinic acid (citrovorin factor, leucovorin factor) should be given intramuscularly and repeated for several days. Di-

arrhea and bone marrow aplasia are treated by supportive measures. Recovery usually begins within 3 to 10 days after treatment is stopped, but toxicity may be irreversible. High dose regimens of methotrexate and folinic acid have produced cutaneous vasculitis and renal impairment.

Therapeutic Uses   Methotrexate is used principally in acute myeloblastic leukemia. It produces temporary hematologic and clinical improvement in young children with this disease. Although methotrexate is rarely effective in acute leukemia in adults (which is usually myeloblastic), it may induce hematologic remissions in patients who responded to 6-mercaptopurine and then became refractory to it. It has produced tumor regression and cures in metastatic choriocarcinoma in women. Methotrexate has been effective in the treatment of psoriasis, but because of its severe toxicities, its use is restricted to physicians skilled in antimetabolite therapy.

Preparations   Methotrexate is available in 2.5-mg tablets for oral use and in 5- and 50-mg vials for intravenous or intrathecal use.

Purine Analogues

Among the large number of purine analogues which have been synthesized, mercaptopurine (6-MP) and thioguanine (6-TG) have proved to be the most clinically effective in cancer chemotherapy. Thioguanine is similar in its pharmacologic properties to mercaptopurine. Two other purine analogues are allopurinol, an inhibitor of xanthine oxidase, and azathioprine, an immunosuppressive agent. The structures of these purine analogues are shown in Fig. 34-3.

Mercaptopurine and Thioguanine

Mechanism of Action   There may be two mechanisms involved in the antimetabolite actions of mercaptopurine. First, it has been shown that mercaptopurine inhibits the utilization of hypoxanthine in the synthesis of nucleic acids. The principal site of action of mercaptopurine might be in the conversion of a hypoxanthine-containing compound to an adenine-containing nucleotide; this has been suggested by the finding that mercaptopurine is converted in vivo to its ribonucleotide (6-thioinosinic acid), which is the active form. Once formed, 6-thioinosinic acid inhibits the conversion

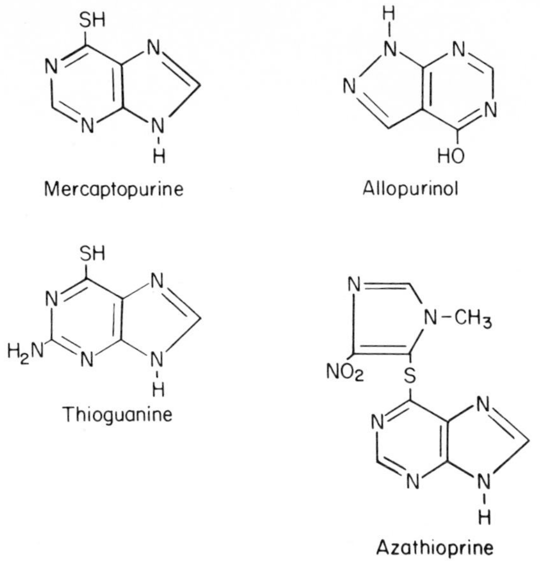

Figure 34-3 Purine antimetabolites.

of inosinic acid to adenylosuccinic acid and xanthylic acid, thus preventing the formation of guanylic acid. Second, mercaptopurine, as the ribonucleotide, interferes with an early step in purine biosynthesis, the conversion of phosphoribosyl pyrophosphate to phosphoribosylamine, which is needed for RNA and DNA synthesis. These actions of mercaptopurine, as with other antimetabolites, are not unique for leukemic cells but may also affect rapidly proliferating normal cells such as bone marrow and intestinal epithelium.

Although thioguanine appears similar to mercaptopurine in chemotherapeutic activity, its mechanism of action is somewhat different. Thioguanine is reported to be incorporated into RNA and DNA by substituting for guanine. This effect leads to abnormal nucleic acid formation.

Physiologic Fate and Distribution Mercaptopurine and thioguanine are well absorbed after oral administration and are distributed in the total body water. Both compounds penetrate the blood-brain barrier. Mercaptopurine is extensively converted by the enzyme xanthine oxidase to 6-thiouric acid, and mercaptopurine half-life in the blood has been estimated at 90 min. Thioguanine undergoes methylation to become 2-amino-6-methylthiopurine. The metabolites of both purine analogues are rapidly excreted in the urine.

Toxicities Some patients, after continued treatment with mercaptopurine or thioguanine, complain of nausea and epigastric distress, probably due to an early toxic effect on the intestinal tract. However, thioguanine causes fewer gastrointestinal side effects than does mercaptopurine. Bone marrow depression is the chief toxic action of both drugs, and excessive dosage produces leukopenia, thrombocytopenia, and bleeding, which may be fatal. Although jaundice occurs frequently in patients taking mercaptopurine, patients requiring treatment with a purine analogue possess very complicated clinical pictures and the evidence for liver toxicities is incomplete.

Therapeutic Uses Mercaptopurine has been of value principally in the treatment of acute lymphoblastic leukemia in children. It is effective in chronic granulocytic leukemia and may be particularly helpful in patients who have become refractory to other agents. Since the mechanism of action of mercaptopurine is different from that of the folic acid antagonists, it may produce remissions in some cases of acute leukemia which have not responded to methotrexate and vice versa. Thioguanine is effective in the treatment of the same types of leukemia as is mercaptopurine.

Preparations and Dosage Mercaptopurine (Purinethol) is available in 50-mg tablets for oral administration. The usual dosage range is 2.5 to 5.0 mg/kg daily.

Thioguanine is available in 40-mg tablets for oral administration. The usual dosage is 2.0 mg per kg of body weight once a day.

Allopurinol Allopurinol is a potent inhibitor in vitro and in vivo of xanthine oxidase, which is responsible for the conversion of hypoxanthine to xanthine to uric acid. Consequently, allopurinol is used to treat diseases which are characterized by excessive production of uric acid—for example, gout, leukemia, and lymphoma—particularly where treatment results in the rapid dissolution of neoplastic cells with liberation of their nucleic acid purines and subsequent oxidation of these purines to uric acid. Since mercaptopurine is also a substrate for xanthine oxidase, the concurrent administration of allopurinol delays the oxidative degradation of mercaptopurine and markedly increases its toxicity. The dose of mercaptopurine should therefore be reduced to one-third to one-fourth of the usual dose if allopurinol is to be given concurrently. Since thioguanine is degraded by other pathways not dependent on xanthine oxidase, its toxicity is not enhanced by allopurinol and, therefore, it may be used more safely than mercaptopurine in clinical situations where allopurinol is needed.

Allopurinol produces little toxicity, although about 5 percent of patients develop an allergic rash, promptly responsive to withdrawal of the medication.

Preparation and Dosage Allopurinol (Zyloprim) is supplied in 100- and 300-mg tablets. The usual oral dosage is 10 mg/kg daily in 3 or 4 divided doses.

Azathioprine Azathioprine, a widely used imidazole derivative of mercaptopurine, has been found to produce clinical responses in leukemia patients and toxicities similar to those produced by mercaptopurine and thioguanine. This compound is used as an immunosuppressive agent and is important as a pharmacologic adjunct in organ transplantation in humans.

Preparation and Dosage Azathioprine (Imuran) is available in 50 mg tablets. The usual dose is initially 3 to 5 mg/kg daily, then a maintenance dose of 1 to 4 mg/kg daily.

Pyrimidine Analogues

A large number of fluorinated pyrimidine analogues were synthesized as potential anticancer drugs. The most intensively studied of these have been fluorouracil (FU, 5-FU) and floxuridine (FUdR, 5-FUdR). The structure of fluorouracil is shown in Fig. 34-1 and the structure of floxuridine is as follows:

Floxuridine

Fluorouracil and Floxuridine

Mechanism of Action Probably the most important mechanism of action of the fluorinated pyrimidines is the inhibition of thymidylate synthetase and thus interference with DNA production. This action is accomplished by formation of an active metabolite, 5-fluoro-2'-deoxyuridine-5'-phosphate (FUdRMP), from both fluorouracil and floxuridine. In clinical use, it is important to watch carefully for early signs of toxicity since continued administration of fluorouracil and floxuridine beyond that point can result in severe, sometimes fatal, gastrointestinal ulcerations and bone marrow aplasia.

Therapeutic Uses Fluorouracil and floxuridine have had extensive trials against cancer in humans. Clinical responses have been reported in a variety of cancers, including those of the large bowel, breast, stomach, ovary, thyroid, pancreas, cervix, pharynx, and urinary bladder. Even among the most responsive cancers (breast, large bowel, liver, stomach, cervix, ovary), there has been considerable variation in the reported response.

Preparations and Dosage Fluorouracil is supplied in ampuls containing 0.5 gm/10 ml. Fluorouracil can be injected rapidly directly into a vein with no undesirable local or immediate systemic side effects. The usual dosage of fluorouracil is 12 mg/kg given daily for 5 consecutive days, followed by 6 mg/kg on alternate days until some evidence of oral, gastrointestinal, or bone marrow toxicity occurs. Floxuridine is given in a dose of 30 mg/kg daily for 5 days, followed by 15 mg/kg on alternate days until toxicity occurs.

Idoxuridine Another pyrimidine analogue is idoxuridine (IUdR). Inhibition of thymidylate synthetase by FUdRMP reduces the methylation of 2'-deoxyuridylic acid to form thymidylic acid. This

Idoxuridine

thymidine deficiency produced by thymidylate synthetase inhibition is presumably the main action of fluorouracil and floxuridine that causes cellular injury and death.

Physiologic Fate and Distribution   Fluorouracil is absorbed irregularly from the gastrointestinal tract and may be degraded to some extent when ingested. The activity is therefore more predictable when given intravenously: it is broken down to dihydrofluorouracil and then to urea. These metabolites appear in the urine. Fluorouracil is incorporated into RNA but not into DNA, although it is not certain that the incorporation into RNA is related to the biologic effects of fluorouracil. It appears that fluorouracil is converted to its ribonucleotide derivatives, in which form it is active. Floxuridine is active at a dose similar, on a molar basis, to that of fluorouracil, and it is thought that it is degraded to fluorouracil. The biologic activity of fluorouracil and floxuridine is dependent on the rate of administration. Slow intravenous infusion markedly *decreases* the toxicity of fluorouracil but markedly *increases* the toxicity of floxuridine.

Toxicity   The effects of fluorouracil and floxuridine are most prominent on the rapidly proliferating tissues, bone marrow, and gastrointestinal tract. The earliest signs of toxicity in humans are glossitis, diarrhea, and a fall in the leukocyte and platelet counts. Because of its incorporation into DNA and its ability to inhibit the growth of DNA viruses, it is used successfully in the topical treatment of herpes simplex infections of the cornea in humans.

Cytarabine   Cytarabine, cytosine arabinoside, is an active antimetabolite effective in the treatment of leukemias. It affects bone marrow and gastrointestinal epithelium most prominently. Although it has been suggested that cytarabine inhibits the enzymatic reduction of ribonucleotides, it appears that its major effect is in inhibiting DNA polymerase.

Cytarabine produces temporary complete remissions in acute granulocytic, acute lymphocytic, and other forms of acute leukemias. It disappears rapidly from the blood following intravenous injection. Its major disposition is by enzymatic deamination to uracil arabinoside, which is inactive in man.

Preparation and Dosage   Cytarabine (Cytosar) is available in 100- and 500-mg vials. The usual dosage range is 1 to 4 mg/kg daily. Maintenance is 1 mg/kg once or twice a week.

ALKYLATING AGENTS
Nitrogen Mustards and Related Compounds

Bis(β-chloroethyl) sulfide (mustard gas) was the most effective war gas used during the First World War. In 1935, a nitrogen-containing analogue of sulfur mustard, tris(β-chloroethyl)amine, was prepared, and this and the related series subsequently prepared have been called *nitrogen mustards*. Many analogues of nitrogen mustard and related agents have been synthesized and tested in various biologic systems. An important stimulus to this work is the parallelism in the biologic effects of alkylating agents and x-rays. The alkylating agents are chemicals that replace the hydrogen in a reacting chemical by an alkyl group. The alkylating agents react with water and with many organic substances; they react with the carboxyl and amino groups in proteins and with the phosphate groups and nitrogen atoms of nucleic acids.

Chemistry   The structures of the alkylating agents used most commonly in cancer chemotherapy are shown in Fig. 34-4. Note that they all contain two or three alkylating groups and are thus known as *polyfunctional* alkylating agents. Despite the differences in structure and chemical reactivity, the pathologic effects of the polyfunctional alkylating agents are fairly uniform in vivo. Representative chemical reactions are shown in Fig. 34-5.

Mechanism of Action   Agents with a monofunctional alkylating group may have a slight biologic effect similar to that of nitrogen mustard itself, but compounds with two or more functional groups are at least 50 to 100 times more active. It has been postulated, therefore, that the polyfunctional compounds are cross-linking agents; their effects are accomplished by the two reactive arms of the molecule bridging across two chromosomal strands or reacting at two points on the chromosome, or by becoming attached at one point on a structure, with the unattached group polymerizing with the free end of another attached alkyl group.

General Toxicity   The effects of the polyfunc-

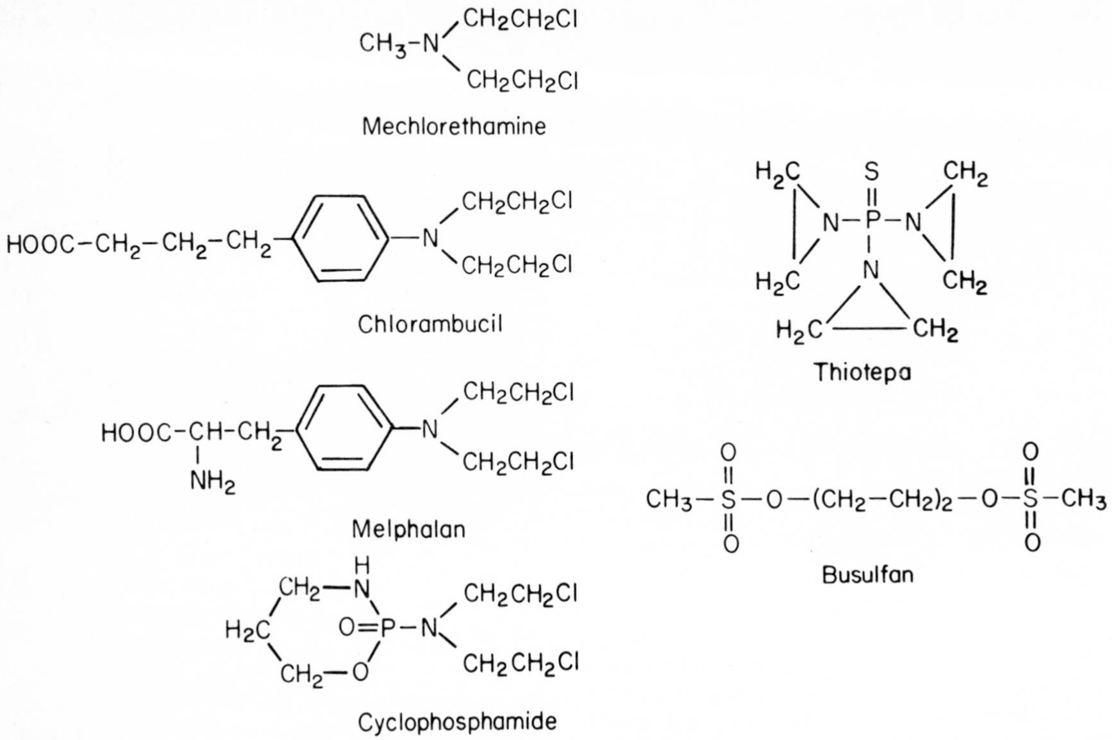

$$CH_3-N \begin{matrix} CH_2CH_2Cl \\ \\ CH_2CH_2Cl \end{matrix}$$

Mechlorethamine

$$HOOC-CH_2-CH_2-CH_2-\bigcirc-N\begin{matrix} CH_2CH_2Cl \\ \\ CH_2CH_2Cl \end{matrix}$$

Chlorambucil

$$HOOC-\underset{\underset{NH_2}{|}}{CH}-CH_2-\bigcirc-N\begin{matrix} CH_2CH_2Cl \\ \\ CH_2CH_2Cl \end{matrix}$$

Melphalan

Thiotepa

$$CH_3-\overset{\overset{O}{\|}}{\underset{\underset{O}{\|}}{S}}-O-(CH_2-CH_2)_2-O-\overset{\overset{O}{\|}}{\underset{\underset{O}{\|}}{S}}-CH_3$$

Busulfan

Cyclophosphamide

Figure 34-4 Alkylating agents.

tional alkylating agents are similar in many respects to those of total body irradiation. When given parenterally at toxic doses, these drugs induce: (1) involution in the size of the lymph nodes, thymus, and spleen; (2) progressive fall in the leukocytes and platelets in the peripheral blood, associated with aplasia of the bone marrow; (3) diarrhea, associated with ulceration and sloughing of the intestinal mucosa; (4) decrease in antibody production and increase in susceptibility to infection; (5) decrease in spermatogenesis; and (6) venous thrombosis.

In humans, occasional patients treated with alkylating agents during pregnancy have had live, normal infants. Nevertheless, it is wise to avoid, if possible, the use of alkylating agents or any other drug capable of inhibiting cell growth during pregnancy—particularly in the first trimester, the period in which organ development is concentrated.

Preparations and Dosage The usual dose and

route of administration of the alkylating agents are shown in Table 34-1.

Mechlorethamine (Nitrogen Mustard, Mustargen) Mechlorethemine acts directly on susceptible tissues; on intravenous injection its action is probably completed within 2 to 3 min.

Chlorambucil (Leukeran) This drug is a useful bis(β-chloroethyl)amine for oral use and is normally well tolerated. Chlorambucil is usually given regularly over a period of several weeks or longer; the therapeutic response may be gradual, and may be sustained by maintenance therapy. Dosage must be carefully regulated, since excessive dosage or prolonged administration can induce severe bone marrow depression. Intermittent courses of treatment may be safer in the lymphomas.

Cyclophosphamide (Cytoxan) Cyclophosphamide has achieved wide clinical use. It requires activation in vivo to achieve a cytotoxic effect. When injected directly into tumor or other tissue, cyclophosphamide does not produce necrosis as do

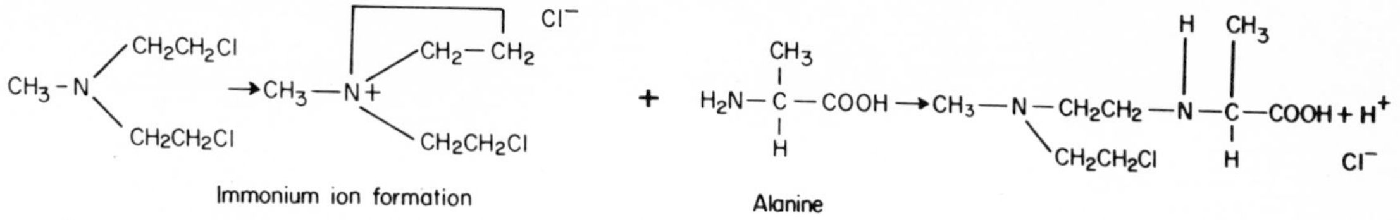

Immonium ion formation   Alanine

β-Chloroethyl group forms a cyclic immonium linkage in an alkaline medium, and this reacts with water or with organic molecules, e.g., alanine.

Figure 34-5 Reactions of an alkylating agent with an amino acid.

other alkylating agents, and when incubated in vitro with leukemia cells, it fails to sterilize them, in contrast to other alkylating agents. However, when given systemically, it is changed, presumably in the liver of the host, to an active form with properties similar to those of other alkylating agents. It has the disadvantages of producing a high incidence of alopecia, severe hemorrhagic cystitis, testicular atrophy, sterility, and ovarian fibrosis.

Melphalan (Alkeran) This compound has had wide use in multiple myeloma, but it is unlikely that it has any specific effects on that disease. Cyclophosphamide has been reported to produce similar responses. Its biologic and toxic effects are the same as those of other alkylating agents.

Thiotepa (Triethylene Thiophosphoramide) This drug has received considerable clinical attention. It is well tolerated, but excessive dosage produces severe bone marrow depression, as is the case with all alkylating agents.

Busulfan (Myleran) This is a poorly soluble material, available only for oral use. It is reported to have selective toxicity for granulocytes and is used principally in chronic granulocytic leukemia, although therapeutic effects have been obtained in

Table 34-1 Clinically Useful Alkylating Agents

Compound	Route	Usual dosage, mg
Mechlorethamine	IV	0.4/kg
Chlorambucil	Oral	10–15/day
Cyclophosphamide	Oral	100–200/day
	IV	40–60/kg
Melphalan	Oral	1–10/day
Thiotepa	Oral	5–10/day
	IV	0.8–1.0/kg
Busulfan	Oral	4–8/day

chronic lymphatic leukemia. Busulfan is well tolerated by mouth. It is a bone marrow depressant, in common with the other alkylating agents. This is the chief hazard in its use, so it should be given under careful hematologic control. It has produced hyperpigmentation in the creases of the skin, particularly on the hands. Pulmonary fibrosis has been observed as a late complication of the prolonged use of busulfan.

Therapeutic Uses In general, the cytotoxic alkylating agents have similar toxicologic and therapeutic effects, and it is likely that they produce cellular injury by a common mechanism. These agents are used principally in generalized diseases of the lymph nodes and blood-forming organs, when systemic symptoms are not being readily or satisfactorily controlled by x-ray therapy. They produce temporary improvement, when given in proper dosage, in suitable cases of Hodgkin's disease, lymphosarcoma, chronic granulocytic and lymphocytic leukemia, polycythemia vera, and mycosis fungoides. They can also produce temporary benefit in some carcinomas, particularly of the lung and ovary. Except for cyclophosphamide, the alkylating agents have not been beneficial in acute leukemia. These drugs must be used with great care, and under careful hematologic control, in order to obtain the maximum therapeutic response without irreversible bone marrow depression.

STEROID HORMONES

In contrast with other chemotherapeutic agents which act indiscriminately on rapidly proliferating cells, the steroid hormones are much more specific in their effects on cells. Each hormone acts on specific tissues and, depending on the tissue involved, stimulates or inhibits its growth. The importance of the steroid hormones in cancer chemotherapy lies in the fact that cancer arising from tissues modified by the steroid hormones may retain some of the hormonal responsiveness of their tissue of origin. Thus, alterations in the hormonal environment may increase the growth rate or cause the cancer to regress, depending on the cancer's primary site and the properties it retains from its tissue of origin. The agents of clinical interest are androgens, estrogens, progestins, and corticosteroids.

Mechanism of Action

The mechanisms by which the steroid hormones produce their effects have not yet been fully clarified. A large body of experimental work has yielded evidence of several possible modes by which the steroid hormones may affect cell growth: peptide bonding in protein synthesis; RNA production; NADPH, NADH, ATP, and GTP levels; ATPase activity; state of aggregation of intracellular enzymes; and permeability of the cell membrane or of subcellular organelles.

Large doses of corticosteroids have many profound effects on normal tissues, which are classically described as Cushing's syndrome in humans. In addition to their well-known effects on salt and water balance, intermediary metabolism, and connective tissue, they produce atrophy of thymic and other lymphoid tissue, lymphopenia, eosinopenia, and neutrophilia. Corticosteroids may exert a direct lymphocytolytic effect, as well as cause suppression of mitosis of lymphocytes.

A steroid hormone is presumed to act on responsive normal and neoplastic tissue in an identical manner. Attempts to alter the steroid molecules in order to dissociate the undesirable effects (for example, masculinization) on responsive normal tissues from inhibitory effects on cancer cells have not been successful.

Therapeutic Uses

Estrogens are effective in the treatment of carcinoma of the prostate and in metastatic mammary cancer in postmenopausal patients. They may also accelerate the growth of mammary cancer, especially in patients who are premenopausal or less than 5 years postmenopausal.

Androgens cause objective temporary regression in patients with breast cancer, but sometimes they accelerate the growth of breast and prostatic cancer.

Progestational agents in large dosage cause temporary objective improvement in patients with inoperable carcinoma of the endometrium.

Corticosteroids sometimes cause striking regression of disease in patients with lymphoma or leukemia. Acute lymphoblastic or undifferentiated leukemia in children responds most favorably, but even in cases where complete remissions occur, frequently with disappearance of all detectable leukemic cells from the blood and bone marrow, the leukemic cells ultimately become resistant to the drugs and the disease recurs.

The corticosteroids may also produce marked effects on the immune response, both in preventing the development of immunity and in suppressing established immunity. The hemolytic anemia which often accompanies chronic lymphocytic leukemia can frequently be alleviated by the use of corticosteroids.

Preparations and Dosage

A summary of the large number of steroid hormone preparations available is given in Table 34-2.

Table 34-2 Clinically Useful Steroid Hormones

Agents	Principal route of administration	Usual dosage, mg
Androgen		
Testosterone propionate	IM	50–100, 3 times/week
Fluoxymesterone	Oral	10–20/day
Calusterone	Oral	200/day
Estrogen		
Diethylstilbestrol	Oral	1–5, 3 times/day
Ethinyl estradiol	Oral	0.1–1.0, 3 times/day
Progestogen		
Hydroxyprogesterone caproate	IM	500, 3 times/week
Corticosteroids		
Cortisone acetate	Oral	50–300/day
Hydrocortisone acetate	Oral	50–200/day
Prednisone	Oral	20–100/day

MISCELLANEOUS AGENTS

Plant Alkaloids

Vincristine and Vinblastine Vincristine and vinblastine are antimitotic alkaloids derived from the periwinkle plant (*Vinca rosea*). Vinblastine shows a wide spectrum of antitumor activity. However, its clinical use is in the treatment of solid tumors, Hodgkin's disease, and other lymphomas. The adverse effects of vinblastine are leukopenia and thrombocytopenia, with evidence of metaphase arrest in the bone marrow. Other toxic manifestations include nausea, vomiting, diarrhea, paresthesias, loss of deep tendon reflexes, alopecia, and mental depression.

Vincristine is more active by weight and, in contrast to vinblastine, can induce remissions in acute leukemia in children. This agent is also indicated in the treatment of solid tumors, Hodgkin's disease, and other lymphomas. Its neurotoxic and gastrointestinal effects can cause more severe injury than its action on normal bone marrow. The neurotoxicity consists of paresthesias, loss of deep tendon reflexes, cranial nerve palsies, peripheral neuritis, and severe constipation with paralytic ileus. Vinblastine produces less neurotoxicity than does vincristine.

Mechanism of Action Vincristine and vinblastine produce nuclear changes in a variety of cells. With metaphase arrest, a range of nuclear effects have been observed in vivo and in vitro, consisting of condensed nuclei, multinucleated cells, and nuclear cleavage and blebbing.

The mechanism of action probably resides in a reversible mitotic arrest, and inhibition of RNA synthesis by effects on DNA-dependent RNA polymerase systems. More extensive work is needed to determine whether these drugs act on the dividing cell through a common mechanism, and whether there is a clear dissociation between their antimitotic activity and their pharmacologic and antitumor activity.

Preparations and Dosage Vinblastine (Velban) is available in 10-mg vials, and vincristine (Oncovin) in 1- and 5-mg vials. The usual dose range for vinblastine is 100 μg to a maximum of 500 μg/kg once a week. Vincristine is usually given in a dose range of 50 to 150 μg/kg once a week.

Antibiotics

A number of compounds obtained from *Streptomyces* have been examined in various laboratory systems and used in patients with cancer.

Dactinomycin (Actinomycin D)

Mechanism of Action Dactinomycin has been shown to form a complex with DNA involving selective binding at the guanine-cytosine segments, with a specific block in DNA-dependent RNA synthesis. This block results in cell injury and death.

Toxicity Dactinomycin causes damage to the bone marrow, lymphoid tissues, and intestinal epithelium. This is associated with diarrhea, dehydration, and bone marrow aplasia. Although these effects on rapidly proliferating tissues are similar to those produced by the alkylating agents, their evolution following dactinomycin administration appears to be more rapid. The toxic effects differ somewhat from those of the alkylating agents: there is definite redness and ulceration of the oral mucosa; occasional abdominal pain and diarrhea may occur; alopecia is more common; and in relation to the degree of damage to the digestive tract, bone marrow depression is less severe than that with the alkylating agents.

Therapeutic Uses Dactinomycin has been used primarily in Wilms's tumor in children, in the lymphomas, in choriocarcinoma, and in testicular tumors in combination with methotrexate and chlorambucil. Dactinomycin may produce striking but temporary responses in Wilms's tumors, and prolonged responses, possibly cures, in choriocarcinomas in females.

Preparation and Dosage Dactinomycin is available in 500-μg ampuls. The usual dosage is 500 μg intravenously once a day for 5 days.

Mithramycin Mithramycin is another antibiotic derived from *Streptomyces*. Its mechanism of action is similar to that of dactinomycin. Mithramycin is recommended in the treatment of testicular carcinoma and trophoblastic neoplasms. The untoward reactions produced by this compound are nausea, vomiting, malaise, hepatotoxicity, bone marrow depression, and hypocalcemia.

Preparation and Dosage Mithramycin (Mithracin) is available in 2.5-mg vials. The usual dose is

25 to 30 μg/kg of body weight given over a 4- to 6-h period.

Bleomycin Bleomycin is a polypeptide antibiotic obtained from *Streptomyces*. The major clinical indications are malignant lymphomas and squamous-cell carcinoma. Its mechanism of action is probably similar to that of dactinomycin, inhibiting the progress of cells through phases of the cell cycle.

Major adverse reactions include nausea, vomiting, fever, edema, pulmonary fibrosis, and cutaneous lesions.

Preparation and Dosage Bleomycin (Blenoxane) is available as a powder in a vial containing 15 units. The usual dosage is 0.25 to 0.5 units/kg once or twice a week.

Doxorubicin Doxorubicin is an anthracycline consisting of a pigmented aglycone joined to an amino sugar by a glycosidic linkage. This compound, as do the other inhibitors of DNA-dependent RNA synthesis, complexes to DNA. Evidence demonstrates that doxorubicin binds to DNA localizing in the cell nuclei and produces a distinctive orange-red nuclear fluorescence. In doing so, doxorubicin elicits cytotoxic and antimitotic activity. Nuclear and nucleolar lesions are observed at toxic drug concentrations. The primary route of elimination is biliary excretion following hepatic metabolism.

The major toxicity of doxorubicin in humans has been in the bone marrow with depression of all marrow elements. In children with solid tumors, thrombocytopenia occurs slowly and is less severe. However, in childhood leukemia, platelet transfusions have been required at the nadir of the depression to prevent severe bleeding. A manifestation of clinical toxicity is the appearance of congestive heart failure, which is usually fatal, in some patients receiving a total dosage greater than 550 mg/m². Thus far this reaction is unexplained. Other manifestations of doxorubicin toxicity are nausea, vomiting, occasional alopecia, fever, and mucositis.

Doxorubicin is used to induce remissions in acute lymphoblastic leukemia, but because of the uncertainty of the cardiopulmonary syndrome, it is not given as maintenance therapy. It is also temporarily effective in neuroblastoma.

Preparation and Dosage Doxorubicin (Adriamycin) is available in 10- and 50-mg ampuls. The recommended dosage schedule for adults is 60 to 75 mg/m² of body surface at 21-day intervals.

l-Asparaginase (Elspar)

The development of *l*-asparaginase followed the observation that a substance in guinea pig serum inhibited the growth of certain transplanted tumors in mice. It was discovered that the active component was *l*-asparaginase, and that its activity is due to the fact that certain neoplastic cells are dependent on exogenous *l*-asparagine, a nonessential amino acid. Exposure to the enzyme *l*-asparaginase eliminates exogenous *l*-asparagine in vivo and results in inhibition of growth of these dependent cells. In contrast, normal cells, which are capable of synthesizing their own asparagine, are not influenced by the presence of asparaginase. Aside from its immediate practical implications, this observation is important because it represents a specific biochemical difference between normal cells and certain neoplastic cells. This biochemical difference has been exploited to inhibit the growth of neoplastic cells.

l-Asparaginase has produced temporary remissions in patients with acute lymphoblastic leukemia. The responses in other forms of leukemia are much less frequent, and thus far, it has not been effective in other forms of cancer. Although no requirement for exogenous asparagine by normal cells has been demonstrated, some host toxicity has occurred with the administration of *l*-asparaginase. Abnormalities of liver function tests, hypoalbuminemia, hypolipidemia, and inhibition of fibrinogen synthesis have been seen regularly. Allergic reactions have developed in occasional patients to whom *l*-asparaginase has been given in a second course following a prolonged period without therapy. Careful desensitization procedures must be followed to avoid anaphylactic reactions. Other toxic effects, such as chills, fever, nausea, and vomiting, have been attributed to bacterial contaminants.

To date, *l*-asparaginase is available for clinical investigation only.

Procarbazine

This compound is one of a large series of hydrazines which have been found to have tumor-inhibitory properties. Procarbazine depresses mitosis, apparently by prolongation of interphase, and the effect of procarbazine on growing cells is due to a direct effect on DNA. It also interferes with transmethylation, and this has been proposed as the principal mechanism of action.

$$CH_3-NH-NH-CH_2-\langle\bigcirc\rangle-CO-NH-\underset{\underset{CH_3}{|}}{\overset{\overset{CH_3}{|}}{C}}H$$

Procarbazine

Procarbazine is effective in Hodgkin's disease but not in other neoplastic disease. Mild nausea and vomiting are regular side effects. Other toxic manifestations include central nervous system depression, bone marrow damage, and, occasionally, gastrointestinal ulceration. It appears to be useful in some cases of Hodgkin's disease which are no longer responsive to other agents, and it is therefore a useful addition to the drugs available for treating this disease.

Preparation and Dosage Procarbazine (Matulane) is available for oral use in 50-mg capsules. The usual dose range is 50 to 300 mg/day.

Part Ten

Anti-infective Agents

Chapter 35

Mechanisms of Action of Antibiotics

All clinically useful antibiotics are selectively toxic to bacterial cells. The nature and degree of this selectivity determines whether an antibiotic is essentially nontoxic for mammalian cells (like benzylpenicillin) or exhibits definite toxic potential for certain specific mammalian tissues (as do the polymyxins). Thus, the clinical toxicity of antibiotics can be best understood by reference to their molecular mechanisms of action. Also, the spectrum of activity of an antibiotic against different types of bacteria is determined, at least in part, by the nature of its action. Finally, some antibiotics produce effects in bacteria which are lethal, and others simply inhibit multiplication without destroying the viability of the individual cell. Antibiotics in the former category are *bactericidal*, whereas those in the latter group are *bacteriostatic*. Whether an antibiotic is bactericidal or only bacteriostatic is determined by the specific effects of the drug on biochemical processes within the organism.

All clinically useful antibiotics exert their antibacterial effects through one of three fundamental mechanisms: (1) inhibition of cell wall synthesis, (2) inhibition of protein synthesis, or (3) interference with the function of the cytoplasmic membrane.

INHIBITION OF CELL WALL SYNTHESIS

The Bacterial Cell Wall and Its Synthesis

The bacterial cell wall is a structure which has no counterpart in mammalian cells. It is composed of a number of complex and unique macromolecular substances. In gram-positive organisms it is largely made up of mucopeptides (65 to 95 percent by weight) and teichoic acids which are polymers of ribitol phosphate or glycerophosphate. Cell walls of gram-negative bacteria are much more complex and contain in addition to mucopeptide (1 to 10 percent) complex lipopolysaccharides and lipoproteins. The mucopeptide of gram-positive bacteria is a linear polymer composed of alternating units of *N*-acetylglucosamine and *N*-acetylmuramic acid (a lactic acid ether of *N*-acetylglucosamine). To each molecule of *N*-acetylmuramic acid is attached (in *Staphylococcus aureus*) a tetrapeptide consisting of L-alanine, D-glutamic acid, L-lysine, and D-alanine. In the complete cell wall mucopeptide of gram-positive bacteria, these polymer strands are cross-linked by amino acid bridges of glycine which connect the L-lysine (or other dibasic amino acid) of one tetrapeptide to the D-alanine of another (Fig. 35-1). This cross-linking is of great importance because it imparts rigidity and determines the shape of the cell.

Penicillins

The mechanism of action of penicillins is limited solely to the inhibition of a specific reaction in the synthesis of the bacterial cell wall, and therefore penicillins are virtually nontoxic for mammalian organisms. They combine with and inactivate the transpeptidase normally responsible for cross-linking. The result of their action is a bacterium without a rigid cell wall, which cannot survive under the conditions prevailing in most body fluids and tissues. Thus penicillins are bactericidal antibiotics.

Cephalosporins

Penicillins and cephalosporins compete with one another for binding sites on sensitive bacterial cells, and this along with much other evidence suggests that the mechanism of antibacterial action of cephalosporins is identical with that of penicillins.

Cycloserine

D-Cycloserine prevents formation of the complete muramic acid pentapeptide, exerting its action at an earlier stage of cell wall synthesis than penicillin.

Vancomycin and Ristocetin

These two antibiotics inhibit the utilization in cell wall synthesis of the lipid-bound intermediate form of the muramic acid pentapeptide. These drugs do not compete with penicillin for binding sites and thus differ from penicillin in site and mechanism of action. In addition to their effects on cell wall synthesis, vancomycin and ristocetin appear to damage the cytoplasmic membrane.

Bacitracin

This is a peptide antibiotic which also contains a structure strikingly similar to the thiazolidine-β-lactam ring system of penicillin. It competes with penicillin for binding sites on sensitive cells. Unlike penicillin it kills bacterial protoplasts and L-forms (bacterial variants with absent or deficient cell walls) at low concentration, and therefore evidently has an effect on the integrity of the cytoplasmic membrane in addition to its inhibition of cell wall synthesis.

Novobiocin

This antibiotic interferes with cell wall synthesis, but in addition has effects on nucleic acid synthesis, protein synthesis, and permeability of the cytoplasmic membranes.

INHIBITION OF PROTEIN SYNTHESIS

Antibiotics Inhibiting Protein Synthesis

The commonly used antibiotics which interfere with protein synthesis in bacteria include: (1) chloramphenicol; (2) erythromycin; (3) lincomycin; (4) the tetracyclines; (5) streptomycin; (6) kanamycin; and (7) neomycin. The end result of interference

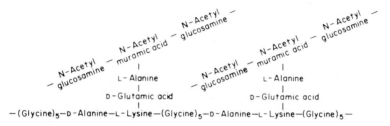

Figure 35-1 Cell wall mucopeptide of *Staph. aureus.*

with protein formation in bacteria may be quite different depending on the antibiotic; some drugs have a bacteriostatic effect while others are bactericidal.

Chloramphenicol, erythromycin, the tetracyclines, and lincomycin are bacteriostatic in their action. Streptomycin, kanamycin, and neomycin have a bactericidal action.

Protein Synthesis in Bacteria

Protein synthesis in the bacterial cell requires not only enzymes but also ribosomal particles (ribosomes); messenger ribonucleic acids (mRNA); transfer ribonucleic acids (tRNA); and amino acids.

The synthesis of proteins in bacteria may be viewed as occurring in two stages. In the first, the information which ultimately determines protein specificity is "transcribed" from the genetic material, DNA, of the bacterium into smaller mRNA molecules. In the second stage, which takes place in the cytoplasm, the information contained in mRNA molecules is "translated" into the appropriate sequence of amino acids which give proteins their specificity (see Fig. 35-2).

The events leading to formation of new proteins are known in considerable detail. The transcription of information concerning protein specificity takes place when single-stranded ribonucleic acid mole-

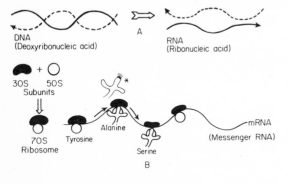

DNA
(Deoxyribonucleic acid)

A

RNA
(Ribonucleic acid)

30S   50S
Subunits

70S   Tyrosine   Serine
Ribosome

Alanine

mRNA
(Messenger RNA)

B

tRNA
Amino acid
(transfer RNA)

Figure 35-2 Protein synthesis. A illustrates the *transcription* of DNA into RNA; B illustrates the *translation* of mRNA into the appropriate sequence of amino acids which comprise polypeptides.

cules are synthesized as complementary copies of portions of one strand of DNA in the nuclear organelle of the bacterium. The sequence of nucleotides in mRNA reflects the nucleotide order in DNA and thus contains the information determining the sequence in which amino acids will be joined to form a specific protein.

The building of protein actually occurs in the cytoplasm of cells with the ribosomal particle acting as a frame. The ribosome is composed of ribonucleic acid and protein and it may be separated into two parts, one subunit having a sedimentation constant of 30 svedbergs (30S) and a larger subunit of 50S size. The mRNA apparently attaches to the 30S subunit of the ribosome.

Amino acids are brought to the ribosome by tRNA molecules. Each amino acid in essence has its own tRNA since the enzyme that binds them is specific for only one tRNA and one amino acid. Each tRNA is in turn also specific for one specific nucleotide sequence (nucleotide triplet or *codon*) in the mRNA. The tRNA is thus a *two-ended* molecule in which one end is specific for an amino acid and the other end specific for a region of three nucleotides in the mRNA.

The tRNA carrying an amino acid (aminoacyl-tRNA) attaches to a ribosome containing an mRNA molecule. The attachment is made to the 30S subunit of the ribosome. The order of attachment of the aminoacyl-tRNAs is determined by the nucleotide sequence (codon sequence) in the mRNA moving along the ribosome. Two or more aminoacyl-tRNA molecules attach to a ribosome at a time. The amino acids are linked by a peptide bond, and eventually a protein is formed by repetition of this process.

The process may be disrupted by antibiotics in any of the several steps by inhibiting:

1 Attachment of mRNA to ribosomes: chloramphenicol
2 Attachment of tRNA to the ribosome: tetracycline
3 Formation of the peptide bond between the amino acid on tRNA and the growing peptide chain: chloramphenicol, erythromycin, and lincomycin
4 Recognition between the aminoacyl-tRNA and its specific codon on mRNA: streptomycin, kanamycin, and neomycin

The Action of Chloramphenicol, Erythromycin, and Lincomycin

The site of action of these drugs is the ribosomal particle, and all attach to the 50S subunit.

Chloramphenicol Chloramphenicol apparently may inhibit protein synthesis in several ways, but it functions primarily by blocking the formation of the peptide bond between the amino acid on the tRNA and the peptide of the peptidyl-tRNA. Thus the growth of the peptide chain ceases under the influence of the drug.

Another effect of chloramphenicol that has been noted indicates that under certain conditions the drug may inhibit the formation of a stable bond between aminoacyl-tRNA and the ribosome. It is very likely that this effect is secondary to blocking of mRNA attachment. The differences in the effect of chloramphenicol on bacterial cells versus its effect on mammalian cells might be explained by one of the postulated modes of action of the drug. The turnover of mRNA in bacterial cells is considerably more rapid than mRNA turnover in most animal cells, and thus bacterial cells should be more susceptible to a drug which blocks mRNA attachment to ribosomes. Mature reticulocytes, in which mRNA turnover is very slight, are not susceptible to chloramphenicol, but young reticulocytes having high turnover are very susceptible to the drug.

Chloramphenicol also may inhibit protein synthesis by blocking the attachment of mRNA to the ribosome.

Erythromycin Erythromycin attaches to the 50S subunit of the ribosome and inhibits the production of active protein by blocking the formation of the peptide bond at the terminus of the growing protein chain.

Lincomycin Lincomycin also inhibits protein synthesis by blocking the formation of the peptide bond. Present evidence indicates that lincomycin probably acts at the same site as does chloramphenicol.

Tetracyclines

The tetracyclines are all similar in their action; they are bacteriostatic for susceptible organisms. These antibiotics interfere with protein synthesis by blocking the attachment of aminoacyl-tRNA to ribosomes.

Streptomycin

Streptomycin inhibits respiration and RNA and DNA synthesis, and impairs the cell membrane with resultant loss of internal ions and nucleotides into the surrounding medium. All these actions appear to be a result of the effect of streptomycin on protein synthesis.

Streptomycin acts directly on the ribosome to inhibit protein synthesis. The antibiotic binds to the 30S subunit of the ribosome and occasionally causes an aminoacyl-tRNA to bind with the wrong codon on mRNA. This results in the insertion of an amino acid in the wrong order in a protein being synthesized. Proteins containing improper sequences of amino acids ("missense" proteins) are often nonfunctional.

Kanamycin and Neomycin

These drugs are also bactericidal. They, too, bind to the 30S subunit and can cause a misreading in the information in mRNA determined by nucleotide sequence.

ACTION ON THE CYTOPLASMIC MEMBRANE

Clearly distinct from the bacterial cell wall is a lipid-rich fragile structure known as the *cytoplasmic membrane*. This structure consists of a monolayer of protein and a monolayer of lipid, primarily phospholipid. The primary function of this bacterial cytoplasmic membrane is to control the internal composition of the cell by action as a selectively permeable barrier to numerous low-molecular-weight substances such as amino acids, nucleotides, and inorganic ions. This allows the bacteria to selectively concentrate certain of these substances within the cell to 400 to 500 times the concentration in the external medium, leading to high osmotic pressures within the cell. It has been shown that damage to the cytoplasmic membrane is followed by release of the concentrated internal solutes. In addition to its function as an osmotic barrier, the membrane is also rich in enzymes and is a site for the biosynthesis of other cell components.

Several antimicrobial agents injure bacteria by directly affecting the function of the cytoplasmic membrane as an osmotic barrier. Amphotericin B, tyrocidine, nystatin, and perhaps novobiocin act in this fashion. The most commonly used antibiotics which act on the cell membrane are the polymyxins.

The polymyxins are a group of closely related cyclic polypeptides. They contain lipophilic and lipophobic groups separated within the molecule; thus the antibiotic is able to become oriented between lipid and protein films of the cytoplasmic membrane and in this way to disorient the lipoprotein membrane of bacteria.

The cell lysis caused by polymyxin, an antibiotic acting on the cytoplasmic membrane, is different in several ways from the cell lysis caused by penicillin, an antibiotic acting on the cell wall. Unlike penicillin, polymyxins produce a lysis which occurs even in appropriate hypertonic media and occurs when bacteria are in either the static or logarithmic phase of growth. Furthermore, the action is extremely rapid.

In contrast to the immediate effect of the surface-active antibiotics on the osmotic barrier, other antibiotics may act by inhibiting the synthesis of the cytoplasmic membrane. It has been shown that streptomycin affects the incorporation of amino acids and glycerol into the membrane fraction of whole protoplasts. The alteration of the cytoplasmic membrane by drugs like streptomycin may reflect the ability of this drug to inhibit protein synthesis and secondarily to impair the function of the cytoplasmic membrane.

Table 35-1 summarizes the mechanisms of action and effects on bacteria of antibiotics.

Table 35-1 Mechanisms of Action and Effects of Antibiotics

Antibiotic	Process or structure affected	Effect on bacteria
Penicillins	Cell wall synthesis	Bactericidal
Cephalosporins	Cell wall synthesis	Bactericidal
Cycloserine	Cell wall synthesis	Bactericidal
Vancomycin	Cell wall synthesis (and cytoplasmic membrane)	Bactericidal
Ristocetin	Cell wall synthesis (and cytoplasmic membrane)	Bactericidal
Bacitracin	Cell wall synthesis (and cytoplasmic membrane)	Bactericidal
Novobiocin	Cell wall synthesis (also nucleic acid synthesis, and cytoplasmic membrane)	Bacteriostatic
Chloramphenicol	Protein synthesis	Bacteriostatic
Erythromycin	Protein synthesis	Bacteriostatic
Lincomycin	Protein synthesis	Bacteriostatic
Tetracyclines	Protein synthesis	Bacteriostatic
Streptomycin	Protein synthesis	Bactericidal
Kanamycin	Protein synthesis	Bactericidal
Neomycin	Protein synthesis	Bactericidal
Polymyxins	Cytoplasmic membrane	Bactericidal

Chapter 36

Antibiotics

PENICILLINS

Penicillin G, the first antibiotic discovered, is still the most important and widely used antibiotic and indeed possesses many of the properties of an ideal antibiotic. It is the drug of choice against virtually all gram-positive bacteria except penicillinase-producing staphylococci and is also highly effective against gram-negative cocci and a few gram-negative bacilli. It is rapidly bactericidal in its effect on susceptible organisms. It is virtually nontoxic for mammalian cells and can be given in almost unlimited dosage if necessary. It is widely distributed in body fluids and tissues and is not rapidly inactivated by metabolic processes of the host. Finally, it is relatively inexpensive.

Chemistry

All penicillins are derivatives of 6-aminopenicillanic acid (6-APA) (Fig. 36-1), a molecule which contains a fused double-ring structure consisting of a β-lactam (Fig. 36-2) and a thiazolidine ring. 6-APA may be obtained from penicillins by hydrolytic cleavage of the amide linkage catalyzed by enzymes from various bacteria and fungi. 6-APA itself possesses significant antibacterial activity against some gram-negative organisms.

The most important way in which bacteria may destroy penicillins is by elaboration of β-lactamases (penicillinases), which hydrolytically open the β-lactam ring at the site indicated in Fig. 36-1. This results in the formation of a penicilloic acid which is virtually devoid of antibacterial activity.

The nature of the acyl group has a profound effect upon the properties of a penicillin. Resistance to destruction by gastric acid and absorption, and resistance to bacterial penicillinases and the spectrum of antibacterial activity, are all determined to a large extent by the nature of this group. In addition, salts may be formed by substitution at the carboxyl group attached to the thiazolidine ring, such as salts with procaine or benzathine which are poorly soluble.

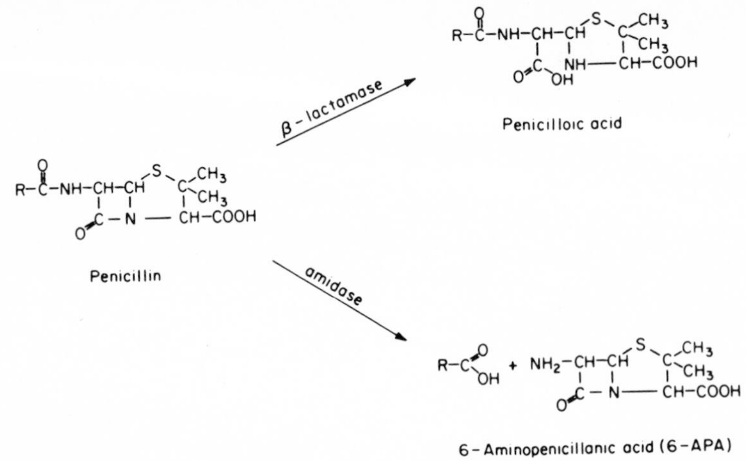

Figure 36-1 Structure of a penicillin and products of its enzymatic hydrolysis.

Some important penicillins in clinical usage are listed in Fig. 36-3. As described in the previous chapter, penicillin exerts its action on bacteria by blocking the final step in the assembly of the mucopeptide of the cell wall. The result is an organism which is unable to survive in ordinary environments; thus the action of the penicillins is bactericidal in nature. Since penicillin can exert its action only when cell wall synthesis is taking place, it is active against growing—but not against resting —cells. Gram-positive bacteria, which have a higher proportion of mucopeptide in their cell walls and also a higher internal osmotic pressure, are much more susceptible as a group to the action of penicillin than are gram-negative bacilli. Although penicillins are effective against susceptible bacteria in extremely low concentrations, they are almost completely nontoxic for mammalian cells, presumably because the synthetic process which they inhibit has no counterpart in mammalian cells.

Pharmacology

Penicillin G   Following oral administration, approximately one-third of a dose of penicillin G is

Figure 36-2 β-Lactam ring.

absorbed from the gastrointestinal tract; therefore, the dose administered must be from 3 to 5 times that which would be given parenterally to yield comparable amounts in the blood. Penicillin G is susceptible to inactivation by gastric acid, but this is not the major factor accounting for the poor absorption. Most of the absorption takes place in the duodenum, and that fraction of the drug which passes through the upper small intestine unabsorbed passes into the colon where it is largely destroyed by bacteria. *In order to achieve maximum absorption, oral penicillin must be taken at least 1 h before or 2 to 3 h after a meal.*

Crystalline penicillin G (sodium or potassium) in aqueous solution is absorbed extremely rapidly following intramuscular (or subcutaneous) injection, and peak plasma levels are reached within 15 min. Renal excretion of aqueous penicillin is so rapid that plasma levels are barely detectable at the end of 5 h. In order to prolong the blood level of penicillin within the body and thus increase the interval between doses, two approaches have been taken: (1) the use of repository preparations such as procaine penicillin or benzathine penicillin to delay absorption from the injection site; and (2) concomitant administration of probenecid to reduce the rate of renal excretion. Probenecid blocks renal tubular transport of penicillin, and its administration results in higher and more prolonged blood levels following a given dose of penicillin. Probenecid may produce undesirable side effects, how-

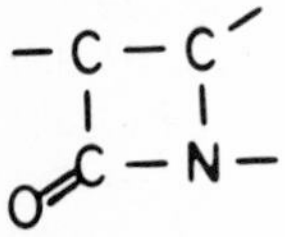

Figure 36-3 Chemical structures and names of various penicillins.

Side Chain	Chemical Name	Generic Name
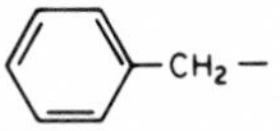	Benzyl penicillin	Penicillin G
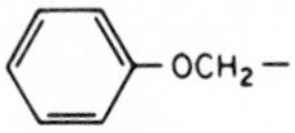	Phenoxymethyl penicillin	Penicillin V
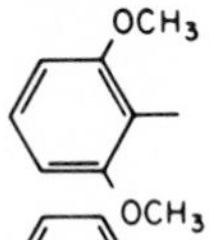	2,6-Dimethoxyphenyl penicillin	Methicillin
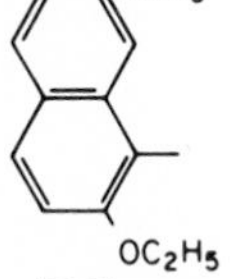	2-Ethoxy-1-naphthyl penicillin	Nafcillin
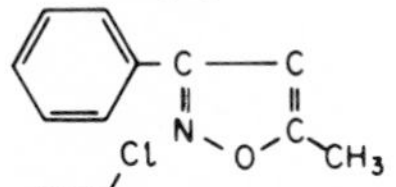	5-Methyl-3-phenyl-4-isoxazolyl penicillin	Oxacillin
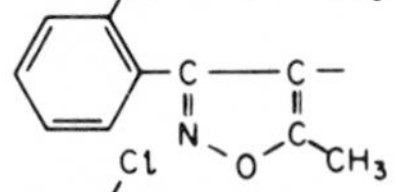	5-Methyl-3-O-chlorophenyl-4-isoxazolyl penicillin	Cloxacillin
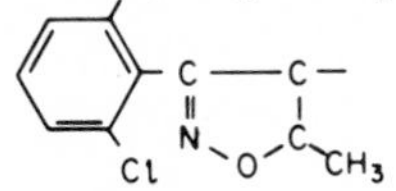	5-Methyl-3-(2,6-dichlorophenyl)-4-isoxazolyl penicillin	Dicloxacillin
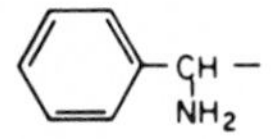	α-Aminobenzyl penicillin	Ampicillin
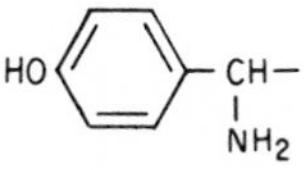	α-Amino(p-hydroxy-)benzyl penicillin	Amoxicillin
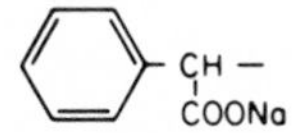	α-Carboxybenzyl penicillin	Carbenicillin

ever, and from a practical standpoint it is usually better simply to increase the dosage of penicillin than to attempt to raise the serum level with probenecid.

Penicillin is widely distributed in the body, and adequate therapeutic levels will be obtained in most tissues if the plasma penicillin level exceeds the minimum inhibitory concentration of the infecting organism by severalfold. However, in the absence of inflammation, only relatively small amounts penetrate into joints, ocular tissues, brain, and cerebrospinal fluid.

Preparations and Routes of Administration Al-though a large variety of formulations of penicillin G have been made available since the discovery of this drug, at present there are four basically different preparations available: (1) penicillin G in aqueous solution for parenteral injection; (2) procaine penicillin G suspension for parenteral injection; (3) benzathine penicillin G suspension for parenteral injection; and (4) penicillin G for oral use.

Penicillin V This penicillin is much more stable than penicillin G in an acid medium and is therefore more completely absorbed (about 65 percent) from the gastrointestinal tract. Following equivalent dosage, penicillin V yields blood levels 2 to 5 times greater than penicillin G. In addition, absorption of penicillin V appears to be subject to less variability and is not readily affected by proximity to meals. In its antibacterial spectrum, distribution within the body, and excretion, it can be considered for practical purposes as equivalent to penicillin G. Penicillin V is available as the potassium salt, which is significantly better absorbed than the free acid.

Methicillin This drug, the first of the penicillinase-resistant penicillins to be introduced, is unstable in the presence of acid; therefore, it cannot be administered orally. It is usually given intramuscularly or intravenously but has also been given by intraarticular, intraspinal, and subconjunctival injection. It is rapidly and quite well absorbed following intramuscular injection. Approximately 75 percent of an injected dose is excreted in the urine, mainly during the first 4 h. Intramuscular injections of methicillin are somewhat painful, and when large doses are required, the intravenous route is preferable. Currently available methicillin preparations are buffered, and can be added to intravenous infusions. Since it is less active than penicillin G against non-penicillinase-producing staphylcocci and other gram-positive cocci, methicillin should be used only in the treatment of infections due to penicillinase-producing staphylococci. It is somewhat less active than the newer penicillinase-resistant penicillins (nafcillin and the isoxazolyl penicillins).

Nafcillin In terms of its antibacterial spectrum and effectiveness, nafcillin can be considered equivalent to the isoxazolyl penicillins (for example, oxacillin) when administered parenterally. It is active against gram-positive organisms, including penicillinase producers. However, it is less well absorbed following oral administration than are the isoxazolyl penicillins. Because of their high degree of activity against both *Staph. aureus* and other gram-positive cocci, nafcillin and the isoxazolyl penicillins are the preferred agents for initial therapy in the treatment of serious infections due to gram-positive cocci pending definitive identification of the organism.

Isoxazolyl Penicillins (Oxacillin, Cloxacillin, and Dicloxacillin) Oxacillin, cloxacillin, and dicloxacillin are isoxazolyl penicillins which contain, respectively, unsubstituted, monochloro- and dichloro-substituted phenyl groups. The activity of these three penicillins against staphylococci and other gram-positive organisms is approximately equal to that of nafcillin. All are very highly bound to serum albumin (oxacillin 94 percent, cloxacillin 95 percent, dicloxacillin 98 percent). The significant difference among these penicillins lies in the height and duration of serum levels achieved after equivalent oral dosage. Cloxacillin and dicloxacillin are available only for oral use. Oxacillin is available for both oral and parenteral use. It is very well absorbed following intramuscular injection and in parenteral usage may be considered equivalent to nafcillin in potency and spectrum of antibacterial activity.

Ampicillin This was the first among the semisynthetic penicillins to exhibit a useful degree of activity against some gram-negative as well as gram-positive bacteria. The sodium salt is about as well absorbed following oral administration as is penicillin V. Following intramuscular or intravenous injection, distribution within the body is probably similar to that of penicillin G. Ampicillin is excreted primarily by the kidney but not so rapidly as penicillin G. Although ampicillin is acid-stable, it is rapidly destroyed by staphylococcal penicillinase, and the drug should not be used for the treatment of infections due to penicillinase-producing staphylococci. In soft-tissue infections due to gram-positive cocci or infections of the gastrointestinal or urinary tracts due to sensitive gram-negative bacilli, oral dosage usually provides adequate concentrations at the site of infection. In the treatment of bacterial meningitis or bacterial endocarditis due to enterococci, a daily dosage of at least 2 to 5 times the oral dosage should be given by the intravenous route.

Amoxicillin Amoxicillin is a semisynthetic penicillin available only for oral use. It closely resembles ampicillin in chemical structure (Fig. 36-3) and antibacterial activity (Table 36-1). It is rapidly absorbed, achieves high blood levels, and has ad-

Table 36-1 Some Characteristics of Penicillins

Name	Route of administration	Sensitivity of organism*		Penicillinase resistance*
		Gram (+)	Gram (−)	
Penicillin G	Parenteral, oral	++	±	0
Penicillin V	Oral	++	±	0
Methicillin	Parenteral	+	±	++
Nafcillin	Parenteral, oral	++	±	++
Oxacillin	Parenteral, oral	++	±	++
Cloxacillin	Oral	++	±	++
Dicloxacillin	Oral	++	±	++
Ampicillin	Parenteral, oral	+	+	0
Carbenicillin	Parenteral, oral	++	++	0
Amoxicillin	Oral	+	+	0

* Effectiveness: ++, high; +, moderate; ±, weak; 0, none.

verse effects similar to ampicillin. Since amoxicillin has an antibacterial spectrum similar to ampicillin, its recommended use is similar to oral ampicillin. It is better absorbed and may cause less diarrhea than ampicillin. Its effectiveness in the treatment of most infections appears to equal that of oral ampicillin.

Carbenicillin This drug has an antibacterial spectrum similar to that of ampicillin except that it shows a high degree of activity against indole-positive species of *Proteus* (*vulgaris, morganii, rettgeri*) and moderate activity against many strains of *Pseudomonas aeruginosa*. A modest synergistic effect has been demonstrated against some strains of *Pseudomonas* using the combination of carbenicillin and gentamicin. Disodium carbenicillin is available for parenteral administration. For oral use carbenicillin indanyl sodium is given.

Characteristics Table 36-1 summarizes some of the characteristics of the various penicillins used in therapy.

Toxicity and Allergic Reactions

Allergic Reactions Despite the inherent nontoxicity of penicillins, allergy to penicillin has become a problem of great importance. Although sensitization to penicillin can theoretically occur by exposure to naturally occurring penicillin in the environment, the incidence of penicillin allergy has definitely increased during the antibiotic era, and allergic reactions to penicillin are much more common in individuals who have been treated with the drug previously, indicating that therapeutic or prophylactic administration of penicillin is the chief means by which sensitization occurs.

Allergic reactions to penicillin may be of several types depending upon clinical manifestations and postulated mechanisms of development. The severity of the adverse reactions ranges from urticaria to anaphylactic shock.

Treatment of acute anaphylactic reaction to penicillin does not differ from treatment of anaphylactic reactions in general.

Other Untoward Reactions Administration of penicillins causes a diminution in the numbers of sensitive bacteria on the skin and in the respiratory and gastrointestinal tracts, followed by an increase in the numbers of bacteria resistant to penicillin, especially *Staph. aureus* and gram-negative bacilli. Penicillins are less likely than the tetracyclines to lead to such an overgrowth. A very small number of cases of nephropathy have been reported following administration of some penicillins. All the patients were receiving large doses of the drug, and signs of renal insufficiency developed several days after initiation of therapy.

Clinical Usage

Table 36-2 shows the effectiveness of penicillins against selected organisms.

CEPHALOSPORIN ANTIBIOTICS

The cephalosporin antibiotics are derivatives of 7-aminocephalosporanic acid, a close relative of 6-aminopenicillanic acid, from which it differs mainly by having a six-membered sulfur-containing ring. As the penicillins are 6-acylaminopenicillanic acids, so the cephalosporins are 7-acylaminocephalosporanic acids. The structural formulas of some cephalosporin antibiotics are shown in Fig. 36-4.

It is interesting that both the penicillins and the cephalosporins contain a β-lactam ring fused with a sulfur-containing ring, and both have a common mechanism of antibacterial activity and a similar spectrum of microorganisms affected.

Table 36-2 Effectiveness of Some Penicillins

Organism	Primary drug
Gram-positive cocci	
Staphylococcus	Penicillin G (P)*
(non-penicillinase-producing)	Penicillin V (O)*
Staphylococcus	Methicillin, nafcillin,
(penicillinase-producing)	oxacillin (P)
	Dicloxacillin, cloxacillin (O)
Streptococcus pneumoniae	Penicillin G (P)
	Penicillin V (O)
Streptococcus (group A,	Penicillin G (P)
β-hemolytic)	Penicillin V (O)
Gram-negative cocci	
Neisseria meningitidis	Penicillin G (P)
Neisseria gonorrhoeae	Penicillin G (P)
	Procaine penicillin G (P)
Gram-positive bacilli	
Bacillus anthracis	Penicillin G (P)
	Penicillin V (O)
Gram-negative bacilli	
Hemophilus influenzae	Ampicillin (P)
(meningitis)	
P. aeruginosa	Carbenicillin (P) (O)
(urinary tract infection)	
Spirochetes	
Treponema pallidum	Penicillin G (P)
	Procaine penicillin G (P)

* P = parenterally; O = orally.

A comparison of the various dosage forms and routes of administration of the cephalosporin antibiotics is presented in Table 36-3.

The cephalosporin derivatives are often considered alternative drugs for patients who are sensitive to penicillins, but the cephalosporins are themselves capable of inducing allergic reactions, including anaphylaxis, in such patients. In one study, 40 percent of patients allergic to penicillins were also allergic to the cephalosporins. The use of cephalosporins in patients allergic to the penicillins, therefore, should only be initiated with great caution because of evidence of partial cross-allergenicity of the penicillins and the cephalosporins.

Sensitivity to β-Lactamase (Penicillinase)

All the cephalosporins are susceptible to β-lactamase, but to varying degrees depending upon the bacterial species involved, the size of the inoculum, and perhaps other factors. However, these agents do exhibit an adequate degree of effectiveness against penicillinase-producing organisms.

Cephalothin

Cephalothin is not significantly absorbed from the gastrointestinal tract and must be administered parenterally. Because of local pain which accompanies intramuscular injection, it is often given intravenously, especially when the patient requires large doses or prolonged therapy. Excretion is rapid; serum levels are often undetectable by 6 h, and 60 to 90 percent of the dose appears in the urine. The administration of probenecid blocks tubular secretion of cephalothin as well as penicillin

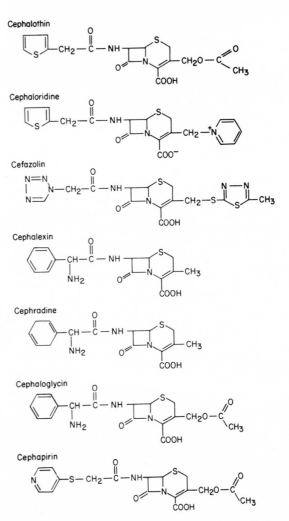

Figure 36-4 Structural formulas of some cephalosporin antibiotics.

Table 36-3 Comparison of Various Cephalosporin Antibiotics

Generic name	Trade name	Routes of administration	Dosage forms
Cephalothin	Keflin	Intravenous Intramuscular	1-, 2-, 4-g vials
Cephaloridine	Loridine	Intravenous Intramuscular	250-mg, 500-mg, 1-g vials
Cefazolin	Ancef Kefzol	Intravenous Intramuscular	250-mg, 500-mg, 1-g vials
Cephalexin	Keflex	Oral	250-, 500-mg capsules; 125, 250, 500 mg/5 ml suspensions
Cephradine	Anspor Velosef	Oral	250-, 500-mg capsules; 125, 250 mg/5 ml suspensions
Cephaloglycin	Kafocin	Oral*	250-mg capsules
Cephapirin	Cefadyl	Intravenous Intramuscular	1-, 2-, 4-g vials

* Intended for treatment of urinary tract infections only.

and results in unpredictable but significantly higher serum levels.

Cephalothin also penetrates other body fluids in a manner similar to penicillin. Cephalothin readily crosses the placenta in either direction. Levels in cord serum are almost one-half those of maternal serum.

In renal failure, the cephalothin level is increased slightly, but its half-life in serum is only minimally prolonged even in the presence of severe renal failure.

Toxicity, Side Effects, and Complications Cephalothin shares the low level of toxicity enjoyed by penicillin. A reversible leukopenia has been described. Positive Coombs's tests have followed cephalothin therapy in azotemic patients but without overt hemolytic anemia. Allergic reactions manifested chiefly by skin rash are encountered in a small percentage of patients. Thrombophlebitis is a common complication of intravenous therapy. The safety of cephalothin in pregnancy has not been established.

Superinfection by cephalothin-resistant gram-negative bacilli, especially *P. aeruginosa,* has been noted by several observers. Cephalosporins should not be used where a narrow-spectrum antibiotic will do as well.

Therapy Cephalothin has been successfully used in the treatment of pneumococcal infections including pneumonia and meningitis; in infections due to *Streptococcus pyogenes*; non-penicillinase-producing *Staph. aureus*; and other penicillin-susceptible gram-positive organisms. In such cases, however, penicillin G or Penicillin V is the preferred agent because of lower cost and narrower spectrum. Even when penicillin allergy is present, the risk of hypersensitivity reactions cannot be entirely eliminated by using cephalothin. Against penicillinase-producing staphylococci, cephalothin is about on a par with the semisynthetic penicillinase-resistant penicillins.

Cephaloridine

Like cephalothin, cephaloridine is not significantly absorbed from the gastrointestinal tract and must be given parenterally. After injection of 0.5 g intramuscularly, peak serum antibiotic levels are achieved at about 30 min. In contrast with cephalothin, appreciable serum levels of cephaloridine are still present after 6 h.

Cephaloridine penetrates tissues and body fluids well except for brain and cerebrospinal fluid. In the presence of acute meningeal inflammation, spinal fluid levels become therapeutically significant. Cephaloridine also readily crosses the placenta and into the fetal circulation, but its safety for use in pregnant women has not yet been established.

Toxicity, Side Effects, and Complications Cephaloridine differs from other members of the penicillin-cephalosporin family in possessing a potentially serious nephrotoxicity. The effect is most likely to occur in patients having already reduced renal function, but large doses may provoke it even in those with apparently normal kidneys. The nephrotoxicity of cephaloridine may be enhanced in the presence of furosemide.

Other side effects are similar to those of cephalothin. Rarely neutropenia and agranulocytosis have been noted. Allergic reactions manifested chiefly by skin rashes occur in approximately 4 percent of patients treated.

Superinfection with resistant gram-negative organisms, principally *P. aeruginosa*, has been a significant problem. Because of cephaloridine's toxicities its use should be restricted.

Cefazolin

Cefazolin differs chemically from cephaloridine in having a tetrazole ring rather than a thiophene ring, and a methylthiadiazolylthio group rather than a piperidinium ring. Pharmacologically, cefazolin is a cephalosporin antibiotic recommended for respiratory infection, skin and soft tissue infections, and urinary tract infections caused by susceptible organisms. Unlike cephalothin it does not produce severe pain on intramuscular injection. Also, it does not induce kidney impairment, as is the case with cephaloridine. This drug is available for parenteral administration only. The side effects of cefazolin are similar to the other cephalosporins discussed.

Cephalexin

Another cephalosporin antibiotic is cephalexin, the desacetoxy form of cephaloglycin. It is so well absorbed from the gastrointestinal tract that cephalexin serum levels exceed those following an equal amount of cephalothin given intramuscularly. Cephalexin is useful in urinary and respiratory infections of susceptible organisms. The most common side effects associated with cephalexin are associated with the gastrointestinal system; diarrhea is particularly common. Allergic reactions are relatively rare.

Cephradine

A cyclohexadien analogue of cephalexin, cephradine is intended for oral administration. Its pharmacologic characteristics are almost identical to those of cephalexin. The most common adverse reactions are similar to those of other cephalosporins.

Cephaloglycin

This antibiotic is a phenylglycine analogue of cephalothin with essentially the same antibacterial spectrum. One major feature is that it is absorbed from the gastrointestinal tract sufficiently well to provide significant antibiotic levels in the urine. Serum levels are generally too low to permit confident treatment of infections in other locations. A side effect not encountered with injectable cephalosporins is the occurrence of gastrointestinal symptoms including severe diarrhea.

Cephapirin

This antibiotic is a pyridylthioglycolyl analogue of cephaloglycin. Cephapirin is intended for intramuscular and intravenous administration. This semisynthetic cephalosporin is equal in effectiveness to other parenteral cephalosporins, and the adverse reactions associated with its use are similar to those of other cephalosporins.

OTHER IMPORTANT ANTIBIOTICS

The antibiotics discussed in this section include some which are sometimes called *broad-spectrum* antibiotics. This designation may be misleading, since all antibiotics have limitations of their antimicrobial spectra. Even an antibiotic with a spectrum as broad as that of chloramphenicol is often ineffective against *Enterobacter, Proteus, Pseudomonas,* and many strains of *Staph. aureus.*

These antibiotics may be grouped into three categories: (1) agents used primarily in the therapy of infections due to gram-positive bacteria; (2) broad-spectrum antibiotics; and (3) antibiotics used primarily in the treatment of infections caused by gram-negative bacteria. The characteristics of the antimicrobial agents discussed in this section are summarized in Table 36-4.

Table 36-4 Characteristics of Selected Antimicrobial Agents

Name	Route of administration	Effectiveness against organism*		Special consideration†
		Gram (+)	Gram (−)	
Erythromycin	Parenteral Oral	++	0	Mycoplasma
Lincomycin	Parenteral Oral	++	0	
Clindamycin	Parenteral Oral	++	+	Anaerobes
Vancomycin	Parenteral	++	0	
Bacitracin	Topical	++	0	
Chloramphenicol	Parenteral Oral	++	++	Salmonella typhi
Tetracyclines	Parenteral Oral	++	++	Rickettsia Mycoplasma
Gentamicin	Parenteral	+	++	Pseudomonas Serratia
Neomycin	Topical	+	++	
Kanamycin	Parenteral	+	++	Proteus except P. mirabilis
Streptomycin	Parenteral	+	++	Mycobacterium tuberculosis
Polymyxins	Parenteral	0	++	Pseudomonas

* ++, high; +, moderate; 0, none.

† These organisms are particularly susceptible to the antimicrobial agent listed.

Antibiotics Used Against Gram-positive Organisms

Erythromycin Erythromycin is highly effective against gram-positive bacteria including such pathogens as *Diplococcus pneumoniae* and group A *Strep. pyogenes,* although resistant strains of both have been reported. It is also effective against *Neisseria gonorrhea* and *N. meningitis,* the clostridial species *Treponema pallidum,* and other gram-positive bacteria.

The mechanism of action of erythromycin appears to be partly inhibition of protein synthesis. Its lack of effectiveness against gram-negative bacilli is thought to be due to inability to penetrate the cell wall. It is an intermediate on the bactericidal-bacteriostatic scale; that is, it is bacteriostatic in lower concentrations but bactericidal at higher concentrations.

Absorption and Distribution Erythromycin is absorbed adequately from the gastrointestinal tract but because gastric juice destroys the antibiotic, it is better absorbed when the stomach is empty. The serum level achieved depends upon the form used. Oral administration of 250-mg erythromycin stea-

rate results in peak serum levels of about 1 μg/ml after 2 h.

Erythromycin diffuses well into tissues, including the pleural and peritoneal spaces and the inflamed meninges. It crosses the placenta and produces detectable fetal plasma concentrations.

The drug is excreted in high concentration in the bile and in smaller quantities (2 to 5 percent) in the urine; the remainder is presumably metabolized.

Therapeutic Uses and Toxicity Erythromycin is mainly used as a substitute for penicillin when oral therapy is appropriate and when the organism to be treated is susceptible. Erythromycin may be substituted for penicillin G in individuals who are allergic to penicillin; for practical purposes this means mild infections due to *D. pneumoniae* or group A *Strep. pyogenes.* This drug is not recommended for widespread use against *Staph. aureus.*

Erythromycin base has a low degree of toxicity with mild gastrointestinal upset and rare skin sensitization. However, since the introduction of erythromycin estolate, numerous reports have appeared describing a cholestatic hepatitis.

Dosage Forms Erythromycin is available as the free base for oral and topical use and as salts of organic acids for oral, intramuscular, and intravenous use (Erythrocin, Ilotycin); it is also available in the form of the propionic acid ester (Ilosone) for oral use (the esterified form is best absorbed orally). The dosage for any of the forms of erythromycin in adults is 250 to 500 mg every 6 h and 20 to 30 mg/kg daily in children. In severe infections, up to 4 g can be given to adults daily.

Lincomycin Lincomycin's antibacterial spectrum and other pharmacologic properties are similar to those of erythromycin. Principally a bacteriostatic agent, lincomycin exerts its antibacterial action by inhibiting tRNA binding to the ribosome. Absorption of lincomycin from the gastrointestinal tract is only moderately complete and amounts to 20 to 35 percent of the administered oral dose. It reaches peak serum levels in 2 to 4 h. Lincomycin diffuses well into tissues, including the pleural and peritoneal spaces and the inflamed meninges. Since lincomycin levels in bone appear to be excellent, this agent may prove very effective in the therapy of chronic staphylococcal osteomyelitis. Lincomycin is excreted unchanged from the biliary and urinary systems.

Toxicity and Side Effects Lincomycin has been associated with deaths reportedly attributed to lincomycin-induced colitis termed *pseudomembranous colitis*. The drug also produces gastrointestinal effects such as abdominal pain, vomiting, bleeding, and severe diarrhea. Superinfection, granulocytopenia, and jaundice have occurred. A large intravenous dose (exceeding 4 g) has been associated with cardiopulmonary arrest. Lincomycin should therefore be used with extreme caution, but when oral antibiotic therapy is desirable and allergy prevents the use of penicillin, lincomycin may be a choice.

Dosage Forms Lincomycin (Lincocin) is available for oral use in 250- and 500-mg capsules as well as a pediatric syrup containing 250 mg/5 ml. For parenteral use it is supplied in vials at a concentration of 300 mg/ml.

Clindamycin Clindamycin resembles lincomycin in its antibacterial spectrum, mechanism of action, and other pharmacologic properties. It should be used primarily in anaerobic infections caused by susceptible organisms and may be considered a substitute for penicillin G in patients allergic to penicillin. As with lincomycin, this antibiotic has been reported to cause the colitis known as pseudomembranous colitis, which is occasionally fatal. Therefore, extreme caution should be exercised in using this agent. However, gastrointestinal side effects may be fewer for clindamycin compared to lincomycin. Thrombophlebitis is possible on intravenous administration. Following drug therapy of 10 days or longer, superinfection can result from nonsusceptible organisms.

Dosage Forms Clindamycin (Cleocin) is available for oral use in 75- and 150-mg capsules as well as a pediatric oral solution containing 75 mg/5 ml. For intramuscular and intravenous use it is supplied in ampuls at a concentration of 150 mg/ml.

Vancomycin The structure of vancomycin is not precisely known. Its antibacterial spectrum includes streptococci, pneumococci, many enterococci, and gonococci, but the drug's marked and consistent effectiveness is against serious staphylococcus infections which are resistant to penicillins.

The mechanism of action of vancomycin appears to be twofold: an immediate inhibition of cell wall synthesis and a somewhat delayed effect on cytoplasmic membrane so that the drug is lethal to both normal cells and spheroplasts.

Intestinal absorption of vancomycin is limited. Because of local pain and frequent necrosis at intramuscular injection sites, vancomycin must be administered intravenously. Vancomycin diffuses well into the pleural, peritoneal, and synovial spaces and, to a limited degree, through inflamed meninges. The antibiotic is excreted primarily by the kidney.

In patients with impaired renal function, there can be considerable accumulation of vancomycin in the serum. In such instances the drug may produce ototoxicity, including permanent deafness, and nephrotoxicity, which is usually reversible. Thrombophlebitis at the injection site is a frequent and troublesome problem of prolonged therapy. Vancomycin rarely causes serious hypersensitivity, but transient chills, fever, urticaria, and macular rash occur in 5 to 10 percent of patients.

Bacitracin Bacitracin's spectrum of antibacterial activity is restricted to gram-positive organisms and the neisseriae. Almost all strains of *Staph. aureus* are susceptible, and this drug was used to treat severe penicillin-resistant staphylococcal infections before other agents became available.

Bacitracin is a bactericidal antibiotic. Its mechanism of action appears to be primarily interference with bacterial cell wall formation leading to suppressed cell wall and protein synthesis.

Nephrotoxicity is a major problem which complicates and limits the usefulness of bacitracin. Skin hypersensitivity or other allergic reactions are rare, however, so its use is now restricted almost entirely to topical application. Its poor percutaneous absorption is also a virtue for a topical agent.

Broad-Spectrum Antibiotics

Chloramphenicol After the initial widespread usage of chloramphenicol, indications for its use have now been markedly restricted. Chloramphenicol is primarily a bacteriostatic agent whose mechanism of action is to inhibit protein synthesis. Chloramphenicol is active against most *E. coli*, *Klebsiella*, *Enterobacter*, *Hemophilus*, *Pasteurella*, *Bacteroides*, *Salmonella*, *Neisseria*, *Shi-*

gella, *Brucella, Vibrio comma, Staphylococcus, Streptococcus, D. pneumoniae, Listeria,* and *Actinomyces.* Whenever possible, antibiotic sensitivity testing should be performed, since there is considerable variation in the sensitivity of different strains of organisms within the same species. *P. aeruginosa* is almost uniformly resistant to chloramphenicol.

Chloramphenicol is rapidly absorbed unchanged from the gastrointestinal tract, and significant plasma levels of the metabolically active form are obtained within 30 min after ingestion. Peak levels in plasma are reached in about 2 h and disappear within 12 to 18 h. Satisfactory blood levels can be maintained with an oral dose every 6 h. About 60 percent of chloramphenicol is bound by plasma albumin. The drug is inactivated by hepatic conjugation to the monoglucuronide, which is highly water-soluble and therefore rapidly excreted in the urine, and in which the concentration of drug is approximately 20 times higher than in the plasma. Chloramphenicol is also excreted by the liver but is so well reabsorbed from the bowel that the eventual path of excretion is also via the kidneys.

Side Reactions and Toxicity Mild gastrointestinal disturbances may occur, but allergic skin rash and drug fever are quite uncommon. Acute necrosis of the liver has occurred after chloramphenicol therapy, and peripheral neuritis associated with optic neuritis has been reported during the prolonged administration of relatively large doses. Acute hemolytic anemia may occur.

The most important effect of chloramphenicol toxicity is that of bone marrow depression. Of all the drugs responsible for aplastic anemia and pancytopenia, chloramphenicol is the most common cause.

A manifestation of serious toxicity of chloramphenicol known as the *gray-baby syndrome* has been noted in newborn infants, especially prematures given large doses of chloramphenicol (usually more than 100 mg/kg). This often fatal syndrome consists of vasomotor collapse, cyanosis, abdominal distention, rapid and irregular respirations, diarrhea, later flaccidity, an ashen-gray color, and hypothermia. This syndrome is related to failure of chloramphenicol conjugation with glucuronic acid because of the immature hepatic conjugating mechanism of the neonate and because of an inadequate renal mechanism for excretion of unconjugated

chloramphenicol in the newborn. As a result, when chloramphenicol must be given to this age group, great care must be exercised to limit the dose administered.

Therapeutic Uses The following general rules concerning utilization of chloramphenicol appear justified:

1 The antibiotic should never be used indiscriminately.
2 It should be used only in serious illness when other antimicrobials would be less effective.
3 Therapy should be stopped if leukopenia supervenes.
4 Chloramphenicol should be used primarily for hospitalized patients and not clinic patients.
5 Chloramphenicol is the treatment of choice for typhoid fever. In many other infections it acts as an excellent antimicrobial but is not utilized because other less toxic antibiotics are equally as effective.
6 The drug is *contraindicated* for prophylactic use.
7 It should *never* be utilized in the treatment of minor infections, upper respiratory infections, or when careful follow-up is not possible.

Preparations Chloramphenicol (Chloromycetin) is available for oral administration in 50-, 100-, and 250-mg capsules and in the liquid form as suspension chloramphenicol palmitate of 125 mg/teaspoonful. Chloramphenicol succinate is the preferred form for parenteral administration and should be given by the intravenous route.

Tetracyclines Chlortetracycline, oxytetracycline, tetracycline, demethylchlortetracycline, doxycycline, rolitetracycline, minocycline, and methacycline constitute the tetracycline family of antibiotics.

The tetracyclines are effective against many gram-positive and gram-negative bacteria, *Rickettsia, Mycoplasma,* and *Bedsonia.* Certain spirochetes (*Leptospira* and *Treponema*), protozoa (*Entamoeba histolytica*), and fungi (*Actinomyces*) are also susceptible. *Proteus* and *Pseudomonas* are generally resistant. Complete cross-resistance is the rule among the various tetracycline preparations. Organisms resistant to one are resistant to all, and thus only one of the tetracyclines need be employed in antibiotic-susceptibility testing. All the tetracyclines are bacteriostatic except in very high concentrations. Although claims have been made suggesting the superiority of one tetracycline over another, the antimicrobial properties are similar enough to discuss this group as a whole.

Tetracycline

Absorption, Distribution, and Excretion All tetracyclines are readily but incompletely absorbed from the gastrointestinal tract. Absorption is impaired by food, milk, or milk products and especially by the concomitant administration of aluminum hydroxide gels and calcium and magnesium salts. These cations form insoluble complexes, with the tetracycline preventing gastrointestinal absorption. Tetracycline is not destroyed by gastric juice or by microorganisms in the colon.

The blood levels which may be achieved are similar for all the tetracycline family except demethylchlortetracyline which, because of delayed excretion, provides higher levels from equal doses of drug by weight.

Peak serum concentrations after single doses of the tetracyclines are reached in 2 to 4 h and decrease slowly over the next 12 to 24 h except in the case of demethylchlortetracycline, methacycline, and doxycycline, which may persist 48 to 72 h after the last dose. Administration of tetracyclines every 6 h produces reasonably constant serum concentrations, the height of which depends upon the dose. Doses of 250-mg tetracycline, chlortetracycline, or oxytetracycline every 6 h produce a mean serum level of about 3 μg/ml.

The tetracyclines are widely distributed in the body fluids and tissues. Concentrations in the cerebrospinal fluid, however, are much lower than those in serum, rarely achieving more than 15 to 20 percent of serum levels unless the meninges are inflamed.

All the tetracyclines are removed from the blood by the liver where they are concentrated and then excreted by way of the bile into the intestine from which they are reabsorbed. This provides an enterohepatic cycle which maintains small amounts of tetracycline in the body and delays its ultimate removal. High levels of tetracyclines are found in the bowel.

All tetracyclines are excreted in both the urine and feces. Renal clearance of tetracyclines is by glomerular filtration.

Any patient with considerably impaired renal function requires a reduction in the dosage of tetracycline to avoid serious side effects.

Side Reactions and Toxicity The most common side reactions encountered clinically with tetracyclines are gastrointestinal: epigastric burning, nausea, vomiting, and diarrhea. Proctitis and stomatitis develop frequently. It is also possible that tetracyclines may injure the liver when given in large doses.

Allergic reactions including skin rash and drug fever may develop with tetracycline therapy, but their occurrence is infrequent. Intravenously administered tetracycline is highly irritating and frequently causes thrombophlebitis.

Photosensitivity has been demonstrated with several of the tetracyclines, especially demethylchlortetracycline. Children receiving long- or short-term therapy with the tetracyclines may develop yellow-brown discolorations of the teeth and bones. This process is caused by the deposition of tetracyclines in the bones and teeth at sites of active calcification. This deposition occurs primarily when infants and young children are treated and may cause not only discoloration of the teeth but also some delay in bone growth. When used in pregnant women after the fourth month of gestation discoloration of the first teeth may occur in the child. Patients taking outdated and degraded tetracycline may develop a form of the Fanconi syndrome. This clinical picture includes proteinuria, glycosuria, gross aminoaciduria, polyuria and polydipsia, and nausea and vomiting. Manifestations of this syndrome disappear about 1 month after therapy. Vestibular reactions may develop following use of minocycline.

Therapeutic Uses Despite the wide range of antibacterial action of the tetracyclines, these drugs now are considered to be the drug of choice in only a few clinical situations. A tetracycline is used in the treatment of infections due to the following: *Rickettsia, Bedsonia* (psittacosis or lymphogranuloma venereum), *Brucella,* many anaerobic streptococci and bacteroides, *Hemophilus ducreyi, Donovania granulomatis* (granuloma inguinale), *Vibrio fetus, V. cholera,* and *Borrelia recurrentis.* The tetracyclines are used in the treatment of urinary tract infections caused by gram-negative organisms shown by in vitro testing to be sensitive to this group of drugs. If the urine is not kept acid, the tetracyclines may be inactivated. The drug is also sometimes recommended for the treatment of gonorrhea, shigellosis, and pulmonary infections caused by *H. influenzae.* The tetracyclines are thought to be helpful in the therapy of acne vulgaris, perhaps because they decrease the concentration of free fatty acid in the sebum.

Preparations, Routes of Administration, and Dosage In general, when a tetracycline is indicated, an oral preparation should be used. Adult doses range from 250 to 750 mg every 6 h for most preparations. Demethylchlortetracycline is given in amounts of 150 to 300 mg every 6 h. Methacycline is given in doses of 150 mg every 6 h or 300 mg every 12 h orally.

The tetracycline family is represented by so many dosage forms for each member that a detailed description of each is not possible here. Beside the major dosage forms there are ophthalmic and otic solutions and ointments, powders, tablets, and troches.

Antibiotics Used Against Gram-negative Organisms: I, Aminoglycosides

Gentamicin Gentamicin sulfate is bactericidal in vitro against over 95 percent of *Staph. aureus,* including strains resistant to penicillin G. It is also effective against many strains of *E. coli, Klebsiella, Enterobacter, Salmonella, Proteus* (indole-positive and -negative), *Herellea,* and *Pseudomonas.* This antibiotic is not effective against enterococci, nor is it very effective against many *Streptococcus, D. pneumoniae, N. meningitides,* or *Providence.* Organisms do not readily develop resistance to gentamicin as they do to streptomycin.

Absorption and Excretion Gentamicin is not significantly absorbed from the gastrointestinal tract. Intramuscular injection of gentamicin sulfate in a dose of 0.4 mg/kg produces a peak plasma level of about 2 μg/ml at 1 h; antibiotic activity persists for 8 to 12 h.

Gentamicin is almost completely excreted in un-

changed form by glomerular filtration. Most of the drug can be recovered from the urine within a 24-h period following parenteral injection. As with neomycin and kanamycin, gentamicin accumulates in the tissues of patients with renal failure and must be given with extreme caution in these circumstances.

Toxicity Vestibular damage, the most important side effect of gentamicin, occurs most often in patients with uremia but can afflict patients with normal renal function. It is related to excessive plasma levels but not to duration of therapy or total quantity of drug given. Symptoms may appear during administration of this drug or within 2 weeks after the drug has been stopped. Damage may be irreversible. Ototoxicity with loss of hearing may also occur but is rare.

Transient proteinuria, azotemia, oliguria, and elevation of transaminase may develop. Gentamicin should not be given to uremic patients, neonates, and pregnant women, or to individuals receiving other ototoxic drugs, except under dire circumstances.

Therapeutic Uses Gentamicin ointment has been useful for local treatment of wounds, especially burns, because of its marked antipseudomonal activity. Severe systemic infections due to sensitive gram-negative microorganisms have been treated successfully by gentamicin administered parenterally. Of particular importance has been the successful treatment of *Pseudomonas* septicemia complicating burns, which is generally fatal without therapy. The drug has a role in the therapy of *Pseudomonas* infections and gram-negative bacteremia caused by organisms resistant to other antibiotics. It is advocated by some for the treatment of gram-negative bacteremia until results of blood cultures and sensitivities are reported and a less toxic agent can be selected.

Preparations, Routes of Administration, and Dosage Gentamicin (Garamycin) is available as a 0.1 percent cream or ointment for topical use against skin infections caused by either gram-positive or gram-negative bacteria. The intramuscular dose of gentamicin is 0.5 to 1.5 mg/kg 2 to 3 times a day. The total daily dose must not exceed 5 mg/kg.

Kanamycin Kanamycin possesses activity against gram-negative bacteria and is also effective against tubercle bacilli and some gram-positive organisms as well. However, because of increasing bacterial resistance, kanamycin is being replaced by gentamicin.

Ototoxicity and nephrotoxicity are the two most important side effects of kanamycin. Kanamycin is thought to have less vestibular and more auditory toxicity than streptomycin. Part of the reason for kanamycin ototoxicity may be that kanamycin reaches very high concentrations in the labyrinthine fluids and is eliminated very slowly from this region. Kanamycin, like neomycin, has been reported to cause neuromuscular blockade.

Preparations and Dosage Kanamycin sulfate (Kantrex) is available for parenteral and oral use. The oral dose is 6 to 8 g/day. Intramuscular injection is used for treatment of systemic infections. Adults are given 0.5 g every 8 to 12 h. Adult dosage should be limited to 1.5 g/day for no more than 1 week if possible. Children should receive 15 mg/kg/day divided equally and given at 6-h intervals. Patients with renal insufficiency should receive markedly reduced doses.

Neomycin Neomycin sulfate is generally used topically but is also available for oral and parenteral administration. At present, gentamicin has essentially replaced neomycin as a parenteral antibiotic. As with kanamycin and gentamicin, ototoxicity and renal damage are the two major complications of parenteral usage. Contact dermatitis is an untoward effect in about 10 percent of patients when neomycin is used topically. A high rate of sensitization occurs with long-term topical use.

Streptomycin Streptomycin has been discussed in detail in the chapter concerning antituberculous drugs. Streptomycin is also used to treat infections due to many gram-negative bacteria. Because of marked vestibular toxicity and rapid development of resistance to this drug by sensitive bacteria, streptomycin is not often the drug of choice for many bacterial infections. Indeed, gentamicin has largely replaced streptomycin in most clinical situations. Streptomycin should be used alone (as the sole antibiotic) in only two situations—the treatment of tularemia and plague. Whenever streptomycin is used, careful monitoring of the renal status is indicated, and the dose of streptomycin must be reduced if renal function is abnormal. Careful neurologic examinations must be performed to deter-

mine signs of early vestibular damage so that streptomycin can be discontinued or its dosage reduced.

Antibiotics Used Against Gram-negative Organisms: II, Polypeptides

Polymyxin B and Colistin Polymyxin B and colistin are bactericidal for many gram-negative bacteria including most *Pseudomonas* and *E. coli*, as well as many *Klebsiella, Enterobacter, Salmonella, Shigella,* and *Hemophilus*. Very few *Proteus* strains and no gram-positive organisms are affected by these drugs. Polymyxin is rapidly bactericidal as would be expected by its mechanism of action. Polymyxin and colistin act by disrupting the cytoplasmic membrane, thereby causing immediate cell death. The development of bacterial resistance to these agents is not frequent, but when it occurs there is complete cross-resistance among all the polymyxins. When these agents are given orally, absorption does *not* occur. The daily administration of 2 to 4 mg/kg intramuscularly to adults yields blood concentrations of 1 to 8 μg/ml, peaking 2 h after injection. The rate of excretion requires that the drug be given every 6 to 8 h to maintain bactericidal concentrations in the blood.

Untoward Effects After parenteral therapy, fever, dizziness, ataxia, dysarthria, and unpleasant paresthesia may occur. Occasional transient azotemia, proteinuria, cylindruria, and hematuria occur. Neurotoxicity and nephrotoxicity occur more frequently in patients with preexisting renal diseases, and in such patients reduced dosage is indicated. There is no satisfactory evidence to suggest that polymyxin B is less nephrotoxic than colistimethate or vice versa. Superinfection with organisms resistant to polymyxin may also occur.

Another form of neurotoxicity, neuromuscular blockade, has been reported following therapeutic doses of polymyxin B or colistimethate and is not commonly seen in patients with preexisting renal disease.

Therapeutic Uses The prime indication for polymyxin B and colistin is in the treatment of gram-negative infections, especially those caused by *Pseudomonas*. Although many other gram-negative organisms are somewhat sensitive to polymyxin B, other antimicrobials are usually considered the drug of first choice in infections due to *E. coli, Klebsi-*

ella, or *Enterobacter* organisms. *Pseudomonas* bacteremia and urinary tract infections may respond well to polymyxin or colistin, but metastatic infections in organs are difficult to treat because of poor tissue diffusion. Topical polymyxin B may be useful in the local therapy of gram-negative infection, especially if *Pseudomonas* is the responsible agent.

Preparations Polymyxin B sulfate (Aerosporin Sulfate) is available for topical use as an ophthalmic ointment, and as an otic solution and tablets. Polymyxin B is also prepared in vials for parenteral usage. It may be given by the oral, intramuscular, intravenous, and intrathecal routes as well as topically. Colistin sulfate is marketed for oral use. Sodium Colistimethate (Coly-Mycin M Parenteral) is marketed for intramuscular and intravenous injection. Colistimethate may be given in doses varying from 2 to 5 mg/kg per day for adults with normal renal function depending on site of infection.

ANTIFUNGAL AGENTS

Nystatin

Nystatin was isolated in 1949 from a *Streptomyces* and was the first antifungal antibiotic to be discovered. The precise mechanism by which nystatin inhibits fungi has not been clarified, but available data indicate that the antibiotic binds to sterols in the membrane of fungi and inhibits endogenous respiration and utilization of glucose in the cells. Additional data show that intracellular protein synthesis is impaired by interference with phosphate utilization and the accelerated degradation of ATP.

Therapeutic Uses Lack of absorption of the antibiotic when administered orally and the significant toxicity it produces when given systemically preclude treatment of systemic fungal infections. Therapy is therefore confined to the prevention and topical treatment of superficial *Candida* infections of the skin and mucous surfaces.

Dosage Forms Nystatin (Mycostatin) is available in oral tablets containing 500,000 units of antibiotic for treating intestinal moniliasis and recalcitrant cases of monilial vaginitis with local vaginal therapy. It is also available in vaginal tablets, a powder for reconstitution for oral use, and in both an ointment and dusting powder for topical use.

Amphotericin B

Antimicrobial studies with amphotericin B show that it inhibits a wide variety of fungal species including those organisms responsible for the common superficial and systemic fungal infections of humans. The antibiotic has also been shown to inhibit strains of *Leishmania braziliensis, L. donovani, Mycobacterium leprae, Schistosoma mansoni,* and *Candida albicans.* The precise means by which amphotericin B inhibits sensitive fungi is not known, but the similarity in structure with that of nystatin strongly suggests that the mode of action of these two antibiotics is comparable.

Side Effects Few patients receiving intravenous amphotericin B escape the side effects associated with this form of administration: fever, chills, headache, nausea, vomiting, anorexia, abdominal pain, flushing, sweating, fatigue, and drowsiness. In most instances, repeated intravenous use of amphotericin B is associated with a reduction in the incidence and severity of side effects, and patients can then tolerate the medication for weeks or months of therapy. Apart from a reduction in hemoglobin, amphotericin B does not appear to interfere with hematopoietic system function.

Dosage Forms An intravenous form of amphotericin B (Fungizone) is available for systemic fungal disease, and a 3 percent concentration for topical use in the management of superficial candidiasis.

Flucytosine

Flucytosine is a new antifungal agent for systemic infections caused by *Cryptococcus neoformans* and *C. albicans.* It is reportedly less toxic than amphotericin B and is absorbed from the gastrointestinal tract. The side effects associated with flucytosine are nausea, vomiting, diarrhea, skin rash, and blood dyscrasias; some instances of vertigo, headache, hallucinations, and confusion have occurred. This agent is recommended in patients who cannot tolerate amphotericin B, particularly in systemic infection of *C. albicans* and cryptococcus meningitis or pneumonia. It should be noted that resistant strains of cryptococcus develop during therapy with flucytosine.

Dosage Forms   Flucytosine (Ancobon) is available for oral administration in 250- or 500-mg capsules.

Griseofulvin

The spectrum of antifungal activity of griseofulvin includes those dermatophytes which predominantly cause cutaneous infection; it is inactive against yeast organisms, bacteria, and those fungi causing deep mycotic infections.

The exact means by which griseofulvin produces inhibitory action on fungi has not yet been determined. In certain concentrations, griseofulvin has been shown to retard oxidative phosphorylation of sensitive fungi, and to inhibit nucleic acid synthesis. Light and electron microscopic studies show that in the presence of griseofulvin the fungal mycelia become swollen and ballooned, the cell wall loses its integrity, and the cytoplasm disappears, leaving remnants of cytoplasmic membrane and large lipid storage granules. The available data indicate that growing fungal cells which are metabolically active are killed by griseofulvin, whereas the dormant metabolically inactive cells are only inhibited.

Toxicity   Adult humans have been maintained on daily oral doses of griseofulvin up to 2 years, and critical studies of the hematopoietic system and renal and testicular function have failed to show any interference with normal function of these organs. Standard biochemical studies for liver function have also been within normal limits. However, griseofulvin interferes with the liver metabolism of the anticoagulant coumarin compounds and should not be used in patients on coumarin therapy.

Extensive clinical usage of griseofulvin in humans has failed so far to reveal any significant changes in organ function, and no case of true agranulocytosis has yet been reported. There have been, however, associated side effects of varying magnitude, including gastrointestinal upsets, headache, skin lesions, irritability, thirst, fatigue and insomnia, urticaria, and pruritus. In rare instances the use of griseofulvin has been associated with potentiation of the effects of alcohol. In isolated patients, it has been reported to be a photosensitizing agent.

Dosage Forms and Therapeutic Use   Griseofulvin (Fulvicin-U/F, Grifulvin V) is available for oral administration in management of superficial dermatophytic infections as 125-, 250-, and 500-mg tablets. Duration of therapy with griseofulvin depends on the time required for normal replacement of the infected tissues. Medication should ideally be continued until the pathogens cannot be isolated from the site of infection. Infection of the body usually clears in 2 to 4 weeks, and tinea capitis responds to griseofulvin in 3 to 5 weeks. Infection of the palms takes approximately 6 weeks to clear, whereas infection of the soles requires approximately 6 to 8 weeks of therapy. Ringworm of the fingernails requires 3 to 6 months, and infection of the toes needs 8 to 12 months. The response of individual lesions is variable, and in some instances, extended periods of therapy are required. Although griseofulvin has been found to be an effective therapeutic agent in the majority of cases, a certain number of cases remain in which the lesion does not respond; responds initially but fails to clear on therapy; is clinically cured and relapses; or is mycologically cured with reinfection occurring at a later date.

Additional Antifungal Compounds: Topically Applied Agents

The use of orally administered griseofulvin has greatly advanced the means of treating superficial dermatophytic infections. However, a number of such infections, especially those of the nails and the toe clefts, frequently fail to respond to adequate griseofulvin therapy and may then be treated with the commonly utilized topically applied agents that are effective against the dermatophytic fungi. Such compounds having useful therapeutic value against dermatophytes are 2 to 5 percent undecylenic acid, and more recently 1 percent *O*,2-naphthyl *m*,*N*-dimethylthiocarbanilate (Tolnaftate). In cases of superficial infections due to *Candida* species, the polyene antibiotics such as candicidin have effectively been used topically in doses comparable to those used for nystatin. In addition, such anticandidal agents as 1 percent tincture of gentian violet, 1 percent hydroxyquinoline, 1 percent chlorhydroxyquinoline, 3 percent iodochlorhydroxyquinoline, and 1 percent chlordantoin may be used as alternatives for the antifungal antibiotics.

Chapter 37

Sulfonamides, Sulfones, and Antituberculosis Agents

SULFONAMIDES

Chemistry

Sulfonamides are derivatives of sulfanilamide (Fig. 37-1) which have antibacterial activity. All sulfonamides are partially acetylated in the body, although the percentage of acetylation varies considerably. The conjugated sulfonamide may be either more or less soluble in water than the unconjugated sulfonamide. In addition, the long-acting sulfonamides (for example, sulfadimethoxine) may be conjugated to form a glucuronide. This conjugate by and large is more soluble than the

Sulfanilamide

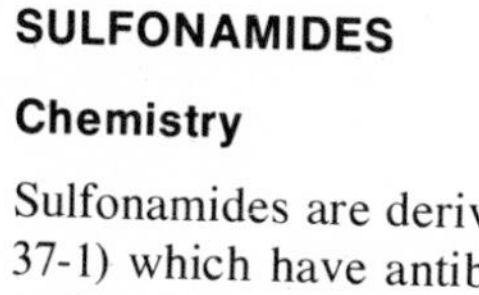

Figure 37-1 Structure of sulfanilamide (p-aminobenzenesulfonamide) with N-1 and N-4 positions indicated.

parent compound. The formulas of representative sulfonamide drugs grouped according to their half-life and absorbability from the gastrointestinal tract are listed in Figs. 37-2 and 37-3.

Mechanism of Action

The sulfonamides are primarily bacteriostatic in concentrations which are normally useful in controlling infections. The sulfonamides restrain bacterial growth, allowing the normal phagocytic cells of the body to engulf and destroy the invading organism. Only when concentrations of the drug are extremely high, as in the urine, are bactericidal concentrations occasionally obtained.

The action of sulfonamides against many microorganisms is the result of interference with the utilization of p-aminobenzoic acid, PABA (Fig. 37-4A). In the presence of sulfonamides, PABA is not incorporated into folic acid, which is essential in reduced forms for certain single-carbon-unit transfers (Fig. 37-4B). However, since humans

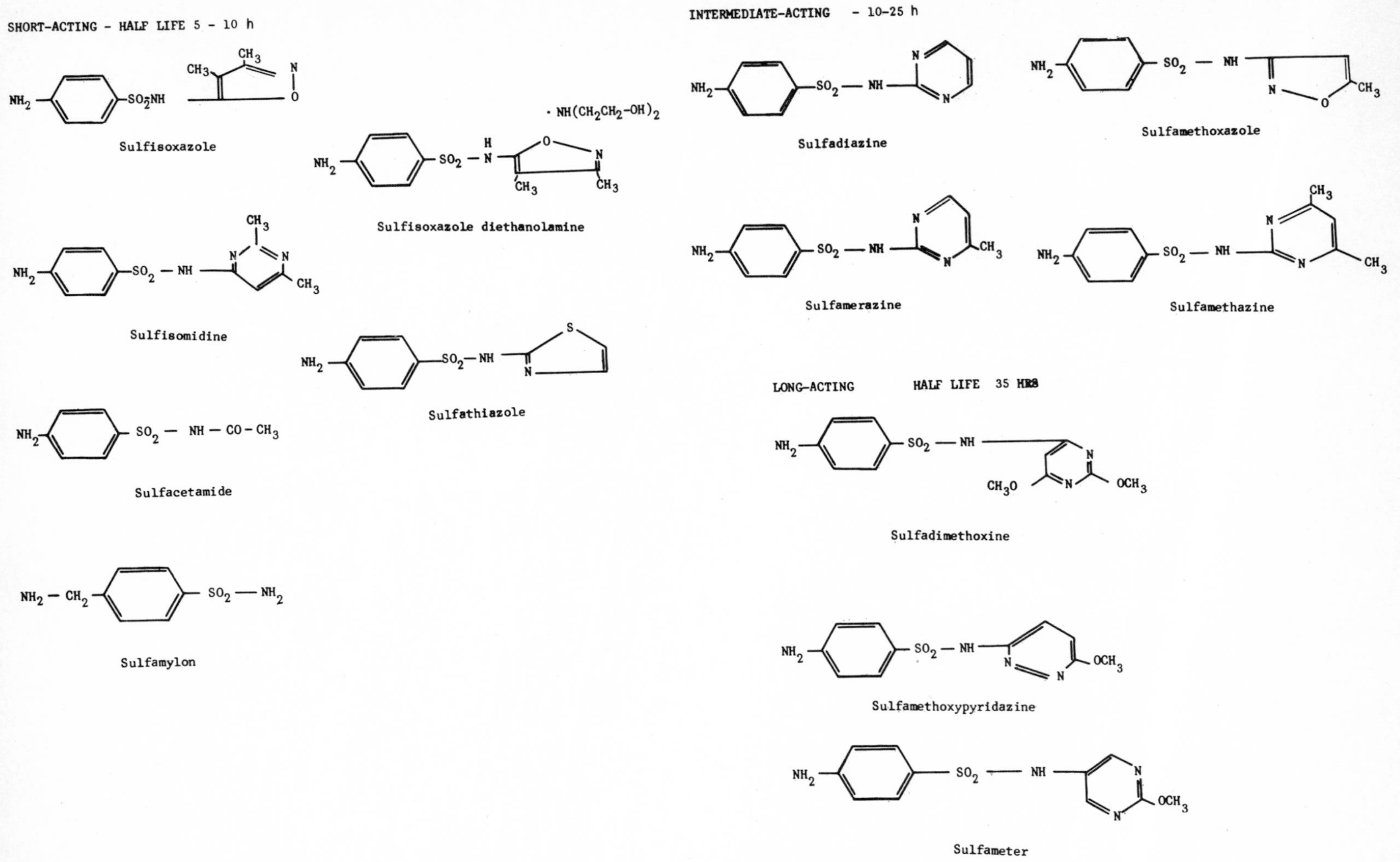

Figure 37-2 Chemical formulas of representative systemic sulfonamides (readily absorbed from the gastrointestinal tract).

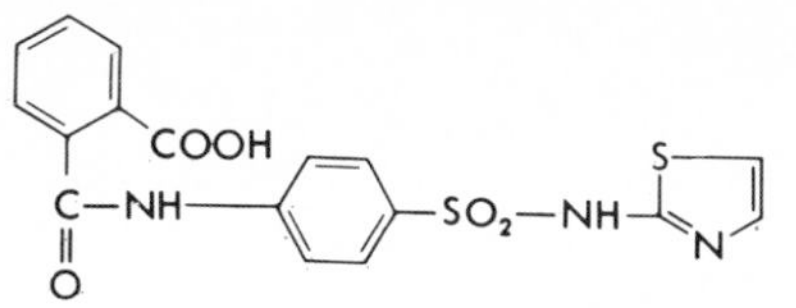

Phthalylsulfathiazole (Sulfathalidine) 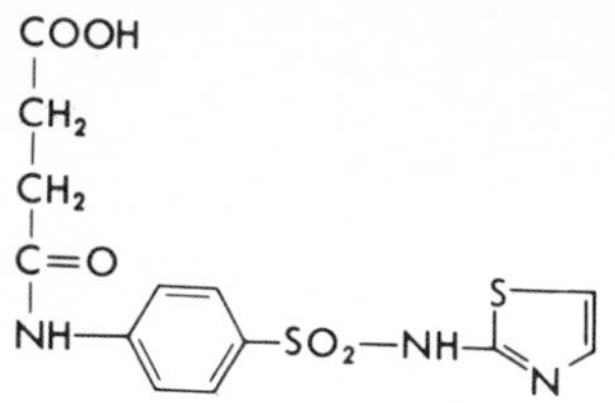   Succinylsulfathiazole

Figure 37-3 Chemical formulas of representative nonsystemic sulfonamides (poorly absorbed from the gastrointestinal tract).

utilize preformed folic acid, the sulfonamides are not particularly toxic to human hosts.

Resistance

A major problem with antibacterial agents is the eventual development of resistant organisms. It is well known that the action of the sulfonamides is essentially bacteriostatic; therefore, the organisms are subjected to a *sublethal* concentration of the sulfonamide. However, in most bacterial populations a few organisms continue to reproduce. Eventually a population of resistant organisms emerges which continues to grow even in concentrations of the sulfonamide which are toxic to the host. It has been observed that once an organism has become resistant to one of the sulfonamides, it will usually be resistant to other sulfonamides.

Bacterial Susceptibility

Sulfonamides are primarily effective against certain gram-positive cocci and diplococci, gram-negative diplococci, and gram-negative bacilli. Although sulfonamides control certain infections satisfactorily, in most infections an antibiotic is even more effective; consequently, sulfonamides are being employed less frequently. At present they may be used for individual prophylaxis of streptococcus infections, group prophylaxis and treatment of *Shigella* enteritis, treatment of urinary tract infections caused by *E. coli* and *Proteus mirabilis*, treatment of nocardiosis and chancroid, and preoperative suppression of intestinal flora. Because they diffuse into the cerebrospinal fluid, they may also be used in combination with antibiotics in the treatment of meningeal infections caused by sulfonamide-sensitive bacteria.

Routes of Administration

Substances used for systemic effect are usually administered orally; however, the sodium salts and acetyl and diethanolamine derivatives of several sulfonamides are available for intravenous use. It is rarely necessary to resort to intravenous medication, since the agents used to treat systemic infections are readily absorbed from the gastrointestinal tract. The alkalinity of most salts precludes subcutaneous or intramuscular administration; however, diolamine salts such as sulfisoxazole diolamine may be given intramuscularly. Certain insoluble poorly absorbed sulfonamides (succinylsulfathiazole and phthalylsulfathiazole), are only used orally for preoperative intestinal sterilization. Sodium sulfacetamide and sulfisoxazole diolamine are recommended for local ophthalmic use because in solution they are less alkaline than the other sulfonamide salts and therefore less injurious to the conjunctiva.

Absorption

On the basis of the degree to which sulfonamides are absorbed, they can readily be divided into two groups: those which are *readily absorbed* (Fig. 37-2) and those which are *poorly absorbed* (Fig. 37-3).

Among the readily absorbed agents, sulfisoxazole and sulfamerazine are absorbed more rapidly than sulfadiazine and sulfamethazine. Four sulfonamides used at the present time—sulfisoxazole, trisulfapyrimidines, sulfamethoxazole, and sulfadiazine—are all rapidly absorbed. Their principal advantage is a high solubility in acid media, reducing the danger of intrarenal precipitation. Sulfadimethoxine, sulfameter, and sulfamethoxypyridazine are absorbed somewhat more slowly but

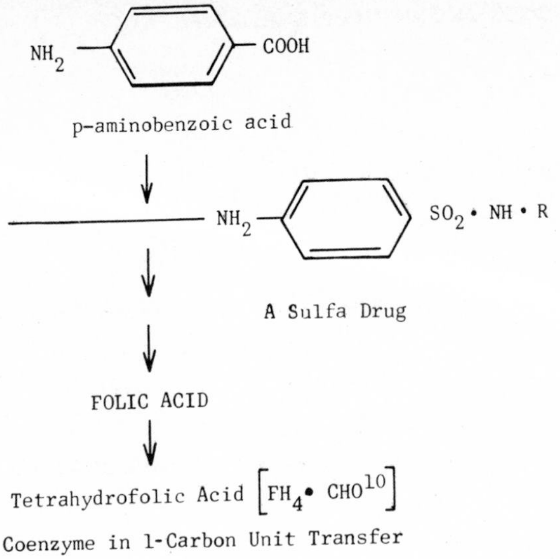
NH2
COOH
p-aminobenzoic acid
NH2
SO2 • NH • R
A Sulfa Drug
FOLIC ACID
Tetrahydrofolic Acid [FH4• CHO10]
Coenzyme in 1-Carbon Unit Transfer

A

$$HS\text{-}CH_2\text{-}CH_2\text{-}CH(NH_2)\text{-}COOH \xrightarrow{FH_4 \cdot C^*HO^{10}} CH_3^*\text{-}S\text{-}CH_2\text{-}CH(NH_2)\text{-}COOH$$

HOMOCYSTEINE — METHIONINE

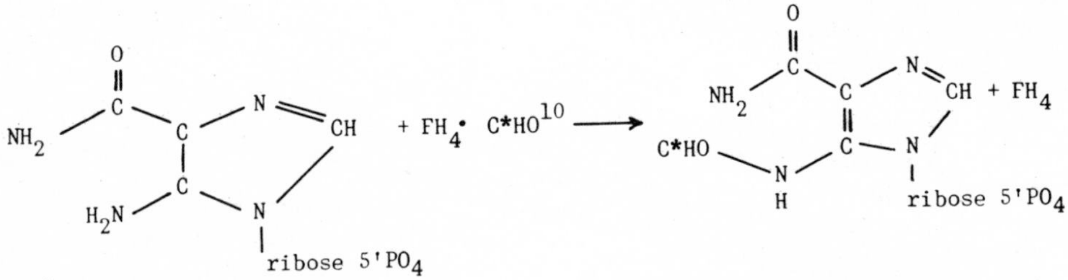
+ FH4• C*HO10
ribose 5'PO4
+ FH4
C*HO
ribose 5'PO4

5-AMINO-4-IMIDAZOLCARBOXAMIDE RIBOTIDE — 5-FORMAMIDO-4-IMIDAZOLE CARBOXAMIDE RIBOTIDE

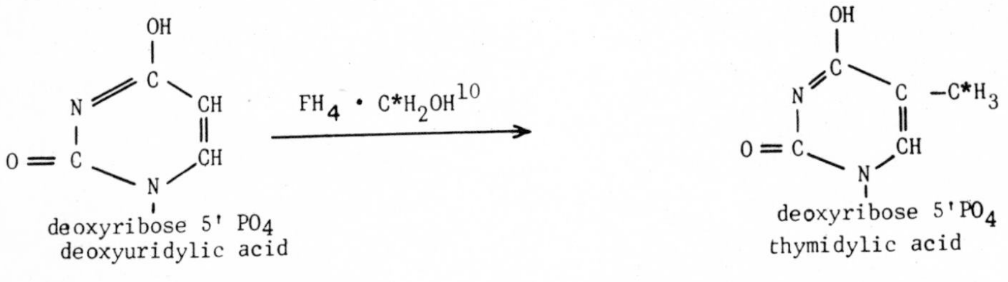
FH4 • C*H2OH10
deoxyribose 5' PO4
deoxyuridylic acid
deoxyribose 5'PO4
thymidylic acid

$$FH_4 \cdot C^*H = N^5H + H_2O \rightleftharpoons FH_4 \cdot C^*HO^{10} + NH_3$$

N^5 Formimino tetrahydrofolic acid — N^{10} Formyl tetrahydrofolic acid

$$OH\text{-}C^*H_2\text{-}\underset{NH_2}{CH}\text{-}COOH + FH_4 \rightleftharpoons N^5N^{10}\ C^*H_2 \cdot FH_4 + NH_2\text{-}CH_2\text{-}COOH$$

Serine + Tetrahydrofolic acid — glycine

B

have the potential advantage of being more slowly eliminated by the kidneys. However, the extended durations of high concentrations of long-acting sulfonamides in the serum contribute to the frequency, severity, and persistence of adverse reactions.

Distribution

Sulfacetamide, sulfadiazine, and sulfamerazine appear to cross the cell membranes freely. Sulfonamides are distributed to brain, red blood cells, lung, liver, pancreas, muscle, and nerve. Sulfonamides readily pass through the human placenta; fetal concentrations reach approximately the plasma concentrations of the mother.

One of the principal advantages of the sulfonamides is their ready diffusion into all the fluids of the body. This property is of particular importance in the treatment of meningitis, because most sulfonamides penetrate into spinal fluid in concentrations of 35 to 75 percent of the blood concentrations. The inflamed meninges offer less of a barrier than the normal meninges. In the presence of infection, therefore, higher spinal fluid levels are observed. Sulfadiazine and sulfacetamide penetrate readily into aqueous humor. The pK_a value and the group which is substituted on the N-1 position determine the degree of conjugation and its lipid solubility.

Biotransformation

Following absorption, a portion of the drug may either be bound to plasma albumin or metabolized. Depending upon the radical substituted on the N-1 or N-4 position of the molecule (Fig. 37-1), the degree to which these reactions occur varies.

The characteristic alteration in sulfonamides is an acetylation on the N-1 position which results in loss of activity. The conjugate may either be more or less toxic than the parent substance, depending largely upon the solubility of the acetylated compound in the urine. Acetylation in humans takes place primarily in the liver, although it may occur to a lesser extent in the other tissues of the body.

Some of the sulfonamides (sulfisoxazole, sulfisomidine, and sulfacetamide) are quite soluble in acid urine at pH 5.5 to 6.5; in addition, the acetylated drug is soluble at these acid pH's. Because of

the potentially pathologic renal changes due to sulfonamide therapy, the solubility of both the sulfonamide and its conjugates in the urine is a matter of primary concern in the therapeutic use of these agents.

Excretion

The kidney is the main route by which all sulfonamides are eliminated from the plasma. They are excreted in both the conjugated and free forms. Excretion may occur by either glomerular filtration or tubular secretion.

A variety of tissue fluids acquire appreciable amounts of sulfonamide. The intestinal juices contain very high concentrations of sulfonamide, approximately two-thirds the concentration of that in blood. Effective concentrations of these drugs are eliminated by the bile. Although the soluble sulfonamides are excreted into the upper intestinal tract, they are largely reabsorbed, since only small quantities (0 to 8 percent) are found in the feces. Other secretions which contain appreciable quantities of sulfonamide are the prostatic fluid, salivary secretion, and bronchial secretion. Relatively small amounts (1 to 2 percent) are found in the milk.

Toxicity

Acute toxicity in individuals receiving sulfonamides for the first time is rarely observed; however, if sulfonamides have been previously administered, toxic manifestations may appear within the first 24 or 48 h after institution of therapy. The manifestations of toxicity fall roughly into two categories: (1) allergies or idiosyncrasies, and (2) renal toxicity. Hypersensitivity reactions are usually encountered after the drugs have been administered for several days to several weeks.

Nausea and vomiting are the most common side effects and may occur in 5 percent of patients. This probably represents a central nervous system action; other less common central effects may be headache, dizziness, ataxia, depression, irritability, and restlessness. A microscopic hematuria is observed in the occasional patient; with the more soluble sulfonamides now in general use, a gross hematuria is rare. Sensitivity to sulfonamides may result in glomerular nephritis. In general, the ap-

Figure 37-4 (A) Schema showing the point of competition of sulfonamide for PABA. (B) Examples of single-carbon unit transfers.

pearance of toxic symptoms bears a direct relationship to the blood level attained, except for idiosyncratic reactions.

Other toxic reactions to sulfonamides observed after a few days to 2 weeks of therapy include fever, anemia, leukopenia, dermatitis, and inhibition of 6-glucose phosphate dehydrogenase.

All sulfonamides, especially the long-acting sulfa drugs, sulfadimethoxine and in particular sulfamethoxypyridazine, have been implicated in the etiology of Stevens-Johnson syndrome.

The toxic manifestation which has perhaps received more careful study than any other is renal damage. This has been shown to be the result of precipitation of crystals in the collecting tubules of the kidney and, in severe toxicity, even in the pelvis of the kidney itself. The concretions formed may obstruct the flow of urine in addition to injuring the tubular epithelium or the epithelial lining of the pelvis of the kidney. These concretions are more frequently observed if the solubility of the drug in the urine is low, if the pH of the urine is low, or if the concentration of the drug in the urine is high.

Prevention of this renal complication is more satisfactory than its treatment once it has become evident; however, treatment usually involves discontinuing administration of the offending agent, increasing the volume of the urine, and increasing the pH of the urine. It has been demonstrated that the presence of one sulfonamide in water or urine does not diminish the solubility of another sulfonamide in the same solution. Employing this principle makes it possible to use a mixture of two or three sulfonamides, each at one-half or one-third the usual concentration; by this method, adequate bacteriostatic concentrations in the blood are obtained without risking serious renal complications.

Therapeutic Uses

The primary use of sulfonamides is in the treatment of acute uncomplicated urinary tract infections.

Depending upon the presence or absence of complications, therapy should be continued at full maintenance dosage for 6 weeks to 3 months, or even longer.

E. coli and gram-positive cocci, except enterococci, are the pathogens most susceptible to sulfonamides. *Klebsiella aerogenes, Pseudomonas aeru-*ginosa, *Alcaligenes faecalis,* and *Proteus* species rarely respond favorably to sulfonamide therapy. Enterococci are notably resistant to all sulfonamide compounds.

Combination Therapy The combination of a sulfonamide and an inhibitor of dehydrofolate reductase is capable of synergistic antibacterial activity. Sulfonamides are competitive inhibitors of PABA and thus prevent the synthesis of folic acid by bacteria. Trimethoprim is a potent inhibitor of bacterial dehydrofolate reductase compared to the mammalian enzyme, and thus prevents the conversion of folic acid to folinic acid, effectively blocking utilization of this vital element in the eventual synthesis of nucleic acids (Fig. 37-5). Sulfonamides are not particularly toxic in the host since humans do not synthesize folic acid. On the other hand, the inhibitors of dehydrofolate reductase are more toxic to humans because they do prevent utilization of preformed folates. Another factor which enhances selective toxicity for the bacteria is the fact that as a rule many lower organisms cannot use preformed folates.

Preparations and Dosage

Sulfonamides for Systemic and Topical Use

Sulfadiazine Available as 250-, 300-, or 500-mg tablets. Sterile sulfadiazine sodium may be used for intravenous injection and is supplied as 2.5 g in a 50- or 10-ml volume. The usual intravenous dose, 4 g in 5 percent solution, may be repeated in 8 h; the usual dose range is 500 mg to 4 g. Initial adult dose is 2 to 4 g; maintenance dose is 4 to 6 g/day in divided doses.

Trisulfapyrimidines Available in oral suspension and tablets, this combination contains sulfamerazine, sulfamethazine, and sulfadiazine. Each 100-ml or oral suspension contains not less than 9.3 g and not more than 10.7 g of total sulfapyrimidines; 3.0 to 3.7 g of each of the three drugs is present in this amount. Trisulfapyrimidine tablets contain 95 to 105 percent of the labeled amount of total sulfapyrimidines, each equal to 31.5 to 35.0 percent of the total labeled sulfapyrimidines. The tablets usually available contain 500 mg of total sulfapyrimidines (167 mg each of the three drugs). Initial adult dose is 4 g. Maintenance dose is 4 to 6 g/day in divided doses.

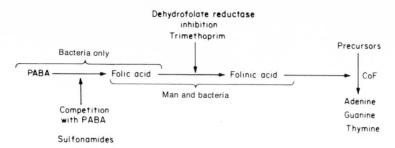

Figure 37-5 The diagram shows the site of action of competitors of PABA in contrast with inhibitors of dehydrofolate reductase in the chain of synthesis and utilization of folic acid by bacteria and humans.

Sulfacetamide Sodium Available for ophthalmic use both as a 0.1 g/g ointment and as a solution containing 0.3 g/ml.

Sulfisoxazole (Gantrisin) Supplied as 0.5-g tablets. Initial adult dose is 4 g; maintenance dose is 4 to 8 g/day in divided doses.

Acetyl Sulfisoxazole (Gantrisin) Available in oral suspension containing not less than 9.3 and not more than 10.7 g sulfisoxazole/100 ml. The usual adult dose is the same as for sulfisoxazole.

Sulfisoxazole Diethanolamine Injection (Gantrisin) Contains the equivalent of 2 g sulfisoxazole base in 5 ml and can be repeated if necessary after 8 to 12 h. Sulfisoxazole diethanolamine ophthalmic ointment, ophthalmic solution, and nasal and ear solutions are also available.

Sulfamethoxazole (Gantanol) Supplied in 0.5-g tablets. For mild infections the initial adult dose is 2 g; maintenance dose is 1 g each morning and evening. For severe infections the initial adult dose is 2 g, and maintenance dose is 1 g every 8 h. It is also available as an oral suspension.

Sulfamethoxypyridazine (Midicel) Available as 0.5-g tablets. Initial adult dose is 1 g; maintenance dose is 0.5 g/day.

Sulfadimethoxine (Madribon) Available as an oral suspension containing 0.05 g/ml and as 0.5-g tablets. Initial adult dose is 2 g; maintenance dose is 1.0 g/day.

Sulfonamides for Local Intestinal Use These compounds are administered orally. They are absorbed so poorly that the blood levels seldom go above 2 mg/100 ml.

Succinylsulfathiazole Available in 500-mg tablets. The initial dose is 0.25 g/kg body weight followed by 0.25 g/kg body weight daily in six divided doses.

Phthalylsulfathiazole (Sulfathalidine) Available in 500-mg tablets. The initial dose is 0.125 g/kg body weight followed by 0.125 g/kg body weight daily in three to six divided doses.

Combinations Sulfamethoxazole and trimethoprim (Bactrim, Septra) is available in tablets containing sulfamethoxazole 400 mg and trimethoprim 80 mg. The usual adult dosage is two tablets every 12 h for 10 to 14 days.

SULFONES

The sulfones have proved reasonably effective in the treatment of leprosy, a disease which has not responded satisfactorily to any other therapeutic agent.

Of the large number of sulfones which have been synthesized, only a limited number have received adequate clinical trial. Those which have been studied most extensively are dapsone (diaminodiphenylsulfone, DDS, Avlosulfon), and sulfoxone sodium (Diasone).

$$NH_2-\!\!\!\!\!\bigcirc\!\!\!\!\!-SO_2-\!\!\!\!\!\bigcirc\!\!\!\!\!-NH_2$$

Dapsone

$$CH_2-NH-\!\!\!\!\!\bigcirc\!\!\!\!\!-SO_2-\!\!\!\!\!\bigcirc\!\!\!\!\!-NH-CH_2$$
$$SO_2Na \qquad\qquad\qquad\qquad\qquad SO_2Na$$

Sulfoxone sodium

Mechanism of Action

p-Aminobenzoic acid partially antagonizes the action of many of the sulfones, suggesting that they interfere with the nutrition of bacteria in a manner similar to that of the sulfonamides. Infections which arise in patients under sulfone therapy are usually sulfonamide-resistant, further suggesting a mechanism of action similar to the sulfonamides.

Route of Administration and Dosage

The sulfones are administered orally. Dapsone is rapidly and almost completely absorbed from the gastrointestinal tract. It is excreted rather slowly. The oral dose of dapsone for lepromatous leprosy, first and second weeks, 25 mg twice weekly; third and fourth weeks, 50 mg twice weekly; thereafter 50 mg/day.

Sulfoxone has been administered orally in a dose of 0.3 g/day the first week, 0.6 g/day the second week, and 0.9 g/day thereafter, provided that no serious side reactions occur.

Toxicity, Idiosyncrasies, and Therapeutic Use

With doses producing a concentration of 2 mg/100 ml or greater in the blood, acute toxic effects, including acute hemolysis of the blood and liver damage, are observed frequently. With blood levels between 1 and 2 mg/100 ml, chronic toxic effects including hemolytic anemia, liver damage, and psychoses are observed. The red blood cell count is often depressed at the start of therapy with sulfones. Iron salts help to counteract the anemia. After continuous therapy with the sulfones, the red cell count tends to return to normal.

Erythema nodosum leprosum is the commonest reaction to the sulfones—a reaction which is believed to be nonallergic. Patients who develop this lesion show a greater diminution of bacilli than do nonreacting individuals. Allergic reactions such as drug fever, dermatitis, and hepatitis have occasionally been seen. At present, sulfones find their primary area of clinical usefulness in the treatment of leprosy and malaria.

ANTITUBERCULOSIS AGENTS

Tuberculosis is usually treated with drugs for 12 to 36 months, depending on the severity of the dis-

ease. This prolonged treatment poses two problems. First, a number of drugs which are effective against the tubercle bacillus and can be administered for a short period of time may produce toxic effects over longer periods. If such drugs must be used, dosage and time intervals between doses must be carefully regulated. Second, the chance of emergence of drug-resistant organisms increases with the length of treatment, a difficulty compounded by the fact that adequate drug concentrations may not be obtained in cavities and caseous lesions. Drugs are therefore given initially in the highest tolerated doses, usually two or more simultaneously, to delay the emergence of resistance.

Currently, streptomycin and/or isonicotinic acid hydrazide combined with ethambutol are the drugs of first choice because they are most effective and least toxic. Following therapeutic failure with these, rifampin (Rifadin, Rimactane), cycloserine (Seromycin), viomycin (Vinactane, Viocin), kanamycin (Kantrex), pyrazinamide, ethionamide (Trecator-SC), capreomycin (Capastat), and p-aminosalicylic acid (PAS) are used in a variety of combinations.

Streptomycin

Mechanism of Action　Streptomycin inhibits protein synthesis. It penetrates into the cell body and combines with the 30S ribosomal particles; since it does not interfere with the attachment of mRNA to the ribosome, it must alter the function of the ribosome *after* the mRNA is attached. The ribosome is altered so that the code is misread and nonfunctional, or nonsense proteins are synthesized by the cells, leading to metabolic alteration and cell death.

Streptomycin

Bacterial Susceptibility Streptomycin is effective chiefly against gram-negative organisms. Occasionally streptomycin is employed in the treatment of gram-positive infections that do not respond to penicillin or other drugs. It may also be used in combination with penicillin in the treatment of resistant strains.

Absorption, Distribution, and Excretion Streptomycin is not absorbed to an appreciable extent by the intestine following oral administration. Streptomycin is well absorbed when injected intramuscularly, and from 25 to 40 percent of the drug is protein-bound. The antibiotic is distributed throughout the body, but the rate of distribution is fairly slow. In general, streptomycin is widely distributed in extracellular fluids, both normal and pathologic, but it does not penetrate into cells. Thus tubercle bacilli in macrophages are not affected by the drug.

Excretion by the kidney is slow. The drug is concentrated only by the kidney and not by the liver, which excretes some of it in the bile. Streptomycin is therefore useful for urinary tract infections caused by certain gram-negative bacteria, despite the fact that high electrolyte concentrations interfere with its action.

Toxicity Streptomycin produces the usual allergic reactions in sensitive patients. Erythema, rashes, urticaria, and purpura may occur, as may a fall in blood pressure accompanied by headache, nausea, and vomiting. Large doses may cause albuminuria and liver damage. Specific toxicity is manifested by damage to the eighth nerve and labyrinth, the symptoms of which appear after 2 or 3 weeks of therapy. The injury is related both to duration of treatment and dosage and is the result of degeneration of the hair cells in the organ of Corti and the semicircular canals. Vertigo and tinnitus, diplopia after rapid movement of the head, and finally permanent deafness may occur following prolonged therapy for tuberculosis. Such severe damage does not follow briefer use, for example, for periods of 5 to 10 days in acute infections. Streptomycin has a curarelike effect on skeletal muscle which must be taken into account if patients treated with the drug are given neuromuscular blocking agents in conjunction with anesthesia.

Therapeutic Uses Streptomycin is chiefly effective against gram-negative bacteria, although occasionally gram-positive organisms that are resistant to penicillin may be susceptible to streptomycin.

Preparations and Dosage Streptomycin is available as the sulfate, the hydrochloride, or a calcium chloride complex in 1- or 5-g vials. For systemic infections, streptomycin is given intramuscularly or subcutaneously in doses of 0.5 to 1.0 g 2 to 4 times a day. The dosage schedule in tuberculosis is adjusted to the severity of the disease and the other drugs administered.

Isonicotinic Acid Hydrazide (Isoniazid)

Mechanism of Action Isoniazid decreases transaminase activity and other pyridoxine-linked enzymes. In mammalian tissues it inhibits NADase (glycohydrolase), while in *Mycobacterium tuberculosis* it stimulates increased NADase production. This action of isoniazid interferes with the viability of the bacilli.

Isonicotinic acid hydrazide

Absorption, Distribution, and Excretion Isoniazid is rapidly absorbed from the intestine. It is distributed throughout the body, including in the cerebrospinal fluid. Peak serum levels occur 1 h after administration, and at this time the cerebrospinal-fluid concentration is about one-fifth that of the serum. In general, the concentration in the tissues is somewhat higher than in the blood. In humans, 75 to 90 percent of the dose is excreted in the urine in 24 h as unchanged drug, isonicotinic acid, N^1-isonicotinyl acetyl hydrazide, N-methyl isonicotinic acid hydrazide, and an unidentified fraction, possibly the isonicotinyl hydrazide of pyruvic acid. The rate of metabolism varies greatly, and three general types of patients have been identified: the rapid metabolizers, who have no drug in the serum 6 h after dose, and who excrete more of the drug in the acetylated form; the slow metabolizers, who excrete less in the acetylated form and who have about one-third of the peak level 6 h after the dose; and an intermediate group. These differences appear to be genetically determined.

Toxicity In therapeutic doses, peripheral neuritis is the main toxic symptom. This may be the result of pyridoxine deficiency since it can be controlled by daily administration of the vitamin which, however, does not interfere with the therapeutic effect. Other toxic symptoms are minor, consisting of constipation, difficulty in starting micturition, orthostatic hypotension, eosinophilia, slight anemia, and albuminuria. Fatty infiltration of the liver, if it occurs, has been attributed to the disease and not to the drug. Very high doses produce hyperglycemia.

Dosage and Administration Usually 2 to 8 mg/kg is given twice daily, but higher doses are necessary for miliary tuberculosis and tuberculous meningitis. The dose should be determined by the 6-h serum level and adjusted accordingly. All routes of administration are feasible, but the drug is usually given by mouth. Pyridoxine in a dose of 50 to 100 mg may be given daily to prevent peripheral neuritis. Isoniazid is supplied in 50- and 100-mg tablets and in a 10 percent solution for injection.

Ethambutol

Mechanism of Action Chelation of divalent metals may be important for some of the therapeutic and toxic effects of the drug. Magnesium and also spermidine antagonize its action on strains of tubercle bacilli in vitro, and its inhibition of RNA synthesis may be the result of magnesium chelation. DNA and protein synthesis are not directly affected.

Ethambutol

Use and Toxicity Growth of various strains of tubercle bacilli and some atypical strains is inhibited by 1 to 4 μg/ml ethambutol. Resistance to the drug develops fairly rapidly. It can be used with most of the other antitubercular drugs.

The most serious toxic effects are on the eye. There is a decrease in visual acuity and loss of green-red perception suggesting retrobulbar neuritis. With a daily dose of 25 mg/kg visual toxicity occurs in approximately 3 percent of patients, but toxicity is not generally manifested with doses of 5 to 10 mg/kg. Ethambutol (Myambutol) is supplied in 100- and 400-mg tablets.

p-Aminosalicylic Acid (PAS)

Mechanism of Action It is probable that PAS acts by interfering with the utilization of PABA by the tubercle bacillus. Resistance to the drug develops, but more slowly than to streptomycin.

p-Aminosalicylic acid

Absorption, Fate, and Excretion The rate of absorption from the intestine is more rapid if the drug is given in solution than if given as a solid. About 50 to 60 percent of the drug in the serum is protein-bound. The principal metabolites are acetylaminosalicylic acid and p-aminosalicyluric acid, which are formed in the liver and are inactive. Most of the dose is rapidly excreted by the kidney; as much as 50 percent of an oral dose may appear in the urine in 2 h.

Toxicity Gastrointestinal irritation with vomiting and diarrhea are common, but severe toxic reactions are rare. Agranulocytosis, allergic reactions, and crystalluria may occur. There may also be hepatitis, although the incidence is low, occurring 8 times in a series of 3,000 patients. With prolonged therapy hypernatremia or hyperkalemia may develop because of the high dosage of sodium or potassium salts required. A prolonged prothrombin time and some suppression of thyroid activity, by interference with iodine uptake, are sometimes seen. Unlike salicyclic acid, PAS is not an antipyretic.

Dosage and Administration Up to 20 g/day of the sodium or potassium salt of *p*-aminosalicylic acid can be given orally over a prolonged period of time. It is now generally given with streptomycin or isoniazid, because this delays the appearance of resistant organisms, and the two drugs together are more effective than either alone. Moreover, PAS inhibits the growth of streptomycin- or isoniazid-resistant strains. PAS (Pamisyl) is available in 0.5-g capsules, tablets, and enteric-coated tablets, or as a syrup or lyophilized sterile powder.

Rifampin

Mechanism of Action This semisynthetic antibiotic inhibits the initiation of transcription, pre-

Rifampin

sumably by combining with DNA-dependent RNA polymerase and therefore reducing RNA synthesis in the microorganism.

Use and Toxicity The antibacterial spectrum of rifampin includes both gram-positive and gram-negative organisms. Rifampin is indicated for the treatment of pulmonary tuberculosis and asymptomatic carriers of *Neisseria meningitidis*. It may be indicated in the initial treatment or retreatment of pulmonary tuberculosis in combination with other antitubercular agents because resistant organisms develop in a high percentage of patients if given alone. When treating asymptomatic *N. meningitidis*, the purpose is to eliminate meningococci from the nasopharynx.

Rifampin is well absorbed from the intestine, and adverse reactions are infrequently observed. This agent should be used with caution in patients with liver disease because transient abnormalities in liver function test results, as well as fatalities, have occurred in patients with preexisting liver disease. Gastrointestinal disturbances have at times been severe enough to necessitate discontinuance of the drug. Thrombocytopenia, leukopenia, hemolytic anemia, and decreased hemoglobin have been reported. Central nervous system abnormalities have also been noted. Urine, feces, saliva, sputum, sweat, and tears may be colored red-orange by rifampin. The usual oral adult dosage of rifampin is 600 mg in a daily administration. Rifampin (Rifadin, Rimactane) is supplied in 300-mg capsules.

Part Eleven

Metals

Chapter 38

Heavy Metals and Chelating Agents

LEAD

Lead forms two well-defined series of compounds in which its oxidation states are bivalent and tetravalent, respectively. It is a soft metal having little tensile strength, and it is the heaviest of the common metals except gold and mercury. In air which contains moisture and carbon dioxide, lead becomes oxidized on the surface, forming a protective layer which is both compact and adherent.

Lead is found in practically all foods as well as in the air. Industrial uses of lead such as the manufacture of batteries, cables, and ceramics provide potential sources of lead exposure. Paint pigments also contain lead–white lead (basic lead carbonate) and red lead (lead oxide). Formerly, paints used for interior purposes contained lead pigments. Even though this application of lead has largely been discontinued, the hazard still remains, especially in dilapidated dwellings where peeling of multicoated walls and woodwork constitutes a major source of lead poisoning in young children. It is small wonder that lead is found in the bodies of all humans and animals.

Absorption, Distribution, and Excretion

The average daily American dietary intake of lead may vary from 0.12 to 0.35 mg. About 0.04 mg lead is inhaled daily. Of this amount, 30 to 50 percent is retained by the lung and readily absorbed. Only about 10 percent of ingested lead is absorbed. Some of the absorbed lead is excreted via the bile into the alimentary tract and passes out in the feces with the unabsorbed portion. Thus the fecal excretion of lead approximates that which is ingested with food. The remainder of the absorbed lead is excreted in the urine. Therefore, the daily intake of lead is equal to the daily output under normal conditions.

Lead is a bone-seeker. Over 90 percent of the human body burden of lead is found in bone. Of the soft tissues, liver, muscle, skin, dense connective tissues, and hair contain the largest amounts, in that order.

Blood and urinary lead levels have been determined in people from all parts of the world. The worldwide ''average'' urinary and blood lead levels are 35 μg/liter and 17 μg/100 ml, respectively. The urinary level of lead indicative of a hazardous exposure is 150 μg/liter urine, while 80 μg/100 ml blood indicates dangerous exposure.

Acute Lead Poisoning

Acute lead poisoning is rare but may result from the massive inhalation of large quantities of finely divided lead or lead fumes. The symptoms include sweet metallic taste, salivation, vomiting, intestinal colic, lowered body temperature, and cardiovascular collapse.

Chronic Lead Poisoning

The signs and symptoms of chronic lead poisoning can be divided into four categories: (1) hematologic, (2) neurologic, (3) gastrointestinal, and (4) other.

Hematologic Signs   A sign of lead intoxication may be the appearance of stippled cells in the peripheral blood. These juvenile forms of erythrocytes are not in themselves diagnostic since basophilic stippling can occur in a variety of blood dyscrasias. Furthermore, stippling is observed in only 60 percent of childhood lead intoxications. Basophilic stippling, however, is an indication that lead interferes with hemoglobin synthesis. An important chemical clue to the effects of lead on the hematopoietic system is the appearance of coproporphyrin III in the urine. This finding alone may be misleading, since coproporphyrinuria occurs in a large variety of other diseases and poisonings. An excellent correlation exists, however, between the amount of lead in the urine and the appearance of urinary coproporphyrins.

Another consistent finding in lead poisoning is the appearance of δ-aminolevulinic acid in the urine. This results from an inhibition by lead of the enzyme aminolevulinic acid dehydrase, which converts δ-aminolevulinic acid to porphobilinogen. Urinary lead and coproporphyrin levels have been shown to correlate well with the appearance of δ-aminolevulinic acid. Some evidence has been presented that a raised urinary δ-aminolevulinic

acid level provides an earlier sign of lead exposure than a raised coproporphyrin level. Lead also interferes with the incorporation of iron into protoporphyrin to form heme. Protoporphyrin levels rise in bone marrow and erythrocytes.

A scheme of the loci of lead's toxic action in hemoglobin synthesis is shown below:

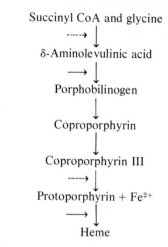

$\longrightarrow$ Steps inhibited by lead.

$----\rightarrow$ Steps at which lead is thought to act but evidence is inconclusive.

The anemia associated with lead poisoning is of the hypochromic, normocytic type and is seldom severe. Hemoglobin values rarely fall below 60 percent or the red cell count below 4×10^6/ml.

Neurologic Signs   The central nervous system manifestations of lead poisoning are termed *lead encephalopathy*. Today, these symptoms occur rarely in adults and only after very high doses of lead; they are of more importance and of higher frequency in children. The early symptoms include irritability, headache, insomnia, restlessness, and ataxia. Later, confusion, delirium, convulsions, and coma may develop. Morphologic changes appear as nonspecific lesions in the cerebrum and cerebellum. Accumulations of serous fluid which distort the normal architecture, and capillary damage and hemorrhages of the meninges, are evident. It is believed that these changes are secondary to increased cranial pressure due to edema.

In addition, there are peripheral neurologic effects known as *lead palsy*. This peripheral neuropathy leads to muscle paralysis which involves primarily the extensor muscles of the wrist and foot. In advanced cases the antigravity muscles may atrophy. Contraction of the flexors produces a limb which is immovable and extremities with a clawlike appearance.

Gastrointestinal Signs Lead stimulates the smooth muscle of the gut, giving rise to intestinal symptoms such as distention after meals, constipation, nausea, and vomiting. Appetite loss leads to loss of body weight and easy fatigability. Dull pains in various parts of the abdomen precede colic. Colic is important diagnostically, since it constitutes a symptom for which the patient seeks relief. Characteristically, the onset of lead colic is sudden and usually occurs at night with severe pain.

Other Signs Another nonspecific sign of lead intoxication is the appearance of a lead line at the margin of the gums. Today, the lead line is infrequent because of better dental hygiene. A black or purplish line is formed when lead sulfide is precipitated at the gingival borders; sulfides produced by bacteria react with lead in the saliva. Other metals, for example, bismuth, mercury, tin, and arsenic, produce similar precipitates at the gingival border, illustrating the nonspecificity of the lead line in diagnosing lead intoxication.

Lead poisoning invariably produces changes in skin coloration known as *lead hue* or *lead pallor*. The patient takes on a pale or ashen-gray appearance.

A summary of the clinical signs and symptoms of lead intoxication in the order of their occurrence is given in Table 38-1.

Tetraethyllead and Tetramethyllead

Tetraethyllead and tetramethyllead are oily lipid-soluble compounds used as antiknock additives in gasoline. Although they are absorbed through the skin, appreciable time is required to achieve a toxic level by this route. Organic lead compounds gain entry into the body mainly via the respiratory tract, usually in handling and during tank cleaning operations. Because of close and skillful industrial hy-

Table 38-1 Lead Intoxication

Reactions	Signs and symptoms
Subjective	Weakness
	Anorexia
	Fatigue
	Nervousness
	Tremor
	Nausea
	Loss of body weight
	Headache
	Gastrointestinal
	Constipation
	Gastric pain
	Colic
	Weakness of extensor muscles
	Impotence, amenorrhea
Objective	Pallor (constricted arterioles), loss of weight
	Increased δ-aminolevulinic aciduria
	Porphyrinuria (coproporphyrin III)
	Constipation
	Blood
	Increased lead content
	Possible slight increase in serum bilirubin and serum iron
	Anemia (basophilic stippling)
	Bone marrow
	Basophilic stippled erythroblasts
	Binucleated erythroblasts
	Possible increase in erythropoiesis
	Lead line
	Weakness of extensor muscles
	Tremor

gienic supervision, intoxication by these compounds is rare. In contrast to inorganic lead intoxication, tetraethyllead produces symptoms which are referable predominantly to the CNS. The patient is irritable, suffers from insomnia, has wild nightmares, and is emotionally unstable. In later stages, the patient hallucinates, becomes hyperexcitable, and requires restraint. Also seen are anorexia, vomiting, and mild diarrhea. There is no effect on porphyrin metabolism. Blood-lead levels remain near normal in tetraethyllead intoxication, whereas urine-lead levels increase markedly, exceeding those found in inorganic lead poisoning.

Calcium Disodium Edathamil in the Treatment of Lead Poisoning

Chemistry Calcium disodium edathamil (calcium disodium versenate) is the calcium chelate of the disodium salt of ethylenediaminetetraacetic acid (EDTA). EDTA binds cations preferentially. Sodium and potassium are held most weakly. Calcium, magnesium, and barium are bound more tightly but can be displaced by cobalt, chromium, cadmium, copper, nickel, and lead, whose chelates have higher stability constants.

Ethylenediaminetetraacetic acid (EDTA)

Calcium disodium EDTA (calcium disodium edathamil)

Absorption, Fate, and Excretion Practically all of a parenterally administered dose of calcium disodium edathamil appears unchanged in the urine within 24 h. Fifty percent of an intravenously administered dose is excreted by 1 h. The absorption of the calcium chelate of EDTA after oral administration is poor. Calcium disodium edathamil distributes exclusively in the body water. In blood, all of the drug is found in the plasma.

Mechanism of Action The therapeutic action of calcium disodium edathamil in lead intoxication is due solely to its ability to form soluble metal chelates. It is generally held that calcium disodium edathamil mobilizes lead from the soft tissues. Sub-

sequently, the soft tissue stores are replenished by the redistribution of lead from bone. The lead chelate formed by EDTA is represented structurally below.

Administration The intravenous route of administration is preferred for calcium disodium edathamil in the treatment of lead intoxication. In treating lead intoxication in children, the mortality rate is about 25 percent when acute encephalopathy is treated with calcium disodium edathamil alone. Because of this, it has been suggested that by administering equimolar amounts of calcium disodium edathamil and dimercaprol (BAL, British antilewisite, or 2,3-dimercaptopropanol) it would be possible to double the ratio of chelators to lead. When this BAL-EDTA treatment was followed, the rate of urinary lead excretion was enhanced and the treatment was more effective than by calcium disodium edathamil alone.

Toxicity The toxicity of calcium disodium edathamil is probably due to the binding of essential metal ions. Large doses have been shown to produce nephrotoxicity.

An excessive chelation syndrome may be produced by large doses or prolonged administration of calcium disodium edathamil. This is an acute febrile state with marked myalgia, headache, nasal congestion, nocturia, and chills. The symptoms subside upon removal of the drug.

Preparations and Dosage Calcium disodium edathamil is available as a 20 percent solution (injection), or as 500-mg tablets. For the treatment of lead intoxication, it is administered by slow intravenous drip in either isotonic sodium chloride solution or 5 percent dextrose solution, in a concentration not to exceed 3 percent by diluting 5 ml of a 20 percent solution (1 g/33 ml). The maximum dose per 4.5 kg (10 lb) of body weight is 170 mg/h, or 330 mg/day, or 1.67 g/week, or 2.5 to 4.5 g/4.5 kg body weight during each course of treatment.

MERCURY

Mercury exists in three states of oxidation: as the element, in a monovalent (mercurous) form, and as a divalent (mercuric) form. Divalent mercury can form covalent bonds with carbon atoms, and mercury in this form is usually referred to as "organic" mercury. The organomercurial diuretics and many of the mercurial fungicides contain mercury covalently bound to carbon.

Elemental or metallic mercury is a somewhat volatile liquid. Human exposure to mercury vapor is mainly occupational and has been noted since antiquity. Mercurous chloride or calomel is the best known of the mercurous compounds. It is still used in some skin creams as an antiseptic and was once frequently employed as a cathartic. The mercuric salts are the most irritating and acutely toxic forms of mercury. Mercuric salts have wide application in industry—as catalysts in the production of vinyl plastics and to suppress the growth of slime molds in paper pulp manufacture. It has recently been observed that microorganisms in river water can synthesize methylmercury from the inorganic forms of mercury such as are discharged from industry. Therefore, discharge of mercury into rivers from industries has led to problems of environmental pollution in Japan, Sweden, and the United States.

All the organomercurials in use today contain mercury having only one covalent link to a carbon atom. From a pharmacologic standpoint, they cannot be considered as a single group. The mercurial diuretics have the lowest toxicity of the organic mercury compounds. Next in order of increasing toxicity are the phenylmercury salts. Phenylmercuric acetate is used in contraceptive jellies and as a fungicide in seed dressing. Phenylmercuric nitrate is used in some hemorrhoidal preparations and in a proprietary throat lozenge. Methoxyethylmercury chloride belongs to a new group of mercury fungicides whose toxicity is similar to that of the phenylmercury compounds. The alkylmercury salts are by far the most dangerous of all the compounds of mercury. The simple salts such as methylmercury chloride and ethylmercury chloride are sufficiently volatile to produce serious toxic effects by inhalation. Methylmercury dicyandiamide is less volatile. All the alkyl mercurials produce characteristic and usually irreversible damage to the CNS. They have had extensive use as fungicides.

Mechanism of Action

Mercury has the property of forming strong chemical bonds with the sulfur atom in thiol compounds. It is probable that this uniquely high affinity for sulfur is ultimately responsible for the toxicity of all compounds of mercury. The organic moiety of the organomercurials and the dissociable anion in the mercuric salts undoubtedly account for the differences between the compounds, such as the degree and type of toxic symptoms, and the differences in hazardous properties associated with volatility, solubility, and so on.

Absorption, Distribution, and Excretion

Mercury may be absorbed into the body via the respiratory and gastrointestinal tracts, the skin, and in the case of contraceptive preparations, across the vaginal surfaces. In general, most compounds of mercury, both organic and inorganic, are well absorbed except calomel, mercurous chloride ($HgCl$). Mercurous chloride is poorly absorbed by the gastrointestinal tract because of its low solubility; an equivalent dose of mercuric chloride would be lethal.

The pattern of deposition of mercury is an important consideration in the toxicology of this metal. Both organic and inorganic mercury compounds, if present at a sufficient concentration, will poison any cell with which they come in contact. Irrespective of the route of administration, mercury is distributed to all organs of the body. The mercury in plasma is protein-bound, and the mercury present in red blood cells is bound to the cysteine residues of hemoglobin.

Mercury is excreted by the kidney, by the liver in the bile, by the intestinal mucosa, by the sweat glands, and by the salivary glands. Urinary and fecal routes of excretion are the most important for elimination.

The biologic half-life in humans for methylmercury is close to 70 days, corresponding to an excretion of about 1 percent/day of the body burden. The decrease in blood mercury follows a similar time course. The half-life of clearance from the brain is about 20 percent longer than the clearance from the whole body.

Normal Levels of Mercury

For mercury, the intake rate roughly balances the total urinary and fecal excretion. A statistical analysis of over 800 samples from 15 countries indicates that 84 percent of the general population have urinary concentrations of less than 5 μg/liter. A zero value, that is, less than 0.5 μg/liter, was found in 79 percent of the samples. The 95 percent confidence limit indicates an upper limit for "normal" mercury in urine of 20 to 25 μg/liter and for blood, 4 μg/100 ml. Fecal excretion was reported in earlier studies to average 10 μg Hg/day.

Chronic and Acute Poisoning from Inorganic Mercury

No clinical distinction has been made between symptoms associated with exposure to mercury vapor and to mercuric salts. The experimental findings of higher brain levels associated with the vapor suggest that central nervous system disturbances would be more pronounced following exposure to this form of mercury.

Symptoms involving the CNS are the most frequently seen, the principal features being tremor and psychologic disturbances (erethismus mercurialis). Proteinuria may occur, and may progress to a nephrotic syndrome. Symptoms related to the mouth such as gingivitis, stomatitis, and excessive salivation often occur. These symptoms may be connected with the secretion of mercury in the saliva. Dermatitis has been observed in some workmen exposed to mercury. Mercurialentis (a colored reflex from the lens) is seen in chronic exposure, but does not indicate intoxication. A number of nonspecific symptoms such as anorexia, weight loss, anemia, and muscular weakness are also associated with chronic exposure.

The symptoms associated with acute oral intake of inorganic mercury salts are acute gastroenteritis, with abdominal pain, vomiting, and some bloody diarrhea. Anuria and uremia are associated with severe kidney damage and may appear a day or more after exposure and frequently precede a fatal outcome. The approximate lethal dose to humans

of mercuric chloride is 1 g. Acute exposure to high concentrations of mercury vapor may give rise to a condition characterized by a metallic taste, nausea, abdominal pain, vomiting, diarrhea, headache, and sometimes albuminuria. A few days later the salivary glands swell, stomatitis and gingivitis develop, and a dark line of mercurous sulfide (HgS) forms on the inflamed gums. The teeth may loosen and ulcers may form on the lips and cheeks.

Chronic and Acute Poisoning from Organomercurial Compounds

The symptoms of chronic and acute exposure to organomercurial compounds are the same. Symptoms may appear weeks to months after an acute exposure, and include ataxia; slurring of speech; numbness and tingling of the lips, hands, and feet; concentric restriction of the visual fields; impairment of hearing; and emotional disturbances. The symptoms are irreversible in cases of severe poisoning.

Mothers ingesting large amounts of methylmercury give birth to babies suffering from palsy, convulsions, and mental retardation. Experimental work indicates that methylmercury compounds are potent inhibitors of cell division and chromosome segregation.

Evidence based on cases of industrial poisoning and ingestion of methylmercury in food indicates that symptoms are first observed at concentrations of 100 μg/100 ml whole blood. Fatalities are associated with brain levels of 10 μg/g wet weight of tissue. It is likely that blood levels of 10 μg/100 ml or less are not associated with toxic symptoms.

Antidote to Mercury Poisoning, Dimercaprol

Dimercaprol remains the only drug routinely used in the treatment of acute mercury poisoning. The properties of dimercaprol and its reaction with mercury have an important bearing on the manner in which dimercaprol is administered. First, mercury and dimercaprol may form two different complexes:

At a molar ratio of dimercaprol to Hg^{2+} of 1, a chelate is formed. When the molar ratio is 2, a complex forms containing two dimercaprol molecules to one atom of mercury. This compound is water-soluble at pH 7.5 and binds mercury more tightly than does the chelate. A high plasma level of dimercaprol favors the formation of the water-soluble compound, which should be rapidly excreted. Second, dimercaprol may produce unpleasant side effects which become more pronounced as the dose is increased. Care should be taken not to greatly exceed the minimal effective plasma level of the drug. Third, dimercaprol is rapidly metabolized to inactive products. Experimental studies indicate that the dimercaprol-mercury complex will dissociate in the body as the dimercaprol level declines. The plasma level must be maintained by repeated doses. Fourth, dimercaprol should be administered as soon as possible after exposure to mercury.

Preparation

Dimercaprol (BAL) is available as a 10 percent solution (100 mg/ml) in peanut oil with 20 percent benzyl benzoate. Benzyl benzoate is added because the compound is more stable in the mixture than in peanut oil alone.

ARSENIC

Arsenic is an active constituent in many fungicides, herbicides, and pesticides. It is used in the paint and dye industry and was at one time used extensively in cosmetics. Organic arsenicals are used today to treat protozoan infections. Arsanilic acid is fed to poultry and livestock to enhance growth rate.

Arsenic exists in the elemental form, and in the trivalent and pentavalent oxidation states. The arsenites—for example, potassium arsenite, $KAsO_2$, and salts of arsenious acid, $H_2As_2O_3$—contain trivalent arsenic. The pentavalent oxidation state is found in the arsenates such as lead arsenate, $PbHAsO_4$. These are salts of arsenic acid, H_3AsO_4. The arsenites have a high affinity for thiol groups and are considerably more toxic than the arsenates. The latter have properties similar to phosphate and have no affinity for thiol groups.

The organic arsenicals contain arsenic linked to a carbon atom by a covalent bond where arsenic exists in the trivalent or pentavalent state. Arsphenamine contains trivalent arsenic; sodium arsanilate contains the element in the pentavalent form. Their structures are given below.

Arsphenamine

Sodium arsanilate

Arsine, AsH_3, is a gas produced by the action of nascent hydrogen on the elemental form of arsenic. It produces toxic effects which are different from those of the other compounds of arsenic.

Uptake, Distribution, and Excretion

Systematic poisoning has been produced by absorption from the lungs, the gastrointestinal tract, and across the skin.

After acute exposure, the deposition in tissues is in the liver, kidney, intestine, spleen, and lungs, in that order. Arsenic appears in hair about 2 weeks after the first exposure, where it is bound to the sulfide linkages in keratin. Chronic exposure leads to accumulation in hair, bone, and skin. Arsenic may be found in high concentrations in the hair years after cessation of exposure and after most of the metal has been removed from the soft tissues.

Arsenic passes the blood-brain barrier only slowly. Brain levels are among the lowest in the body. Arsenic readily crosses the placental barrier, and fetal damage has been reported.

Excretion occurs by all physiologic routes—feces, urine, sweat, and milk. In general, the arsenite salts are lost mainly via the feces and the arsenates via the urine. Arsenate excretion is more rapid than arsenite excretion and probably occurs via the phosphate excretory mechanisms.

Symptoms of Acute Toxicity

Acute poisonings occur because arsenic, especially in the form of As_2O_3, is readily available, practically tasteless, has the appearance of sugar, and is quickly absorbed from the gastrointestinal tract. Oral intake is followed by an asymptomatic period of about 30 min. The victim experiences a tightness in the throat and stomach pains. Vomiting may ensue, which can be life-saving. Other effects quickly follow, such as intensive diarrhea with watery feces containing shreds of mucus, very much like the "rice water" stools in cholera. Depressed urine flow is characteristic of acute arsenic intoxication. Death usually results in 1 to 3 days, with the victim in a state of collapse. Deaths which occur up to 14 days after poisoning are caused by nephritis. Ingestion of 100 μg of As_2O_3 will cause severe poisoning; the minimal lethal dose in humans is quoted as 1 g.

Inhalation of arsine gas leads to rapid hemolysis, which gives rise to anemia, reduced red blood cell count, and hemoglobin in the urine. The released hemoglobin causes jaundice and may block the kidney tubules. Death usually results from anoxemia in 2 to 9 days after exposure. Some symptoms of typical arsenic poisoning may also appear.

Symptoms of Chronic Poisoning

Diarrhea and vomiting occur but are less pronounced than in cases of acute poisoning. The mucous membranes are affected, giving rise to symptoms of the common cold. The horny layer of the skin is stimulated, leading to the appearance of dark brown scales. Peripheral neuritis similar to that associated with chronic alcoholism is observed in approximately 5 percent of the cases of chronic arsenic poisoning. The afferent motor nerves and sensory fibers are affected, especially in the legs. The ankle jerk disappears and the leg muscles atrophy. Tremors have been reported in 10 percent of the cases of chronic exposure.

Continued exposure to arsine gas generally results in symptoms similar to the picture of arsenic poisoning. However, a compensated destruction of red cells takes place, resulting in a steady level of anemia.

Skin keratoses result from prolonged exposure to arsenic, and may become malignant.

Biochemical Aspects of Arsenic Poisoning

Trivalent arsenical compounds, both the inorganic arsenic salts and the monosubstituted organic arsen-

icals, possess a high affinity for vicinal thiol groups. Thus reactions of the type

$$R\!-\!As\!=\!O + \begin{array}{c} HS\!-\!CH_2 \\ | \\ HS\!-\!CH \\ | \\ HO\!-\!CH_2 \end{array} \longrightarrow R\!-\!As\!\!\begin{array}{c} S\!-\!CH_2 \\ | \\ S\!-\!CH \\ | \\ HO\!-\!CH_2 \end{array} + H_2O$$

lead to the formation of stable five-membered rings. It is likely that the affinity of trivalent arsenic for thiol groups of enzymes and other proteins in tissues is ultimately responsible for the toxicity of this class of arsenic compounds.

The Action of Arsenic on Capillaries

Arsenic produces dilation of capillaries, and an increase in permeability of the capillary walls. This results in a fall in blood pressure and tissue edema leading to a state of shock.

Capillary damage is especially pronounced in the splenic area. The loss of plasma proteins into the intestinal areas causes blisters under the mucosal layer. Stimulated intestinal peristalsis leads to diarrhea and the shedding of epithelial cells.

Capillary and epithelial cell damage also occurs in the kidneys. Protein and red blood cells appear in the urine. The depression in urine flow results from both the vascular damage to kidney and the loss of fluid in the capillary beds.

Treatment

Dimercaprol is used in the treatment of chronic arsenic poisoning (see section on Mercury, above).

GOLD

At present, gold compounds have a therapeutic usefulness limited to the treatment of rheumatoid arthritis of the peripheral joints, and of certain rare skin diseases such as discoid lupus. Colloidal radioactive gold, because of its distribution in the body and its short half-life, has been used as a radiation source in the treatment of cancer.

Use of Gold Compounds in Treatment of Rheumatoid Arthritis

Gold compounds are used in the treatment of rheumatoid arthritis. Gold, certainly no miracle drug, nevertheless offers considerable benefit to many individuals subjected to a painful and prolonged disease. Gold compounds are most efficacious in the early stages of the arthritic disease, reducing the inflammatory process but without inducing any repair process in the joints. The mechanism is unknown. There are two disadvantages associated with chrysotherapy. One is that patients who show improvement as a result of treatment may relapse after treatment is discontinued. The second disadvantage is the toxicity: gold compounds should be used with great caution, especially in aged individuals.

Absorption, Distribution, and Excretion

Gold compounds administered by intramuscular injection, either in a watery solution or as an oil suspension, are absorbed very slowly from the site of injection, carried in the blood plasma in a non-dialyzable form, with little in the cells, and distributed throughout the soft tissues of the body. Even after a single injection, gold appears in the blood and urine for months afterward. Of the gold that is absorbed, about 20 percent is rapidly excreted, mostly in the urine in the case of soluble compounds and in the feces in the case of insoluble compounds, and about 80 percent is fixed for long periods in the tissues. After therapeutic doses, the levels in plasma and urine in humans contain about 1 to 2 mg/100 ml.

Toxicity

The most frequent toxic reaction to gold is a dermatitis—an erythema, urticaria, or rash—often with stomatitis. These reactions are usually preceded by pruritus, which is one of the best alarm signals. The skin lesions may last for some time but will eventually disappear after gold therapy has been discontinued. In some cases, severe exfoliative dermatitis results. A temporary nephritis with albuminuria may occur, and occasionally may become serious. Gastrointestinal damage (gastritis, colitis, or stomatitis) and hepatitis have been observed rarely. Blood dyscrasias, such as leukopenia, agranulocytosis, thrombopenia, or aplastic anemia, are rare but very serious when they occur. The severe cases of toxicity respond well to treatment with dimercaprol; penicillamine increases urinary gold excretion, and in a number of cases toxic effects have been successfully treated with ACTH.

Contraindications to the use of gold are organic diseases of the liver or kidney, skin lesions, or abnormalities of the hematopoietic system.

Preparation and Doses

A variety of gold preparations are available for clinical use.

Gold Sodium Thiomalate (Myochrysine) Contains about 50 percent gold and is available in aqueous solution in 10-, 25-, 50-, or 100-mg/ml ampuls.

Aurothioglucose (Gold Thioglucose, Solganal) Supplied as a suspension in sesame oil containing 10, 50, or 100 mg/ml. A dose schedule commonly accepted is 10 to 20 mg biweekly until a total of 200 to 300 mg is reached. Some clinicians use a maximum of 25 mg weekly. There are many variants of this schedule, but it seems clear that weekly doses greater than 50 mg increase the frequency of toxic reactions.

Bibliography

CHAPTER 1

Bliss, C. I.: The Calculation of the Dosage-Mortality Curve, *Ann Appl Biol,* **22**:134–167 (1935).
———: Some Principles of Bioassay, *Am Sci,* **45**: 449–466 (1957).
Furchgott, R. F., S. M. Kirpekar, M. Rieker, and A. Schwab: Actions and Interactions of Norepinephrine, Tyramine and Cocaine on Aortic Strips of Rabbit and Left Atria of Guinea Pig and Cat, *J Pharmacol Exp Ther,* **142**:39–58 (1963).
Gaddum, J. H.: Methods of Biological Assay Depending on a Quantal Response, *Med Res Counc (B) Spec Rep Ser,* **183**:5–46 (1933).
Gold, H., N. T. Kwit, and A. J. Golfinos: A Rapid Quantitative Method for the Comparison of Diuretic Agents in Bed Patients with Congestive Failure, *Am J Med Sci,* **239**:665–680 (1960).
Levine, R. R.: *Pharmacology: Drug Actions and Reactions,* Little, Brown, Boston, 1973.
Loewe, S.: Duration of Drug Action, *Proc Soc Exp Biol Med,* **81**:596–598 (1952).

CHAPTER 2

Albert, A.: *Selective Toxicity,* 5th ed., Halsted Press, New York, 1973.
Ariëns, E. J.: *Molecular Pharmacology,* Academic, New York, 1964.
Beckett, A. H., and A. F. Casy: Synthetic Analgesics: Stereochemical Considerations, *J Pharm Pharmacol,* **6**:986–1001 (1954).
Burgen, A. S. V.: Receptor Mechanisms, *Annu Rev Pharmacol,* **10**:7–18 (1970).
Gero, A.: Graphic Differentiation Between Competitive and Functional Synergism, *Mol Pharmacol,* **1**:312–313 (1965).
Hurwitz, L., and A. Suria: The Link Between Agonist Action and Response in Smooth Muscle, *Annu Rev Pharmacol,* **11**:303–326 (1971).
Portoghese, P. S.: Relationships Between Stereostructure and Pharmacological Activities, *Annu Rev Pharmacol,* **10**:51–76 (1970).
Waud, D. R.: Pharmacological Receptors, *Pharmacol Rev,* **20**:49–88 (1968).

CHAPTER 3

Binns, T. B. (ed.): *Absorption and Distribution of Drugs,* Williams & Wilkins, Baltimore, 1964.

Goldstein, A.: The Interactions of Drugs and Plasma Proteins, *Pharmacol Rev,* **1**:102–165 (1949).

Hogben, C. A. M., D. J. Tocco, B. B. Brodie, and L. S. Schanker: On the Mechanism of Intestinal Absorption of Drugs, *J Pharmacol Exp Ther,* **125**:275–282 (1959).

Levine, R. R.: *Pharmacology: Drug Actions and Reactions,* Little, Brown, Boston, 1973.

——, and E. W. Pelikan: Mechanisms of Drug Absorption and Excretion: Passage of Drugs out of and into the Gastrointestinal Tract, *Annu Rev Pharmacol,* **4**:69–84 (1964).

Schanker, L. S.: Passage of Drugs across Body Membranes, *Pharmacol Rev,* **14**:501–530 (1962).

Stein, W. D.: *The Movement of Molecules across Cell Membranes,* Academic, New York, 1967.

Ther, L., and D. Winne: Drug Absorption, *Annu Rev Pharmacol,* **11**:57–70 (1971).

CHAPTER 4

Albert, A.: Patterns of Metabolic Disposition of Drugs in Man and Other Species, in G. Wolstenholme and R. Porter (eds.), *Drug Responses in Man,* Little, Brown, Boston, 1967, pp. 52–62.

Anders, M. W.: Enhancement and Inhibition of Drug Metabolism, *Annu Rev Pharmacol,* **11**:37–56 (1971).

Brodie, B. B.: Distribution and Fate of Drugs: Therapeutic Implications, in T. B. Binns (ed.), *Absorption and Distribution of Drugs,* Williams & Wilkins, Baltimore, 1964, pp. 199–251.

Conney, A. H.: Pharmacological Implications of Microsomal Enzyme Induction, *Pharmacol Rev,* **19**:317–366 (1967).

Gillette, J. R., D. C. Davis, and H. A. Sasame: Cytochrome P-450 and its Role in Drug Metabolism, *Annu Rev Pharmacol,* **12**:57–84 (1972).

Kuntzman, R.: Drugs and Enzyme Induction, *Annu Rev Pharmacol,* **9**:21–36 (1969).

Parke, D. V.: *The Biochemistry of Foreign Compounds,* Pergamon, New York, 1968.

Remmer, H.: The Fate of Drugs in the Organisms, *Annu Rev Pharmacol,* **5**:405–428 (1965).

Schreiber, E. C.: The Metabolic Alteration of Drugs, *Annu Rev Pharmacol,* **10**:77–98 (1970).

Williams, R. T.: Patterns of Excretion of Drugs in Man and Other Species, in G. Wolstenholem

and R. Porter (eds.), *Drug Responses in Man,* Little, Brown, Boston, 1967, pp. 76–90.

CHAPTER 5

Albert, A.: *Selective Toxicity,* 5th ed., Halsted Press, New York, 1973.

Calesnick, B.: Practical Problems in Drug Dosage, *Semin Drug Treat,* **1**:63–91 (1971).

Irwin, S.: Drug Screening and Evaluative Procedures, *Science,* **136**:123–128 (1962).

Leake, C. D.: The Rational Use of Drugs in Clinical Practice, *Semin Drug Treat,* **1**:1–9 (1971).

McKusick, V. A.: *Medical Genetics, 1958–1960: An Annotated Review,* Mosby, St. Louis, 1961.

Mitscherlich, A., and F. Mielke (trans. by H. Norden): *Doctors of Infamy; The Story of the Nazi Medical Crimes,* Henry Schuman, New York, 1949, pp. 23–25.

CHAPTER 6

Alper, M. H., and Flacke, W.: The Peripheral Effects of Anesthetics, *Annu Rev Pharmacol,* **9**:273–296 (1969).

Brown, E. B., Jr.: Drugs and Respiratory Control, *Annu Rev Pharmacol,* **11**:271–276 (1971).

Cherkin, A.: Mechanisms of General Anesthesia by Non-Hydrogen-Bonding Molecules, *Annu Rev Pharmacol,* **9**:259–272 (1969).

Dobkin, A. B., and J. Po-Giok Su: Newer Anesthetics and Their Uses, *Clin Pharmacol Ther,* **7**:648–682 (1966).

Dundee, J. W.: Clinical Pharmacology of General Anesthetics, *Clin Pharmacol Ther,* **8**:91–123 (1967).

Eger, E. I., II, L. J. Saidman, and B. Brandstater: Minimum Alveolar Anesthetic Concentration: A Standard of Anesthetic Potency, *Anesthesiology,* **26**:756–763 (1965).

Kety, S. S.: The Theory and Applications of the Exchange of Inert Gas at the Lungs and Tissues, *Pharmacol Rev,* **3**:1–41 (1951).

Lambertsen, C. J.: Drugs and Respiration, *Annu Rev Pharmacol,* **6**:327–378 (1966).

Ngai, S. H., L. C. Mark, and E. M. Papper: Pharmacologic and Physiologic Aspects of Anesthesiology, *N Engl J Med,* **282**:479–491, 541–556 (1970).

Seeman, P.: The Membrane Actions of Anesthetics and Tranquilizers, *Pharmacol Rev,* **24**:583–655 (1972).

CHAPTER 7

Campbell, A. H., J. A. Stasse, G. H. Lord, and J. E. Willson: *In Vivo* Evaluation of Local Anesthetics Applied Topically, *J Pharm Sci,* **57**:2045–2048 (1968).

Foldes, F. F., W. M. Foldes, J. C. Smith, and E. K. Zsigmond: The Relation between Plasma Cholinesterase and Prolonged Apnea Caused by Succinylcholine, *Anesthesiology,* **24**:208–216 (1963).

Hodgkin, A. L.: *The Conduction of the Nerve Impulse,* Charles C Thomas, Springfield, Ill., 1964.

Ludena, F. P.: Duration of Local Anesthesia, *Annu Rev Pharmacol,* **9**:503–520 (1969).

Ritchie, J. M., and P. Greengard: On the Mode of Action of Local Anesthetics, *Annu Rev Pharmacol,* **6**:405–430 (1966).

Seeman, P.: The Membrane Actions of Anesthetics and Tranquilizers, *Pharmacol Rev,* **24**:583–655 (1972).

Stewart, D. M., W. P. Rogers, J. E. Mahaffey, S. Witherspoon, and E. F. Woods: Effect of Local Anesthetics on the Cardiovascular System of the Dog, *Anesthesiology,* **24**:620–624 (1963).

Taylor, R. E.: Effect of Procaine on Electrical Properties of Squid Axon Membrane, *Am J Physiol,* **196**:1071–1078 (1959).

CHAPTER 8

Domino, E. F.: Sites of Action of Some Central Nervous System Depressants, *Annu Rev Pharmacol,* **2**:215–250 (1962).

Essig, C. F.: Newer Sedative Drugs That Can Cause States of Intoxication and Dependence of Barbiturate Type, *J Am Med Assoc,* **196**:714–717 (1966).

Freund, G.: Chronic Central Nervous System Toxicity of Alcohol, *Annu Rev Pharmacol,* **13**: 217–228 (1973).

Harger, R. N., and H. R. Hulpieu: The Pharmacology of Alcohol, in G. N. Thompson (ed.), *Alcoholism,* Charles C Thomas, Springfield, Ill., 1956.

Hawkins, R. D., and H. Kalant: The Metabolism of Ethanol and Its Metabolic Effects, *Pharmacol Rev,* **24**:67–157 (1972).

Matthews, V., H. E. Lehmann, and T. A. Ban: A Comparative Study of Thirteen Hypnotic Drugs, *Appl Ther,* **6**:806–809 (1964).

Oswald, I.: Drugs and Sleep, *Pharmacol Rev,* **20**: 273–303 (1968).

Rickels, K., and H. Bass: A Comparative Controlled Clinical Trial of Seven Hypnotic Agents in Medical and Psychiatric Patients, *Am J Med Sci,* **245**:142–152 (1963).

CHAPTER 9

Aghajanian, G. K.: LSD and CNS Transmission, *Annu Rev Pharmacol,* **12**:157–168 (1972).

Brawley, P., and J. C. Duffield: The Pharmacology of Hallucinogens, *Pharmacol Rev,* **24**:31–66 (1972).

Himwich, H. E., and H. S. Alpers: Psychopharmacology, *Annu Rev Pharmacol,* **10**:313–334 (1970).

Hoffer, A., and H. Osmond: *The Hallucinogens,* Academic, New York, 1967.

Hofmann, A.: Psychotomimetic Agents, in A. Burger (ed.) *Drugs Affecting the Central Nervous System,* Marcel Dekker, New York, 1968, chap. 5.

Kalant, H., A. E. Le Blanc, and R. J. Gibbons: Tolerance to, and Dependence on, Some Non-Opiate Psychotropic Drugs, *Pharmacol Rev,* **23**: 135–191 (1971).

Murphree, H. B.: Clinical Effects of Hemp Preparations, *Semin Drug Treat,* **1**:195–206 (1971).

Paton, W. D. M.: Pharmacology of Marijuana, *Annu Rev Pharmacol,* **15**:191–220 (1975).

CHAPTER 10

Ban, T.: *Psychopharmacology,* Williams & Wilkins, Baltimore, 1969.

Berger, F. M.: The Similarities and Differences between Meprobamate and Barbiturates, *Clin Pharmacol Ther,* **4**:209–231; and commentaries by E. F. Domino, 231–233 (1963).

Blackwell, B.: Rational Drug Use in the Management of Anxiety, *Ration Drug Ther,* **9**:1–7 (1975).

Costa, E., and P. Greengard (eds.): *Mechanisms of Action of Benzodiazepines,* Raven, New York, 1975.

Crane, G. E.: Clinical Psychopharmacology in Its 20th Year, *Science,* **181**:124–128 (1973).

Davis, J. M., and W. E. Fann: Lithium, *Annu Rev Pharmacol,* **11**:285–302 (1971).

Domino, E. F., R. D. Hudson, and G. Zografi: Substituted Phenothiazines: Pharmacology and Chemical Structure, in A. Burger (ed.), *Drugs Affecting the Central Nervous System,* Marcel Dekker, New York, 1968, pp. 327–397.

Gardos, G., A. DiMascio, C. Salzman, and R. I. Shader: Differential Actions of Chlordiazepoxide and Oxazepam on Hostility, *Arch Gen Psychiatry,* **8**:757–760 (1968).

Gordon, M.: Phenothiazines, in M. Gordon (ed.), *Psychopharmacological Agents,* Academic, New York, 1967, pp. 1–198.

Schwartz, A., G. E. Lindenmayer, and J. C. Allen: The Sodium-Potassium Adenosine Triphosphatase: Pharmacological, Physiological and Biochemical Aspects, *Pharmacol Rev,* **27**:3–134 (1975).

Snyder, S. H., S. P. Banerjee, H. I. Yamamura, and D. Greenberg: Drugs, Neurotransmitters, and Schizophrenia, *Science,* **184**:1243–1253 (1974).

CHAPTER 11

Akiskal, H. S., and W. T. McKinney, Jr.: Overview of Recent Research in Depression, *Arch Gen Psychiatry,* **32**:285–305 (1975).

Blackwell, B., E. Marley, J. Price, and D. Taylor: Hypertensive Interactions between Monoamine Oxidase Inhibitors and Foodstuffs, *Br J Psychiatry,* **113**:349–365 (1967).

Bunney, W. E., and J. M. Davis: Norepinephrine in Depressive Reactions: A Review, *Arch Gen Psychiatry,* **13**:483–494 (1965).

Cole, J. O.: Therapeutic Efficacy of Antidepressant Drugs: A Review, *J Am Med Assoc,* **190**: 448–455 (1964).

Gessa, G. L., E. Cuenca, and E. Costa: On the Mechanisms of Hypotensive Effects of MAO Inhibitors, *Ann N Y Acad Sci,* **107**:935–944 (1963).

Gyermek, L.: The Pharmacology of Imipramine and Related Antidepressants, *Int Rev Neurobiol,* **9**:95–143 (1966).

Himwich, H. E., and H. S. Alpers: Psychopharmacology, *Annu Rev Pharmacol,* **10**:313–334 (1970).

Schildkraut, J. J.: Neuropharmacology of the Affective Disorders, *Annu Rev Pharmacol,* **13**: 427–454 (1973).

———, S. M. Schanberg, G. R. Breese, and I. J. Kopin: Norepinephrine Metabolism and Drugs Used in the Affective Disorders: A Possible Mechanism of Action, *Am J Psychiatry,* **124**: 54–62 (1967).

CHAPTER 12

Barbeau, A.: Drugs Affecting Movement Disorders, *Annu Rev Pharmacol,* **14**:91–113 (1974).

Cotzias, G. C., G. S. Papavasilion, and R. Gellene: Modification of Parkinsonism: Chronic Treatment with L-DOPA, *N Engl J Med,* **280**:337–345 (1969).

Maynert, E. W.: The Role of Biochemical and Neurohumoral Factors in the Laboratory Evaluation of Antiepileptic Drugs, *Epilepsia,* **10**:145–162 (1969).

Schmidt, R. P., and B. J. Wilder: *Epilepsy: A Clinical Textbook,* Davis, Philadelphia, 1968.

Schwab, R. S., A. C. England, Jr., D. C. Poskanzer, and R. R. Young: Amantadine in the Treatment of Parkinson's Disease, *J Am Med Assoc,* **208**:1168–1170 (1969).

Schwartz, A., G. E. Lindenmayer, and J. C. Allen: The Sodium-Potassium Adenosine Triphosphatase: Pharmacological, Physiological and Biochemical Aspects, *Pharmacol Rev,* **27**:3–134 (1975).

Swinyard, E. A.: Laboratory Evaluation of Antiepileptic Drugs, *Epilepsia,* **10**:107–119 (1969).

Winkelman, A. C., and J. R. DiPalma: Drug Treatment of Parkinsonism, *Semin Drug Treat,* **1**: 10–62 (1971).

Woodbury, D. M.: Role of Pharmacological Factors in the Evaluation of Anticonvulsant Drugs, *Epilepsia,* **10**:121–144 (1969).

Yahr, M. D., R. C. Duvoisin, M. J. Schear, R. E. Barrett, and M. M. Hoehn: Treatment of Parkinsonism with Levodopa, *Arch Neurol (Chicago),* **21**:343–354 (1969).

CHAPTER 13

Blumberg, H., H. B. Dayton, and P. S. Wolf: Counteraction of Narcotic Antagonist Analgesics by the Narcotic Antagonist Naloxone, *Proc Soc Exp Biol Med,* **123**:755–758 (1966).

Foldes, F. F., and T. A. G. Torda: Comparative Studies with Narcotics and Narcotic Antagonists in Man, *Acta Anaesthesiol Scand,* **9**:121–138 (1965).

Fraser, H. F., and L. S. Harris: Narcotic and Narcotic Antagonist Analgesics, *Annu Rev Pharmacol,* **7**:277–300 (1967).

Lewis, J. W., K. W. Bentley, and A. Cowan: Narcotic Analgesics and Antagonists, *Annu Rev Pharmacol,* **11**:241–270 (1971).

Martin, W. R.: Opioid Antagonists, *Pharmacol Rev,* **19**:463–521 (1967).

CHAPTER 14

Allopurinol Symposium, 1966, *Ann Rheum Dis,* **25**:599–718 (1966).

Beaver, W. T.: Mild Analgesics: A Review of Their Clinical Pharmacology, *Am J Med Sci,* **250**:577–604 (1965).

Bland, J. H.: Drug Treatment of Rheumatoid Arthritis, *Semin Drug Treat,* **1**:93–118 (1971).

Dixon, St. J., B. K. Martin, M. J. H. Smith, and P. H. N. Wood (eds.): *Salicylates: An International Symposium,* Little, Brown, Boston, 1963.

Ferreira, S. H., and J. R. Vane: New Aspects of the Mode of Action of Nonsteroid Anti-Inflammatory Drugs, *Annu Rev Pharmacol,* **14**:57–73 (1974).

Flower, R. J.: Drugs Which Inhibit Prostaglandin Biosynthesis, *Pharmacol Rev,* **26**:33–67 (1974).

Kelley, W. N.: Effects of Drugs on Uric Acid in Man, *Annu Rev Pharmacol,* **15**:327–350 (1975).

———, and J. B. Wyngaarden: Drug Treatment of Gout, *Semin Drug Treat,* **1**:119–147 (1971).

Malawista, S. E.: Colchicine: A Common Mechanism for Its Anti-Inflammatory and Antimitotic Effects, *Arthritis Rheum,* **11**:191–197 (1968).

O'Brien, W. M.: Indomethacin: A Survey of Clinical Trials, *Clin Pharmacol Ther,* **9**:94–107 (1968).

Paulus, H. E., and M. W. Whitehouse: Nonsteroid Anti-Inflammatory Agents, *Annu Rev Pharmacol,* **13**:107–125 (1973).

Weiner, M., and S. J. Piliero: Nonsteroid Anti-Inflammatory Agents, *Annu Rev Pharmacol,* **10**:171–198 (1970).

Winters, R. W., J. S. White, M. C. Hughes, and N. K. Ordway: Disturbances of Acid-Base Equilibrium in Salicylate Intoxication, *Pediatrics,* **23**:260–285 (1960).

CHAPTER 15

Epstein, S. S. (ed.): *Drugs of Abuse: Their Genetic and Other Chronic Nonpsychiatric Hazards,* M.I.T., Cambridge, Mass., 1971.

Martin, W. R., and D. R. Jasinski: Physiological Parameters of Morphine Dependence in Man: Tolerance, Early Abstinence, Protracted Abstinence, *J Psychiat Res,* 19–28 (1969).

Nahas, G. G.: *Marihuana: Deceptive Weed,* Raven, New York, 1973.

Wikler, A. (ed.): The Addictive States, *Res Publ Assoc Res Nerv Ment Dis,* vol. 46, 1968.

Wittenborn, J. R., H. Brill, J. P. Smith, and S. A. Wittenborn (eds.): *Drugs and Youth,* Charles C Thomas, Springfield, Ill., 1969.

CHAPTER 16

Andén, N., A. Carlsson, and Häggendal: Adrenergic Mechanisms, *Annu Rev Pharmacol,* **9**:119–134 (1969).

Patil, P. N., D. D. Miller, and U. Trendelenburg: Molecular Geometry and Adrenergic Drug Activity, *Pharmacol Rev,* **26**:323–392 (1974).

Rubin, R. P.: The Role of Calcium in the Release of Neurotransmitter Substances and Hormones, *Pharmacol Rev,* **22**:389–428 (1970).

Shore, P. A.: Transport and Storage of Biogenic Amines, *Annu Rev Pharmacol,* **12**:209–226 (1972).

Smith, A. D.: Subcellular Localisation of Noradrenaline in Sympathetic Neurons, *Pharmacol Rev,* **24**:435–457 (1972).

Symposium: Regulation of Catecholamine Metabolsim in the Sympathetic Nervous System, in *New York Heart Association Symposium,* Williams & Wilkins, Baltimore, 1972.

Triggle, D. J.: Adrenergic Receptors, *Annu Rev Pharmacol,* **12**:185–196 (1972).

Volle, R. L.: Ganglionic Transmission, *Annu Rev Pharmacol,* **9**:135–146 (1969).

Weiner, N.: Regulation of Norepinephrine Biosynthesis, *Annu Rev Pharmacol,* **10**:273–290 (1970).

CHAPTER 17

Davies, B. N., and P. G. Withrington: The Actions of Drugs on the Smooth Muscle of the Capsule and Blood Vessels of the Spleen, *Pharmacol Rev,* **25**:373–413 (1973).

Furchgott, R. F.: The Pharmacological Differentiation of Adrenergic Receptors, *Ann N Y Acad Sci,* **139**:553–570 (1967).

Himms-Hagen, J.: Sympathetic Regulation of Metabolism, *Pharmacol Rev,* **19**:367–436 (1967).

Northrop, G.: Effects of Adrenergic Blocking Agents on Epinephrine and 3′, 5′-AMP-induced Responses in the Perfused Rat Liver, *J Pharmacol,* **159**:22–28 (1968).

Patil, P. N., D. D. Miller, and U. Trendelenburg: Molecular Geometry and Adrenergic Drug Activity, *Pharmacol Rev,* **26**:323–392 (1974).

Robison, G. A., R. W. Butcher, and E. W. Suther-land: Adenyl Cyclase as an Adrenergic Receptor, *Ann N Y Acad Sci,* **139**:703–723 (1967).

Shore, P. A.: Transport and Storage of Biogenic Amines, *Annu Rev Pharmacol,* **12**:209–226 (1972).

CHAPTER 18

Blinks, J. R.: Evaluation of the Cardiac Effects of Several Beta Adrenergic Blocking Agents, *Ann N Y Acad Sci,* **139**:673–685 (1967).

Davies, B. N., and P. G. Withrington: The Actions of Drugs on the Smooth Muscle of the Capsule and Blood Vessels of the Spleen, *Pharmacol Rev,* **25**:373–413 (1973).

Lucchesi, B. R., L. S. Whitsitt, and J. L. Stickney: Antiarrhythmic Effects of Beta Adrenergic Blocking Agents, *Ann N Y Acad Sci,* **139**:940–951 (1967).

Patil, P. N., D. D. Miller, and U. Trendelenburg: Molecular Geometry and Adrenergic Drug Activity, *Pharmacol Rev,* **26**:323–392 (1974).

Shore, P. A.: Transport and Storage of Biogenic Amines, *Annu Rev Pharmacol,* **12**:209–226 (1972).

Stone, C. A., and C. C. Porter: Methyldopa and Adrenergic Nerve Function, *Pharmacol Rev,* **18**:569–575 (1966).

CHAPTER 19

Brimblecombe, R. W.: *Drug Actions on Cholinergic Systems,* University Park Press, Baltimore, 1974.

Davies, B. N., and P. G. Withrington: The Actions of Drugs on the Smooth Muscle of the Capsule and Blood Vessels of the Spleen, *Pharmacol Rev,* **25**:373–413 (1973).

Greenblatt, D. J., and R. I. Shader: Anticholinergics, *N Eng J Med,* **288**:1215–1219 (1973).

Higgins, C. B., S. F. Vatner, and E. Braunwald: Parasympathetic Control of the Heart, *Pharmacol Rev,* **25**:119–155 (1973).

Kabachnik, M. I., A. P. Brestkin, N. N., Godovikov, M. J. Michelson, E. V. Rozengart, and V. I. Rozengart: Hydrophobic Areas on the Active Surface of Cholinesterases, *Pharmacol Rev,* **22**:355–388 (1970).

Karczmar, A. G.: Pharmacologic, Toxicologic, and Therapeutic Properties of Anticholinesterase Agents, in *Physiological Pharmacology,* vol. 3, Academic, New York, 1967, pp. 163–322.

Koelle, G. B.: Acetylcholine: Current Status in Physiology, Pharmacology and Medicine, *N Engl J Med,* **286**:1086–1090 (1972).

Volle, R. L.: Ganglionic Transmission, *Annu Rev Pharmacol,* **9**:135–146 (1969).

CHAPTER 20

Colquhoun, D.: Mechanisms of Drug Action at the Voluntary Muscle Endplate, *Annu Rev Pharmacol,* **15**:307–326 (1975).

Hubbard, J. I., and D. M. J. Quastel: Micropharmacology of Vertebrate Neuromuscular Transmission, *Annu Rev Pharmacol,* **13**:199–216 (1973).

Riker, W. F., Jr., and M. Okamoto: Pharmacology of Motor Nerve Terminals, *Annu Rev Pharmacol,* **9**:173–208 (1969).

Waud, D. R.: The Nature of Depolarization Blocks, *Anesthesiology,* **29**:1014–1024 (1968).

CHAPTER 21

Bentley, J. D., G. H. Burnett, R. L. Conklin, and R. H. Wasserburger: Clinical Application of Serum Digitoxin Levels, *Circulation,* **41**:67–76 (1970).

Braunwald, E., and P. E. Pool: Mechanism of Action of Digitalis Glycosides, *Mod Concepts Cardiovasc Dis,* **37**:129–133 (1968).

Cohn, J. N., F. E. Tristani, and J. M. Khatri: Cardiac and Peripheral Vascular Effects of Digitalis in Clinical Cardiogenic Shock, *Am Heart J,* **78**:318–330 (1969).

Doherty, J. E.: The Clinical Pharmacology of Digitalis Glycosides: A Review, *Am J Med Sci,* **255**:382–414 (1968).

Fisch, C., B. Surawicz, with S. B. Knoebel, K. Greenspan, and L. N. Katz: *Digitalis,* Grune & Stratton, New York, 1969.

Lee, K. S., and W. Klaus: The Subcellular Basis for the Mechanism of Inotropic Action of Cardiac Glycosides, *Pharmacol Rev,* **23**:193–261 (1971).

Mason, D. T.: Digitalis Pharmacology and Therapeutics: Recent Advances, *Ann Intern Med,* **80**:520–530 (1974).

Reiter, M.: Drugs and Heart Muscle, *Annu Rev Pharmacol,* **12**:111–124 (1972).

Roberts, J., and G. J. Kelliher: The Mechanism of Action of Digitalis at the Subcellular Level, *Semin Drug Treat,* **2**:203–220 (1972).

Schwartz, A., G. E. Lindenmayer, and J. C. Allen: The Sodium-Potassium Adenosine Triphosphatase: Pharmacological, Physiological and Biochemical Aspects, *Pharmacol Rev,* **27**:3–134 (1975).

CHAPTER 22

Basset, A. L., and B. F. Hoffman: Antiarrhythmic Drugs: Electrophysiological Actions, *Annu Rev Pharmacol,* **11**:143–170 (1971).

Bigger, J. T., Jr., and R. H. Heissenbuttel: The Use of Procaine Amide and Lidocaine in the Treatment of Cardiac Arrhythmias, *Prog Cardiovasc Dis,* **11**:515–534 (1969).

Davis, L. D., and J. V. Temte: Effects of Propranolol on the Transmembrane Potentials of Ventricular Muscle and Purkinje Fibers of the Dog, *Cir Res,* **22**:661–677 (1968).

———, and ———: Electrophysiological Actions of Lidocaine on Canine Ventricular Muscle and Purkinje Fibers, *Cir Res,* **24**:639–655 (1969).

Mendez, R., and E. Kabela: Cardiac Pharmacology, *Annu Rev Pharmacol,* **10**:291–312 (1970).

Sasyniuk, B. I., and R. I. Ogilvie: Antiarrhythmic Drugs: Electrophysiological and Pharmacokinetic Considerations, *Annu Rev Pharmacol,* **15**:131–156 (1975).

Singer, D. H., and R. E. Ten Eick: Pharmacology of Cardiac Arrhythmias, *Prog Cardiovasc Dis,* **11**:488–513 (1969).

CHAPTER 23

Battack, D. J., H. Alvarez, and C. A. Chidsey: Effects of Propranolol and Isosorbide Dinitrate on Exercise Performance and Adrenergic Activity in Patients with Angina Pectoris, *Circulation,* **39**:157–170 (1969).

The Coronary Drug Project Research Group: The Coronary Drug Project, *J Am Med Assoc,* **214**:1303–1313 (1970); **220**:996–1008 (1972).

Dempsey, P. J., and T. Cooper: Pharmacology of the Coronary Circulation, *Annu Rev Pharmacol,* **12**:99–110 (1972).

Epstein, S. E., and E. Braunwald: Inhibition of the Adrenergic Nervous System in the Treatment of Angina Pectoris, *Med Clin North Am,* **52**:1017–1030 (1968).

Lees, R. S., and D. E. Wilson: The Treatment of Hyperlipidemia, *N Engl J Med,* **284**:186–195 (1971).

Mendez, R., and E. Kabela: Cardiac Pharmacology, *Annu Rev Pharmacol,* **10**:291–312 (1970).

Oliver, M. F.: The Primary Prevention of Ischemic Heart Disease by Means of Atromid-S (Clofibrate), *Bull N Y Acad Med,* **44**:1021–1027 (1968).

Peterson, M. J., C. C. Hillman, and J. Ashmore: Nicotinic Acid: Studies on the Mechanism of Its Antilipolytic Action, *Mol Pharmacol,* **4**:1–9 (1968).

Rowe, G. G.: Pharmacology of the Coronary Circulation, *Annu Rev Pharmacol,* **8**:95–112 (1968).

Weiss, P.: The Treatment of Hyperlipidemia, *Ration Drug Ther,* **6**:1–6 (1972).

Winbury, M., B. B. Howe, and M. A. Hefner: Effect of Nitrates and Other Coronary Dilators on Large and Small Coronary Vessels: A Hypothesis for the Mechanism of Action of Nitrates, *J Pharmacol Exp Ther,* **168**:70–95 (1969).

CHAPTER 24

Burg, M. B., and N. Green: Effects of ethacrynic acid on the thick ascending limb of Henle's loop. *Kidney Int,* **4**:301–308, 1973.

Cafruny, E. J.: The Site and Mechanism of Action of Mercurial Diuretics, *Pharmacol Rev,* **20**:89–110 (1968).

Goldberg, M.: The Renal Physiology of Diuretics, in *Renal Physiology, Handbook of Physiology,* Sect. 8. (J. Orloff, and R. W. Berliner, eds.) American Physiological Society, Washington, D.C., 1973, pp. 1003–1031.

Hutcheon, D. E.: Recent Advances in the Pharmacology of Diuretic Drugs, *Am J Med Sci,* **253**:620–628 (1967).

Landon, E. J., and L. R. Forte: Cellular Mechanisms in Renal Pharmacology, *Annu Rev Pharmacol,* **11**:171–188 (1971).

Mudge, G. H.: Renal Pharmacology, *Annu Rev Pharmacol,* **7**:163–184 (1967).

Natochin, Y. V.: Renal Pharmacology: Comparative, Developmental, and Cellular Aspects, *Annu Rev Pharmacol,* **14**:75–90 (1974).

Schwartz, A., G. E. Lindenmayer, and J. C. Allen: The Sodium-Potassium Adenosine Triphosphatase: Pharmacological, Physiological and Biochemical Aspects, *Pharmacol Rev,* **27**:3–134 (1975).

Suki, W. N., G. Eknoyan, and M. Martinez-Maldonado: Tubular Sites and Mechanisms of Diuretic Action, *Annu Rev Pharmacol,* **13**:91–106 (1973).

CHAPTER 25

Ehrlich, E. N.: Aldosterone, the Adrenal Cortex, and Hypertension, *Ann Rev Med,* **19**:373–398 (1968).

Pettinger, W. A., and H. C. Mitchell: Minoxidil: An Alternative to Nephrectomy for Retractory Hypertension, *N Engl J Med,* **289**:167–171 (1973).

Swartz, C., K. E. Kim, P. Lyons, and G. Onesti: Drug Therapy of Hypertension: Current Management and Future Agents, *Medicine/Genesis,* **1**: 12–17 (1975).

Veterans Administration Cooperative Study Group on Antihypertensive Agents: Effects of Treatment on Morbidity in Hypertension: II. Results in Patients with Diastolic Blood Pressure Averaging 90 through 114 mm Hg, *J Am Med Assoc,* **213**:1143–1152 (1970).

Zimmerman, B. G.: Drug Action on Peripheral Vascular System, *Annu Rev Pharmacol,* **12**:125–140 (1972).

CHAPTER 26

Beck, W. S.: Deoxyribonucleotide Synthesis and the Role of Vitamin B_{12} in Erythropoiesis, *Vitam Horm (NY),* **26**:413–442 (1968).

Beutler, E., V. F. Fairbanks, and J. L. Fahey: *Clinical Disorders of Iron Metabolism,* Grune & Stratton, New York, 1963.

Bothwell, T. H., and C. A. Finch: *Iron Metabolism,* Little, Brown, Boston, 1962.

Friedkin, M.: Enzymatic Aspects of Folic Acid, *Annu Rev Biochem,* **32**:185–214 (1963).

Moore, C. V., and R. Dubach: Iron, in C. L. Comar, and F. Bronner (eds.), *Mineral Metabolism,* vol. 2B, Academic, New York, 1962, pp. 287–348.

Weissbach, H., and R. T. Taylor: Metabolic Role of Vitamin B_{12}, *Vitam Horm (NY),* **26**:395–412 (1968).

Wintrobe, M. M.: *Clinical Hematology,* 6th ed., Lea & Febiger, Philadelphia, 1967, chap. 11.

CHAPTER 27

Friedberg, C.: Anticoagulant Therapy, *Heart Bull,* **17**:27, 33–40 (1968).

Lyon, A. F., and A. C. DeGraff: Indications for Anticoagulant Therapy, *Am Heart J,* **77**:132–136 (1969).

Nagashima, R., R. A. O'Reilly, and G. Levy: Kinetics of Pharmacological Effects in Man: The Anticoagulant Action of Warfarin, *Clin Pharmacol Ther,* **10**:22–35 (1969).

O'Reilly, R. A., and P. M. Aggeler: Determinants of the Response to Oral Anticoagulant Drugs in Man, *Pharmacol Rev,* **22**:35–96 (1970).

Wright, I. S.: Anticoagulant Therapy: Practical Management, *Am Heart J,* **77**:280–286 (1969).

CHAPTER 28

Black, J. W., W. A. M. Duncan, C. J. Durant, C. R. Ganellin, and E. M. Parsons: Definition and Antagonism of Histamine H_2-Receptors, *Nature,* **236**:385–390 (1972).

Brand, J. J., and W. L. M. Perry: Drugs Used in Motion Sickness, *Pharmacol Rev,* **18**:895–924 (1966).

Goth, A.: Histamine Release by Drugs and Chemicals, in M. Schachter (ed.), *International Encyclopedia of Pharmacology and Therapy: Histamine and Antihistamines,* vol. 1, Pergamon Press, New York, 1973.

Rocha e Silva, M.: Histamine and Anti-Histamines: Part I. Histamine, Its Chemistry, Metabolism and Physiological and Pharmacological Actions, in *Handbook of Experimental Pharmacology,* vol. XVIII, Springer-Verlag, New York, 1966.

Wood, C. J., and M. A. Simkins: *International Symposium on Histamine H_2-Receptor Antagonists,* Smith, Kline & French Laboratories Limited, Weleyn, Garden City, 1973.

CHAPTER 29

Copp, D. H.: Calcitonin and Parathyroid Hormone, *Annu Rev Pharmacol,* **9**:327–344 (1969).

———: Endocrine Control of Calcium Homeostasis, *J Endocrinol,* **43**:137–161 (1969).

Hirsch, P. F., and P. L. Munson: Thyrocalcitonin, *Physiol Rev,* **49**:548–622 (1969).

Liberti, P., and J. B. Stanbury: The Pharmacology of Substances Affecting the Thyroid Gland, *Annu Rev Pharmacol,* **11**:113–142 (1971).

Mills, L. C.: Drug Treatment in Thyroid Disease, *Semin Drug Treat,* **3**:377–402 (1974).

Potts, J. T., Jr., and L. J. Deftos: Parathyroid Hormone, Thyrocalcitonin, Vitamin D, Bone, and Bone Mineral Metabolism, in P. K. Bondy (ed.), *Duncan's Diseases of Metabolism,* 6th ed., Saunders, Philadelphia, 1969, pp. 904–1082.

Talmage, R. V., C. W. Cooper, and H. Z. Park: Regulation of Calcium Transport in Bone by Parathyroid Hormone, *Vitam Horm (NY)*, **28**:104–142 (1970).

Wallach, S., J. Aloia, and S. Cohn: Treatment of Osteoporosis with Calcitonin, *Semin Drug Treat*, **2**:21–25 (1972).

CHAPTER 30

American Diabetes Association: Special Report, Classification of Genetic Diabetes Mellitus, *Diabetes*, **16**:540 (1967).

Hamwi, G. J., and T. S. Danowski (eds.): *Diabetes Mellitus: Diagnosis and Treatment*, vol. II, American Diabetes Association, New York, 1967.

Karam, J. H., S. B. Matin, and P. H. Forsham: Antidiabetic Drugs after the University Group Diabetes Program (UGDP), *Annu Rev Pharmacol*, **15**:351–366 (1975).

Kryston, L. J., and R. A. Shaw: The Rationale for the Use of Drugs in the Treatment of Diabetes Mellitus, *Semin Drug Treat*, **3**:365–375 (1974).

Pilkis, S. J., and C. R. Park: Mechanism of Action of Insulin, *Annu Rev Pharmacol*, **14**:365–388 (1974).

CHAPTER 31

Berczeller, P. H., and H. S. Kupperman: The Anabolic Steroids, *Clin Pharmacol Ther*, **1**:464–482 (1960).

Kupperman, H. S.: *Human Endocrinology*, Davis, Philadelphia, 1963.

Lipsett, M. B., and S. G. Korenman: Androgen Metabolism, *J Am Med Assoc*, **190**:757–762 (1964).

Sohval, H.: The Anatomy and Endocrine Physiology of the Male Reproductive System, in J. T. Velardo (ed.), *The Endocrinology of Reproduction*, Oxford University Press, Fair Lawn, N.J., 1958, pp. 243–312.

Wilson, J. D.: Recent Studies on the Mechanism of Action of Testosterone, *N Engl J Med*, **287**:1284–1291 (1972).

CHAPTER 32

Drill, V. A.: Oral Contraceptives: Relation to Mammary Cancer, Benign Breast Lesions, and Cervical Cancer, *Annu Rev Pharmacol*, **15**:367–385 (1975).

Emmens, C. W.: Antifertility Agents, *Annu Rev Pharmacol*, **10**:237–254 (1970).

Kellie, A. E.: The Pharmacology of the Estrogens, *Annu Rev Pharmacol*, **11**:97–112 (1971).

Kistner, R. W.: The Use of Clomiphene Citrate in the Treatment of Anovulation, *Semin Drug Treat*, **3**:159–175 (1973).

Odell, W. D., and M. E. Molitch: The Pharmacology of Contraceptive Agents, *Annu Rev Pharmacol*, **14**:413–434 (1974).

Turksoy, R. N.: Induction of Ovulation with the Use of Human Menopausal Gonadotropins in Anovulatory Infertile Women, *Semin Drug Treat*, **3**:177–187 (1973).

CHAPTER 33

Bland, J. H.: Drug Treatment of Rheumatoid Arthritis, *Semin Drug Treat*, **1**:93–118 (1971).

Fries, J. F., and H. O. McDevitt: Systemic Corticosteroid Therapy in Rheumatic Diseases, *Ration Drug Ther*, **6**:1–5 (1972).

Melby, J. C.: Assessment of Adrenocortical Function, *N Engl J Med*, **285**:735–739 (1971).

O'Malley, B. W.: Mechanisms of Action of Steroid Hormones, *N Engl J Med*, **284**:370–377 (1971).

Schwartz, A., G. E. Lindenmayer, and J. C. Allen: The Sodium-Potassium Adenosine Triphosphatase: Pharmacological, Physiological and Biochemical Aspects, *Pharmacol Rev*, **27**:3–134 (1975).

Thorn, G. W.: Clinical Considerations in the Use of Corticosteroids, *N Engl J Med*, **274**:775–781 (1966).

CHAPTER 34

Carter, S. K., and M. Slavik: Chemotherapy of Cancer, *Annu Rev Pharmacol*, **14**:157–183 (1974).

Chabner, B. A., C. E. Myers, C. N. Coleman, and D. G. Johns: The Clinical Pharmacology of Antineoplastic Agents, *N Engl J Med*, **292**:1107–1113, 1159–1168 (1975).

Gerebtzoff, A., P. H. Lambert, and P. A. Miescher: Immunosuppressive Agents, *Annu Rev Pharmacol*, **12**:287–316 (1972).

Young, C. W., and J. H. Burchenal: Cancer Chemotherapy, *Annu Rev Pharmacol*, **11**:369–386 (1971).

CHAPTER 35

Davis, B. D., R. Dulbecco, H. N. Eisen, H. S. Ginsberg, and W. B. Wood, Jr.: Chemotherapeutic Actions on Bacteria, in *Microbiology,* Harper & Row, New York, 1967, pp. 301–334.
Goldberg, I. H.: Mode of Action of Antibiotics: II. Drugs Affecting Nucleic Acid in Protein Synthesis, *Am J Med,* **39**:722–752 (1965).
Hash, J. H.: Antibiotic Mechanisms, *Annu Rev Pharmacol,* **12**:35–56 (1972).
Newton, B. A.: Mechanisms of Antibiotic Action, *Annu Rev Microbiol,* **19**:209–240 (1965).
Strominger, J. L., and D. J. Tipper: Bacterial Cell Wall Synthesis and Structure in Relation to the Mechanism of Action of Penicillin and Other Antibacterial Agents, *Am J Med,* **39**:708–721 (1965).
Weisblum, B., and J. Davies: Antibiotic Inhibitors of the Bacterial Ribosome, *Bacteriol Rev,* **32**:493–528 (1968).

CHAPTER 36

Bennett, J. E.: The Treatment of Systemic Mycoses, *Ration Drug Ther,* **7**:1–4 (1973).
Caldwell, J. R., and L. E. Cluff: The Real and Present Danger of Antibiotics, *Ration Drug Ther,* **7**:1–5 (1973).
Johnson, A. H.: Adverse Effects of Antibiotics, *Semin Drug Treat,* **2**:331–351 (1972).
Newberry, W. M.: Drug Treatment of the Systemic Mycoses, *Semin Drug Treat,* **2**:313–329 (1972).
Pittinger, C. B., and R. Adamson: Antibiotic Blockade of Neuromuscular Function, *Annu Rev Pharmacol,* **12**:169–184 (1972).
Thrupp, L. D.: Newer Cephalosporins and "Expanded-Spectrum" Penicillins, *Annu Rev Pharmacol,* **14**:435–467 (1974).
Tilles, J. G.: Antiviral Agents, *Annu Rev Pharmacol,* **14**:469–489 (1974).
Stewart, G. T.: Allergy to Penicillin and Related Antibiotics: Antigenic and Immunochemical Mechanism, *Annu Rev Pharmacol,* **13**:309–324 (1973).

CHAPTER 37

Browne, S. G.: Drug Treatment of Leprosy, *Trans R Soc Trop Med Hyg,* **61**:265–271 (1967).
Fox, W.: Changing Concepts in Chemotherapy of Pulmonary Tuberculosis, *Am Rev Respir Dis,* **97**:767–790 (1968).
Place, V. A., and H. Black (eds.): New Antituberculous Agents: Laboratory and Clinical Studies, *Ann N Y Acad Sci,* **135**:681–1120 (1969).
Shepard, C. C.: Chemotherapy of Leprosy, *Ann Rev Pharmacol,* **9**:37–50 (1969).
Weinstein, L., M. A. Madoff, and C. M. Samet: The Sulfonamides, *N Engl J Med,* **263**:793–799, 842–849, 952–957 (1960).

CHAPTER 38

Bland, J. H.: Drug Treatment of Rheumatoid Arthritis, *Semin Drug Treat,* **1**:93–118 (1971).
Chisolm, J. J., Jr.: The Use of Chelating Agents in the Treatment of Acute and Chronic Lead Intoxication in Childhood, *J. Pediatr,* **73**:1–38 (1968).
Ciaccio, E. I.: Mercury: Therapeutic and Toxic Aspects, *Semin Drug Treat,* **1**:177–194 (1971).
Clarkson, T. W.: The Pharmacology of Mercury Compounds, *Annu Rev Pharmacol,* **12**:375–406 (1972).
deBruin, A., and H. Hoolboom: Early Signs of Lead Exposure: A Comparative Study of Laboratory Tests, *Br J Ind Med,* **24**:203–211 (1967).
Ferm, V. H., and S. J. Carpenter: Malformation Induced by Sodium Arsenate, *J Reprod Fertil,* **17**:199–201 (1968).
Gibson, S. L. M., J. C. Mackenzie, and A. Goldberg: The Diagnosis of Industrial Lead Poisoning, *Br J Ind Med,* **25**:40–51 (1968).
Schroeder, H. A., and J. J. Balassa: Abnormal Trace Metals in Man: Arsenic, *J Chronic Dis,* **19**:85–106 (1966).

INDEX

In an effort to conserve space no attempt is made in this index to mention all the tradenames of various drugs. When tradenames are cited, they have been chosen because by prior usage they have become established in the parlance of physicians.